WORK WITH DISPLAY UNITS 92

WORK WITH DISPLAY UNITS 92

Selected Proceedings of the
Third International Scientific Conference on
Work with Display Units
Berlin, Germany, September 1–4, 1992

edited by

HOLGER LUCZAK

Institut für Arbeitswissenschaft
Technische Universität Berlin
Berlin, Germany

AHMET ÇAKIR
GISELA ÇAKIR

ERGONOMIC Institut
für Arbeits- und Sozialforschung
Forschungsgesellschaft mbH
Berlin, Germany

1993

NORTH-HOLLAND
AMSTERDAM • LONDON • NEW YORK • TOKYO

NORTH-HOLLAND
ELSEVIER SCIENCE PUBLISHERS B.V.
Sara Burgerhartstraat 25
P.O. Box 211, 1000 AE Amsterdam, The Netherlands

Library of Congress Cataloging-in-Publication Data

International Scientific Conference on Work with Display Units (3rd : 1992 : Berlin, Germany)
Work with display units 92 : selected proceedings of the Third International Scientific Conference on Work with Display Units, Berlin, Germany, September 1-4, 1992 / edited by Holger Luczak, Ahmet Çakir, Gisela Çakir.
p. cm.
Includes bibliographical references and index.
ISBN 0-444-89759-3 (acid-free paper)
1. Video display terminals--Health aspects--Congresses. 2. Human engineering--Congresses. I. Luczak, H. (Holger) II. Çakir, A. III. Çakir, Gisela. IV. Title.
RC965.V53I57 1992
363.18'9--dc20 93-19702
CIP

ISBN: 0 444 89759 3

This book is printed on acid-free paper.
Transferred to digital printing 2006

Preface

It is with great pleasure that we present this volume, and we would like to take this opportunity to thank all the authors who contributed to.

The volume presents the most significant articles from each of the fields represented at the Conference. Presentations were evaluated by the Conference´s Scientific Committee, and selected for inclusion on the basis of their significant contributions to the body of knowledge of VDU use. The Committee was aided in its evaluation of the scientific quality of the presentations by specialists in the various fields represented at the Conference as well as by the chairmen of the sessions.

At this point, we would like to take the opportunity to thank the members of the International Scientific Advisory Committee for their work, especially in the preliminary stages of the Conference, as well as the Session Chairs, who organized parts of the Conference and invited experts to contribute.

We acknowledge with gratefulness the organizational and financial support by our sponsors and co-sponsoring organizations. They enabled us among other things to invite several delegates from the new East European countries.

We thank too all the participants for their engagement and the fruitful interdisciplinary discussion.

Last but not least, we would like to sincerely thank all those who were involved in all aspects of the organization and contribution of the Conference in front and behind the scenes, particularly Gisela Çakir, Johannes von Moltke, Thomas Müller, Peter Ortmann and Martina Szymon.

President WWDU'92
Holger Luczak
Technische Universität Berlin
Institut für Arbeitswissenschaft
Ernst-Reuter-Platz 7-9
D - 1000 Berlin 12

Secretary General WWDU '92
Ahmet Çakir
ERGONOMIC Institute
for Social and Occupational Sciences
Research Co., Ltd.
Soldauer Platz 3
D - 1000 Berlin 19

PATRONAGE

Federal Minister of Labour and Social Affairs, Dr. Norbert Blüm

SUPPORT

The Conference is kindly supported by

DFG Deutsche Forschungsgemeinschaft (German Research Foundation)

Federal Ministry of Labour and Social Affairs

Commission of the European Communities, Directorate-General for Employment, Industrial Relations and Social Affairs

SPONSORS

IBM Deutschland GmbH, Stuttgart, FRG

ICL Data Kista, Schweden

Siemens AG, SNI AG München, Nürnberg, FRG

Tandberg Data A/S Oslo, Norway

Vitra GmbH Weil am Rhein, FRG

Waldmann Lichttechnik GmbH VS-Schwenningen, FRG

CO-SPONSORING ORGANIZATIONS

Berliner Bank AG

CIE - Commission Internationale de l' Eclairage

GfA - Gesellschaft für Arbeitswissenschaft e. V.

IEA - International Ergonomics Association

IIID - Internationales Institut für Informations-Design

Japan Ergonomics Research Society

Japan Institute of Human Posture Research

MATSUSHITA electric industrial co., ltd.

NEC Corporation

Oki Electric Industry Company

REFA - Verband für Arbeitsstudien und Betriebsorganisation e. V.

TOSHIBA corporation

VDI-EKV, VDI- Gesellschaft Entwicklung Konstruktion Vertrieb

VDMA - Verband Deutscher Maschinen- und Anlagenbau e. V.

VW Volkswagen AG

The "Brandenburger Tor"-Logo was kindly provided by the publisher of Der Tagesspiegel.

INTERNATIONAL INDUSTRIAL ADVISORY COMMITTEE

INTERNATIONAL SCIENTIFIC ADVISORY COMMITTEE

CONTENTS

WORKLOAD, STRESS AND STRAIN

OPENING SESSION

WORK WITH DISPLAY UNITS 92
H. Luczak, A. Çakir and G. Çakir (Editors)

Welcome Address

Holger Luczak*, Ahmet Çakir**

* Technische Universität Berlin, Institut für Arbeitswissenschaft, Ernst-Reuter-Platz 7-9, D - 1000 Berlin 12, F.R. Germany

** ERGONOMIC Institute for Social and Occupational Sciences, Research Co., Ltd. Soldauer Platz 3, D - 1000 Berlin 19, F. R. Germany

It is the right of the President not only to open the conference, but to say a few words about the conference over which he presides. I believe, I should let you know my thoughts about the concept and the process of conference preparation, to involve you in our spirit of breaking up to new shores of science and technology in "Work With Display Units", and to explain to you our responsibilities for highlights and weaknesses in the topics and selection of structure for this conference. When I say "our", I mean, the cooperative effort of the chiefs and coworkers in the institutes of the Secretary General and the President of WWDU III.

1. CONCEPTUAL MODEL

In principle the organization of a conference is the design of a service product. In so far a conceptual model of "service quality" might help to derive the basic quality relevant features of conference organization. I hope for your understanding for this perspective, but since some time I am not merely professor of ergonomics and industrial engineering at a university, but the managing research director of a federal rationalization research institute. This position helps me sometimes to solve organizational problems, but it biases to a certain extent the working style. So let me report, how we cooked the menu Work With Display Units III for you. This report will give me the opportunity to confront you with some ideas and concepts, that may show to you, that an international scientific conference is not only an organizational problem of considerable dimensions, but it is a seducing and interesting scientific task, which implies the meta-scientific approach of structuring disciplines and bringing an order or systematization in the field of divergent and vast knowledge.

According to this model of service quality one of the first and first ranking tasks of a provider, that is the conference organizer, is to close Gap 1: This is the difference between consumer expectations and management perception of consumer expectations. So the provider is well advised, if he tries to get as much knowledge as possible about criteria, that consumers perceive and evaluate as high quality of a service delivery.

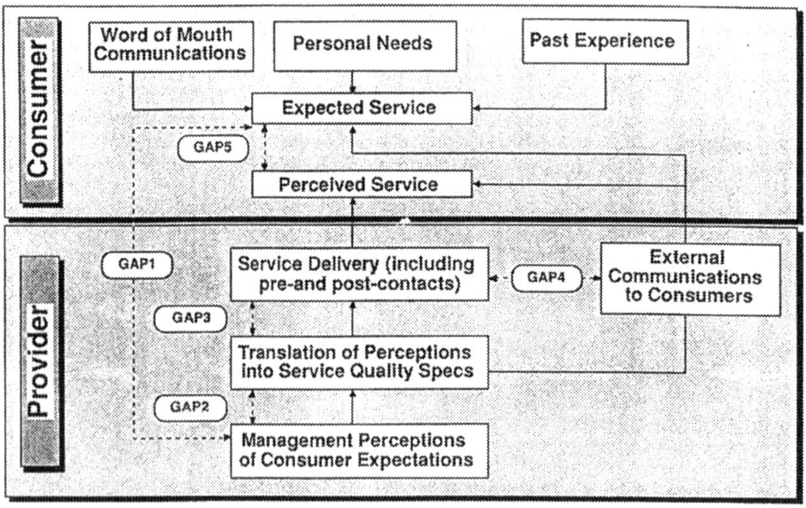

Figure 1. Conceptual model of service quality

2. EMPIRICAL BASIS

To know, what kind of conference you possibly expect, we can or could use at least 3 approaches: The *first* approach is to look into the past. No doubt, that if we plan a conference WWDU III we have to ensure a scientific heritage of the first and the second international WWDU-conferences in Stockholm and Montreal. Their programme was an interesting interdisciplinary mixture for attendees with a professional interest in occupational health, occupational hygiene, image quality and vision, work physiology, work place design, work organization, and human computer interaction. On the whole the topics centered around health and well-being at work with display units were the kernel of the conferences. Taking this experience of the past as guide-line would have the disadvantage to neglect recent developments, for instance in cognitive ergonomics, in computer tools and other themes, which have come up shortly. At that, it is not very interesting for a scientist and conference organizer to plan a copy of earlier events.

A *second* approach to find out something about "expected services" is to communicate with people of similar interests to get an impression of the atmosphere, "how the wind blows". The opinion in different circles, like the international commission on human aspects of computing - for example - is not very favourable for a WWDU conference organizer: Most people say, there are too many conferences in this scientific field, and especially the competitors from HCI - Human Computer Interaction - as well as CHI - Computer Human Interfaces - do not hesitate to declare, that WWDU is simply superfluous! As you see we did not follow this word of mouth communications! We think that WWDU has its specific function in our scientific world! But what are the functions derived from "personal needs" for this conference?

What is the *message* of WWDU'92? There is no doubt, that we are "underway", but everybody on this path, seeing the landscape under his perspective. So it is impossible to formulate the one and only message. Nevertheless I try to extract some principles, some mottos, at least tasks for you and me from thoughts and discussions with numerous competent people. These mottos are coupled to interests, interests of detection of the new, interests of application, interests of use and misuse. So it seems to be appropriate to assign the mottos to specific interests, which may be the outcome of "personal needs".

Because WWDU is planned as a scientific conference, I begin with the interest of the ***pure scientist***. His motto might be: *Initiate the "right" diagnosis with clear logical relationship to the "real" causes by the development of valid and reliable methods, and introduce consequent therapies on this basis!*

The ***applied scientist*** would construct the focus of his formulation a bit differently and say: *Proceed from descriptive-analytical approaches to prescriptive-synthetical measurements!*

If we separate the scientists into different disciplines, the mottos may become more specific.

The ***occupational physician*** might pronounce: *Either accept fears for potential dangers and health risks or definitely discard the fears by intelligent epidemiological studies!*

The ***psychologist*** would shift the perspective and might formulate: *Use chances of individual self-fulfilment by learning and working in computer-assisted tutorials and tools!* Or more critically and pessimistically: *Take up the discussion on social and individual consequences of computerization and detect personality-changing and societal impacts!*

The ***ergonomist*** brings another point into focus in his mottos: *Check the promised support functions of computer systems and evaluate software packages for their efficiency!* Or, more task-related: *Gain insights into the functional complexity of technological processes and formulate appeals for appropriate human actions!*

The ***design engineer*** would prefer another formulation and say: *Support the development of new physical and technical principles of display design and configuration as well as of all input devices!* Or, to phrase his approach more generally: *Close the gap between design necessities and actual design intentions and design efforts!*

The ***public health practitioner*** would intervene with his motto: *Enforce the offset of research before standardization and thus remove deficits in theory and respective regulations!*

The ***employer*** and perhaps the ***economist*** would say: *Use rationalization potentials of WWDU-technology and increase cash flows and incomes!* Or: *Direct the way to new products and an innovative market of workplace equipment!*

The ***unionist*** would object partially and bring in his view: *Avoid decreases of qualification and fight for the interests of workforce affected by computer-oriented rationalization!* Adding, perhaps: *Make transparent the deregulation of standards for working conditions and respective measurements of employers and state authorities!*

The ***representative of the political and social sciences*** would summarize this in his motto on a more general level: *Develop strategies to avoid risks in physiological and physical, but in social and organizational contexts too! Provide arguments for political action!*

Perhaps you have your own motto and respective "personal needs" yourself. Thus you may perceive, that it is somewhat difficult to form a coherent concept of "perceptions of consumer expectation" and to transform them into "service quality specifications".

The task to fill GAP 2 requires something more than bringing together different empirical results. A theoretical framework is needed, which means a third approach to fill in consumer expectancies.

3. PARADIGM

The preparation of a scientific conference is a scientific process in itself. To give you an insight in the "philosophy" of the conference and how it was developed by you, the Çakir group, and my crew to its actual status, I dare to analyze this process. This analysis may show you, how a specific profile of WWDU III was generated.

The nomination "Work With Display Units" has only two "Starting positions" for conference design, namely "work" and "display units". So a first idea was to define, what we did not want to do: Taking into account existing congresses in the field of action we should not orient WWDU III to purely technical aspects of display units and lighting, not to purely ergonomical design of input-output-devices, not only to possible hazards of occupational health and physiology a.s.o. In all these specific disciplinary approaches the market of scientific communication shows congresses, conferences, symposia, meetings a.s.o. with mostly one separate scientific perspective. So if WWDU should have a specific value in the scientific land-scape, it should have a cross section character, centered around "work" in all its facets, which have to do with the technological help, or frictions, or frustrations caused by something, that lies in or behind the "display units".

What was the basic idea and basic theory for the structure of the conference, its topics and its contributions to our scientific field?

Theories, methods and design principles depend upon the context, they are built in. To systematize this broad, cross-section oriented context, a paradigm is needed, that guarantees, that the whole problem field is covered and that the separate problems can be seen in their coherence.

The paradigm divides working processes and working structures into 7 levels, the highest level representing work related to its societal impacts (level 7), the lowest (level 1) representing elementary physiological processes. The 3 lower levels distinguish between a subject-oriented (human) approach and an object-oriented (work-environment, workplace, work means related) approach.

Interests of the lowest level (1) are anatomical and physiological basics, like biomechanics of the workplace, metabolism and effects of the working environment, rhythmological functions related to working hours etc.

Interests of the second level (2) are the elementary human functions in physical and psychical terms: Anthropometrical workplace design, the investigation of movements and movement control and the physical design of displays and controls are dominating.

Object of level 3 are those psychical processes on the one hand, which allow and steer a senseful sequence of operations; on the other hand the system analysis and

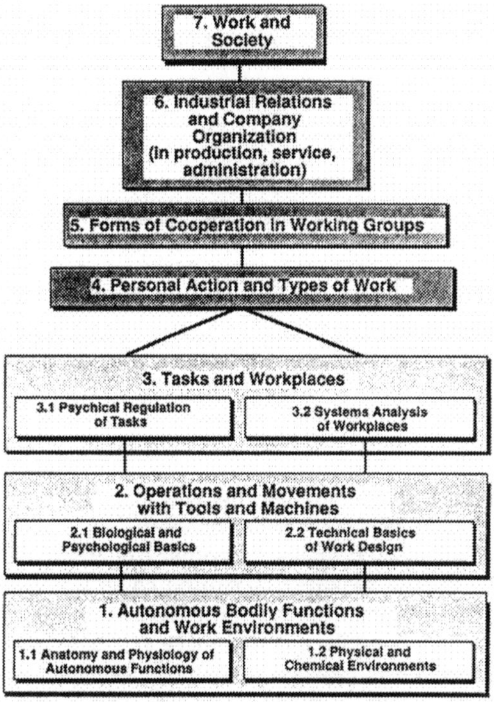

Figure 2. Levels for the description of working processes

system evaluation of workplaces, in other words the functional and time-line oriented cooperation of humans and technical means to fulfill a purpose (that is for instance production of a good or delivery of a service).

On the central level 4 the worker, the human being as individual working person, is focussed; The typical approach on this level is a holistic view of human work as an entity of motivational, voluntative, qualification-based and social elements. On this level and all higher levels a distinction between a subject-oriented and object-oriented approach is no longer necessary.

The level 5 brings into focus the working groups and group work, which means the cooperation of individual working persons with their specific tasks. This implies work/labour partition, hierarchical aspects, behaviour of crew-leaders, participation as well as questions of communication and information transfer, with respect to human relations.

Level 6 describes industrial relations of employers and employees' representatives. Questions of codetermination with respect to new information technologies, questions of organization of work in enterprises and other strategical decisions with respect to human work in computer integrated systems are brought up.

According to this scheme level 7 is oriented to comprehensive sociopolitical and societal contexts of work. Typical questions on this level deal with work regulation and standardization, work in the national economy, structural and economical components of employment, working market and activities of employers and unions in sociopolitics.

A special advantage of this paradigm is, that it brings together the different disciplinary approaches with respect to their contribution to the analysis and design of "work". So it seems to be a good basis for the structuring of a conference on *Work* With Display Units. The other advantage is, that the scheme especially refers to an object-oriented side, which means working equipment and so comprises especially "displays", and all scientific problems, that lies in or behind display-technology.

Coming back to the service quality model, we see, that a GAP 3 and a GAP 4 has to be closed. Gap 3 represents the possible difference between service quality specifications and the service actually delivered, Gap 4 the difference between service delivery and what is communicated about the service to the customers.

4. SPECIFICATION

Having an idea about the broadness of the problem field and its structuring, does not guarantee a useful conference in the sense of "service delivery".

A conference like WWDU, which has to compete with other conferences and congresses, has to develop a unique profile to attract scientific communications and communicators and to fulfil a specific function in scientific discussion and the process of development of scientific knowledge. In a competitive world with lots, perhaps too many conferences, any conference may become superfluous quickly, which can not demonstrate its specific attraction to the potential costumers.

A priori WWDU is not in a very stable position with respect to a stable group of customers. If I compare WWDU, for instance, to the congresses of IEA, the International Ergonomics Association, I conclude, that IEA can rely on the different national ergonomics research societies, which bring together a certain amount of people for IEA-events, whatever might be the programme of the gettogether, and where it is planned to take place, even at the end of the world. In comparison to this WWDU has not an a-priori basis of international or national groups of scientists, who by their cooptation or membership to a society or group demonstrate their interest in a disciplinary/discipline-oriented event. WWDU is free, free of difficult processes of finding a consensus, but free of stable support structures, too.

A support structure, we could really rely on, was our scientific advisory committee. An inner circle of persons, who later organized themselves as WWDU-group, looked around in the world to find scientists of reputation in at least one of the fields of our scheme with a worldwide and regional standing. The idea was, to have different perspectives from different persons and different countries. In a process of discussion and communication with these persons we identified the most important features of WWDU, as they were actually en vogue in science and technology.

The result was the overview "*Ideas and Proposals for Conference Topics ... as advised by the International Scientific Advisory Committee*", which was published in the "2. *Call for Participation*". You clearly identify the "paradigm" behind the systematization of the conference topics.

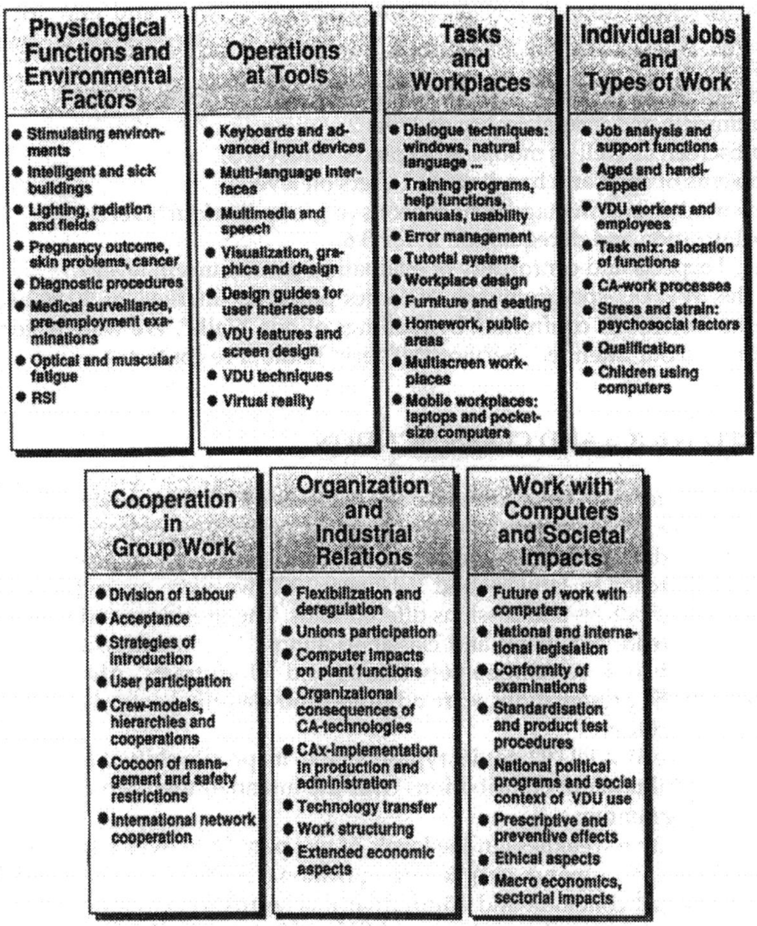

Figure 3. Ideas and proposals for conference topics as advised by the International Scientific Advisory Committee

No doubt, a lot of classical and permanent problems of Work With Display Units were named, such as

* lighting and radiation as well as medical surveillance in level 1,
* keyboards and visualization in level 2,
* dialogues and workplace design in level 3,
* job analysis and qualification in level 4,
* acceptance and user participation in level 5,
* work structuring and implementation difficulties in level 6,
* standardization and legislation in level 7.

But, to our pleasure and satisfaction, new problem areas and new topics were brought up, which until then were not yet discussed on conferences to a considerable extent, such as

* stimulating environments and sick building syndromes on level 1,
* multimedia and virtual reality on level 2,
* multiscreen as well as mobile workplaces on level 3,
* problems of aged and handicapped users on level 4,
* crew models and management cocoons of group work in level 5,
* flexibilization and deregulation in level 6,
* ethical aspects and conformity of evaluation procedures in level 7.

With this WWDU-specific bunch of topics potential "market" of 30.000 scientists all over the world was confronted by mailings of our "Calls". We were eager to hear the response to our intended "Service Delivery" in the "Pre contacts".

5. OFFERED TOPICS AND CLASSIFICATION

The response to a call for papers is a clear signal from the research units, how the intentions of the conference organizers and their scientific-advisory committee on the one hand and the actual research work in terms of results and possible presentations can be matched.In January and February 1992 we were overwhelmed by the quantity of presentations and sessions offered to us. The president and secretary general of WWDU read, evaluated and classified almost 500 abstracts, any member of the scientific advisory committee between 20 and 70 abstracts. After this filtering process almost 350 presentations were admitted and classified according to the introduced systematization:

The conference WWDU'92 got its typical shape, its profile shifted from the "ideal" of an equal distribution of contributions over the intended topics to the "real" of the preliminary programme:

It shows a relative weakness in the levels of our paradigm, which deal with societal impacts, with performance oriented organizational measures and group work approaches. We must conclude and admit, that this seems to be the field of action of some other conferences and congresses, which get their reputation and their customers from these research areas. In a competitive world anybody must find his segment of the market and we found ours in the levels 1 to 4 of our scheme: The conference is very strong in the object-oriented fields of workplaces and environments as well as in the 'subject-oriented field of physiological, psychophysical and health-related analysis and diagnosis'. We have another center of gravity in user related and user friendly design approaches, which are connected partially with workload considerations and stress-strain-measurements. From the point of view of application of the research results work protection measurements, respective standardization and legislation procedures are in the focus as well.

From the point of view of continuity we can conclude that WWDU III lies directly in the topic-line of WWDU II and WWDU I. WWDU has become a "brand" with specific criteria of function and quality. So if it is a brand, a market analysis of customer response might be useful too.

6. RESPONSE OF PARTICIPANTS

One possibility to make the market-place of communications more transparent in advance, is to ask the participants, in which topics and sessions they are interested in, beneath perhaps the session they present their own communication. This is a necessary condition to have an unbiased picture of interests. Apparently in the last years and decade, the character of conferences has changed a bit. In former times participants came to hear the famous "preachers" in their discipline. Nowadays almost everybody who wants to go to a conference, has to "preach" himself because otherwise he would not have the chance to raise the funds for his travel expenses and conference fees from his university, his organization or his research foundation. So most participants are presenters themselves, which is a difficulty in separating an interest

Workload, Stress and Strain	Applications in Office and Industry	Work Analysis, Design and Structuring	Strategies for future WWDU
• Critical Organizational and Job Design Issues in Work with VDT and Stress I+II • Stress Considerations in Computer Networks • Health Aspects and Stress Symptoms • Assessment of Stress and Strain Factors • Effects of Electronic Performance Monitoring on VDT User Stress • Longitudinal Studies of Job Design and VDU Work I+II	• Applications in Miscellaneous Areas • Expert Systems and DSS in Medical Area • Information Ergonomics of Videotex-Systems • Video & Hypermedia for Communication within Groups + Demonstrations • Designing Expert and DSS-Systems • VDUs in Education • Computer Aided Design	• Implementation of Data Systems and Impacts on Job Contents • Work with VDT within Groups • Work Organization Factors of Special Interest to Labor Unions • Implementations I • Implementations II	• Research Methods • Methods • Kansei Engineering • Ergonomics of HCI • Applications of Chaos Science to Organizational Behavior • Strategies of International Standardisation • The Context and Consequences of the VDT Health Debate • Social Aspects of Homeworking in Rural Areas • European Regulations for Work with VDT • National Programmes and Social Context of VDT Use

Environmental Impacts	Psychophysiological Aspects	Input Devices and Workplace Design	Fatigue and Health Hazards	User Interfaces
• Sick Building Syndrom • Radiation, Electrostatic and Electromagnetic Fields • Skin Problems, "Electric Sensivity" and VDU Work • Pregnancy Outcomes and VDU Work • Electric and Magnetic Sanitation of the Office • VDT and Lighting I • VDT and Lighting II	• Oculumotor Functions: Concepts and Practical Consequences I+II • Oculumotor Functions: Vertical Gaze Direction • Psychological Effects of Working With VDU • Psychophysiology in the Workplace	• VDT Features and Techniques • VDT-Filter • Input Devices • Colour and Vision I • Colour and Vision II • Workplace Design in Office Area • Workplace Design in Industrial Area • Video Session Workplace Design • Work with VDUs for the Handicapped • Effective Work with VDU	• Current Issues on Health Effects: Perspectives and Trends + MEPS • Two NIOSH Field Studies on Musculoskeletal Disorders • Field Studies to Visual Fatigue • Aspects of Visual Fatigue • Investigations on Muscular Activity and Postures • Field Studies to Muscular and Neuropsychic Fatigue • Strategies for Prevention • Medical Surveillance I+II	• Error Management • Dialoque Techniques • User Interfaces I • User Interfaces II • User Interfaces for Process Control • Usability Evaluation • Multi-modal Interfaces I+II • User Involvement in Development Process • Training and Help

Figure 4. Structure of programme

of presenters, and an interest of the auditory. Nevertheless we tried to get an overview over the relationship between offers and demands: A questionnaire was distributed in our preliminary programme, which was meant to help us in the allocation of rooms with different sizes to sessions. This material can be used to identify the potential interest in conference topics.

The different conference streams are related to the level of interest, they found in the evaluation of those participants, who answered to our question. As expected, the distribution is far from equal. The clear leadership can be assigned to fatigue and health hazards, followed by environmental impacts, psychophysiology, devices and workplaces, workload and strategies on a quite similar level, whereas user interfaces, organizational and performance oriented applications in office and industry as well as work structuring with computers rank comparatively lower in WWDU-contexts.

If we compare the structure of WWDU'92 with that of WWDU'89 and '86 we can diagnose a certain stability. A stability of topics which can be assigned to streams, that are quite similar to those of the past. This indicates, that the problems in WWDU at least grow at a speed, that is even comparable to the generation of solutions by scientific processes.

To a certain extent the scientific and practical problem "Work With Display Units" is coupled to the development of the industrial application of hardware and software technology. No doubt, we can diagnose an explosion of knowledge in the sense of available tools for working processes and a simultaneous decrease of the "half-life" of use of newly introduced products. The cycles of innovation in this field come thick and fast. So a strategy of research for WWDU, which is oriented to an analysis and evaluation of existing tools and structures, is in the bad position of running behind a technological development, which cannot be defined precisely in scientific terms. The "pudding" is flowing away, if you try to nail it to the wall. The strategy has to be oriented to something like an "in process control" of technological development under the aspect of human-oriented and work-related criteria. "Simultaneous Engineering" of the design process with human engineering and social sciences based criteria, a toolbox of methods for evaluation and design seems to be the only alternative to get to the heals or even to pass the high-speed development process of software and hardware technology. We should try to reach this speed of innovation in our perspective of Work With Display Units. We need a spirit of enterprise if we are to overcome our difficulties.

Another stability can be diagnosed in customer demands. As you could see in our theoretical concept of conference planning, our approach to broaden the field of scientific interest which is covered by WWDU, failed to a certain degree. The offers for presentations as well as the interests of the auditory are centered around the "classics" of WWDU.

This stability gives hope and a perspective for future WWDU-conferences: The childhood of the problem field is finished, the maturity of the problem field is signalized by decreasing growth rates, but the possibility to activate more than 700 people for a WWDU conference under the financial restrictions of a worldwide flaw economical situation and activity, gives a clear sign, that WWDU is in its best age, not in position of retiring from the scientific field of action, neither in front of death nor in the position of being suck up by other congress activities.

WORK WITH DISPLAY UNITS 92
H. Luczak, A. Çakir and G. Çakir (Editors)

Occupational Safety and Health and the New Technologies

R. Kraus

Federal Ministry of Labour and Social Affairs, Postfach 14 02 80, 5300 Bonn-Duisdorf, Federal Republic of Germany

1. Invasion of industry and administration by the new technologies

Over the last years industry and administration have virtually been 'invaded' by the new technologies. This also includes the office world being 'invaded' by information technology. A good example in this context is the design engineer. In the past the drawing board was his workplace. Today it is the CAD workplace. In the past he worked with ruler and pencil. Today he uses keyboard and light pen. New technologies liberate employees from burdensome activities, open up more freedom of action and new opportunities. But there is no joy without sorrow.

The introduction of new technologies, also of display screen equipment, first of all triggers of scepticism on the part of the persons concerned which often turns into fear and rejection. The reasons for this reaction are multiple and complex.

The introduction of new technologies may involve social risks. In the beginning jobs may be lost as the monitoring of complicated automated installations and machines requires fewer staff than 'manual work'. The employees concerned have to assume great responsibility which is often accompanied by isolated work to be performed by one staff member only. These technology-linked working conditions put a great strain on the employee's psyche and his physical condition. At first 'only' health problems occur which may develop into diseases once the human body's resistance is lowered.

2. Human work design

The introduction of new technologies requires the broad consent of the persons concerned. Early information and involvement of works council members and concerned employees already during the planning stage are indispensable.

Discussions at the company level must begin at an early stage as only transparency can counteract fears.

Also in the world of technology man must be the measure of all things. This measure is occupational safety and health.

New technologies are always met with acceptance if they are designed in a human way. This leads to high motivation and personal identification of the employees with their work. As a rule this does not only lead to a reduction of working days lost due to illness but also to a reduction of absenteeism and labour turnover. Every employer knows that his employees' ability to perform, their motivation, creativity and of course their health is his most valuable capital in tough international competition.

Human work design is an important basis for a company's success. It is also the basis for a - in the true meaning of the word - 'healthy' national economy. 'Work makes you ill' - this slogan must never be applicable in the modern world of work.

New technologies allow for a more flexible organization of production processes. In order to make full use of this opportunity new roads must be embarked upon when organizing working hours. The planned Law on Working Time takes account of increased flexibility and self-determination with respect to working time organization. In this context the principal prohibition of work on Sundays must not be compromised. Moreover, there must be no doubt that a flexibilisation of working hours has to go hand in hand with improved occupational safety and health. Here night work is a good example. It cannot be generally avoided, but it is in contradiction with man's natural time rythm. Therefore night work has to be linked to an increased protection of the employees' health.

3. Challenges to occupational safety and health

'Those who want to have healthy enterprises must seek to have healthy employees.' This slogan presents a great challenge to all persons concerned which can only be coped with jointly.

For this purpose researchers must also in future process their new findings, instruments and their knowledge so as to accommodate company practice in occupational safety and health. It is important that this knowledge is increasingly incorporated into training and further training.

Design engineers and designers should take account of these research results already when developing and designing products. There is no better approach to a human work design.

Occupational safety and health is a managerial task - just as quality policy is. Opportunities missed today will have to be paid for dearly tomorrow.

Therefore it is necessary to build up an effective and comprehensive system of occupational safety and health at the company level. Occupational safety and health is no social burden. It depends on practice-oriented research. This requires, however, that employers admit researchers to their companies.

4. Occupational safety and health must not stop at country borders

On January 1st, 1993 the European Single Market becomes a reality. It does not only provide for a free movement of goods and persons but also for a European-wide exchange of good ideas.

Further developments in the area of occupational safety and health must not stop at country borders. Occupational health must apply at a transitional level.

Already today it is becoming clear that among the various social policy fields the area of safety and health at the workplace is most strongly governed by Community legislation. A set of directives which lays down binding minimum occupational safety and health requirements on a European-wide basis is already in existence. The so-called occupational safety and health framework directive is of central importance in this context.

It is the future legal basis for occupational safety and health in Europe. Its provisions include all measures that contribute to protecting the lives and health of people in employment, to maintaining ther ability to work and to designing work humanly.

5. Work at with display screen equipment

The Council Directive on minimum provisions concerning the safety and health for work with display screen equipment of May 29th, 1990 is one of the individual directives under the framework directive. It governs the design of these workplaces in a comprehensive manner: from an analysis of the risks involved with working with display screen equipment and the elimination of these risks, the requirements for work organization, the right to eye examinations to minimum requirements for work equipment and hardware, to the working environment and to the man/machine interface.

In the Federal Republic of Germany this directive will be implemented by means of an ordinance which will be based on the new Law on Safety and Health at Work. It is intended to adopt the high protection level provided for by the directive. The accident insurance funds will have the task to lay down more detailed branch-specific provisions. This is necessary because an ordinance cannot on its own govern all applications of the work with display screen equipment finally and definitely.

Work with display screen equipment is constantly gaining in importance. It is estimated that by the year 2000 all in all 4 million display units will be found in German offices. 10 to 15 years ago they amounted to a few hundred units only.

Also in case of work with display screen equipment the safety and health of employees must of course have first priority. All too often employees complain about back pains, eye problems and headaches. These health problems must be identified and remedied as early as possible in order to prevent them from turning into diseases. As examples for factors causing such pains the following may be mentioned:

- adaptation and adjustment problems as well as the fear of technology as a consequence of insufficient employee qualification as well as

- design of computer programmes which is not user-friendly.

In the area of work with display screen equipment there is still a lot of research to be carried out. But a lot has been done already. In the mid-seventies already, the Federal Ministry of Labour and Social Affairs commissioned a detailed research project on work with display units. At the time it included the design of hard- and software as well as the working environment which was a novelty then. The research report was for years the basis for a human design of the work with display screen equipment, also for the subsequent activities of the European Communities.

But the translation of research studies into laws and ordinances alone is not sufficient. Their application at the company level is the key to successful occupational safety and health.

WORK WITH DISPLAY UNITS 92
H. Luczak, A. Çakir and G. Çakir (Editors)
1993 Elsevier Science Publishers B.V.

WORK WITH DISPLAY SCREENS

G. GOUVRAS
Health and Safety Directorate
Commission of the European Communities
Jean Monnet Building
L - 2920 LUXEMBOURG

On behalf of the Commission of the European Communities I wish to extend a warm welcome to the participants of this conference.

The Commission's Health and Safety Directorate, which I represent here, is particularly pleased and honoured by the invitation to take part in the preparation and holding of this event, which it considers to be of a major importance:

Firstly, because it permits the enquirers into the ever-growing field of work with visual display screens to come together and share information on advances in pertinent knowledge.

Secondly because it represents, by its scope, its objectives, its quality, its foreseeable impact, the most vivid vindication of the bold move taken by the Commission of the European Communities, several years back, to make manufacturing industry, regulatory authorities and the social partners to look hard into the consequences of the everyday application of modern technology, of which the display screen was the spearhead, and take the measures needed to ease the adverse impact, allay the fears, and ensure the well-being of users, and in particular workers.

It is my educated guess that no other single piece of human ingenuity has been the object of so much learned study, from so many angles, by so many professionals and researchers, as the display screen. Not the wheel, not pen and paper, not the typing machine ! But, no matter how much was accumulated in knowledge, the quest for new data, more precise information, confirmatory evidence, and unshakeable proofs concerning the human-screen system and its effects on humans continues unabated.

Yet and despite what was going on at the workplace, at the universities and laboratories, and at many a home, the lessons as regards the well-being of those working on display screens were hardly formulated, still less learnt.

Four years ago, the problems and concerns over the display screen surfaced at the political level. The decision-makers and administrators were forced to listen, first to the users, then to the physicians, the scientists and the engineers. The users spoke of eyestrain, difficulties in perception, headaches, skin irritation, back pain, stress, numbness and strain in the hands and arms. More, they related their fears of radiation, of toxic gas emissions, of being spied upon, of being dismissed for not coping with the pace or the system.

The experts unrolled the evidence and guidance that was hitherto available, and advised on the technical, physiological and psychological requirements needed to ensure a symptom-free performance during work with display screens. It all amounted to a solid base from which to launch sets of measures addressing the various aspects of the working environment around the display screen.

The timing and the circumstances were just right when the Commission seized the initiative and proposed legislation, in the form of a Council of Ministers directive on work with display screens.

Indeed, the opening up of the social dimension of the internal market in 1987 privileged occupational health and safety more than any other social issue. The Commission devised a programme in which organisation and management of safety, the arrangement of the workplace, and the application of ergonomics were given the prominence they had long deserved. The directive on display screens, perhaps the most well known of the series of occupational health and safety directives proposed by the Commission as part of its programme, followed a parent directive, which contained the frame for occupational health and safety to be established in the European Community, and two daughter directives dealing with the workplace and work equipment in general.

The directive on display screens not only went further than those in the detail of their common points, but also introduced sound ergonomic principles, including work organisation techniques and software requirements, as well as eye and eyesight examinations. This legislative proposal proved to be too much for many, including, it is true to say, for at least an initial period following the publication of the proposal, some experts. What has happened since the promulgation of the directive though, seems to indicate the Commission's judgement: the matter has been taken seriously by all, set in its right proportion and made the subject of more, multi-disciplined, and rigorous investigation, the main results of which we are about to hear and see during this conference.

I will conclude by stating that the public, the authorities, and most of all those who win their bread working on screens are relying on practitioners such as those assembled here for this conference for their protection and well being; in their endeavour they will find the European Communities a good listener, a friend and a supporter.

WORK WITH DISPLAY UNITS 92
H. Luczak, A. Çakir and G. Çakir (Editors)
1993 Elsevier Science Publishers B.V.

Welcome Address to the Members of the 3rd International Conference, WORK WITH DISPLAY UNITS '92, Berlin, Germany, 1 - 4 September 1992

Prof. Dr.-Ing. D. Severin

Dean of Department 11, Design and Manufacturing,
Technical University of Berlin,
Straße des 17. Juni 135, 1000 Berlin 10.

Mr. President
Mr. Gouvras
Ladies and Gentlemen

On behalf of the President of the Berlin Technical University, who has suddenly fallen ill, and on behalf of my collegues of the Faculty of Mechanical Engineering, I have the honour of welcoming you to Berlin.

This town is changing and developing as fast as the ambitious problems you will be dealing with in the next few days, and I hope the president of this meeting makes enough time available for you to visit the town to get an impression of Berlin history, culture and the special Berlin air at night.

We are happy that this international conference is being held in Berlin, because you can find deep roots of your science in our University, let me say, in our faculty.

I remember Georg Schlesinger. He was one of the first scientists who thought about the connection of science, work und technology.

In 1918, he founded the institute for "Industrial Psychotechnics". He included the human being in his consideration and he introduced his scientific theory.

Schlesinger was convinced of the advantage of the division of labor, and he saw the possibility for rationalization by this means. He anticipated the future changes in work und technology.

At the same time, he was aware of the disadvantages of the separation of mental und manual work. Aware of the loss of knowledge and experience in the field of skilled workers, Schlesinger warned employers. They should consider these people as highly skilled experts, whom all engineers should regard with admiration.

The current state of debate on work organization still bears distinct traits of the reorientation initiated by Schlesinger.

Today, we work for shorter periods of time and with higher productivity. We have more spare time. And our performance has increased.

At the same time, we attempt to redesign technology through innovative concepts of work, not only to overcome the negative consequences of taylorism by avoiding monotony and unskilled tasks, but also by regenerating and mobilizing valuable human resources.

Teamwork, job enlargement, job rotation, job enrichment, workshop-programming, assembly and design islands, lean production, these are some of the main concepts.

And if we think about working with display units, we have to raise the question whether in the age of mechanical reproduction, work has not already become obsolete as an object for studies in the science of technology.

It is my belief that the range of topics offered by this conference is ideally suited to emphasize the interdisciplinary quality of technological science. In the next few days, you will have sufficient opportunity to discuss a wide range of different approaches to work with display units. Experts from different fields will debate the conclusions of their research and applications as we do in our university.

The Berlin Technical University offers a wide range of technical disciplines. In this circumstances, scientific exchange and cooperation can be kept alive in any number of areas, promoting the development of new approaches in research and teaching.

More than ever, we need the cooperation of engineers and colleagues of the human and social sciences.

One of the projects of the German Research Council, which includes a considerable contribution from our University, is dedicated to change conditions of machine design.

The project is entitled "Non-technological components of design under increasing implementation of CAD". It provides a wide field of research for the disciplines of ergonomics, design-technology and psychology. Its aim is to acquire new information about the special demands by using computers and displays. I believe we may expect some important contributions on this topic during this conference.

Ladies and gentlemen, I hope you enjoy your stay in Berlin. I also hope you get a lot of new impressions and experiences during this conference and I would like to say thank you to professor Luczak and his staff, who have organized this meeting so well.

PLENARY SESSIONS

WORK WITH DISPLAY UNITS 92
H. Luczak, A. Çakir and G. Çakir (Editors)

Evaluative research on the prevention of occupational health problems related to the use of VDU

D. Berthelette, Ph.D.

Department of Administrative Sciences, University of Quebec in Montreal, P.O. Box 6192, Station A, Montreal (Quebec), Canada H3C 4R2

Abstract

Despite the large dissemination of ergonomic recommendations on VDU workstation design, there is unsufficient scientific knowledge on their implementation process. Moreover, very few studies have tried to evaluate their effectiveness to prevent VDU operator's health problems. We emphasize the importance of evaluative research in this area and we discuss related methodological issues.

1. INTRODUCTION

Many authors have published various recommendations and a number of standards have been adopted in order to improve the design of VDU workstations and workplaces, and ultimately prevent health problems among VDU operators. The interventions proposed in the literature to improve the workers' well-being and performance, are mainly based on ergonomic theories. Unfortunately, work organization has received less attention. Moreover, the prevention of operators' health problems is more than the simple application of rules. However very few attention has been paid by the scientific community, to the complexity of the ergonomic reform which might have been implemented in the workplace [1]. Despite the need to reduce prevalent symptoms among workers, and the cost of ergonomic reform, very few studies have tried to evaluate the effectiveness of the recommendations published. Further data is needed on this subject if we hope to optimize the outcome of the information and training activities which often ensue from our research project.

2. THE CONTRIBUTION OF EVALUATIVE RESEARCH TO THE STUDY OF VDU

2.1 Historical development of evaluative research

Most definitions of evaluative research seem to share the conviction that its ultimate aim is to produce scientific results which could be used to make a value judgement on an activity, a service, a program or any of its components. Evaluation can be approached in different ways, notably according to the aim of the intervention and to its stage of development. It can serve three immediate goals: a) help plan and develop an intervention, b) provide information for the improvement of the intervention (formative goal) and c) determine the results (outcomes) and consequences (impact) of the intervention (summative goal). In practice, evaluation goals translate into questions which the evaluator wants to answer . Each of these questions correspond to a particular type of evaluation. Table 1 summarizes Champagne's taxonomy of evaluative research [2].

Table 1
Taxonomy of evaluative research

Strategic evaluation	Adequacy between the intervention's objectives and the health problems to be solved
Evaluation of structure	Adequacy of human, physical and financial resources invested
Process evaluation	Adequacy and completeness of the intervention
Evaluation of outcome	Relationship between the intervention and its expected effects
Evaluation of impact	Direct / indirect, desired / undesired changes related to the intervention
Efficacy	Relationship between the outcomes and the intervention process in a controlled optimal environment
Effectiveness	Relationship between the outcomes and the intervention process in a real life setting
Efficiency	Relationship between the program resources and its outcomes

Program evaluation emerged as a discipline in the United States, in the 1960s. Two main factors seem to be related to its emergence: the rapid growth of governmental funding of social programs [3] and the increase of formal rationality and accountability [4]. The stakeholders were mainly concerned with the efficiency of the programs in producing their expected outcomes. The evaluators primary focus was to assess wether or not the programs worked. In this context, the experimental paradigm dominated the discipline: programs were conceptualized as dichotomous variables. Moreover, evaluators were mainly concerned with the development of scientific methods which could maximize the internal validity of their study [5-6]. However, atheoretical evaluation referred as "black box evaluation", fails to produce scientific knowledge on the underlying mechanisms of programs success or failure. Consequently, it provides little useful information for program design and improvement [4].

During the last decade some authors have stressed the importance of theory-oriented evaluation which takes into account the complexities of program components. Moreover, it can help clarify the role of contextual variables which can accompany the program under study, or interact with its components for the production of its outcomes [4]. According to this perspective the "black box" needs to be opened. Since the relative contribution of the program components and context is evaluated, it can provide useful information to improve program development. Our work is in line with this approach.

2.2 Previous evaluative studies on VDU

Most of the evaluative studies on VDU design are laboratory experiments. They put the emphasis on the efficacy of specific recommendations: in general, the researchers attempt to compare the effect of one specific VDU workstation attribute on work performance, some physiological characteristics and/or satisfaction and comfort. The main variables used in these studies are listed in tables 2 and 3.

Table 2
Dependent variables used in evaluative studies about VDU

Physiological measurements	Subjective measurement
• Visual function tests	• Comfort/ discomfort
• Muscle activity	• Worker well-being
	• Fatigue
VDU task performance	• Body complaints
• Time	• Preferences / perceptual quality
• Accuracy	• Satisfaction
• Lost of productive time	

Table 3
Independent variables used in evaluative studies about VDU

Screen quality	Workstation setting
• Type of screen	• Table
• Display size	• Chair
• Screen luminance	• Arm / wrist support
• Screen luminance contrast	• Line of sight angle
• Image polarity	• Viewing distances
• Colors	
• Filters / antireflection coatings	
Lighting	Keyboard
• Direct / indirect	• Conventional/ flat
• Office / workstation	• Optimal configuration
Ophtalmic lenses	Postures
	• 90° upright/backward/forward leaning
	• Standing / sitting
	Work organization
	• Kind / number of breaks
	• Learning
	Gymnastic

[1] References are available from the author upon request.

Although experimental studies are useful, their scope is limited. Since they are done in a controlled environment, their internal validity is increased. However, this is at the expense of external validity: we cannot be sure that their results could be reproduced in a real work environment. For one thing, sample size is small and subjects are not representative of usual VDU operators. In addition, these studies do not allow us to evaluate operators' utilization of the modifications brought to the VDU workstation design. For example, in laboratory experiments, the workstation is already appropriately set by the observer for the subject, whereas in a real life situation, not all operators will know how to set the potential complex adjustment of its workstation. Finally, experimental studies do not allow for an evaluation of the relative effect of simultaneous modifications made to VDU workstations, to job design and to work organization on operators' well-being and performance.

2.3 Analysis of implementation

Field studies are the only means of assessing the degree to which the prevalence of the operator's health problems have been reduced by the implementation of various recommendations. However, given the potential diversity of the different strategies developed by the firms, evaluation of results is unsufficient to identify the specific recommendations which are producing the best results. Analysis of implementation is a type of evaluative research which can help to achieve this goal. It is based on a theoretical framework which includes independent variables both on the intervention process and resources, and the organizational context in which the intervention is implemented [7-8]. The internal validity of this type of study is closely related to the theoretical framework complexity and exhaustivity. In the case of VDU, since we possess little information on the ergonomic reforms implemented by different worksettings, a grounded theory approach would be cost-effective: an exploratory study should be done, prior to the evaluative research, in order to build the theoretical framework i.e. to identify the many dimensions of both the recommendations actually implemented in the worksettings and the organizational context in which they took place. Moreover the theoretical framework should include variables on the VDU operators characteristics. Finally, cross-sectional design would be recommended, the workstation being the unit of analysis. The sample size should be 6 to 10 times the number of independent variables in order to obtain an adequate statistical power. Albeit analysis of implementation requires much effort, we believe it can enhance our knowledge and our capacity to identify efficient interventions.

3. REFERENCES

1 S. Sauter, M. Dainoff and M. Smith (eds.), Promoting Health and Productivity in the Computerized Office: Models of Successful Ergonomic Interventions, Taylor and Francis, London, 1990.

2 F. Champagne, A.P. Contandriopoulos and R. Pineault, Health Care Program Evaluation, Health Management Forum, Vol.7 (1986): 57-65.

3 W.R. Shadish Jr., T.D. Cook and L.C. Leviton, Foundations of Program Evaluation, Sage Publications, Inc., Newbury Park, 1991.

4 H.T. Chen, Theory-Driven Evaluations, Sage Publications, Inc., Newbury Park, 1990.

5 D.T. Campbell and J.C. Stanley, Experimental and Quasi-Experimental Designs for Research, Houghton Mifflin Company, Boston, 1966.

6 T.D. Cook and D.T. Campbell, Quasi-Experimentation: Design and Analysis Issues for Field Settings, Houghton Mifflin Company, Boston, 1979.

7 J.-L. Denis and F. Champagne, Analyse de l'implantation: rôle et méthode, La Revue canadienne d'évaluation de programme, Vol.5 (1990): 45-65.

8 F. Champagne and J.-L. Denis, Pour une évaluation sensible au contexte: l'analyse d'implantation, Service social, Vol. 41 (1991): 143-163.

WORK WITH DISPLAY UNITS 92
H. Luczak, A. Çakir and G. Çakir (Editors)

Organizational design and management (ODAM) in HCI

H. W. Hendrick

Institute of Safety and Systems Management, University of Southern California, Los Angeles, CA 90089-0021, USA

Abstract

The concept of macroergonomics is reviewed, including its historical development and relation to other ergonomics technologies. The sociotechnical systems model is summarized, and its use in macroergonomically improving HCI systems is discussed. The relating of macro- to micro-ergonomic design to achieve synergism is proposed as a means for *exponentially* improving HCI productivity, operator health and job satisfaction.

1. INTRODUCTION

As a practice, ergonomics has tended to focus on the design of specific jobs and related human-machine interfaces, or at the *micro-ergonomic* level. Conceptually, it is entirely possible to do an outstanding job of micro-ergonomically designing a system's work stations and environments, yet fail to reach relevant system effectiveness goals because of inattention to human factors activities at the *macro-ergonomic* level (Hendrick, 1984). No where is this failure more prevalent than in WWDU jobs. One need only review the proceedings from the previous WWDU conferences to gain an appreciation of this failure. Indeed, widespread problems with both operator health and job satisfaction were the motivation for these WWDU conferences.

2, HISTORICAL DEVELOPMENT OF MACROERGONOMICS

ODAM was first given formal recognition in ergonomics by the U.S. "Human Factors Society Select Committee on the Future of Human Factors, 1980-2000" (Hendrick, 1991). Papers based on the Committee's work were presented at the HFS Annual Meeting in 1980, including my own on *Human Factors in Management*. Based on my research of organizational trends, I noted the following which were of particular relevance to WWDU's.

2.1 Technology

The rapid development of new technology in the computer and telecommunications industries would fundamentally alter the nature of work in offices and factories during the 1980-2000 time frame. In general, we were entering a true information and automation age that would profoundly affect work organization and related human-machine interfaces.

2.2 Demographic shifts

During the next two decades the work force will become progressively older, more experienced, and professionalized. As professionalism increases, it becomes important for work systems to become less formalized, tactical decision-making to become decentralized, and management systems to similarly accommodate.

2.3 Value changes

Beginning in the late '60s, a fundamental shift in the value systems of the work force has been occurring internationally. Briefly, workers now both value and expect to have greater control over the planning and pacing of their work, greater decision-making responsibility, and jobs that enable a greater sense of responsibility and accomplishment (e.g.,see Argyrus, 1971;Yankelovich,1979). Collectively, these findings indicate that effective future ergonomic design will require consideration of ODAM factors as an integral part of work systems design.

2.4 The failure of traditional (micro) ergonomics

Early attempts to incorporate ergonomics into the design of VDU work stations and software have been disappointing in their effectiveness. Better designed work stations and software clearly are an improvement, but less than expected gains in productivity, continued symptoms of high job stress, and poor intrinsic job satisfaction remain the norm rather than the exception. [More recent WWDU evidence comes from a NIOSH (1992) study: Upper extremity disorders of VDT users were found associated with seven psycho-social variables of the type typically addressed by macro-, rather than micro-ergonomic design.]

Based upon these and other observations, I concluded in my 1980 paper that for the ergonomics profession to be truly effective in the future, there was a strong requirement to integrate ODAM factors into our research and practice. It is interesting to note that all of these predictions from 1980 have come to pass, and are continuing. I believe these same factors explain why the ODAM focus of ergonomics has enjoyed such rapid growth, including the new technology of *macroergonomics*.

3. THE CONCEPT OF MACROERGONOMICS

One way to define, the nature of any field of science and practice is by noting the nature of its *technology*. I have proposed that the unique technology of ergonomics is *human-system interface* technology (Hendrick, 1991). At present, this technology has at least four identifiable major components. Ranging from the earlier to the most recently developed, they are: *Human-machine interface technology* or hardware ergonomics; *human-environment interface technology* or environmental ergonomics; *user-system interface technology* or software ergonomics (also known as cognitive ergonomics); and *organizational-machine technology* or macroergonomics.

Conceptually, *macroergonomics is a top-down sociotechnical systems approach to organizational and work system design, and the design of related human-machine, user-system, and human environment interfaces.* In order to gain an understanding of macroergonomics, one first must have a familiarity with the key components of organizational structure and a grasp of the empirically derived sociotechnical systems model.

3.1 The components of organizational structure

The structure of an organization can be conceptualized as having three major components: *complexity, formalization,*and *centralization* (Robbins, 1983). *Complexity* refers to the degree of *differentiation* and *integration* inherent in the systems structure. Three major types of differentiation exist in organizations: *Horizontal differentiation*, or the degree of departmentalization and specialization; *vertical differentiation*, or the number of hierarchical levels; and *spatial differentiation* or the number of units geographically separated from the headquarters, proportion of employees not in the headquarters, and the extent of geographical dispersion. *Integration* refers to the number of integrating mechanisms required to ensure effective coordination and control of the differentiated elements. As differentiation increases, the number of integrating mechanisms needed for effective functioning also increases.

Formalization refers to the extent to which work processes are controlled by rules, procedures and detailed job descriptions, and employee discression is limited by the design of software and hardware interfaces. As education and training (professionalism) requirements increase, formalization needs to be decreased for effective functioning.

Centralization is the extent to which decision-making is concentrated in an individual or unit, usually high in the organization. It should be noted that system requirements may be different for *tactical* and *strategic* decision-making.

3.2 The sociotechnical systems model

To more adequately convey the nature of complex human-machine systems, Emory and Trist (1960) coined the term "sociotechnical system". The sociotechnical system concept views organizations as open systems engaged in transforming inputs into desired outputs. Organizations bring two major components to bear on the transformation process: Technology in the form of a *technical subsystem,* and people in the form of a *personnel subsystem* These two subsystems interact with one another at every human-machine and user-system interface. They thus are interdependent and operate under *joint causation*, meaning that both are affected by causal events in the environment.

Joint causation gives rise to an important related sociotechnical concept of particular importance to ergonomics: *joint optimization.* Joint optimization means that since both the technical and personnel subsystems respond jointly to causal events, optimizing one subsystem and then fitting the other to it will result in suboptimization of the joint *system.* Joint optimization thus requires *joint design* of the two subsystems.

3.3 Sociotechnical system considerations in work system design

As inferred from the above, the design of an organization's

structure involves consideration of the key elements of three socio-technical system components: (a) the technological subsystem, (b) the personnel subsystem, and (c) the relevant external environments. Each of these three major system components has been studied in relation to its effect on the fourth component, organizational structure, and empirical models have emerged that can be used to optimize a system's organizational design. I have summarized a number of these models and how they can be used in macroergonomics (e.g., see Hendrick, 1987; 1991). For example, the (a)information requirements of the technology, (b)professionalism level of employees, and (c)degree of environmental complexity and change all can be assessed and used to determine the optimal levels of the organizational complexity dimensions, integration requirements, formalization, and centralization of decision-making, based on empirically developed models.

3.4 Relation of macro- to micro-ergonomic design

Through a macroergonomic approach to determining the optimal design of an organization's structure, many of the characteristics of the jobs to be designed into the system, and of the related human-machine and user-system interfaces, already have been prescribed. In summary, effective macroergonomic design drives much of the micro-ergonomic design of the system, and thus insures *optimal ergonomic compatability* of the system components with the system's overall structure. In contrast, a purely micro-ergonomic approach has a high probability of creating systems in which the personnel subsystem is forced to adapt to the system's technology and structure in a suboptimal fashion. Beginning with the classic longwall coal mining studies by the Tavistock Institute (Trist and Bamforth, 1951), and carrying though to numerous WWDU studies, including some of those reported in these WWDU conferences, the organizational literature is full of examples which show that this lack of compatibility adversely affects system functioning.

4. MACROERGONOMICS AND ACHIEVING ORGANIZATIONAL SYNERGISM

As we have noted, macroergonomics has the potential to improve the ergonomic design of systems by ensuring that the system's organizational design harmonizes with the system's critical sociotechnical characteristics. Equally important, macroergonomics offers the means to ensure that the design of the entire work system, down to each individual VDU job and work station, harmonizes with the over-all structure of the system.

A widely accepted view among system scientists is that organizations are synergistic: that the whole is more, or less, than the simple sum of its parts. Because of this synergism, when organizational structures are grossly incompatible with their sociotechnical system characteristics, and/or jobs and human-system interfaces are incompatible with the organization's structure, the whole is *less than* the sum of its parts. Under these conditions, we can expect the various indices of organizational functioning to be poor, including WWDUs. In contrast, when organizational structures have been effectively designed macroergonomically, and that effort is carried through to the micro-ergonomic design of WWDU jobs and work stations, then indices of system functioning will be much *greater* than the simple sum of the parts would indicate.

Assuming the above two propositions are indeed true, then *macroergonomic approaches have the potential to improve system functioning exponentially rather than linearly.* For example, indices of productivity, accidents, repetitive strain, and employee job satisfaction among VDU operators should not show the typical 10% to 20% improvement often seen as the result of typical *successful* micro-ergonomic efforts. Instead, improvements of 60% to 80% more typically should occur (and, in some cases, much greater) and be sustainable. Already, there is some empirical support for this expectation. For example, in several recently reported industrial studies in Japan and the U.S. by Nagamachi and Imada (1992) using macroergonomic approaches, reductions in both industrial injuries and motor vehicle accidents by 76% to over 90% were achieved; and, to date, have been sustained.

REFERENCES

Argyris,C.(1971). *Management and Organizational Development.* New York: McGraw-Hill.

Emery,F.E.and Trist,E.L.(1960). Sociotechnical systems. In C. W. Churchman and M. Verhuylst (Eds.), *Management Science: Models and Techniques, Vol 2.* Oxford: Pergamon.

Hendrick,H.W.(1984). Wagging the tail with the dog: Organizational design considerations in ergonomics. *Proceedings of the Human Factors Society 28th Annual Meeting.* Santa Monica, CA: Human Factors Society.

Hendrick,H.W.(1987). Organizational design. In G. Salvendy (Ed.), *Handbook of Human Factors.* New York: Wiley, 470-494.

Hendrick,H.W.(1991). Human factors in organizational design and management. *Ergonomics, 34*,743-756.

NIOSH (1992). Health Hazard Evaluation Report, US West Communications. HETA 89-299-2230.

Nagamachi,M.,and Imada,A.S.(1992). A Macroergonomic approach for improving safety and work design, *Proceedings of the Human Factors Society 36th Annual Meeting*. Santa Monica, CA: Human Factors Society,859-861.

Robbins, S.R. (1983). *Organizational theory:the structure and design of organizations*. Englewood Cliffs, NJ: Prentice-Hall.

Trist,E.L.,and Bamforth,K.W. (1951). Some social and psychological consequences of the longwall method of coal-getting. *Human Relations, 4,* 3-38.

WORK WITH DISPLAY UNITS 92
H. Luczak, A. Çakir and G. Çakir (Editors)

A "Balance" Model for Examining Psychological Job Stress in VDU Work

Michael J. Smith, Pascale Carayon

Dept. of Industrial Engineering, University of Wisconsin, Madison, WI 53706 USA

Abstract

Work organization considerations and job stress factors have been examined at computerized workplaces since the late 1970's (Cakir et al, 1978; Gunnarsson & Ostberg, 1977). Additional attention was given in the 1980's (Smith, et al, 1980, Dainoff, 1982; Johansson & Aronsson, 1984; Aronsson & Johansson, 1986; Stellman et al, 1987; Sainfort, 1989; Smith & Carayon-Sainfort, 1990; Aronsson, 1989; Schleifer & Amick, 1989) and still continues today. However, there have been relatively few work organization and job stress research studies as compared to other VDU considerations. Since the early 1970's, the primary emphasis in examining human-computer interaction at work (including VDU use) has been on the physical safety and ergonomic aspects of the environment, the design of the workstation and technology design and safety (Bergqvist, 1984; Smith, 1987; Smith et al, 1992). This is changing as there becomes increasing recognition that computerization at the workplace has substantial effects on the design of work and work organizations. To examine the potential job stress impact of the VDU at the workplace it is useful to develop a conceptual framework. This paper presents a theoretical perspective termed the "balance" theory (Smith & Carayon-Sainfort, 1989).

INTRODUCTION:

Occupational stress is emerging as a major factor in the health of many employees who work with video display units (VDU's). There are four recognized mechanisms through which VDU work has the potential to affect user stress response and subsequently health. These are (1) sociotechnical influences, (2) psychosocial effects, (3) techno-stress and (4) interactions with ergonomic factors. The following describes some of the effects of work organization and design on employee stress and an approach for achieving better job design for VDU work.

SOCIOTECHNICAL INFLUENCES:

Changes in the structure and nature of work occur when VDU's are introduced into the workplace. These changes are necessary for the efficient utilization of the new technology and the recovery of the costs of the technology. Often, there is an increase in the amount of workload with a decrease in the number of employees. The technology brings about efficiencies that fundamentally change the nature of the work activities. These changes have been shown to affect work satisfaction and mental health (Smith et al, 1981). In addition, a number of "ergonomic" problems have accompanied the introduction of VDU's which have led to physical health complaints regarding vision and upper extremity musculoskeletal disorders (Gunnarsson and Ostberg, 1977; Cakir, Hart and Stewart, 1979). These sociotechnical problems are due to the transition from one technology to another, which creates "change" with all of the associated uncertainty, restructuring, new learning and performance "tension".

PSYCHOSOCIAL:

As already described, there are substantial job task changes that can accompany the use of VDU's at work. Stress considerations in VDU work include changes in workload, workpacing, the complexity of tasks, personal control over the task, participation in decision making, socialization, peer support, supervisory style career advancement potential and job stability (Smith, et al, 1980,1981, 1992; Dainoff, 1982; Johansson and Aronsson, 1984, 1986; Stellman et al, 1987; Sainfort, 1990; Aronsson, 1989). The use of computer technology has tended to produce increased workloads, greater work pressure, loss of personal control, social isolation, decreased social support of peers, less supportive and' more aggressive supervision, less career advancement potential and greater possibility of job loss. While, the nature and extent of these VDU work-related stressors vary from company to company, they have generally been observed in many diverse settings with a variety of management styles and organizational structures.

TECHNO-STRESS:

Brod (1984) has characterized some of the "psychological" disturbances that are unique to using technology such as VDU's. These psychological effects are created from fear that the technology can cause the user serious harm. For instance, many pregnant VDU operators worry about the effects of radiation from the VDU on the developing fetus and themselves. This fear can cause stress that may produce adverse health consequences for the women and the fetuses. Other psychological disturbances that have been defined include equipment phobias and delusions about the equipment. Some VDU users develop a debilitating fear of the VDU such that the employee cannot function normally in the presence of the VDU. Others experience frightening dreams about the VDU having intelligence which wishes to harm them. For a very small proportion of VDU users, these fears may lead to psychotic episodes.

ERGONOMIC:

There is evidence accumulating that the stress associated with VDU use may contribute to cumulative musculoskeletal disorders (Smith, et al, 1981; Bernard et al, 1992; Hales et al, 1992; Smith et al, 1992). The psychological and biological mechanisms by which this may occur have been postulated by Carayon and Smith (1993). At the personal level psychological stress can lead to an increased physiological susceptibility to CTD's by modifying hormonal responses and circulatory responses that exacerbate the influences of the traditional risk factors of repetition, posture and force. In addition, psychological stress can affect employee attitude, motivation and behavior which can lead to risky behaviors that increase CTD risk. At the organizational level, the policies and procedures of a company can affect CTD risk through the design of jobs, the length of exposure to risk, the nature of work-rest cycles, defining the extent of work pressures and establishing the psychological climate regarding socialization, career development and job security. In addition, the organization defines the nature of the task activities (work methods), the level of employee training, the availability of assistance and supervisory relations.

WORK ORGANIZATION, STRESS AND BALANCING:

We have shown how work organization and job stress factors can have an influence on employee psychological and physical health. The mechanisms of action are varied, but they are interrelated. Strategies to research, evaluate and control psychosocial stress factors related to VDU work must be comprehensive to accommodate this huge range of mechanisms. One such approach is the balance theory proposed by Smith and Carayon-Sainfort (1989). This model can be used to establish relationships between job demands, job design factors, work organization and ergonomic loads. The work system has five elements: (1) the person, (2) the work environment, (3) tasks, (4) technology and (5) the work organization.

In this model these various elements interact when work is being done, and the overall physical and psychological effects are defined by the ways in which these elements are integrated. This is a systems concept in that any one element will have an influence(s) on any other element(s). Demands are placed on the individual by the other four elements which create loads that can be healthy or harmful. Harmful loads lead to physical and psychological stress responses that can produce adverse health effects such as CTD's. (See Smith and Carayon-Sainfort, 1989 for a more detailed explanation of how the elements interrelate and the role of specific stress factors).

This model defines the process by which working conditions at different levels (i.e. individual, task, environment, technology, and organization) can produce worker stress. The model is comprehensive enough to address the four mechanisms of VDU related psychological stress, eg, the sociotechnical, psychosocial, techno-stress and ergonomic. It proposes a system that helps balance the loads placed on the employee due to these mechanisms. When balance cannot be achieved through changing the negative elements of the workplace, then it can be improved by enhancing the positive elements to achieve a better "balancing". Thus, the good aspects of work can be used to "counter-balance" the bad. The essence of this approach is to reduce physical and psychological stress and the negative health consequences not only by removing sources of stress, but also by "balancing" the various elements of the work system.

CONCLUSIONS:

A comprehensive model of work design that encompasses various elements of design considerations is required to research and understand the complex mechanisms of job stress in VDU work. This paper has presented such a model. Proper job design can be achieved by providing those characteristics of each work element that meet recognized criteria for physical loads, work cycles and job content that provide for individual physiological and psychological needs. The best designs will eliminate all sources of stress. However, as such a perfect job cannot always be achieved, then using positive work elements to compensate for poor work elements can balance the stress by moderating those factors that reduce the load and potential satisfaction, emotional and physical health consequences. Research should concentrate not only on the critical dimensions of each element, but also on how the elements are integrated to properly characterize job stress and propose effective solutions.

REFERENCES

Aronsson, G., 1989. Changed qualification demands in computerized administrative work, Applied Psychology: An International Review, 38, 57-71.

Aronsson, G. and Johansson, G., 1986. Work content, stress and health in computer-mediated work, in B. Knave & P.G. Wideback (Eds) Work With Display Units 86, Amsterdam: Elsevier, 732-738.

Bergqvist, U., 1984. Video display terminals and health: a technical and medical appraisal of the state of the art, Scandinavian Journal of Work and Environmental Health, 10, 1-87.

Bernard, B., Sauter, S., Peterson, M. and Hales, T., 1992. Upper extremity musculoskeletal outcomes among newspaper employees, in H. Luczak, A. Çakir & G. Çakir (Eds) Work With Display Units 92 Abstracts, Berlin: TUB, D-15.

Çakir, A., Hart, D. and Stewart, T., 1979. The VDT Manual, Darmstadt: Ince-Fry Research Association.

Carayon, P. and Smith, M.J., 1993. Stress and cumulative trauma disorders: a theoretical relationship, Madison: Dept. of Industrial Engineering - University of Wisconsin.

Dainoff, M., 1982. Occupational stress factors in visual display terminal operation: a review of empirical research, Behavior and Information Technology, 1, 141-176.

Gunnarsson, E. and Ostberg, O., 1977. The physical and psychological working environment in a terminal-based computer storage and retrieval system, Stockholm: NBOSH Report 35.

Johansson, G. and Aronsson, G., 1984. Stress reactions in computerized administrative work. Journal of Occupational Behaviour 5: 159-181.

Hales, T., Sauter, S., Peterson, M. & Bernard, B., 1992. Upper extremity musculoskeletal conditions among VDT users in a telecommunications company, in H. Luczak, A. Çakir & G. Çakir (Eds) Work With Display Units 92 Abstracts, Berlin: TUB, D-14.

Sainfort, P. Carayon, 1990. Job design predictors of stress in automated offices, Behavior and Information Technology, 9, 3 -1 6.

Schleifer, L. and Amick, B., 1989. System response time and method of pay: stress effects in computer based tasks, International Journal of Human-Computer Interaction, 1, 23-39.

Smith, M.J., 1987. Mental and physical strain at VDT workstations, Behavior and Information Technology, 6, 243-255.

Smith, M.J., Cohen, B.G. and Stammerjohn, L.W. Jr., 1981. An investigation of health complaints and job stress in video display operations. Human Factors, 23(4): 387-400.

Smith, M.J., Carayon, P. and Miezio, K., 1987. VDT technology: psychosocial and stress concerns. In: Knave, B. and Wideback, P.-G. (Eds.), Work With Display Units 86. Elsevier Science Publishers, The Netherlands. 695-712.

Smith, M.J. and Carayon:Sainfort, P., 1989. A balance theory of job design for stress reduction, International Journal of Industrial Ergonomics, 4, 67-79.

Smith, M.J., Carayon, P., Sanders, K.J., Lim, S-Y and LeGrande, D., 1992. Employee stress and health complaints with and without electronic performance monitoring, Applied Ergonomics, April, 1 - 11.

Stellman, J.M., Klitzman, S., Gordon, G.C. and Snow, B.R., 1985. Air quality and ergonomics in the office: survey results and methodologic issues. American Industrial Hygiene Association Journal 46(5): 286-293.

WORK WITH DISPLAY UNITS 92
H. Luczak, A. Çakir and G. Çakir (Editors)

Externalizing Task Structures for Software Design Purposes

W. Dzida

German National Research Center of Computer Science,System Design Technology Institute, Schloss Birlinghoven, D-5205 Sankt Augustin 1, Germany

Abstract

In designing software the design of user's tasks is implied. The semantic nature of task is conceived as an event structure which is extrapolated from the concept of problem, and is represented in terms of a Petri net, so as to provide a formal model of a task. The model fits in well with the paradigm of action-regulation. Assuming that Petri nets help externalizing valid task representations, they can be applied to test the semantics of software design for compliance with the user's concepts of tasks.

1. Introduction

A well accepted statement is that the design of software can also be conceived as the design of human work tasks (Hacker, 1987). For instance, the separation of computer functions from human functions is a key problem of both the design of tasks and software. Although accepted among specialists in ergonomics the above mentioned statement has rarely been taken seriously by system designers. They almost exclusively conceive software design as a means to automate a work domain according to the potential of software technology.

A rarely recognized statement, however, is that task design should contribute to software design, so as to take the design of tasks as an opportunity to prepare the validation of the software design. Provided the representation of tasks validly externalizes the semantic concepts of users, the mapping of task design to software design should be evaluated for quality assurance purposes.As a preventive measure this validation contributes to the assurance of software quality in a very early stage of the user-centered design process.

This paper argues for a theory-based model of 'task', the semantics of which can be verified. Empirical results in the research of human memory organization (Klix, 1984, 1986) as well as assumptions involved in the psychological paradigm of action-regulation (Volpert, 1982, Hacker, 1985) are taken as a compound platform to establish a model of 'task'. Furthermore, elementary semantic concepts which are assumed to govern human knowledge representation are linked to a well-recognized design language, a class of so-called Petri nets, thereby introducing a formal approach into the design of work tasks.

2. The role of tasks in human-computer interaction

The design of human-computer systems incorporates as an essential element: the task. Prior to the design of the system it is vital to really understand the user's task. Commonly raised questions are: "What are you working upon?" "What means are you using for this purpose?" "What is the result contributing to?" Thus, the user's internally stored concepts of tasks are attempted to be externalized.

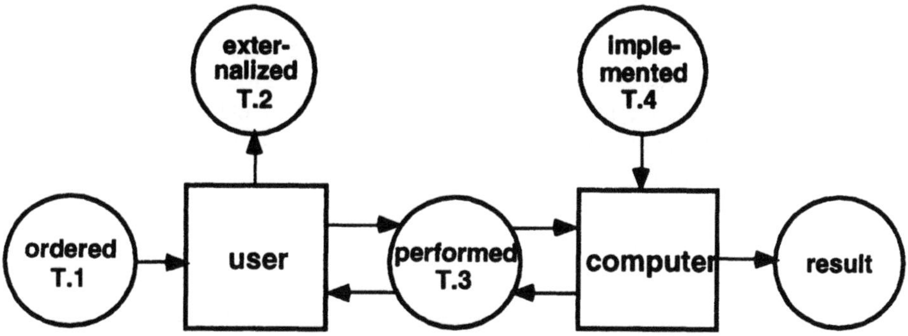

Figure 1: Various aspects of task (T) in a user-computer system

Figure 1 illustrates a user-computer system which particularly directs the attention to the various roles a task (T) can play. User and computer are conceived as active components in the shared execution of a task. The external task (T.1), i.e. an *order* (c.f. Hacker, 1985), is an objective entity, but need not necessarily comply with the user's internally represented task concept, i.e. the mental model of the task which needs to be elicited (T.2). Furthermore, the user's concept of a task may be affected by the features of the user-interface where the task is performed (T.3). Last but not least, it is questionable whether the designer has implemented valid concepts of tasks (T.4).

3. From problem to task

Human beings organize their memory such that nearly all semantic concepts can be reduced to three basic concepts: event, object, and relation (Klix, 1984, 1986). In applying these results to the concept of task the question is raised: "Is a task an event or an object?" It can easily be shown that a task is an event. To give evidence to this postulate I trace back the concept of task to the semantic structure of *problem*. Essential components establishing the concept of problem (i.e. a certain class of problems) are the initial state, the goal state, and a yet unspecified operation working on the initial state to transform its properties. The concepts of problem and task are quite similar. The task evolves from a successfully completed problem solving process. A task appears to be executable due to its specified operation, whilst a problem is somehow inactive, because of the unknown means which are needed to achieve the goal. If the concept of problem is conceived as an event, its core concept is an *activity*, which is yet unspecified. A task is also a typical event structure; the involved activity is aimed at a transformation of an object to yield a result that satisfies a goal. The yet unknown core concept of a problem is associated to a goal (intended object). In that the problem solving process determines a core concept, the goal is semantically transformed into a specific result (the attainable object). Thus, the problem solving process implies a test of realizability. Hence, it is expedient to distinguish goal and result in knowledge representation. - The tool is an essential constituent of the concept of task. A tool is inherently characterized by its capability of causing typical effects on an object. These effects are attainable results which, of course, may serve different goals. The concept of tool determines the core concept of a task, an activity; it also specifies the result. From an activity (called *operation* in cognitive psychology) an operator is extracted to specify the operation and to give evidence for the realizability of a result.

4. A model of the task

The ergonomic and psychological literatur reveals a tremendous confusion about what a task is. The space for this paper does not allow to trace back to these sources. Instead I want to introduce a concept of task which integrates the tradition of thought in cognitive psychology (see e.g. Newell and Simon, 1972) as well as work psychology. From the cognitive perspective the semantic concept of task might be represented as a semantic net composed of a number of sub-concepts (such as tool, object, result) which constitute the task. From the work psychologist's perspective a task might be conceived as a goal directed activity with the goal being represented as a specific result to be achieved. From the designer's perspective the concept of task needs to be represented in terms of a (semi-)formal language, serving as a means for communication between him and the user.These three perspectives contribute to a model of task which is represented in terms of a Petri net (figure 2); for Petri nets see Reisig, 1985.

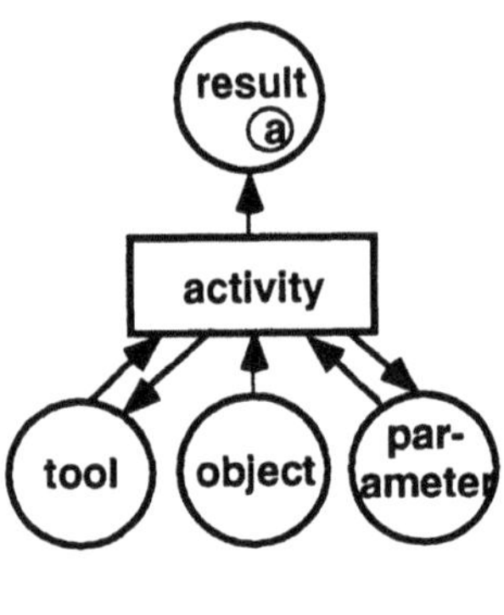

Figure 2: Components of a task

An example may help explain the model in detail: Let us assume that your task is to make a photo with the aid of a camera. To photograph is the *activity* to be carried out. The picture is the intended *result*, the camera is the *tool*, and the film is the *object*. In forming the concept of task it is important to consider the main result, but it may also be relevant to consider additional attributes of this result. The attributes are of secondary importance and may be planned as effects in addition to the main effect. A *parameter* of the camera serves as a means for justification to achieve such additional attributesⓐ for instance, a sharp background can be achieved by adjusting the aperture.

This model of the task has some advantages. It is assumed to represent the user's internal concept of task. For instance, the above mentioned concept 'photograph' can be the semantic core of an *event*, with the core concept being related to a number of objects, e.g. the object 'camera' is associated with photograph and the established relation can be named 'instrument'. Furthermore, the model is in line with fundamental assumptions of the action-regulation theory (see section 5), and it is represented by a formalism which is not at all arbitrary, since the formalism fits in well with empirical results of research in memory organization (see section 6).

5. Task structures

The semantic concept of task can properly be integrated in the action-regulation theory. Figure 3 illustrates a graph which represents an *action-unit*. This is a portion within a complex of action-units organized hierarchically and sequentially (Volpert, 1982).

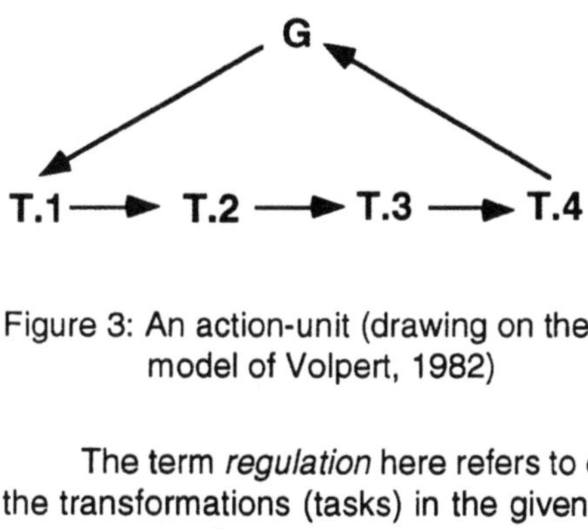

Figure 3: An action-unit (drawing on the model of Volpert, 1982)

Each action-unit is generated as a sequence of goal-directed *transformations* (T) starting with an initial one (T.1), continued by mediating transformations which contribute to the accomplishment of the unit. A check of the final result for compliance with the goal (G) completes the unit. Taking each transformation as a *task* one can say that the concept of action-unit is *refined* by a sequence of tasks.

The term *regulation* here refers to cognitive control governing the performance of the transformations (tasks) in the given order. Further regulation functions govern the performance of the whole action structure, the action-unit being a component of it. Figure 4 illustrates the hierarchical order of an action. The decomposition is controlled by a *specification* of the action into sub-actions up to action-units. Ideally one can assume that the performance of an action is regulated top down. The leaves of the tree structure represent elementary tasks. All higher order nodes represent action-units (or sub-actions) which are refined by higher level tasks. Hence, in externalizing knowledge on an action, people 'vertically' *specify* an action on different levels of abstraction, and on each level an action is 'horizontally' *refined* in terms of tasks.

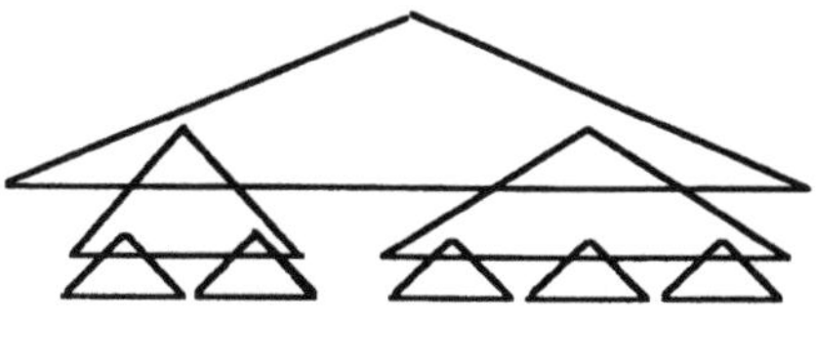

Fig. 4: Hierarchical order of an action (c.f. Volpert, 1982)

Thus, tasks are externalized in more or less concrete terms depending on the level within the action structure. These structural features are in line with empirical results of memory research, where *refinement* and *specification* are found as fundamental mechanisms in memory organization (Klix, 1984).

6. Externalized task structures

The structural features of an action can be utilized when eliciting the users knowledge on his tasks. A representation of the externalized task structures in terms of Petri nets is recommended. Figure 5 illustrates fragments of nets to show, how tasks are arranged on different levels of specification. On the top level an organized conference is completed, if the conceptualized programme (see fig. 5) has been delivered as a result among four results which complementarily contribute to the general goal. Below the action level one of four action-units is *specified*. The conceptualized programme (a sub-goal) requires four task results to be delivered, one of which is the invitation of a speaker (see).To achieve the sub-sub-goal of ' invitation' a sequence of tasks needs to be accomplished on the activity level where they are represented as a *refinement* of the action-unit. In terms of the Petri net, the tasks on the activity level can be *folded* to attain the representation of the higher order task 'invite speakers' (located on the action-unit level).

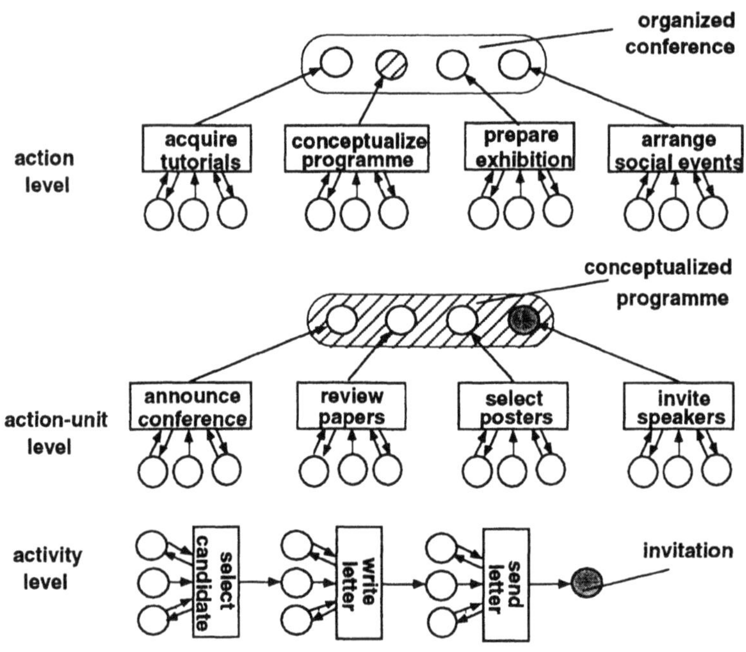

Figure 5: Hierarchical-sequential arrangement of taks to organize a conference

On higher levels the semantics of tasks need not be determined by tools in the common sense; a 'tool' on the action-unit level can be conceptualized in terms of a *rule* (e.g. rules for reviewing papers); on the action level a 'tool' can be a *role* (e.g. a chairman).

It is not claimed that human beings use to *internally* store the complex of tasks as presented in figure 5. Nevertheless, the user's externalized task knowledge is by no means arbitrarily presented, since it satisfies theoretical postulates.

Basic semantic concepts	Elements of a Petri net
event object relation	active passive flow relation

Table 1: Semantic resemblances

Furthermore, a formal representation in terms of Petri nets is apparently advantageous, since the knowledge presented rests on elementary semantic concepts which are assumed to govern human knowledge representation. To provide evidence for this postulate, the striking resemblance of the formal semantic elements to the basic semantic concepts of human knowledge representation is uncovered here (see table 1).

Externalized knowledge on tasks lacks detail, since the user knows more than he/she is aware of knowing. The acquisition of knowledge, however, can be aided by the action-regulation theory as well as the Petri net formalism to identify the lacking details. Accordingly, the designer of software can utilize the task representations to validate and upgrade the semantic concepts involved in the design. The match between the user's semantic concepts and the semantics presented at the user interface can also systematically be tested on the basis of the externalized task structures. Of course, the validation method for software design and user-interfaces has yet to be developed.

7. References

W. Hacker, Activity: A fruitful concept in industrial psychology, In: M.Frese and J. Sabini (eds.), Goal Directed Behavior. Lawrence Erlbaum, Hillsdale N.J. (1985) 262.

W. Hacker, Computerization versus computer aided mental work. In: M. Frese, E Ulich and W. Dzida (eds.), Human Computer Interaction in the Work Place, Elsevier, Amsterdam (1987) 115.

F. Klix, Über Wissensrepräsentation im menschlichen Gedächtnis. In: F. Klix (Hrsg.), Gedächtnis, Wissen, Wissensnutzung, Deutscher Verlag d. Wiss., Berlin (1984) 7.

F. Klix, Memory research and knowledge engineering. In: F. Klix and H. Wandke (eds.), Man-Computer Interaction Research. North-Holland, Amsterdam (1986) 97.

A. Newell and H.A. Simon, Human Problem Solving, Prentice Hall, Englewood, 1972.

W. Reisig, Petri Nets - An Introduction, Springer, Berlin, 1985.

W. Volpert, The model of the hierarchical-sequential organization of action, In: W. Hacker et al (eds.), Cognitive and Motivational Aspects of Action. North-Holland, Amsterdam (1982) 35.

ENVIRONMENTAL IMPACTS

WORK WITH DISPLAY UNITS 92
H. Luczak, A. Çakir and G. Çakir (Editors)

Why do gender, job stress, job satisfaction, perceived indoor air quality and VDT use influence reports of the sick building syndrome in offices?

Alan Hedge[a], William A. Erickson[a], and Gail Rubin[b]

[a] Department of Design and Environmental Analysis, NYS College of Human Ecology, Cornell University, Ithaca, NY 14853, U.S.A.

[b]Biometrics Unit, Cornell University, Ithaca, NY 14853, U.S.A.

Abstract

The relationship between the sick building syndrome (SBS), indoor air quality, individual and occupational variables, was investigated in a survey of 4,479 workers in 27 air-conditioned office buildings. The number of SBS symptoms reported by each worker was not significantly associated with worker's age, smoking status, or job grade, or with concentrations of the indoor air contaminants which were measured. The number of SBS symptoms reported by each worker was significantly associated with gender, perception of indoor air quality, hours of daily VDT use, and ratings of job satisfaction and job stress. It is suggested that these variables affect symptom reports by influencing individual susceptibility to work environment conditions.

1. INTRODUCTION

The sick building syndrome (SBS) is comprised of symptoms of eye, nose, and throat irritation, headache, lethargy, respiratory difficulties and skin irritation, which are experienced by workers when at work but which are alleviated on days when workers are away from their workplace [1]. When there is a high incidence of SBS symptoms among workers in a building, usually more than an average of 2 symptoms per worker, then the building may be a "sick" building [2]. Because reports of the SBS have increased since the mid-1970s and because there are consistent differences in prevalence rates between buildings with different types of ventilation systems [3], it is widely believed that poor indoor air quality and inadequate rates of outdoor air ventilation are primarily responsible for the symptoms. However, research on the SBS conducted in North America [4], in Europe [5,6,7,8,9,10], and in Australia [11] and Canada [12] challenges this assumption.

A U.K. survey showed that SBS symptoms are more prevalent among women than men [5]. A nationwide survey of 4,373 office workers in 47 office buildings in the U.K. showed an overall difference in the prevalence of the SBS between air-conditioned and unconditioned offices, but also found that individual variables (gender, age, perceived control, attitudes to environmental conditions), occupational variables (VDT use, job stress), and organizational variables (organization type, office type) influenced symptom reports [6]. Unfortunately, these U.K. surveys did not measure environmental conditions, and therefore the degree to which the SBS symptoms were a consequence of exposure to polluted indoor air cannot be gauged. However, another U.K. study compared an air conditioned building where the SBS was more prevalent than in the adjoining naturally ventilated building [7], and found no significant differences in air temperature, globe temperature, air velocity, negative and positive air ion concentrations, formaldehyde, carbon monoxide, and ozone between the two buildings.

Danish researchers surveyed 4,369 office workers in 14 Danish town halls and 14 associated office buildings and measured environmental conditions [8,9]. Although there was considerable variation in the prevalence of the SBS among buildings, apart from total dust and air temperature, indoor air pollutant concentrations generally were not associated with symptoms, although the highest prevalence of the SBS was in the building with the highest level of total volatile organic compounds. There was also an effect of a fleece factor (the area of material surface divided by the room volume), and a shelf factor (the area of open-shelving divided by the volume of the room), and effects of worker's gender, drinking coffee at work, and length of use of a VDT. Similar effects of individual and occupational variables have been reported in a Dutch survey of 7,000 workers in 61 offices [10]. Research in Australia [11] and Canada [12] has found that increasing the ventilation rate, which should improve indoor air quality, did not reduce complaints of the SBS.

The results of these studies question the assumption that the SBS occurs solely because of exposure to poor indoor air quality. To further investigate the etiology of this syndrome, a field experimental study was undertaken to systematically examine the relationship between the SBS and individual variables (age, gender, smoking status), occupational variables (hours of VDT use, job grade, job stress, and job satisfaction), workers' perceptions of indoor air quality, and measured environmental conditions.

2. METHODS

2.1 Office Buildings

Twenty seven air-conditioned buildings with either variable air volume (VAV) or constant air volume (CAV) ventilation systems were studied. The buildings were occupied by 17 organisations representing typical office work (insurance, finance, sales and marketing, etc.). Fifteen of these organisations were private companies occupying 25 of the 27 buildings. One building was occupied by a federal agency, and one by a municipality. Buildings were grouped by their smoking policy into smoking prohibited, smoking restricted to rooms with local electrostatic air filtration units, smoking restricted to areas with no local air treatment, smoking restricted to rooms ventilated by a separate ventilation system, smoking restricted to enclosed offices and open plan cubicle workstations. Prior to the study one building was thought to have an indoor air quality problem, otherwise the environmental conditions in the buildings were unknown to the investigators.

2.2 Indoor Air Quality and Questionnaire Surveys

Buildings were surveyed in the winter/springtime for two consecutive workdays, although one building was surveyed for one day because a census of workers was achieved. Each day, two areas were measured in the morning and two different areas in the afternoon, giving 8 areas over the two day survey. All office areas were open office locations. In total, 117 smoking and 95 nonsmoking areas were surveyed. The indoor air quality survey measured formaldehyde, nicotine, respirable particulates (<2.5 μm and <3.5 μm), ultraviolet particulate mass (particulates from tobacco smoke), carbon monoxide, carbon dioxide, air temperature, relative humidity, and illumination. The detailed indoor air quality survey protocol is available [4].

A questionnaire survey was conducted along with the indoor air quality survey. The questionnaire asked about workers' perceptions of environmental conditions, occupational variables, work-related SBS symptoms, and personal details. Questionnaires were distributed to about 30 workstations in each indoor air quality survey area. Investigators manually distributed and collected questionnaires on the same day, apart from 3 buildings where this was done by in-house staff. A pre-addressed return envelope was given to workers unable to complete the questionnaire in time. Less than 2% of workers refused to participate. Of the 6,335 questionnaires distributed 4,479 were returned (average 72% return rate: minimum 58%, maximum 88%). The detailed questionnaire survey method is available [13].

2.3 Statistical Design and Analysis

Environmental data were analyzed using analysis of variance to test the effect of smoking policy on indoor air quality. Concentrations of carbon monoxide, carbon dioxide, and formaldehyde were lognormally distributed, and analyses were performed on natural log transformed data. For computational purposes a value of 10^{-4} was added to each carbon monoxide reading because of zero readings, and zero readings for formaldehyde were replaced with the detection limit of the method. The detailed statistical design and analysis of the environmental data is available [4]. Responses to the perceived environmental conditions, and the job stress and job satisfaction questions were analyzed using factor analysis with varimax rotation. Multiple regression analysis was used to model the relationships between occupational and personal variables, and the total number of SBS symptoms reported by each worker.

3. RESULTS

Although significant differences in nicotine and particulates related to environmental tobacco smoke were found between smoking policies, the levels of all pollutants generally were low and the environmental findings will not be discussed here. Smoking policy had only a marginally significant effect on the average number of SBS symptoms ($F_{4,22}=2.62$, $p=0.0627$: average of 4.71 symptoms per worker in smoking prohibited buildings compared with between 3.04 and 3.83 symptoms per worker for other policies). Evidence that indoor air quality differences accounted for variations in SBS reports was not found.

Factor analysis of the perceived environment conditions yielded a 3 factor solution and items with factor loading > 0.45 on the first factor were used to create a perceived indoor air quality (PIAQ) scale comprised of 7 questions: insufficient ventilation, too little air movement, too warm, too dry, unpleasant odors, stale air, and dusty air. Positive responses to these questions (i.e. the worker reported having experienced this condition at least once during the previous month) were summed for each respondent.The reliability of this scale was estimated using Cronbach's standardized alpha (α), which is a measure of the average inter-item correlation. Values of $\alpha > 0.67$ indicate acceptable internal consistency, and α for the PIAQ scale was satisfactory ($\alpha= 0.85$).

Factor analysis of the occupational questions confirmed two orthogonal factors which together explained 55.8% of the common factor variance (see Table 1). Six questions loaded highly on the job satisfaction factor, and five questions loaded highly on the job stress factor. Items with negative wording were reversed scored and α was calculated for the job stress items (α= 0.72), and for the job satisfaction items (α= 0.90). The average scores for the five job stress questions, or six job satisfaction questions, for each person were used as the job stress or job satisfaction measures.

Table 1
Factor analysis of the job stress and job satisfaction questions

Question	Job satisfaction	Job Stress
My job is usually interesting	0.83	0.16
I'm happy in my job	0.89	-0.06
I dislike my job	-0.83	0.09
I am satisfied with my job	0.81	-0.06
I'm enthusiastic about my job	0.85	0.03
My job is rather monotonous	-0.67	-0.13
My job is not very stressful	-0.05	-0.51
I usually have to work fast	0.06	0.68
I often feel stressed at work	-0.18	0.82
My job demands a lot of concentration	0.31	0.58
I often feel overworked	-0.11	0.79
Eigenvalue	4.23	2.47
% Common Variance	35.20	20.60

Relationships between occupational and personal variables, and the total number of SBS symptoms per worker were modelled using multiple regression analysis. Data first were checked for collinearity by calculating tolerance values (the closer the tolerance value is to unity the greater the independence of variables), and this confirmed that the variables were not collinear. Results showed that the best regression model for the total number of SBS symptoms per worker (adjusted $R^2 = 0.32$; $F_{(5,4389)} = 343.06$, $p=0.0000$) has separate intercepts for men (parameter estimate = 0.07 ± 0.31) and women (parameter estimate = 0.35 ± 0.31); common slopes for hours of VDT use (parameter estimate = 0.12 ± 0.02), job stress (parameter estimate = 0.64 ± 0.06), and job satisfaction (parameter estimate = - 0.45 ± 0.05); and separate slopes for the PIAQ for each sex (parameter estimate for men = 0.57 ± 0.03 and for women = 0.71 ± 0.02). Reports of SBS symptoms were not affected by workers' smoking status, age, or job grade. In 9 buildings samples of settled dust were taken and a significant correlation between the number of mineral fibers per unit area and the number of SBS symptoms was found ($r=0.89$, $p=0.0015$). Scanning electron microscopy confirmed that man-made mineral fibers were in settled dust on the computer screens.

4. DISCUSSION

This study confirms findings from previous research that reports of SBS symptoms are affected by workers' gender, with men reporting an average of 2.83 ± 0.14 SBS symptoms compared with 4.00 ± 0.13 SBS symptoms for women. The study also confirms that reports of the SBS increase with increasing hours of VDT use, increasing job stress, and decreasing job satisfaction (i.e. increasing job dissatisfaction). There is also a pronounced effect of workers' perceptions of indoor air quality on their reports of the SBS, even though adverse conditions were not indicated by the measures of environmental conditions. These results are similar to those previously reported which suggests that the SBS does not arise from direct exposure to indoor air pollutants alone. We think it unlikely that the symptoms reported by workers were manifestations of psychosomatic problems, rather we tentatively suggest that gender, perceived indoor air quality, job stress and job satisfaction may influence SBS reports because they may modify a workers' susceptibility to environmental stressors in the workplace. Such a change in susceptibility should be reflected by changes in physiological measures of stress, but as yet we have no direct evidence of such physiological changes. We also suggest that the correlation found between the SBS and hours of VDT use may arise because of a separate process whereby the VDT acts as an electrostatic precipitator attracting physical irritants, such as man-made mineral fibers and particles capable of causing eye, nose, throat and skin irritation, into each worker's micro-environment. Further research on these effects is needed.

5. REFERENCES

1 W.H.O., Indoor Air Pollutants: Exposure and Health Effects, EURO Reports and Studies 78, World Health Organisation, Copenhagen, 1983.

2 G. Raw M.S. Roy and A. Leamon, Indoor Air '90: Precedings of the 5th Int. Conf. on indoor Air Quality and Climate, 1 (1990) 231.

3 M. Mendell and A. Smith, Amer. J. Pub. Health, 80 (1990) 1193-1199.

4 A. Hedge W.A. Erickson and G. Rubin, Healthy Buildings-IAQ '91, ASHRAE (1991) 151.

5 A. Hedge, J. Arch. and Plan. Res., 1 (1984) 163.

6 A.S. Robertson et al., Brit. Med. J., 291 (1985) 373.

7 A. Hedge et al., Environ. Int., 15 (1989) 143.

8 P. Skov et al., Scand. J. Work Environ. Health, 15 (1989) 286.

9 P. Skov et al., Environ. Int. 13 (1987) 339.

10 T. Zweers et al., Indoor Air '90: Precedings of the 5th Int. Conf. on Indoor Air Quality and Climate, 1 (1990) 495.

11 D. Rowe and S.E. Wilke, Paper presented at Indoor Air Quality, Ventilation, and Energy, Montreal, (1992) October.

12 R. Menzies et al., Healthy Buildings-IAQ '91, ASHRAE (1991) 90.

13 A. Hedge W.A. Erickson and G. Rubin, In J.C. Quick, L.R. Murphy, and J.J. Hurrell, Jr. (eds.), Work and Well-Being: Assessments and Interventions for Occupational Mental Health, Washington, D.C. Amer. Psych. Assoc. (1992) 286.

Acknowledgement

Work was conducted under contract to the Center for Indoor Air Research, Linthicum, Maryland, U.S.A.

WORK WITH DISPLAY UNITS 92
H. Luczak, A. Çakir and G. Çakir (Editors)

A LONGITUDINAL STUDY OF SYMPTOMS IN OFFICE VDU-WORK AT DIFFERENT ROOM TEMPERATURES. A PRELIMINARY REPORT.

L. Jorulf[1], N-H. Andersson[1], L. Barregård[2], Stig Hagberg[2], A-L. Krogstad[3], A. Ran[1].

1 Volvo Truck Corp and Volvo Data, 405 08, Gothenburg, Sweden
2 Dept Occup Medicine, Sahlgrenska Hospital, 412 66, Gothenburg, Sweden
3 Dept Dermatology, Sahlgrenska Hospital, 413 45, Gothenburg, Sweden

1. INTRODUCTION

It is probable that our office environment has become increasingly warm in recent years as a result of the growing use of office equipments which produce heat, such as computer monitors. As a matter of fact we often find room temperatures today in the range of 22-24°C in Swedish offices, even during the winter.

In the same years, working with VDU has been discussed as the possible cause of facial skin symptoms. One interesting aspect which links facial skin symptoms to warm office climate, is the fact that the places where heat from the body can be emitted, if we are working with surplus heat, are the exposed areas of skin which are not covered, for example the face.

VDU are also sometimes said to cause additional problems - for instance from the mucous membranes in the eyes and respiratory tract, and general symptoms such as fatigue, dizziness, and difficulties to concentrate. These symptoms are also common in the so called "Sick Building Syndrome", SBS.

2. OBJECTIVES

The aim of the study was to investigate the variation of some symptoms, often discussed in connection with work with VDU, within a temperature range of 20-24°C and to see wether there was a temperature optimum in relation to the occurrence of these symptoms.

3. SUBJECTS AND METHODS

100 employees who worked on a permanent basis during the study period in five open-plan offices were selected to participate in the study. The mean age in the population was 41 years, 77% were men, 18% were smokers, 86% worked more or less with VDU. Those who worked with VDUs spent an average of 13 hours a week in front of their computer, with a range of 1-41 h/week.

During a 10-week long period comprising week 42-51 in 1990, the temperature was changed up and down in a predetermined order in the range 20-24°C. The temperature and relative humidity were measured continuously in each office using thermohygrographs, and the mean weekly temperature and relative humidity values based on the thermohygrographs, corrected by using a reference intrument, were calculated for every week and office.

Questionnaires were used to describe the study group prior to the period of temperature variation and at the end of every week. The complaints were based on fifteen symptoms (table 1). The intensity of symptoms was rated using a 0-10 point scale and the mean levels were studied as a function of the room temperatures. The influence of temperature, age, gender, time spent at the VDU, relative humidity and smoking was studied using the multiple regression technique.

TABLE 1
SYMPTOMS

GENERAL:	1)Fatigue; 2)Head feels heavy; 3)Headache; 4) Nausea, dizziness; 5)Difficult to concentrate
MUCOUS MEMBRANES:	6)Eyes itching, burning, irritated; 7)Nose irritated, blocked, running; 8)Throat hoarse, dry; 9) Throat soe; 10)Coughing
SKIN:	11)Facial skin dry; 12)Facial skin flushed; 13)Face itching, prickly, tight, feels hot; 14)Scalp-ears dry, itching; 15)Hand skin dry, itching, red

4. RESULTS

The overall response rate was 74%. There was no systematic non-response for the different temperatures.

We had some difficulties to set the temperatures to the predetermined levels and we got a spectrum of mean weekly temperatures for the different weeks and different offices. In the analyses all persons exposed to the same temperature - sometimes at different weeks - were brought together to form one group.

4.1 UNIVARIATE ANALYSIS

It was possible to fit significantly a second degree equation for the dependence on temperature of seven symptoms. For these symptoms bar diagrams of proportions and of mean intensities are shown in figure 1. There was a rather large inter-individual variation of intensities both for warmer and colder temperatures. For three symptoms there was also a significant temperature optimum at 21.0-21.1°C.

FIGURE 1
Bar diagrams of symptoms with significant squared functions

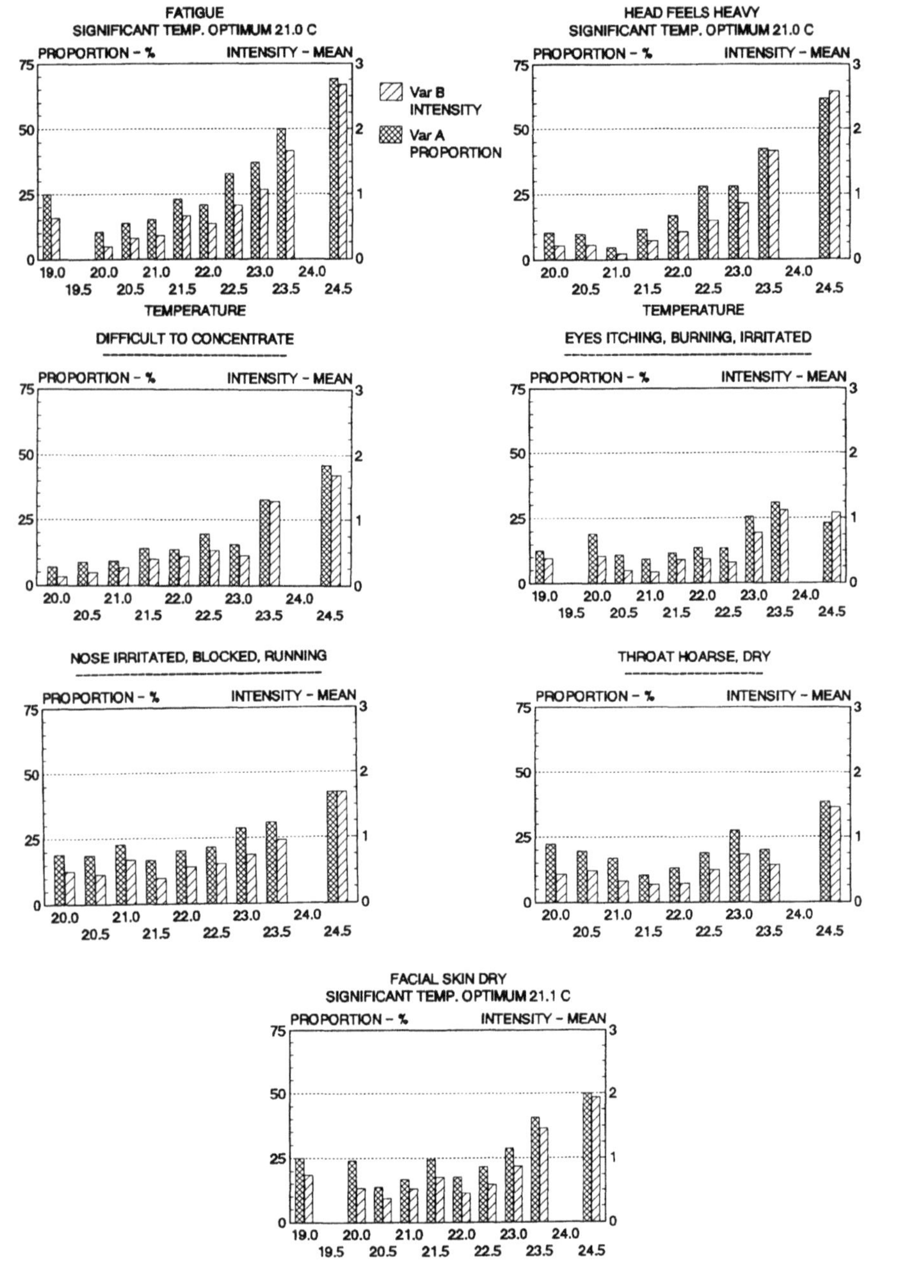

"Facial skin dry" was the only skin symptom where it was possible to fit a squared function. A significant optimum was also observed at 21.0°C. For the other two facial skin symptoms - "Facial skin flushed" and "Face itching/prickly/tight/feels hot" - there was, however, a tendency towards an increase above 22.5°C (figure 2).

FIGURE 2
Bar diagrams of facial skin symptoms.

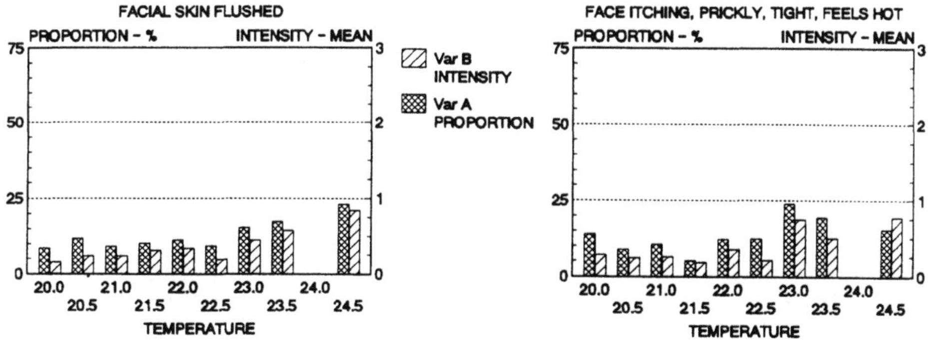

The humidity in the offices was relatively normal for the time of the year and varied within a narrow range. No relationship between humidity and the mean severity of problems was found in the univariate analysis.

4.2 MULTIPLE REGRESSION ANALYSIS
In the multiple regression model, temperature showed the strongest covariance with the general symptoms, while skin symptoms were more associated to gender, and the mucous membrane symptoms to gender and the time spent at the VDU. When, however, in the next step, the material was analysed by gender the regression showed that temperature contributed significantly to all three skin symptoms in the face for men but for women only for "Dry skin in the face".

5. SUMMARY
When summing up the influence of temperature on symptoms we got table 2. From this you can see that temperature played a role for many symptoms both reported from work with VDU and from sick buildings.

TABLE 2
Associations with temperature in univariate and multivariate analyses (+ indicates statistically significant increase of symptoms with increasing temperature)

	GENERAL					MUCOUS MEMBR.					SKIN				
Symptom number (see table 1)	1	2	3	4	5	6	7	8	9	10	11	12	13	14	15
UNIVARIATE	+	+			+	+	+	+			+				
MULTIVARIATE	+	+	+	+	+	+	+	+	+		+	+M	+M		

The multiple regression showed an influence of working time spent at the VDU on the mucous membrane symptoms and on some skin symptoms but not on the facial skin symptoms. So the study did not support the hypothesis that work at VDU may influence facial skin symptoms but indicates that these symptoms rather may be affected by gender and temperature.

The results indicate that there was an optimum temperature for certain symptoms within the given range. This optimum temperature was 21°C and was found for the symptoms "Fatigue", "Head feels heavy" and "Facial skin dry".

In the case of other symptoms, a lower occurrence of symptoms and their severity was seen when temperature was reduced below a threshold temperature of about 23°C. Above this threshold the severity of problems tended to increase.

We concluded that there may be much to gain by reducing high room temperatures in offices, and that this is true especially for the general symptoms. In our opinion the temperature in ordinary office workplaces should not exceed 22°C. The optimum seems to be around 20-21°C.

WORK WITH DISPLAY UNITS 92
H. Luczak, A. Çakir and G. Çakir (Editors)

JOB STRESS, VDU-WORK AND SKIN SYMPTOMS

BB. Arnetz[a], M. Berg[b] and S. Lidén[b]

[a]Department of Stress Research, Karolinska Institute, Box 60205, S-104 01 Stockholm, Sweden

[b]Department of Dermatology, Karolinska Hospital, S-104 01 Stockholm, Sweden

Abstract
We followed 47 VDU-workers with or without work-associated skin complaints during one regular work-day and one day of leisure. Employees with skin symptoms had a selective neuroendocrine stress reaction during work, but not during leisure time. They experienced more extreme job stress at the same time as they had higher control over work-processes. We postulate that employees suffering from cognitive failure during VDU-work develop "techno-stress". A model is proposed in which physiological signals act as unconditioned stimuli and the VDU-environment as the conditioned stimulus.

1. INTRODUCTION

One of the more common complaints among VDU-users concerns the skin (1-3). Despite much research, little is known about the etiology behind VDU-associated health problems (3, 4). The purpose of this study was to assess the possible etiological importance of psychophysiological and environmental factors in the precipitation of VDU-associated skin problems.

2. METHODS

The study group consisted of a randomized selection from a larger cohort (2,5) of those reporting facial skin symptoms associated with their work (n=19) and those who had no such symptoms (n=28). The subjects were studied during a typical work-day as well as during a day off (i.e. a day of leisure) in the employees regular work-environment. Psychosocial and psychophysiological measurements were made during a regular work-day as well as a day of leisure. Itching behavior was registered by specially-trained nurses. Blood samples were analyzed for serum cortisol, prolactin, testosterone, thyroxin, and growth hormone. Urinary concentrations of adrenalin and noradrenalin were also determined. The physical work-environment was also characterized in detail, as was exposure to passive and active smoking. Subjects with or without VDU-associated skin symptoms were compared using non-paired t-test and two-way analysis of variance. Finally, stepwise logistic regression was applied using the two skin groups as dependent factors. Results were age- and sex-adjusted and significance levels were set at a p-value of less than .05.

3. RESULTS

Persons with VDU-associated symptoms had more authority over work-content and work-organization than those without symptoms (7.9 vs 6.3 on a scale from 2 to 10, $p<0.05$) and experienced more occupational stress ($p=0.01$). Furthermore, during a work-day those with symptoms showed a tendency for higher global occupational stress perception, with no differences during leisure time (Figure 1).

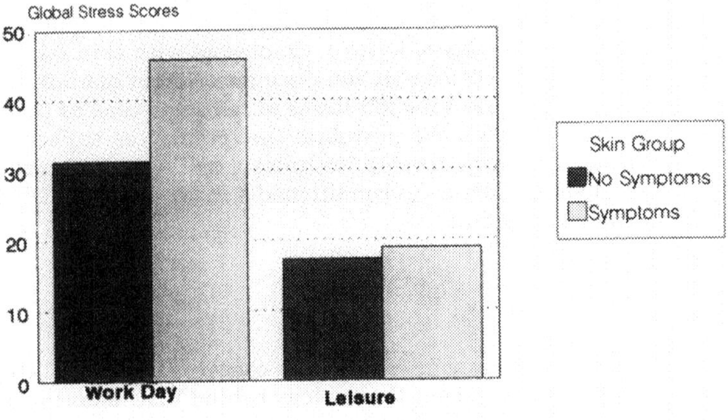

Figure 1. Global stress scores by skin symptoms grouping during work and leisure.

There were no differences between groups in intellectual discretion, i.e. the development of new skills in one's job. In contrast, compared to the control group, they exercised significantly less ($p<0.05$). In the stepwise logistic regression analyses the following variables were significant independent predictors of skin symptoms: itching behaviour ($p<0.01$) and authority ($p<0.01$). In the logistic regression analysis it was found that serum testosterone, prolactin (Figure 2) and thyroxin were significant predictors of skin symptoms during work, but not during days off. Thus, the anabolic hormone testosterone was decreased, while the stress hormones prolactin and thyroxin were elevated. There were no significant group differences in serum levels of growth hormone or cortisol. Even though there was no clinical difference in skin conditions between the groups, those with symptoms had a more frequent itching behavior (Anova $p<0.05$, mean value 14 vs .1 arbitrary visual analogue units). Those with skin symptoms also complained significantly more often of eye strain (Anova, $p<0.05$).

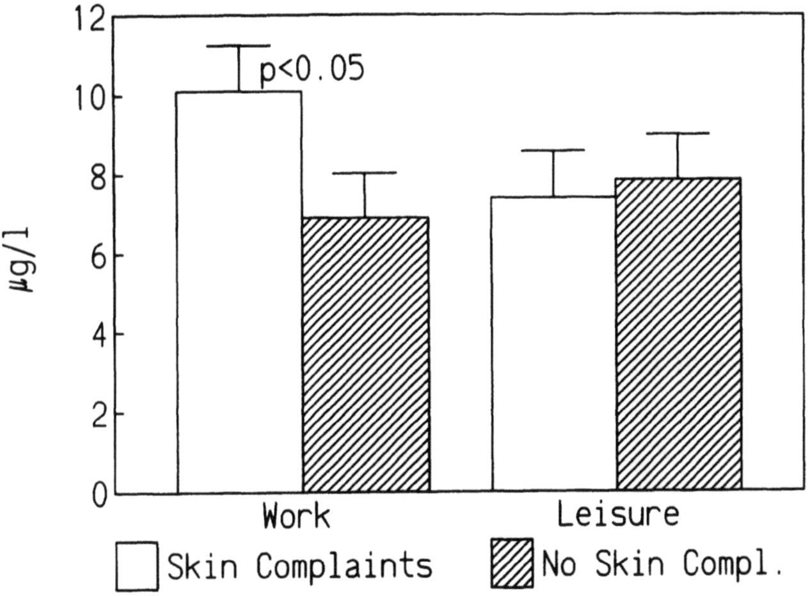

Figure 2. Serum prolactin by skin symptoms grouping during work and leisure (mean +/- S.E.M.)

There were no systematic differences between groups with or without skin symptoms respectively with regard to age, gender, job functions, alcohol and coffee consumption or smoking habits. On the average, subjects with skin symptoms had been involved in computer-work 7.7 years compared to 8.6 for the reference group (n.s.). The groups did not differ with regard to neuroticism, extrovertness, psychiatric morbidity, pigmentation ability, prior and ongoing allergies or skin diseases, moodiness or occurrence of headache. The physical work-environment was similar, as was the average distance between the employee and the VDU-screen (63.5 cm +/- 3.5 S.E.M.). There was a near three-fold increase in urinary excretion of noradrenalin during work (Figure 3) compared to a day of leisure without any significant group differences.

4. DISCUSSION

Our findings show that employees with skin symptoms suffer from more occupational stress compared to healthy controls working under similar objective physical indoor environmental and electromagnetic fields conditions. This is reflected in higher stress hormone levels as well as increased subjective feelings of occupational stress and decreased levels of the stress-protective anabolic hormone testosterone. Subjects with skin complaints also suffered more frequently from eye-strain and scratched themselves more frequently. Since both groups were using VDUs to the same extent, our findings imply that there must be factors other than electromagnetic fields contributing to the development of VDU-associated skin symptoms. Based on our results to date, we postulate the following hypothesis: Many employees working with computer technologies suffer from occupational stress. This results in physiological changes characterized by elevated metabolism and increased dermal blood-flow. This response acts as an unconditioned stimulus. The conditioned stimulus in this case is the VDU-environment. Once the conditioned response has been learned, the psychophysiological response is elicited purely by the conditioned stimulus, i.e. the VDU-environment.

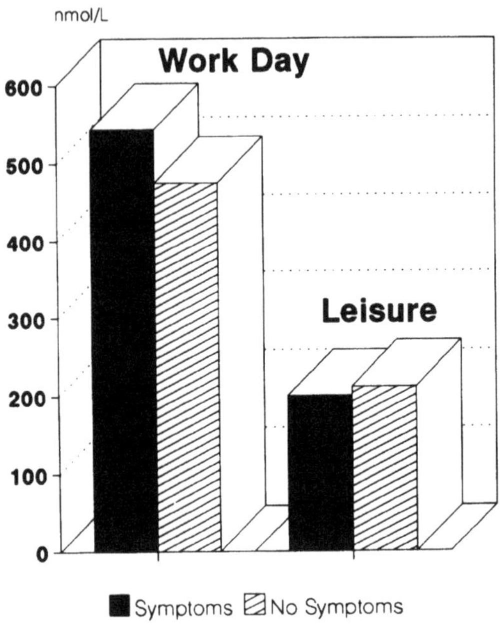

Figure 3. Urinary excretion of noradrenalin by skin grouping.

The introduction of new technologies has resulted in major changes in work-content and work-organization. These changes have too often resulted in sub-optimal organization, discrepancy between mental capacity and goals of the employee and what is achievable by the software programs. The result of this discrepancy is a psychophysiological "techno-stress", as employees actively try to cope with feelings of cognitive failure resulting from poor man-machine interface (6-8). Occupational health aspects should be an integrated part of all systems implementations (9-11).

In conclusion, our study has found psychophysiological differences between persons with or without VDU-associated skin complaints. These differences were limited to work-days only. We believe that the whole implementation strategy related to information technology needs to be reassessed. Specification requirements for new software systems should take human issues into consideration. Corrective measures must entail many more factors than merely installing "low-emitting" VDUs. We have now launched a state-of-the-art research and treatment center offering VDU-employees psychophysiological treatment and testing as for sensitivity to electric and magnetic fields.

Acknowledgement

This work was supplied by the Swedish Work Environment Fund.

References

1 M. Berg. Skin Problems in Workers Using Visual Display Terminals; A Study of 201 Patients. Contact Dermatitis 1988;19:335-341.

2 M. Berg, S. Lidén and O. Axelson. Skin Complaints and Work at Visual Display Units; An Epidemiological Study of Office Employees. J. Am. Acad. Dermatol., 1990;22:621-5.

3 M. Berg. Facial Skin Complaints and Work at Visual Display Units. Epidemiological, Clinical and Histopathological Studies. Acta Dermatovenereol. (Stockholm). Suppl 150, 1989.

4 G. Swanbeck and T. Bleeker. Skin Problems from Visual Display Units. Acta Dermatovenereol. (Stockholm) 1989;69:46-51.

5 M. Berg, BB. Arnetz, S. Lidén, P. Eneroth and A. Kallner. "Techno-Stress"; A Psychophysiological Study of Employees with VDU-Associated Skin Complaints. J. Occup. Med. 1992;34:698-701.

6 BB Arnetz and JE Arnetz. "Hypersensitivity to Electricity and Video Display Units". A Controlled Occupational Health Survey in a Hightech Work Environment. Submitted 1992.

7 A. Smith, D. Peck, and T. Clatworthy. After-Effects of Working at Visual Display Units. Work & Stress 1989;3:195-201.

8 DE. Broadbent, PF. Cooper, P. FitzGerald and KR. Parkes. The Cognitive Failures Questionnaire and its Correlates. Br. J. Clin. Psychol. 1982;21: 1-16.

9 Work With Visual Display Terminals: Psychosocial Aspects and Health. Report on a World Health Organization meeting. JOM 1989;31:957-969.

10 G. Johansson. Growth and Challenge vs Wear and Tear of Humans in Computer Mediated Work. In: B. Knave and P.-G. Widebeck: Work with Display Units 86, pp 725-731, Elsevier Science Publishers B.V. (North-Holland), 1987.

11 G. Johansson and G. Aronsson. Stress Reactions in Computerized Administrative Work. J. Occup. Behav. 1984;4:159-181.

WORK WITH DISPLAY UNITS 92
H. Luczak, A. Çakir and G. Çakir (Editors)
1993 Elsevier Science Publishers B.V.

Skin diseases, symptoms and complaints at VDU work - investigating the impact of electric and magnetic fields

U. Bergqvist and J. E. Wahlberg

Departments of Neuromedicine and Dermatology
National Institute of Occupational Health, S-171 52 Solna, Sweden

Abstract

A cross-sectional study of 353 office workers with and without VDU work was performed, with data obtained from questionnaires, a dermatological examination and work-station measurements of various physical factors. No associations were found between skin problems and exposures to various electric and magnetic fields at the VDU work station.

1. INTRODUCTION

We have investigated the possible involvement of VDU work on skin problems in a 6-year study based on employees in seven Stockholm-based companies. In a 1981 cross-sectional investigation, skin complaints were more common among VDU users than non-users [1, 2]. Between 1981 and 1987, the cumulative incidence of skin complaints were, however, similar for VDU and non-VDU users [3]. In a 1987 cross-sectional investigation, VDU work was, in combination with some work load parameters, associated with erythema and skin complaints. There were no such associations between diagnosed skin diseases and VDU work [4].

Here, we report on the association between skin problems and electric and magnetic fields due to the VDU work station, with data from the 1987 cross-sectional investigation.

2. MATERIALS AND METHODS

353 office workers in seven Stockholm companies formed the basis for this investigation. A questionnaire (92% response rate) gave information on skin complaints, work descriptions and several individual and organisational variables. 299 individuals were subjected to a dermatological examination and a first work-place investigation. Later - by at least a year - various electric and magnetic field exposures were measured among 216 VDU users, and skin complaints were again solicited.

The dermatological examination, which was carried out in a blind manner - the dermatologist did not know if the subject was a VDU user or not - resulted in several diagnoses which were specifically subjected to analysis; seborrhoic eczema, acne, rosacea and lentigo, as was also the presence of any diagnosis. Unspecific erythema - not included in any diagnosis - were also recorded. The questionnaire provided data on skin complaints on the face, neck or hands within the last 12 months. Similar questions were again asked at the time of the second workplace investigation.

The use, weekly extent of use, and 5-year cumulative amount of VDU use were obtained from questionnaires. VDU models, both current and previous, were noted. Variables describing the individual (age, sex, smoking, stress reactions etc) and perceived organisational conditions (influence, peer contacts, rest breaks, flexibility, work pace and work load etc) were also used in the analysis.

The first work-place investigation provided data on the relative humidity and electrostatic variables. The static charge of the operators performing specific movements were recorded, and electrostatic fields from the VDUs were measured, using a "field mill" (ELTEX Q 475C), in general accordance with the methods used by Sandström et al [5].

The second work-place investigation provided data on humidity, temperature and rms electric and magnetic fields at the VDU work stations, using a Holaday instrumentation (HI-3600, HI-3601, HI-3602 and HI-3615). Recordings were made both for ELF net/image frequencies (~50-80 Hz) and VLF line frequencies (~15-35 kHz). The instrument was oriented so as to maximize the field from the VDU at a standard distance and at facial position (operator absent) and was not grounded during measurements. The electric and magnetic field level data obtained for the VLF band were also used to calculate an accumulated dose (field level x accumulated VDU work hours) during the five years preceeding the dermatological examination. This calculation was based on each individual´s accumulated working hours at specific VDU models and the average VLF electric and magnetic fields (at 30 cm distance) for those models - and also took account of changes between VDU models.

For each endpoint - diagnosis, erythema or complaints - a multivariate model was obtained which (generally) included VDU work, individual, organisational and physical variables [4]. The different electric and magnetic fields were introduced in these models, in order to estimate associations between field exposures or doses and skin problems. Unconditional maximum likelihood estimates of the odds ratios and their 95% confidence intervals were obtained from these multivariate logistic regression analysis [6].

3. RESULTS

The outcome of these analyses are shown in tables 1-4. For all tables, the odds ratio comparisons are made with the category assigned the odds ratio 1.00. For the other categories, adjusted odds ratios (and their 95% confidence intervals) are presented. Adjustments for possible confounding by other variables have been made in multivariate logistic regression models. Outcomes of analyses of specific diagnoses are not shown, but estimates exceeding unity are commented on in the text. The low number of individuals with specific diagnoses resulted in rather broad confidence intervals for these analyses.

There were no associations between skin problems and the propensity for static charging (table 1). For seborrhoic eczema and lentigo, excess odds ratios were found, though; 2.52 (0.26-24.6) and 4.93 (0.73-33.1).

Table 1. Associations between the static charge of the operators and skin problems.

	Diagnoses n=231	Erythema n=221	Complaints n=243
Low (<1 kV)	1.00	1.00	1.00
High (≥1 kV)	0.99	0.97	0.64
	(0.52-1.88)	(0.31-3.10)	(0.34-1.18)

Table 2 shows associations between electrostatic fields (expressed as the equivalent surface potential) and skin problems. Seborrhoic eczema showed an excess odds ratio of 1.32 (0.42-4.12) in comparison b/ (cf table 2). The electrostatic fields were in some cases reduced due to the application of external grounded filters. Measuring the fields after removal of such filter resulted in an odds ratio of 1.04 (0.53-2.03), compared to the 0.66 (0.35-1.26) ratio presented in table 4, comparison b/.

Table 2. Associations between the electrostatic field from a VDU and skin problems.

	Diagnoses		Erythema		Complaints	
	n=245	n=208	n=236	n=199	n=268	n=215
	a/	b/	a/	b/	a/	b/
No VDU usage	1.00	--	1.00	--	1.00	--
VDU with lower	0.97	1.00	3.09	1.00	2.77	1.00
field (<5 kV [1])	(0.37-2.51)		(0.36-26.7)		(1.15-6.68)	
VDU with higher	1.18	1.19	3.38	1.12	1.86	0.66
field (≥5 kV [1])	(0.56-2.49)	(0.59-2.42)	(0.36-31.2)	(0.33-3.76)	(0.71-4.86)	(0.35-1.26)

Odds ratios compare those with different field exposures from VDUs with a/ those without a VDU and b/ within the VDU user group. [1] Equivalent surface potential.

Table 3. Associations between electric and magnetic fields at facial position from the VDU and concurrent skin complaints (n=174).

	Electric fields		Magnetic fields	
	ELF	VLF	ELF	VLF
"Low" exposure	1.00	1.00	1.00	1.00
"High" exposure	0.72	1.41	1.25	0.57
	(0.35-1.48)	(0.67-2.9)	(0.57-2.72)	(0.27-1.22)
Field level separating "low" and "high"	4 V/m	0.06 V/m	125 nT	4 nT

The analysis was restricted to the VDU user group.

Table 4. Associations between exposure to and the accumulated dose of VLF (line frequency) electric or magnetic field from a VDU and skin problems.

	Diagnoses n=229 or 239 [1]		Erythema n=220 or 229 [1]		Complaints n=241	
	electric	magnetic	electric	magnetic	electric	magnetic
Exposure from VDU model, comparisons within the VDU user group						
Low exposure [2]	1.00	1.00	1.00	1.00	1.00	1.00
High exposure [2]	1.13	1.28	0.99	0.84	0.81	0.97
	(0.57-2.24)	(0.67-2.45)	(0.29-3.37)	(0.26-2.71)	(0.44-1.50)	(0.54-1.76)
Accumulated dose, comparisons with non-VDU user group						
No VDU usage	1.00	1.00	1.00	1.00	1.00	1.00
Low dose [3]	0.80	0.82	2.76	4.86	1.09	0.86
	(0.33-1.95)	(0.30-2.29)	(0.28-26.9)	(0.46-51.5)	(0.48-2.46)	(0.32-2.33)
High dose [3]	0.72	0.73	7.14	4.87	1.54	1.48
	(0.31-1.67)	(0.32-1.66)	(0.83-61.7)	(0.59-40.6)	(0.72-3.30)	(0.72-3.07)

Fields were measured at 30 cm distance, and averaged for each VDU model. Changes between models were taken into account - thus exposure was due to the model used at the time of dermatological examination and complaint response. [1] Refer to exposure and dose computations, respectively. [2] Delineations between "low" and "high" are 5 V/m (electric) and 100 nT (magnetic). [3] Delineations are 5 V·year/m (electric) and 125 nT·year (magnetic).

As shown in table 3, there were no appreciable associations between the exposure to any time-varying electric or magnetic field and skin complaints obtained at the time of measuring the fields. The small excess noted (1.25 and 1.41) were eliminated by adjusting for confounding by some organisational variables - but these latter were not obtained at the same time, making their inclusion in the model debatable.

Table 4 shows associations between line frequency (VLF) electric and magnetic exposure or dose and skin problems. For interpretation of the excess odds ratios in table 4, see discussion below. For seborrhoic eczema, the exposure comparison produced an odds ratio of 1.87 (0.63-5.62), and the dose comparison gave odds ratios of 0.89 (0.04-18.2)/"low" and 2.18 (0.22-21.1)/"high".

4. DISCUSSION

A requirement in these analysis was that assocations between exposure and effect should use only concurrent data or evaluations. For VLF fields, estimates of concurrent exposure were based on the recorded model used by the individual at the time of dermatological examination, and the average field for all measured units of that model. The accumulated dose was likewise based on the recorded models used by each individual during 5 years prior to the examination. The underlying rationale was that VLF fields were basically due to the VDUs. Such assumptions could not be made for ELF fields, where other contributing sources are common. This precluded an analysis of associations between skin disorders or signs and ELF fields. Thus, for ELF fields, the findings are restricted to that of skin complaints - which were (again) ascertained at the time of field measurements. Electrostatic fiels and static charges were measured at the same day as the dermatological examination.

Small sizes of certain subgroups (primarily among non-VDU users) resulted in wide confidence intervals, as indicated by erythema (see table 1-4) and specific diagnoses like seborrhoic eczema and lentigo (see text). Within these restrictions, the study was nevertheless unable to demonstrate any associations between the propensity for static charge, or exposure to electrostatic, electric or magnetic fields and examined skin diseases, erythema or complaints. The low odds ratio for electrostatic fields and skin complaints (0.66, table 2) could conceivably be due to the preferential subsequent application of filters to those experiencing skin problems. This interpretation is supported by the finding that measuring the fields after removing the filters changed the odds ratio to close to unity - which mimics a "reconstruction" of fields as they existed before the filter application.

The only noticable excess odds ratios were those found for erythema and complaints in relation to the accumulated dose (table 4, lower part). This is most likely due not to the field component of the dose, but rather to the VDU work hour component. Such an interpretation is supported by a/ the lack of any association with the exposure (table 4, upper part), and b/ the association found between these two endpoints and accumulated hours of VDU work. For e.g.

skin complaints, the adjusted odds ratio for more than 2.5 man-years of accumulated VDU work was 2.46 (1.08-5.63) [4] while the adjusted odds ratio for a high dose (accumulated man-years and magnetic field levels) was 1.48 (0.72-3.07) (table 4).

Few other studies have been made on associations between measured or estimated field levels at VDU work stations and skin complaints. Koh and coworkers [7] did not find any differences in skin complaints between workers using VDUs based on cathode ray tubes and those based on plasma display technologies. (Cathode ray tubes can be assumed to cause - in general - higher exposure levels.) Sandström and coworkers did find a univariate association between ELF magnetic fields at VDU work stations and skin complaints [5], but this association was not confirmed by multivariate analysis [Stenberg, presented at the WWDU conference]. Other fields at the VDU work position - i.e. in front of the VDUs - were not shown to be associated with skin complaints in this study [5].

REFERENCES

1. Knave B, Wibom R, Voss M, Hedström L and Bergqvist U. Work with video display terminals among office employees. I. Subjective symptoms and discomfort. Scandinavian Journal of Work, Environment and Health. 1985, **11**: 467-474.

2. Lidén C and Wahlberg J E. Work with video display terminals among office employees. V. Dermatologic factors. Scandinavian Journal of Work, Environment and Health. 1985, **11**: 489-493.

3. Bergqvist U, Knave B, Voss M and Wibom R. A longitudinal study of VDT work and health. International Journal of Human Computer Interaction. 1992, **4**: 197-219.

4. Bergqvist U and Wahlberg J E. Skin diseases and complaints during work with visual display terminals. In manuscript, .

5. Sandström M, Mild H K, Lönnberg G, Stenberg B and Wall, S. Inomhusmiljö och hälsa bland kontorsarbetare i Västerbotten. Elektriska och magnetiska fält: en fall - referentstudie bland bildskärmsarbetare (The Office Illness Project in Northern Sweden. Electric and magnetic fields: a case referent study among VDT workers, in Swedish.). National Institute of Occupational Health, Solna, Sweden, 1991. Report U-91:12.

6. SAS Users Guide. Statistics, 5th edition. 1985, Cary, NC: SAS Institute Inc.

7. Koh D, Goh C L, Jeyaratnam J, Kee W C and Ong C N. Dermatological Symptoms Among Visual Display Unit Operators Using Plasma Display and Cathode Ray Tube Screens. Annals of the Academy of Medicine. 1990, **19**: 617-620.

WORK WITH DISPLAY UNITS 92
H. Luczak, A. Çakir and G. Çakir (Editors)
1993 Elsevier Science Publishers B.V.

Pregnancy Outcome and VDU Work - A Review

U. Bergqvist

Department of Neuromedicine
National Institute of Occupational Health,
S-171 52 Solna, Sweden

1. HISTORICAL BACKGROUND

The use of a visual display unit (VDU) has been commonplace in certain specific types of workplaces for decades. At the end of the seventies, though, use of VDUs increased dramatically in many common work situations. In e.g. Sweden, it has been estimated that by now (1990), about 30-35% of all employees use a VDU daily, with another 15-20% having some regular use [1]. Following this increase in usage, concerns about possible negative effects began to appear. The primary concerns were centered on possible effects on the eyes - especially in terms of visual fatigue - and on observed or expected changes in work content.

In juli 1980, a Canadian newspaper reported on four pregnant VDU operators who all gave birth to children with malformations. Several other such clusters were at the time or subsequently reported from primarily North America. A possible explanation of these clusters were that they were no more common than what could be reasonably attributed to random variations [2]. The possibility of other, more causal explanations did, however, result in a number of studies being directed towards the question whether a pregnant woman's work with a visual display unit (VDU) is related to increased occurrences of adverse reproductive outcomes - especially spontaneous abortion and serious malformations.

Among other types of explanations was the emission of radiation from VDUs - but careful measurements were unable to detect those at levels compatible with injury. In 1982, a Spanish research team reported on the possible teratogenic effects of low frequency magnetic fields [3], which led to a change in interest from radiations to low-frequency fields. Later, increased attention has also been given other types of factors such as stress and ergonomic conditions.

2. FORMULATION OF HYPOTHESES

The issue of VDU work and pregnancy needs to be more explicitly formulated. In essence, we are considering two different possible scenarios; one in which there is a general influence of VDU work (due to some ubiquitous factors in VDU work situations), and one in which an influence is present only in some specific subgroups of VDU workers. In the latter scenario at least, the factor need not be specific for VDU work. These considerations can be translated into the following operational issues:

1. *Is there a general increase in the occurrence of adverse pregnancy outcome associated with VDU work? If so, can some specific factor(s) be identified as responsible?* This issue is addressed primarily by a number of epidemiological studies, comparing VDU users with non-VDU users. If a difference is established, then the second question should be addressed, by considering both detailed data on specific factors from the epidemiological studies (if such are available) , and knowledge obtained from other (e.g. experimental) studies.

2. *Can subgroups of VDU users be identified - by a specific factor or factors - that have an increased occurrence of adverse pregnancy outcome?* This issue can be considered also from epidemiological data, comparisons being made between different groups of VDU users according to the presence or absence of specific factors. Data from other studies (primarily experimental ones) are also of major interest in this evaluation. Due to the uncertainty of how we characterise certain factors in terms of their possible biological effects, experimental studies on specific factors and teratogenic effects should be performed with the factor(s) being as similar as possible to those appearing in VDU work situations.

Pregnancy outcomes under consideration are primarily those for which the original observations of clusters arose; i.e. spontaneous abortion and (serious) malformations. Indications of reduced growth have been studied in a number of studies, and are thus also summarized. For other outcomes such as early birth, placental weights and fecundity, only limited data exist, seriously limiting the possibility of evaluation.

Secondly, factors of possibly causal interest need to be specified. The evaluation in this review will - apart from a "general" difference between VDU and non-VDU work as described above - be performed for the following factors; 1/ magnetic fields in the net/image frequency region (about 50-100 Hz), 2/ magnetic fields in the line frequency region (about 15-35 kHz), 3/ stress and 4/ ergonomic conditions, with focus on the first two. Other factors will not be considered, due to lack of data and/or plausibility as causal factors.

3. MAGNETIC FIELDS AND TERATOGENIC EFFECTS

A number of studies have been performed on the possible teratogenic effects of magnetic fields on various biological systems; chick embryos, rodents, human cells in vitro etc. For details, see some recent reviews [4, 5] as well as some selected papers from the earlier WWDU conferences. In summary:

- A number of studies have been performed using chick embryos and (mostly) pulsed fields in the 50-100 Hz frequency region. The outcome has been varied, and indicative of the involvement also of other, uncontrolled factors (see e.g. Berman et al [6] and Handcock and Kolassa [7]). There is also an expressed reluctance for relying on chick embryo studies (being non-mammalian) for human pregnancy risk evaluation [8].
- Studies of rats and mice exposed to 50 Hz magnetic fields have not resulted in adverse reproductive outcomes being related to the field exposure [4].
- Studies on human or mammalian cells exposed in vitro to 50 Hz fields have resulted in mixed results [9-11].
- Studies on rats and mice exposed to saw-tooth 18-20 kHz magnetic fields (similar to the line frequency fields from VDUs) have resulted in mixed results. The discussion on causes for this variability has centered on 1/ different species, 2/ other uncontrolled factors (e.g. noise) and 3/ different statistical analyses [4, 5].

4. EPIDEMIOLOGICAL STUDIES

Table 1 lists 16 epidemiological studies that have made comparisons between VDU and non-VDU users. Additional studies have been performed, but details of their design precludes their contributing to the evaluations - small size, low response rate, lack of individual exposure assessment etc. (None suggested a real difference between VDU and non-VDU users.)

Spontaneous abortion was studies in 12 of the 16 studies, generally without any noticable difference between VDU and non-VDU users (see table 1). A few studies did suggest an increase with increased usage (in hours/week), though [12-14]. In two studies, that of McDonald et al [15] and that of Goldhaber et al [13], selection or other types of bias have been identified or strongly suggested as contributing to the observed increased occurrence of spontaneous abortion among VDU users [2, 15, 16].

Serious malformations were investigated in 8 of the 16 studies (table 1). An excess was noted in one [17], but was largely eliminated after controlling for the impact of stress and smoking. For specific malformations, examples of both increased and reduced occurrence for VDU users were noted, but there was little consistency between studies as to which malformation was increased. An increase in one study [18] concerning cardiovascular malformations led to a follow-up study, which failed to verify such an increase [19].

Foetal growth retardation was somewhat increased in one of the studies [16], but not in the other 5 that addressed this issue (table 1). A few other endpoints were studied, such as early birth or perinatal mortality, without evidence of increased occurrence among VDU users [15, 19-21, 25, 29]. In one study, fecundity - expressed as time to pregnancy - was increased among VDU operators working long hours on VDUs [27]. This finding was however only apparent in some analysis, leading the authors to suspect the possibility of recall bias [27].

Two studies have investigated relationships between magnetic fields around VDU units [14] or at VDU workplaces [24]. In the latter, no association between fields and spontaneous abortion could be seen. In the former, though, those who during pregnancy had worked with a VDU model which had - in laboratory measurements - shown high net/image frequency magnetic field levels, were at a significant higher risk of spontaneous abortion compared to those working with a VDU models showing low field levels. See further table 2.

As is apparent from table 2, the comparability of measured values in these two studies are limited, due to differences in where measurements were made, instrumentation etc. It is also noteworthy that interpretation of the results of the Lindbohm et al study are subject to choise of comparison group. The authors argue that a within VDU group comparison appears more appropriate, since this would reduce the heterogenicity of the groups [14]. (This is also consistent with the second hypothesis formulation above.) A number of discussion points were raised at the WWDU meeting, where this study [14] was presented. 1/ What does the value of "0.9 μT" represent - and how common is it?. Some misconceptions did arise due to the apparent confusion in the discussion between peak-to-peak (as given in the report) and the more common rms values (as given here). Comparison with other studies shows that while the levels are fairly high, they are not entirely uncommon. 2/ The fields were not measured at the workplace, which probably - especially since this include 50 Hz fields - would lead to some exposure misclassification. The authors argue [14] that such misclassification is unlikely to be directional, and should thus not be able to cause inflated odds ratios. 3/ All VDUs with the highest fields were from one company. The authors considered this, but were unable to find that other conditions in this company (such as stress conditions) could explain the results [14].

Table 1. Epidemiological studies of VDU work and pregnancy outcomes

Study	Description Type	Size	Results SA	MF	GR	Comment (see further text)	Reference
Kurppa et al 1985	CC	2950	--	no	--		[18]
Ericson et al 1985	Cohort	4347	no	no	no		[20]
Ericson & Källén 1986	CC	1385	no	var	--	stress	[17]
Butler & Brix 1986	Cohort	817	no	--	--	time	[12]
McDonald et al 1988	CC	104649	var	no	no	selection	[15]
Goldhaber et al 1988	CC	1583	yes	no	--	time, bias	[13]
Nurminen & Kurppa 1988	CC	1475	--	--	--	other effects	[21]
Bryant & Love 1989	CC	980	no	--	--		[22]
Brandt & Nielsen 1990 a/	CB	4628	no	no	no	stress, ergonomics	[23, 28-29]
Windham et al 1990	CC	1361	no	--	var		[16]
Tikkanen et al 1990	CC	1555	--	no	no		[19]
Schnorr et al 1991	Cohort	882	no	--	--	fields measured	[24]
Bramwell 1992	Prospektive	7819	no	no	no	stress	[25]
Lindbohm et al 1992	CC	585	no	--	--	time, field measured stress, ergonomics	[14]
Roman et al 1992	CC	447	no	--	--		[26]
Brandt & Nielsen 1992	CB	2252	--	--	--	other effects	[27]

Type: CC=case control, CB=case base. Size: number of pregnancies in the study analysis. Results: SA=spontaneous abortion, MF=serious malformation, GR=foetal growth retardation. yes=a substantial difference between VDU and non-VDU users, no=no such difference noted, var=depending on analysis and/or criteria for "substantial", results could be described both as "yes" or "no". a/ also Nielsen & Brandt 1990 and Nielsen et al 1989.

Table 2. Comparison between two studies [14] and [24] as to associations between spontaneous abortion and net/image frequency magnetic fields.

	No VDU use	VDU with low field	VDU with high field
Lindbohm et al [14]			
Magnetic field a/	Not measured	<0.13 μT	>0.3 μT
Odds ratio/within VDU group	--	1.00	3.4 (1.4-8.6)
Odds ratio/cf with non-VDU group	1.00	0.4 (0.2-0.8)	1.6 (b/)
Schnorr et al [24]			
Magnetic field c/	0.037 μT	0.19 μT	0.25 μT
Magnetic field d/	0.036 μT	0.046 μT	0.050 μT
Odds ratio/cf with non-VDU group	1.00	0.98 (0.58-1.64)	0.92 (0.58-1.47)

a/ Measured in laboratory for appropriate type of VDU, at 50 cm and (for some) 25 cm below screen center. Recalculated into rms. b/ Confidence interval not stated, but given as "not significant". c/ Measured at random selection of workplaces, value assigned to type of VDU. Measured at 30 cm in front of VDU and equivalent for non-VDU workplace. Levels in rms. d/ Same as in c/, but measured in foetal position, with operators present.

5. EVALUATION

Based on these data, the questions formulated above can be partly answered:

1. *Is there a general increase in the occurrence of adverse pregnancy outcome associated with VDU work?* There appear to be no associations between spontaneous abortion, serious malformations or foetal growth retardation and the mother's VDU usage during pregnancy - where the term VDU usage has been given a general meaning.

2. *Can subgroups of VDU users be identified - by a specific factor or factors - that have an increased occurrence of adverse pregnancy outcome?* This question is addressed specifically for the different factors.

For line frequency magnetic fields. There was a lack of association between field levels and spontaneous abortion in the two epidemiological studies that included data on these fields [14, 24], and a varied response in the experimental studies performed. This leads to the conclusion that, at present, an effect of line frequency magnetic fields from VDUs on the risk of spontaneous abortion is not established nor strongly supported.

For net/image frequency fields. Here, the two epidemiological studies present opposing indications [14, 24], whereas little if any support for the suggestion is offered by experimental studies. Furthermore, some points in the positive study [14] do detract from their findings (not workplace measurements, different result dependent on comparison groups and restriction of positive findings to one company). In conclusion, firm evidence for an effect of net/image frequency magnetic fields are at present not available. Nevertheless, the positive association noted in one study motivates an effort for replication.

For stress and ergonomic conditions. Suggestions of a stress involvement were noted in several studies [14, 17, 23 and 25], but there were also indications that this was influenced by recall bias [Lars Brandt, presented at the WWDU conference]. No indications of an involvement of ergonomic conditions were found [14, 28]. These data appear insufficient for definite conclusions to be made.

REFERENCES

1. SCB. Datorvanor 1990 (Computer use 1990, in Swedish). Statistical Central Office, Stockholm, 1990. Report DF1:1990.

2. Bergqvist U. Video display terminals and health. Scandinavian Journal of Work, Environment and Health. 1984, **10**, suppl 2: 1-87.

3. Delgado J M R, Leal L, Monteagudo J L, and Garcia M G. Embryological changes induced by weak, extremely low frequency electromagnetic fields. Journal of Anatomy. 1982, **134**: 533-551.

4. Juutilainen J. Effects of low-frequency magnetic fields on embryonic development and pregnancy. Scandinavian Journal of Work, Environment and Health. 1991, **17**: 149-158.

5. Kavet R, and Tell R A. VDTs: Field levels, epidemiology, and laboratory studies. Health Physics. 1991, **61**: 47-57.

6. Berman E, Chacom L, House D, Koch B A, Leal J, Løvstrup S, Mantiply E, Martin A H, Martucci G I, Mild K H, Monahan J C, Sandström M, Shamsaifar K, Tell R, Trillo M A, Ubeda A, and Wagner P. Development of chicken embryos in a pulsed magnetic field. Bioelectromagnetics. 1990, **11**: 169-187.

7. Handcock M S, and Kolassa J E. Statistical Review of the Henhouse Experiments: The Effects of a Pulsed Magnetic Field on Chick Embryos. Bioelectromagnetics. 1992, **13**: 429-433.

8. Schardein J L. Principles of teratogenesis applicable to human exposure to drugs and chemicals, in Chemically induced birth defects, J.L. Schardein, editor. 1985, Marcel Dekker, Inc: New York.

9. Galt S. Optical fiber scattering and biological electromagnetic effects. Chalmers Technical University, Gothenburg, 1990. Technical Report No 198.

10. Livingston G K, Witt K L, Gandhi O P, Chatterjee I, and Roti Roti J L. Reproductive integrity of mammalian cells exposed to power frequency electromagnetic fields. Environ Mol Mutagen. 1991, **17**: 49-58.

11. Nordensson I, Mild K H, Sandström M, and Mattsson M O. Verkan av lågfrekventa magnetfält på kromosomnivå hos humana amnionceller (The effect of low frequency magnetic fields on human amnion cells at a chromosomal level, in Swedish). National Institute of Occupational Health, Solna, Sweden, 1989. Report U 1989:25.

12. Butler W J, and Brix K A, Video display terminal work and pregnancy outcome in Michigan clerical workers, in Allegations of Reproductive Hazards from VDUs, B.G. Pearce, editor. 1986, Humane Technology: Nottingham. p. 31-52.

13. Goldhaber M K, Polen M R, and Hiatt R A. The risk of miscarriage and birth defects among women who use visual display terminals during pregnancy. American Journal of In-

dustrial Medicine. 1988, **13**: 695-706.
14. Lindbohm M-L, Hietanen M, Kyyrönen P, Sallmén M, von Nandelstadh P, Taskinen H, Pekkarinen M, Ylikoski M, and Hemminki K. Magnetic Fields of Video Display Terminals and Spontaneous Abortion. American Journal of Epidemiology. 1992, **136**: in press.
15. McDonald A D, McDonald J C, Armstrong B, Cherry N, Nolin A D, and Robert D. Work with visual display units in pregnancy. British Journal of Industrial Medicine. 1988, **45**: 509-515.
16. Windham G C, Fenster L, Swan S H, and Neutra R R. Use of video display terminals during pregnancy and the risk of spontaneous abortion, low birthweight, or intrauterine growth retardation. American Journal of Industrial Medicine. 1990, **18**: 675-688.
17. Ericson A, and Källén B. An Epidemiological Study of Work with Video Screens and Pregnancy Outcomes: II. A Case-Control Study. American Journal of Industrial Medicine. 1986, **9**: 459-475.
18. Kurppa K, Holmberg P C, Rantala K, Nurminen T, and Saxén L. Birth defects and exposure to video display terminals during pregnancy. Scandinavian Journal of Work, Environment and Health. 1985, **11**: 353-356.
19. Tikkanen J, Heinonen O P, Kurppa K, and Rantala K. Cardiovascular malformations and maternal exposure to video display terminals during pregnancy. European Journal of Epidemiology. 1990, **6**: 61-66.
20. Ericson A, Källén B, and Westerholm P. Ingen ökad risk för fosterskador hos kvinnor med bildskärmsarbete (No increase in the risk of foetal damage among women working at a VDU, in Swedish). Läkartidningen. 1986, **82**: 2180-2184.
21. Nurminen T, and Kurppa K. Office employment, work with video display terminals, and course of pregnancy. Scandinavian Journal of Work, Environment and Health. 1988, **14**: 293-298.
22. Bryant H E, and Love E J. Video display terminal use and spontaneous abortion risk. International Journal of Epidemiology. 1989, **19**: 132-138.
23. Brandt L, and Nielsen C V. Congenital malformations among children of women working with video display terminals. Scandinavian Journal of Work, Environment and Health. 1990, **16**: 329-333.
24. Schnorr T M, Grajewski B A, Hornung R W, Thun M J, Egeland G M, Murray W E, Conover D L, and Halperin W E. Video display terminals and the risk of spontaneous abortion. New England Journal of Medicine. 1991, **324**: 727-733.
25. Bramwell R. A Prospective Study of the Impact of VDU Work on Women's Reproductive Health, in Work with Display Units, WWDU '92 - Abstracts, H Luczak, A E Çakir and G Çakir, editors. 1992, Technische Universität Berlin. p. A-23
26. Roman E, Beral V, Pelerin M, and Hermon C. Spontaneous abortion and work with visual display units. British Journal of Industrial Medicine. 1992, **49**: 507-512.
27. Brandt L, and Nielsen C V. Fecundity and the use of video display terminals. Scandinavian Journal of Work, Environment and Health. 1992, **18**: 298-301.
28. Nielsen C V, and Brandt L. Spontaneous abortion among women using video display terminals. Scandinavian Journal of Work, Environment and Health. 1990, **16**: 323-328.
29. Nielsen C V, Brandt L, Helsborg L, Waldström B, and Nielsen L T. Effekten av skærmterminalarbejde på svangerskabsforløb - en reproduktionsepidemiologisk undersøgelse (The effect of VDU work on the course of pregnancy - a reproductive epidemiological study, in Danish). Department of Social Medicine, University of Aarhus, 1989.

WORK WITH DISPLAY UNITS 92
H. Luczak, A. Çakir and G. Çakir (Editors)

Electric and magnetic sanitation of the office*

Anna-Christina Blomkvist Department of Human Work Sciences, University of Luleå, 951 87 Luleå, Sweden

Per Erik Boivie Swedish Confederation of Salaried Employees (TCO), 114 94 Stockholm, Sweden

Yngve Hamnerius Department of Microwave Technology, Chalmers University of Technology, 412 96 Göteborg, Sweden

Kjell Hansson Mild National Institute of Occupational Health, Box 7654, 907 13 Umeå, Sweden

Torbjörn Klittervall Swedish Foundation for Occupational Health and Safety for State Employees, 311 87 Karlskrona, Sweden

Olov Östberg Swedish Agency for Administrative Development, Box 34107, 100 26 Stockholm, Sweden

Abstract

The research evidence of hazardousness of long term exposure to 50-60 Hz magnetic fields is growing. It seems to be good advice to avoid such fields already at a level of 0,2 μT. People claiming a general sensitivity to electricity point to the need also to reduce the electric fields, and not to restrict the preventive measures to the low frequency regions. There is still no hypothesis on the mechanisms behind their symptoms. A pragmatic attitude towards prudence in office environments is developing among employers, safety representatives, and employees. The background to such a position is given for Sweden, and some tips are offered on office sanitation and how it can be worked out.

1. THE RATIONALE OF EMF-SANITATION IN OFFICES

The interest in sanitation for Electric and Magnetic Fields (EMFs) has multiple causes. *a)* VDU users are worried about being exposed to radiation; concerns have ranged from X-rays, ionization and UV light over EMFs to static electricity. Gradually, findings from 1979 [1] on the relationships between magnetic fields of extremely-low-frequency (ELF, e.g. 50-60 Hz) and childhood

---

* Equal and shared responsibility is assumed by the authors, who made individual contributions to a session organized and chaired by O. Östberg.

leukemia have gained acceptance. *b)* An increasing number of employees are reporting that their health is impaired by EMFs. A Swedish association of EMF afflicted persons has about 1500 active members claiming experience of sensitivity to electrical equipment. These EMF sensitive people draw their conclusions from their own observations: They react to electrical equipment, and feel better away from such equipment. Corresponding associations exist in e.g. Denmark and Germany. A recent study on electromagnetic field sensitivity supports the hypothesis that there could be an effect on the autonomous nervous system[2]. *c)* Studies on effects of EMFs neither rule out the possibility of hazards nor clarify the mechanisms, leading to conflicting signals to the users of office equipment. In August of 1990, the IEEE US Activities Board stated that there is no convincing evidence that EMFs influence the users of VDUs, but in April of 1991 they published ergonomics layout guidelines for workstations[3] covering the Swedish "MPR recommendations"[4], which in turn is based on the respect for potential hazards from EMFs. *d)* Entrepreneurs advertise and sell EMF reducing equipment. They offer shielding equipment, such as conductive screens to mount in front of VDUs, and other equipment for shielding and grounding of electrical apparatus, conductors, and data connections. Also systems for switching off equipment properly are developed in order to reduce fields from equipment people believe they have switched off already. Aluminium wallpaper and conductive floor coating are other examples of EMF-sanitation products.

Three recent Nordic investigations have added fuel to the sanitation debate. A study from the Finnish Institute of Occupational Health[5] showed that women who had used VDUs with high levels of ELF magnetic fields (> 0,3 μT) had significantly increased odds ratio of spontaneous abortion when compared to those having used low level VDUs (< 0,15 μT). The Swedish National Institute of Occupational Health[6] at the same time reported that industry workers exposed to a *daily average* of > 0,29 μT had a three times higher risk of developing chronic lymphocytic leukemia, compared to workers with an average daily exposure of < 0,16 μT. There was furthermore a significantly increased risk of brain tumors. The Swedish Institute of Environmental Medicine[7] similarly found that children who live within 50 meters of high voltage power lines run 2,9 times the average risk of developing leukemia. In a normal home, the magnetic ELF fields rarely exceed a daily average of 0,1 μT, a level at which the incidence of childhood leukemia was found to be 2,4. The incidence increased to 2,7 when the daily dose increased to 0,2 μT, and to 3,8 when the dose was 0,3 μT.

1.1 Symptoms of EMF sensitivity

There are two main kinds of reactions; one - a lighter form - is skin rashes or a feeling of burning under the skin, the other is neurological reactions such as nausea and sensitivity to light. We have learned from the association of EMF afflicted persons, newspapers and interviews that 1) one can restrain the development of symptoms with sanitation measures at an early stage, 2) there is no constant feeling of illness, but after exposure it can take days or weeks to recover, 3) it is possible to ration exposure so that if you avoid exposure for several days you can risk a dose without getting ill, and 4) reactions are individual; one can not be sure that different people react to the same features of EMFs.

1.2 Risk management agenda for employers

It is becoming increasingly clear that strong magnetic fields at 50-60 Hz should be avoided. The role of higher frequencies, and of electric fields, are less clear-cut. In Sweden, and other countries, it has also become a fact of life that some people seem to develop sensitivity to electric and magnetic fields, but for these cases a scientific explanation is still missing. Explanations or not, employers are forced to address the fact that some employees using VDUs have lowered production and/or have high rates of forced absenteeism.

The emerging, pragmatic employer attitude seems to be that it is prudent to avoid exposing workers to electric and magnetic fields, which, just like noise and pollution, are not needed in the office environment and should thus be as low as reasonably achievable. Low emission VDUs are better than high emission VDUs. Shielded power cables are better than non-shielded. Employers should work from the top in the following general Risk Management agenda, where, for the time being, "Risk" should be read as electric and magnetic fields:

- Identify the risk
- Eliminate the risk
- Modify the risk
- Reduce the exposure
- Reduce the consequences
- Move the risk
- Ensure the risk

1.3 Risk management at a national level

The Swedish Government in 1987 declared that, by 1991, governmental agencies shall provide VDU workplaces free of EMFs, without sacrificing good vision ergonomics. Providing office environments where the EMF levels are "as low as reasonably achievable" begs the questions about what is low (safety and health; physics) and what is reasonable (economics; physics). So, in parallel, the National Board of Occupational Safety and Health and the Swedish Institute for Radiation Protection were asked to work with the National Council for Metrology and Testing (MPR; now renamed SWEDAC) and the parties of the labour market to establish mandatory measurement rules and voluntary guidelines on ergonomics parameters and EMF levels. With regard to EMF, a consensus was reached to the effect that (i) a VDU shall not add more to the background EMF levels than other sources in the offices, and (ii) that the reduction of the EMFs should not deteriorate other important qualities of the VDUs. It can be assumed that this tripartite approach has also given ample room for the economics dimensions of "reasonable and achievable". The EMF guidelines for VDUs today read as follows [4]:

- Electric fields should be, respectively, below 25 V/m (*I*) and 2,5 V/m (*II*).
- Magnetic fields should be, respectively, below 0,25 μT (*I*) and 0,025 μT (*II*).

I and *II* denotes, respectively, the bands of 5 Hz - 2 kHz and 2 kHz - 400 kHz.

2. EXAMPLES OF EMF INITIATIVES IN SWEDEN

Presently several projects on sensitivity to EMF are in progress in Sweden. Two epidemiology studies are being run by the National Institute of Occupational

Health. One project, organized by a private company, is looking for causes and treatments along the lines of "techno stress". Of great importance is a new project principalled by the Ministry of Housing and Physical Planning, and with financial backing of among others Vattenfall (former Swedish State Power Board). Under the acronym HEEM, the project will investigate and remedy "Negative Effects of Electric and Magnetic Fields". *Elkontoro* is a project run by and for governmental agencies, and in the formation of which four of the present authors took an active part. In practice, it takes a starting point in the symptom descriptions above and uses the experiences described below.

2.1 Elkontoro

Elkontoro started in April of 1992. It is a joint project on electric and magnetic sanitation of offices within six Swedish governmental agencies; another five governmental agencies are providing expert help. The project is partly funded by the Working Life Fund and will last for two years. It is not assumed in the project that sanitation is always necessary, but it is assumed that knowledge about sanitation is necessary. The various offices involved will develop "all-embracing" local policies and action plans in parallel with the common activities within the sanitation project. The common goal is to offer employer strategies on how to:

- map out electric and magnetic conditions of workrooms;
- realize sanitation step by step;
- map out the effect of sanitation;
- meanwhile evaluate attitudes and well-being of employees.

2.2 Trade union views

The Swedish Confederation of Professional Employees (TCO) considers sensitivity to electricity to be accompanied by social problems[8]. It causes suffering, absenteeism, and is met with unequal treatment depending on who is affected. The social problem is amplified by research deficiencies, inertia of funding systems, and the conventional demand that a problem has to be understood or that symptoms should be scientifically explained before measures can be taken. Employees, with their concrete experience, contribute to the accumulation of knowledge on which to base activities for change. However, their knowledge has its limitations as a means of prevailing on government and parliament to take action. No matter how formidable the employees' knowledge, according to TCO it is still possible for the authorities to refrain from action on the grounds that scientific evidence is lacking.

Everyone at the workplace can help prevent problems of electrical sensitivity from occurring. Sometimes individual employees ignore their own symptoms. They are so dedicated to their work that they do not recognize warning signs. It is, however, important to be on the look-out for symptoms, both one's own and fellow-employees', so that actions can be taken in good time.

Some TCO hints to everybody at the workplace: Symptoms are not to be trifled with! Take care if someone is affected. Problems can be reduced by prompt action. Individuals affected should begin by approaching their supervisory staff and ask for investigative and other measures to be taken. It is important to ask the following questions:

- **How were the problems made manifest?**
- **When were the problems made manifest?**
- **Where environmental changes made when or just before the symptoms started?**
- **What does the individual affected believe to be a possible cause?**

By finding out as much as possible about the work situation immediately before the symptoms began to show up, one gets data on which to base a choice of practical measures. In this way TCO considers it possible to find common denominators of the environment in which the individual affected has developed the disorders. Researchers, physicians, physicists, safety engineers, union representatives, and, not least, the individuals affected, can all contribute to greater clarity via a dialogue between experts and between experts and practitioners.

3. EMFs IN LOCAL POWER DISTRIBUTION SYSTEMS

Electric equipment emits electric fields when not enclosed in a metal cabinet which is electrically connected to zero potential via a protective ground wire. Even equipment connected to protective earth often has separate metallic parts which are not in electrical contact with the grounded parts and therefore emit electric fields. This is often the case with desk top lamps. Metallic objects which form parts of electrical systems, such as the metallic frame of an office desk, emit electric fields when the metallic structure is capacitively coupled to a power cord. Electric fields can often be reduced by simple means such as shielding and connecting metallic objects to ground potential. By using shielded cables, the electric fields from the building installations can be greatly reduced.

3.1 Vagabonding currents

Power frequency magnetic fields in buildings can have various sources, e. g. power lines outside the house, vagabonding currents and in-house transformer stations. The most common source of elevated magnetic fields in buildings, in Sweden, is vagabonding ground currents. When a four conductor system with a common neutral and protective earth lead is used, the protective earth lead is often in contact with water, gas and heating pipes. Return current can therefore travel in these pipes, and we have measured up to 30 amperes of vagabonding current. This creates increased magnetic fields over the whole building, not just close to the pipes, due to the 1/r dependence of the magnetic field from them. The magnetic fields from other sources fall off more rapidly; from a three phase overhead power line the field decreases as $1/r^2$, and from a point source, such as a VDU, the field falls off as $1/r^3$. In office buildings we have often found vagabonding currents in the computer network, not just creating magnetic fields, but also communication problems. If the magnetic flux density is over 0,5 - 1 μT, the magnetic fields will cause instability of the picture on the VDU screens.

The best way to eliminate these sources is by using a five conductor system with separate conductors for neutral and protective earth all the way from the (supplying) transformer station [9]. The magnetic field levels in buildings with five conductor systems are typically one level of magnitude lower than for buildings with four conductor installations. We have, in practical trials on four conductor systems, shown that the magnetic field can be greatly reduced when the vagabonding return currents are blocked. A vagabonding current in a pipe can be blocked, for example, by replacing a short section of the metallic pipe by a plastic pipe. This technique can easily be used for small buildings. In large buildings, it becomes impractical, due to too many paths for the vagabonding currents. In these cases a five conductor system is the most practical solution. So, to minimize EMF from power distribution systems, all new governmental buildings in Sweden are equipped with such a five conductor systems[10].

3.2 In-house transformers

In-house transformer stations typically give magnetic flux densities in the order of 1 - 10 μT in adjoining rooms. The magnetic fields are proportional to the current, so the low voltage switch gear gives high magnetic fields as the current is high on that side. To reduce the fields from transformers and their switch gears we have used shielding. Magnetic fields can either be shielded by materials which have high magnetic permeability such as steel, or by high conductivity materials like copper or aluminium. Calculations with the finite element method and practical trials have shown that high conductivity materials often give better shielding than steel. Very high permeability materials, such as μ-metal give excellent results, but the costs are usually prohibitive. When the ceiling and walls of a transformer station room is shielded with 5 mm aluminium sheets with all joints welded together, we have measured a magnetic field reduction of 10 to 20 times. The cost for this shielding is considerable, in the order of USD 100 000. Also the phase conductors to the low voltage switch gear are major sources. The phase conductors are often copper bars, and placed in a row at 10-20 cm distance from each other. The separation of the bars means that the magnetic field components from the bars do not cancel each other out. When insulated cables are used instead of bars, the cables can be put close together in a triangle, typically reducing the field by a factor of 10 at no extra cost if built this way to begin with!

4. EMFs FROM OFFICE EQUIPMENT

Electric and magnetic fields in offices have many sources. Examples of electrical equipment in the immediate vicinity of the employee are typewriters, calculators, radios, low voltage lamps and transformers, and equipment associated with computer usage (e. g., CRT display, laser printer, and modem). Fluorescent light systems in the room, or the room underneath, can also be a problem. Furthermore, the usage of electric equipment has a bearing on the fields from the power distribution system, as discussed above, since this will influence the amplitude and the shape of the supply current.

In an investigation covering 150 VDU workplaces[11], the median magnetic flux density was found to be 0,07 μT, and the median electric field 20 V/m. Electrical equipment in the rooms add to the background field. Typically, electric fields in the order of 100 - 500 V/m were found about 10 cm from ungrounded appliances. The magnetic fields could in such situations reach a few μT. Near the VDUs, EMFs are found with frequencies ranging from 50 Hz up to tens of MHz. VDUs are not the dominating source of the electric fields in offices.

Of importance, however, is that the low frequency magnetic field, as measured 50 cm in front of a VDU screen, is three times higher than the background field.

Below follow some tips on how to keep the EMF exposure low without too much investment costs:

[1] Remove all unnecessary electrical equipment such as the typewriter, calculator, and radio. Copiers and printers shall not be located in workrooms.

[2] Make sure that the equipment is properly connected to protective earthing. Sometimes VDUs and other equipments are connected to an ungrounded power outlet. This then leads to very high electric fields near the screen. In fact, the dominant source for electric fields in Swedish offices is modern ungrounded desk top lamps.

[3] Switch off the equipment when it is not in use.

[4] New VDUs should meet the low emission guidelines (see section 1.3 above).

[5] Choose workplace design so that the total exposure from equipment EMF is minimized. Note that magnetic fields are not reduced after passing through a normal wall or a screening between two workplaces.

5. THE ROLE OF OCCUPATIONAL HEALTH SERVICES

The Swedish model of occupational health services for state employees builds on preventive measures. However, when problems or injuries occur, the response is to work at eliminating causes. When VDU users began to complain about facial skin rashes, and in association with these, tingling, burning and red colouring, we had never before had any experience with these types of symptoms. Seemingly without any explanations the symptoms were often connected to dry air and/or high indoor temperatures. Even what has heretofore been called techno stress was believed to have been a factor related to the symptoms. Similar symptoms have been attributed to exposure to fluorescent lighting, and other electric components.

In 1990 all patients of the 118 health care centres covered by Swedish Foundation for Occupational Health and Safety for State Employees were investigated. Criterion for inclusion in the study was that the aforementioned skin symptoms should have been reported during the last three years to any of the centres. In several cases the patients themselves had tried to seek "EMF relief". Based on the severity of the problems, the 1650 patients were cast in the following four simple categories:

Category 1; 1150 patients: Light skin pain during VDU work. Ceases till next day if exposure stops.

Category 2; 350 patients: Skin pain for some duration after work with VDU or exposed other electric equipment, such as fluorescent lighting.

Category 3; 90 patients: General sensitivity to electric and/or magnetic fields. Limited capacity for work. Placed on sick leave or transferred to other work.

Category 4; 60 patients: Serious symptoms from exposure to electric equipment, even at home, involving considerable limitations on life style and on fitness for work.

The attempts at solving these challenging problems began with experiments on shielding the electric fields by equipping the VDUs with various types of filters. If this did not work, measures were also taken to extend shieldings to include all remaining electric equipment in an office area.

Gradually, all the EMF sanitation methods described in section 4 were tried. Through teaching and by comparing experiences, the knowledge of sanitation has now spread among the network of safety and health engineers. This sanitation technology is been successfully practiced by more and more '"EMF sanitation engineers'". As occupational health care is mediating experiences between scientists and practitioners, it is the practical successes which counts. The work of the '"EMF sanitation engineers'" are aimed at getting as many employees as possible to continue their work, and in so doing they practice those afore-mentioned different measures to help the afflicted individuals not to end up as disability cases.

Results from the project *Elkontoro*, from measuring electric and magnetic fields, and from evaluation of "EMF sanitation products", are being compiled and classified to serve as guidelines for all those who need qualified electric and magnetic sanitation in their office environments.

6. REFERENCES

1 Wertheimer, N., & Leeper, E., Electric wiring configuration and childhood cancer. *American Journal of Epidemiology*, *109*, 273-284, 1979.

2 Rea, W. J., Pan, Y., Fenyves, E. J., Sujisawa, I., Samada, N., & Ross, G. H., Electromagnetic field sensitivity. *Journal of Bioelectricity*, *10*, 241-256, 1991.

3 Tips on setting up your workstation. *IEEE Spectrum*, 36-37, April 1991.

4 *User's Handbook for Evaluating Visual Display Units*. Stockholm: Swedish Board for Technical Accreditation, 1990. (MPR 1990:10).

5 Lindbohm, M-L., Hietanen, M., Kyyönen, P., Sallmén, M., *et al.*, Magnetic fields of VDTs and spontaneous abortion. *WWDU '92 Abstract Book*. Berlin, 1992. (A-22).

6 Cancers related to strong electromagnetic fields. (Editorial article on a study by B. Floderus). In the English edition of Forskning & Praktik No. 7/1992: *New Evidence of Cancer from Electromagnetic Fields*. Stockholm: Swedish National Institute of Occupational Health, 1992. (Pp. 3-5).

7 Feychting, M., & Ahlbom, A., *Magnetic Fields and Cancer in People Residing near Swedish High Voltage Power Lines*. Stockholm: Institute of Environment Medicine, 1992. (Report IMM 6/92).

8 *Hypersensitivity to Electricity - An Action Program from TCO*. Stockholm: TCO, 1991.

9 Hamnerius, Y., Electric and magnetic fields in offices. (In Swedish). In P-E. Engfeldt, C. Johansson and L. G. Pärletun (Eds.), *Kontoret, Tekniken och Människan*. Lund: Studentlitteratur, 1992. (Pp. 49-67).

10 *Building Construction Handbook*, Part 92-11-A. (In Swedish). Stockholm: National Board of Public Buildings, 1992.

11 Sandström, M., Hanssson Mild, K., Lönnberg, G., Stenberg, B., & Wall, S., *The Office Illness Project in Northern Sweden*. (In Swedish), Umeå: National Institute of Occupational Health, 1991. (Investigation Report 1992:12).

WORK WITH DISPLAY UNITS 92
H. Luczak, A. Çakir and G. Çakir (Editors)

An investigation on state-of-the-art and future prospects of lighting technology in German office environments

A. Çakir

ERGONOMIC Institute for Social and Occupational Sciences, Research Co., Ltd.
Soldauer Platz 3, D - 1000 Berlin 19, F. R. Germany

Abstract

The impact of the office environment (noise, air quality, lighting) on workers health was assessed in a four part study in German offices. Self-reported health symptoms are significantly correlated with the type of work (VDT-, typewriter-, conventional office work) and environmental factors such as noise, lighting or air quality. In general, VDT-users reported more health disorders than workers performing conventional office work. Artificial lighting has proven to be one major source of health disorders, all complaints increased with growing distance of the workplace from the window.

However, the impact depends on the type of artificial lighting, with overhead lighting with narrow radiating angle (so called "VDT-lighting") being the worst and twin-component-lighting with two sources (an indirect part as general lighting and a direct part as task lighting) the best.

1. PURPOSE AND METHODS

The subjects discussed in this paper represent some of the results of the project "Light and health" which was conducted by the Ergonomic Institute in Berlin with the aim of determining the effects of work environment on the workers. Office employees in the Federal Republic of Germany were selected as the target group, since these have enjoyed the special protection of the "Ordinance on Workplace Conditions", the "Safety Regulations for Display Work Places" and effective lighting standards for more than five decades. This group was therefore particularly suitable for a study which was intended to establish the positive effects of artificial lighting. In addition, a particularly large number of changes had occurred in the area of interest over the course of the last 20 years, since the introduction of VDTs led to visual problems. As a result, new standards were drawn up for VDT workplaces, for example, and new lamps and luminaires were put onto the market. A substantial proportion of workrooms has been totally refurbished.

During the project, 2000 workers in 80 organizations, largely working at VDT workplaces, as well as a representative group of 1000 office employees, were questioned about their assessment of disturbing ambient factors and problems related to health and well-being. The study covered a total period of 10 years, with the representative poll taking place at the end of 1989 and the beginning of 1990. In a further phase, more than 300 workers in selected organizations were questioned. In the first and last phases all relevant physical characteristics were measured.

2. RESULTS

The most relevant distracting factors in the physical environment are "*noise and sound*" and "*dry air*", which 60 % assessed to be a regular impairment (fig. 1) and "*lighting*" (57 %).

Surprisingly, almost nobody complains about daylight although more than 40 % of the workplaces are placed within one meter from the next window. The overall rate of 57 % for lighting is increased to more than 80 %, if only workplaces with little daylight are included.

Health and well-being outcomes, surveyed with a modified questionnaire after v. Zerssen (1), show a general trend which is correlated with the distribution of natural light in the workroom (fig. 2); decreased levels of daylight correlate with increased levels of fatigue or other symptoms. The general trend is the same for all types of work, however, the effect is less significant for conventional office work than for VDT-work. The strongest effect was displayed for work with typewriters.

The type of work has no significant effect on health outcomes, if the workplace is located in the vicinity of windows within two meters and becomes significant in the depth of the rooms (2). This result is in contradiction to the generally assumed adverse impact of daylight on VDT-work.

A stepwise regression calculated with the nine variables displayed in fig. 1 as independent variables and health outcomes shows that the variable "lighting" is responsible for the biggest proportion of variance in almost all cases, e.g. for 50 % of common variance for the variable "rapid fatigue". "Noise and sound" and "conversations" as impairing factors do only affect variables like "poor concentration" or "irritability". This is in good agreement with the results of physical measurements, which show that the overall noise level in the offices has declined in the last decade.

The health and well-being outcomes of the representative survey differ significantly depending on the type of artificial lighting used, with table lamps (as the only lighting) having the worst impact, overhead lighting with a negative impact on 60 % and twin-component lighting on only 42 %.

Thus, changing lighting conditions is likely to be the most effective means to reduce adverse health effects, especially at VDT-workplaces. To prove this result of the first and second phase of the study, in two organizations new lighting equipment was installed and further surveys conducted some months after the installation.

In the first case, an overhead lighting was replaced by indirect lighting (approx. 300 lx to 400 lx) and additional task lighting (approx. 500 lx to 700 lx). The task lighting was under the control of each user, while the indirect component was planned as general lighting, representing the technically optimized version of twin component lighting. After eight months, health and and well-being outcomes were significantly improved after six of eight variables (fig. 3).

In the second case, twelve different lighting systems, belonging to five different types, were installed in similar rooms in an office building. The survey was carried

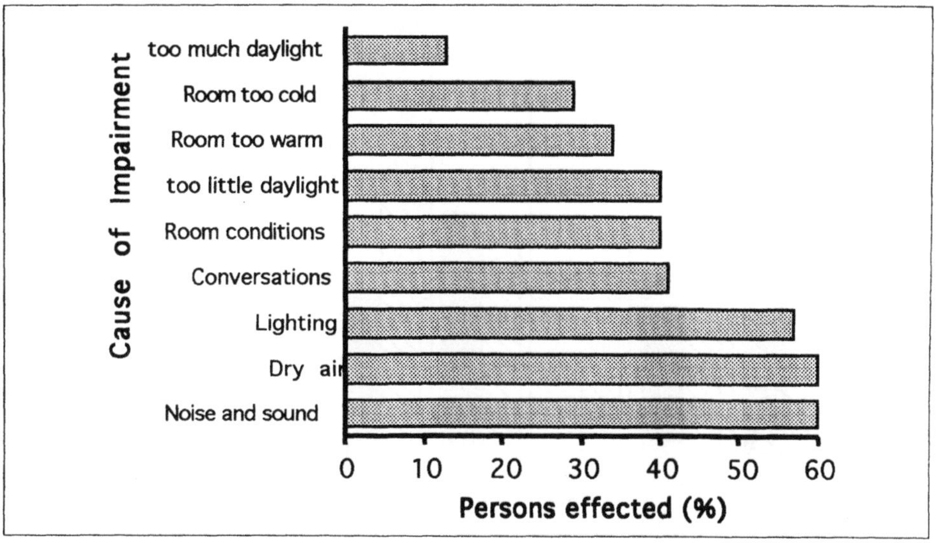

Fig.1 Causes of impairment related to work environment in German offices (multiple answers permitted)

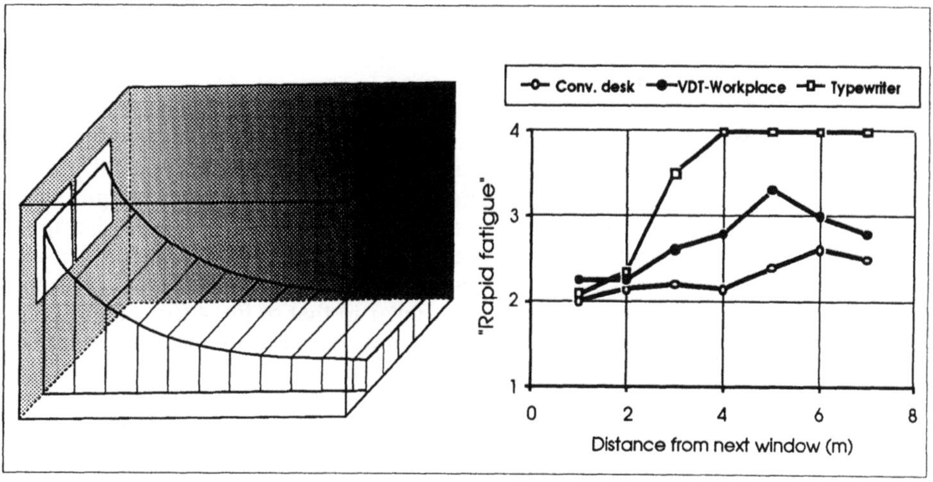

Fig. 2 Typical distribution of daylight in a work room (left) and general trend in health outcomes (right). Reported fatigue levels correspond to 1 = "no" and 4 = "strong".

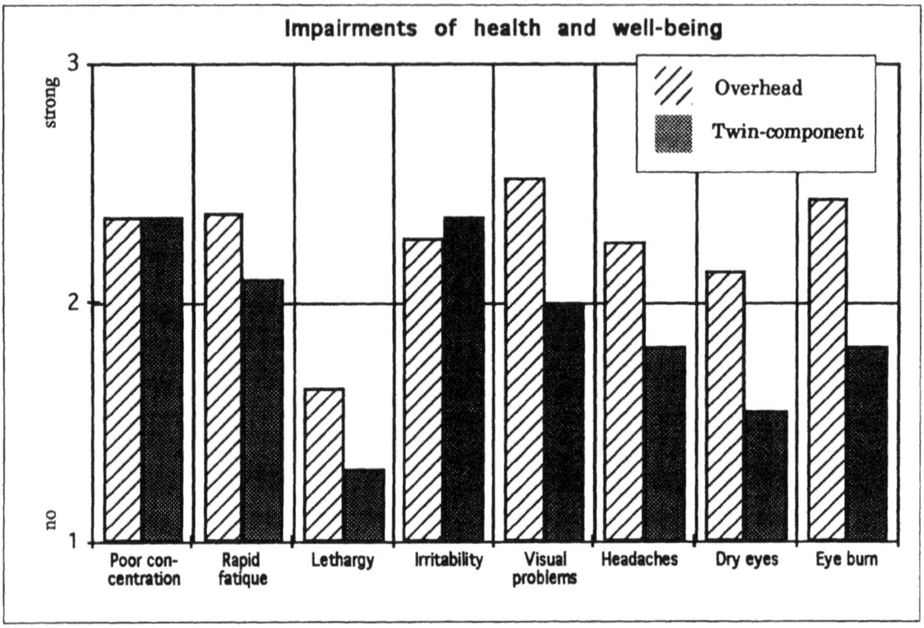

Fig. 3 Impairments of health and well-being under overhead lighting and twin-component lighting

out four months after the installation. The types of lighting have been selected to represent all possible light distributions, from "VDT-lighting" with 100 % direct to 100 % indirect and indirect plus direct task lighting. One result of this survey is displayed in fig. 4. In this figure, the "discomfort glare" caused by different types of lighting as assessed by 30 persons is shown, which is a good approximate to the overall impact of lighting on users. The statistics for the health effects could not be calculated in this case, as the number of the persons in different rooms and also their tasks were too different. However, the general tendency is similar to that of fig. 4 (fig. 5). Only the evaluation of indirect lighting may be worse than it should be due to the fact that in this survey all conditions in the test rooms were unfavorable for the assessment of lighting, e.g., visual tasks, quality of screens, room conditions.

This last survey showed, like the previous investigations, significant effects of the type of lighting on pleasantness, sensation of disturbance, reported health symptoms, etc.

3. DISCUSSION

It is not surprising, that lighting has an impact on workers as this seems to be a well-known fact. Human beings cannot live and work without light, thus, to show an influence of light on humans looks to be an easy task.

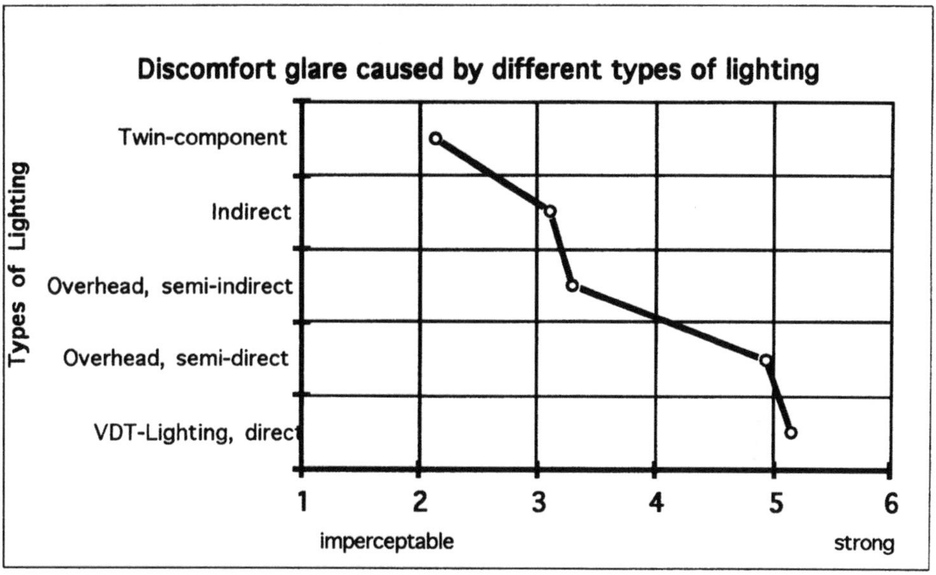

Fig. 4 Discomfort glare caused by different types of lighting in work areas where according to existing standards no glare was accepted

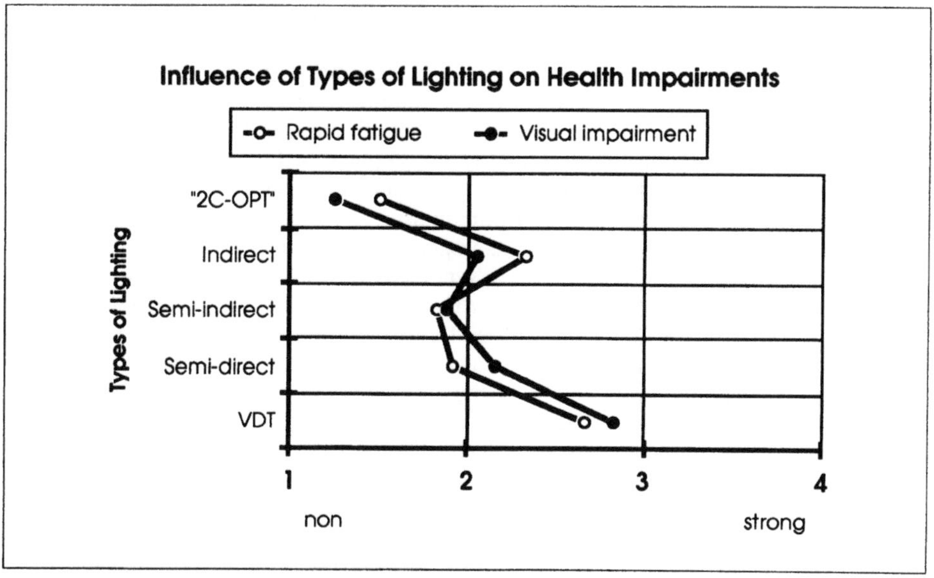

Fig.5 Health effects caused by different types of lighting (Note: The assessment of indirect lighting was effected by many negative factors of the specific test environment)

However, we did not expect that the five decades old belief, artificial lighting was an adequate means to replace daylight, would prove to be wrong. Since the invention of fluorescent lamps, architects and lighting engineers plan work environments like factories or open plan offices assuming that artificial light could fulfil all functions of natural light, many of them even believe that artificial lighting has superficial features. This study shows exactly the opposite. Wherever and whenever natural light is absent instead of being present where needed, workers tend to feel uncomfortable and "sick". Commonly, "fluorescent light" is blamed for such influences. According to our study, the real reason is the absence of daylight at the workplace.

Measured in physical quantities, e.g., uniformity of luminance or illuminance, natural lighting seem to be inferior to artificial lighting. One can never achieve the uniformity of physical quantities like "color temperature", "shadowiness" or "luminance distribution in the visual field" under natural lighting as it is possible under artificial lighting. But most physically measurable quantities do not describe the peoples' feelings about the subjects they should characterize.

Physical measurements and subjective assessments are in good agreement only for some factors like noise; "*conversations of colleagues*" have become a source of distraction where noise of equipment has disappeared. But in the case of dry air, for example, there is no agreement between measured values and subjective evaluation; the same level of relative humidity, e.g. 40 %, is felt to be "too dry" in air-conditioned rooms but well accepted in naturally ventilated work spaces. For lighting, most of the (engineering oriented) criteria believed to be "quality criteria" for lighting in general have only little significance for workers.

Office environments in Germany belong to working areas where the most elaborate and efficient standardization with respect to health and safety of workers has been effective in recent decades and years; e.g., lighting standards since 1935. Thus, it could not be expected that in such an environment physical factors like lighting or noise could have such significant effects, worst of all, the specific type of lighting developed to be an adequate solution for VDT-workplaces proving itself as an adverse factor on health and well-being. It seems to be the source rather than the solution of visual problems in modern office environments.

Windows seem to have a healthy effect in general, many reasons may be responsible for this. Various studies on sick building syndrome or on daylighting may give good answers to the question "Why?". Whatever the reason may be, the best solution to the "lighting problem" is natural light, and soft and glare-free indirect light, where and when it is not available or sufficient. Having an additional component to it, in form of a self-controlled task light has proven to be the most acceptable, and accepted solution.

The findings of our study are in very good agreement of some recent research conducted in the USA (3). A comparative "before and after" field survey which was designed to evaluate the performance of a parabolic downlighting system (similar to *VDT-lighting*) and an indirect lighting system yielded two main results that are in agreement with the outcome of our study: First, the downlighting system did not reduce the visual problems of computer users. Second, the indirect lighting system resolved glare problems better and gave significantly higher levels of visual comfort and environmental satisfaction. In addition, the survey results also suggest that productivity may be better supported by the indirect lighting system.

4. CONCLUSIONS

Two major conclusions may be drawn from the study:

First: Planning office space in future should aim at maximizing the impact of windows, including the influence of natural light.

Second: Lighting systems, planned for satisfactory environments, should have an indirect component as general lighting and a second component which is under control of the specific user.

As one important result we noted the deplorable circumstance that (lighting) technological concepts dominate those for office architecture and interior design; though this led to technological changes over a long period in which the current appearance of office interiors was defined, the value of these changes for the people at the workplace remains open to question. Lighting of office space represents only one of many goals of ergonomic design of office environments. Thus, lighting engineering should not try to dominate the activities of those who´s objectives are of higher importance.

This study has also shown that health disturbances caused by light are by no means impairments that have to be considered unavoidable due to a lack of alternatives. There exist at least two, possibly more, new lighting concepts which not only help to reduce or avoid such disturbances, but which can indeed also contribute positively to well-being.

Any new lighting concept should always include task lighting as one of its components. As has become clear in this study, even the mere availability of a desk lamp of unspecified quality is sufficient for creating a more favorable influence of artificial lighting. With the help of this second component, a quality of lighting can be obtained which could never be achieved by means of general lighting, no matter what quality. This also facilitates an individualization of lighting, which for a substantial proportion of the working population is not only a question of pleasantness, but rather an indispensable aspect of work safety and productivity.

In the future, conceptual faults in the conversion from theory into practice of the most important goals of lighting technology must be avoided. These goals are as follows:

- ***Based on its quality, lighting has an effect on the visual performance, the degree of activation, the work-safety, and the well-being of humans.***
- ***Consequently, lighting should be designed in a manner which accomplishes the respective tasks and which can be integrated harmoniously into the room.***
- ***Rather than measuring the value of lighting in quantitative (engineering) terms, lighting technology should be concerned primarily with respecting certain qualitative characteristics relevant from the perspective of users.***

5. REFERENCES

1 v. Zerssen, Die Befindlichkeitsskala (Bf-S), Klinische Selbstbeurteilungsskalen aus dem MPI. Beltz Test GmbH, Weinheim, 1975

2 Çakir, A., Light and Health, An investigation on state-of-the-art and future prospects of lighting technology in German office environments. ERGONOMIC, Berlin, 1991

3 Hedge, A., Lighting the computerized office. Cornell University, Ithaca, NY, 1989

WORK WITH DISPLAY UNITS 92
H. Luczak, A. Çakir and G. Çakir (Editors)

Personally-adjustable Daylighting for Display Screen Tasks in Private Office Workplaces

G. E. Sweitzer

Department of Architectural Lighting, The Royal Institute of Technology, S-100 44 Stockholm, Sweden

Abstract

Access to window view and daylight are given high priority by office occupants, including display screen (VDU) users [1]. VDU lighting standards which in effect limit window access thereby conflict with human welfare as well as electricity-saving potentials. This conflict, not surprisingly, involves a web of city, state, national, and international as well as corporate, industry, and political interests. The prevailing response to this dilemma is toward international standards, resulting in compromises. These compromises however dilute not only well-founded local interests, but also global differences in daylight availability and window exposure along with those among VDU equipment, tasks, and – most importantly – users [1,2]. As a result, VDU users are left with lighting standards that are inappropriate as well as unenforceable.

In order to better accommodate these differences, a radical alternative is proposed. This is to discount current VDU lighting standards concerning window access and instead delegate responsibility for visual comfort and elecricity use to office users. The potential for this is readily apparent in daylighted private office workplaces where single occupants hold responsibility for control of both day- and electric lighting. By integrating these controls, lighting can be moreover personally adjusted, for example, from specific task positions where lighting decisions can best be made. Although the hardware to achieve this is considered to be both technically and economically feasible [1], user education is proposed in addition in order to optimize its use.

1. REFERENCE OFFICE

The potential for this alternative approach is explored in the context of a hypothetical daylighted private office workplace that includes VDU tasks. Such offices, although increasingly preferred, are more narrow and smaller (ca 10 -

$12m^2$) in plan than their predecessors in order to optimize the number with window exposures. As a consequence, two limited functional as well as social zones emerge: 1) a semi-public interior zone to accommodate face-to-face meetings and conventional horizontal tasks and 2) a private work area near the window that includes a display screen in the direct or reflected field of view of a window (Figure 1), a worst-case according to current VDU lighting standards.

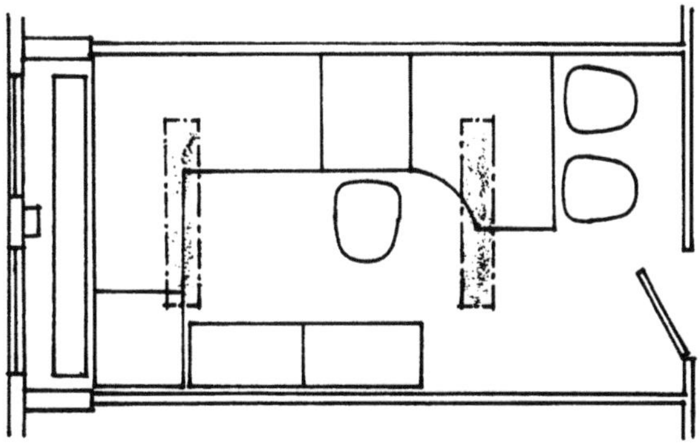

Figure 1. Reference office plan (suspended luminaires shown shaded)

2. LIGHTING CONTROLS

The lighting controls proposed for the reference office integrate both day- and electric lighting. The daylighting controls center on window access while those for electric lighting involve room and task lighting. Together these controls are intended to provide their users alternate means to achieve visual comfort while limiting electric lighting use.

2.1. Daylighting controls

The daylighting controls considered appropriate for this case simultaneously shade direct sun- and skylight from the VDU operator position while directing the same overhead toward interior ceiling and upper wall surfaces. Lower window view is thus preserved while balancing room and task surface luminances in both room zones. The window controls are categorized according to their location relative to the window glazing: exterior, integral, or inter-ior.

The exterior window shading controls can be fixed or operable. Although the shading elements are uniformly opaque or transparent, all include smooth edges in order to avoid projecting sharp shadows on interior surfaces; spaced elements or blinds are therefore not included (here or with integral or interior systems). The operable units meanwhile retract automatically in response to light or wind thresholds as well as (manually) to facilitate maintenance.

The integral window controls meanwhile are limited to insulating glazing surfaces and airspaces. Low-emmissivity surface coatings, for example, can provide increased visible transmittance for a given thermal transfer rate. In the near future, moreover, electrochromic glazings will be available that permit manual or automatic (graduated) shading of both visible and thermal transmission by window area.

The interior window controls include roller blinds and drapes made of translucent materials. These can provide for gradual luminance transitions in both the direct and reflected (display screen) fields of view. Excessive window coverage with any of these however may prompt unnecessary use of electric lighting when daylight is available.

Two or more of these window controls may also be effectively combined. Light shelves, for example, which may be located out- and/or inside of the window glazing, can effectively shade high angle sun- and skylight while directing same to the interior. Likewise, prismatic window panels in conjunction with configured ceiling elements can enhance this effect (Figure 2) [3]. Shading of the lower window for each case meanwhile can be provided by either roller blinds or (switchable) electrochromic glazing.

Figure 2. Reference office section - with prismatic panel system and configured ceiling

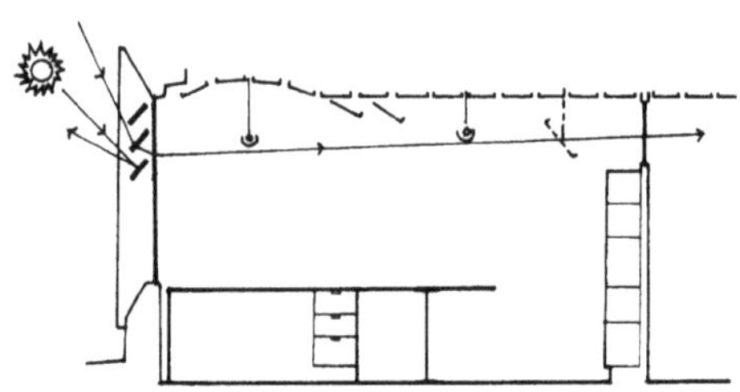

2.2. Electric lighting controls

Electric lighting controls can extend the use of admitted daylight and thereby limit electricity use in two ways. First, room as well as task (electric) lighting can be continuously dimmed in response to preset illuminance and/or luminance ratios [4]. Second, manual on/off lighting controls can be located where switching decisions can be best made from. It is therefore proposed that the suspended luminaires (room lighting) be individually switched from the door as well as from task positions while window controls and task lighting be switched and adjusted only from task positions.

3.0 LIGHTING CONTROL EDUCATION

In order to optimize use of the above described systems, user education is proposed. By empowering the users [5], the failures of previous attempts to introduce advanced or unfamiliar lighting technologies independently may be avoided; these resulted in system disuse, misuse, alteration [6], or even sabatoge. Two educational tools are discussed: individual checklists and breaks.

3.1. Checklists

One current checklist enables individual VDU users to evaluate their own work and workplaces, creating a 'risk profile', and to decide whether further action is necessary. In addition, it then provides them with arguments to improve certain aspects of their jobs [7]. It is proposed to add the above described daylighting control options to such arguments.

Another checklist, made available to white-collar union workers in Sweden, focuses specifically on VDU conditions [8]. Although the display screen measures include reflections, control of window access is not addressed. This addition could well contribute to the original intent of the checklist: to create a feedback loop to aid the development of improved VDU products.

3.2. Breaks

Intermittent breaks are recommended in order to sustain visual task performance despite remaining controversy about their type and frequency. A general conclusion is that VDU workers do not take breaks early enough, long enough, or frequent enough [9].

In order to remind VDU users when to take a break, a software program has been developed to act as an alarm clock. The parameters are individually defined and include the working periods as well as the length of the breaks. In addition, the program does not disturb the active application but freezes it. The user can therefore reactivate the application at any time [10].

As an option to such a program, it is proposed to input sensor-measured illuminance and/or luminance ratios as threshold parameters. Should lighting adjustments be needed, control options could be provided along with break notices. Lighting control could accordingly become integral with breaks.

4. CONCLUSIONS

It is concluded that personally-adjustable lighting controls can be used in daylighted office workplaces to provide user benefits in excess of those delimited by current VDU lighting standards. Improved visual comfort for VDU users can be provided by ready access to (lower) window view and daylight while shading direct sun- and skylight. Electric lighting use meanwhile can be reduced by a combination of selectively-located manual and automatic controls that facilitate response to available daylight. Each may be further optimized through the use of educational tools, for example, individual checklists and periodic breaks.

5. REFERENCES

1 Çakir, A, 1992, "An Investigation On State-of-the-art and Future Prospects of Lighting Technology in The German Office Environment", Presented at Work With Display Units '92, Berlin

2 Boyce, PR, Berman, SM, Collins, BL, Lewis, AL, & Rea, MS, 1989, Lighting and Human Performance: A Review, Lighting Research Institute, Lighting Equipment Division, National Electrical Manufacturers' Association, Washington, DC, and Lighting Research Institute, New York

3 Sweitzer, G, 1991, "Prismatic Daylighting Panel Systems: Daylighting Distribution and Electric Lighting Use Patterns in Perimeter Office Workplaces", Proceedings of the 1st European Conference on Energy-Efficient Lighting 99-108

4 Sweitzer, G, & Bailey, I, 1990, "Adjustable Task Lighting for Visual Display Unit Tasks in Office Workplaces", Work With Display Units '89 Conference Proceedings, Montréal, L Berlinguet & D Berthelette, eds, 81-88

5 Stock, L, 1990, "New Technology and Workers' Health: Strategies for Promoting Worker Involvement in Technological Change", Work With Display Units '89, L Berlinguet & D Berthelette, eds, Elsevier Science Publishers BV (North Holland) 511-516

6 Ne'eman, E, Sweitzer, G, & Vine, E, 1984,"Office Worker Response to Lighting and Daylighting Issues in Workspace Environments: A Pilot Survey", Energy and Buildings 6 (2) 159-171

7 Berndsen, MB, Andries, F, & Vaas, S, 1992, "A 'First-Aid Kit' for VDU Workers", Presented at Work With Display Units '92, Berlin

8 Screen Checker, 1986, TCO (White-collar Labor Organization), Sweden

9 Henning, RA, Alteras, SM, Jacques, P, Killel, Gv, & Sullivan, AB, 1992, "Frequent, Short Breaks During Computer Work: The Effects on Productivity and Well-being in a Field Study", Presented at Work With Display Units '92, Berlin

10 Molnar, M, Urban, E, & Scherzer, A, 1992, "PC-FIT User-Saver: Software for the Ergonomic Structuring of Work at Display Units", Presented at Work With Display Units '92, Berlin

WORK WITH DISPLAY UNITS 92
H. Luczak, A. Çakir and G. Çakir (Editors)

LUMINANCE PATTERNS IN VISUAL DISPLAY UNITS

Craig A. Bernecker, Philip A. Sanders, & Richard G. Mistrick

Department of Architectural Engineering, Penn State University, 104 Engineering Unit "A", University Park, PA 16802 U.S.A.

Abstract

Data for a numerical verification task performed on visual display units was collected for thirty-two subjects for two screen surface types, two screen polarities, four uniform background luminances ranging from 30 to 900 candelas per square meter, and four superimposed patch luminances ranging from a zero luminance patch to 1200 candelas per square meter. Results of the analysis clearly show a difference in performance with polarity, but no statistically significant change in performance across either background luminance or patch luminance. There also was no significant difference with screen surface type.

1. Introduction

Current standards for the lighting of visual display units (VDU's) vary significantly. For example, the standards in Germany, the United Kingdom and those promoted by the International Commission on Illumination are far more stingent than those of the United States - especially in terms of the magnitude of maximum allowable luminance, but also in terms of other criteria such as luminance ratios. These standards, at least in the United States, are based primarily on concensus, and in particular, lack a foundation in performance-based research.

Thus, the overall goal of this project was to begin to develop a scientific basis for recommendations for luminances reflected in visual display terminals. Previous work by the authors (Sanders and Bernecker, 1990) demonstrated that visual performance with VDU's changed as a function of both screen polarity and uniform luminances projected on the screen. The study was limited to a single, specular screen type, a very wide range of completely uniform luminances, and a letter search task with performance measured solely by error count. The present study maintains the variable of screen polarity, but extends this work to include both specular and diffuse screens, and uniform background luminances with a single, superimposed luminance patch which represent a more realistic range of background and luminaire luminances reflected in VDU's in actual environments. Further, a numerical verification task more consistent with typical visual performance studies conducted in the United States was used.

2. Current Experimental Work

As shown in Figure 1, a VDU was positioned facing a backlighted translucent panel designed with 800 ma fluorescent lamps spaced behind it in an attempt to achieve maximum uniformity across the panel face. Additionally, a slide projector was positioned behind the panel for rear-projection of patches of luminance. The uniform background luminance was controlled by dimming the fluorescent lamps, while the slide projector was fitted with neutral density filters to vary the luminance of the patch superimposed on this background luminance. Note that the patch image on the VDU screen was positioned over the shoulder of the subject, whose viewing distance was fixed by a headrest. The background luminance levels were 30, 75, 150, and 300 cd/m2, while the patch luminances superimposed on each of the background luminances provided an additional 0, 60, 300, and 1200 cd/m2, generating a total of sixteen luminance combinations.

Screen finish was changed by treating one of two identical specular monitors with a diffuse coating, while polarity was simply manipulated by the software created for the experiment. Performance data was collected for thirty-two subjects, with a group of eight subjects assigned to each background luminance while all other variables were varied. A numerical verification task, consisting of two lists of numbers requiring identification of errors in the right list when compared to the left, was used as the performance measure. Subjects compared ten number lists, each consisting of ten quasi-randomly-generated five-digit numbers, for each experimental condition.

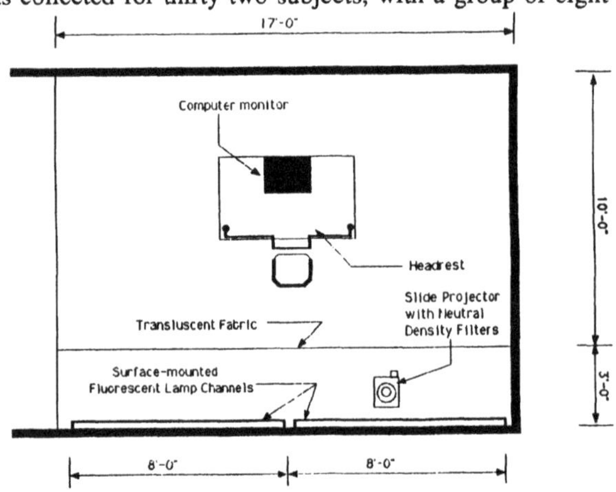

Figure 1. Plan View of Experimental Apparatus

3. Results

An analysis of variance was completed for the thirty-two subjects comparing the mean response time per line item among the subjects between viewing conditions. The factors in the analysis of variance for the background and patch luminance data included screen polarity, screen finish, background luminance, patch luminance, and patch location, that is whether the line item was located within the luminous patch or outside it. This factor was included because differences in performance would be manifested not only relative to the magnitude of the patch, but also between items within the luminous patch versus those outside the luminous patch on the screen. From this analysis, the only statistically significant difference between response times was due to the polarity of the screen. Polarity has an F ratio of 45.921 (df=1,28) which is clearly significant when compared to a critical F of 4.20 at a significance level of 0.05. There were no statistically significant differences due to background luminance (F=1.254, df=3,28) or patch luminance (F=1.863, df=3,84), nor due to screen finish (F=0.027, df=1,28) or patch location (F=1.681, df=1,28).

Figures 2 through 5 show representative plots of the mean response time plotted against patch luminance for each of the other factors included in the analysis of variance. Figure 2 shows the mean response times and confidence intervals per line item within the luminous patch for eight subjects (80 screen lists) plotted against both patch and background luminance for the specular finish screen with the bright background. The lack of effect of patch luminance on response time can readily be seen by the overlap of the confidence intervals on each graph. Although not as apparent for background luminance from the graphs, the omnibus test is indeed non-significant because each background luminance involved a different group of subjects and the variance across all subjects would be larger than represented by the confidence intervals shown here.

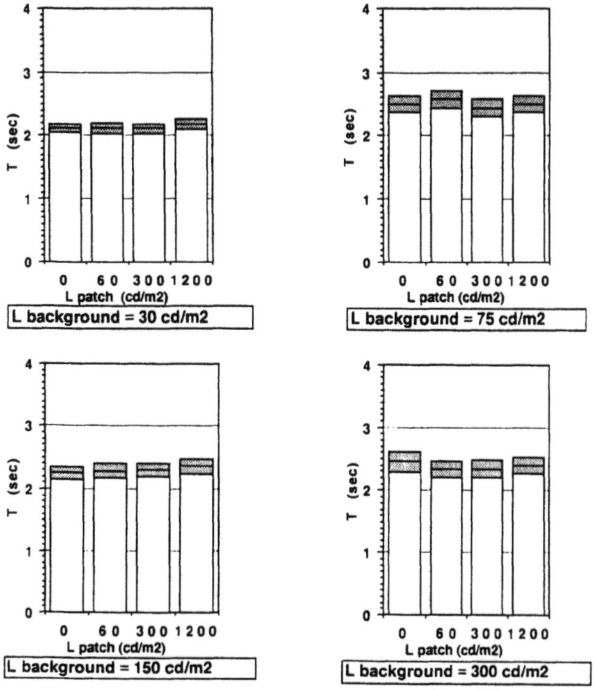

Figure 2. Performance As A Function of Patch and Background Luminance (Time Within Patch) Specular Screen With Bright Background

Figure 3 further substantiates the fact that patch luminance had little effect on performance. The data shown in these graphs compares mean response time within the patch versus mean response time outside the patch for the 150 cd/m^2 background luminance and specular finish screen condition for each of the dark and bright polarity conditions, respectively. If the luminous patch had affected performance, one would expect differences in response time between items within the patch as opposed to those outside the patch, along with any differences as the magnitude of the patch luminance varied. Figure 3 shows no such differences, supporting the results of Figure 2.

Figure 4 portrays the effect of screen finish on performance, in this case at a background luminance of 30 cd/m^2 for the dark background display. Again, as readily seen here and borne out by the statistical analysis, there is no difference in performance due to screen reflectance characteristic.

Figure 5 compares performance for the dark background display versus the bright background display, using the data for both specular and diffuse screens at the 75 cd/m^2 background luminance condition. As is evident here, there is a significant difference due to polarity, with response times greater for dark background screens. This suggests performance is better for VDU screens with dark letters on a bright background.

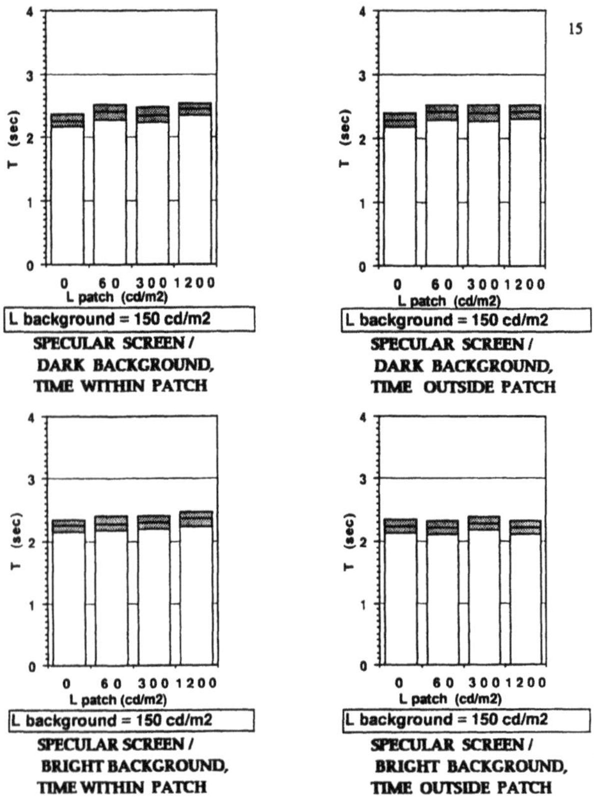

Figure 3. Performance Comparison for Time Within Luminance Patch vs. Outside Patch @ L_b = 150 cd/m2 Specular Screen

4. Discussion

In summary, numerical verification task performance, measured by response time, was collected for thirty-two subjects for two screen surface types, two screen polarities, four uniform background luminances ranging from 30 to 300 cd/m^2, and four superimposed patch luminances ranging from a zero luminance patch (i.e. uniform background luminance) to 1200 cd/m^2. Results of the analysis clearly show a difference in performance with polarity, but no statistically significant change in performance across either background luminance or patch luminance. There also is no significant difference with screen surface type.

The difference due to polarity, specifically better performance with bright background screens, supports the results of several previous studies (Adrian and Flemming, 1989). The lack of difference with either luminance variable suggests that visual performance with visual display units for typical office tasks is not greatly influenced by the luminances usually found in these environments, at least over the short term. It is not until more extreme luminances are present to sufficiently degrade task contrast, or perhaps when a more difficult or critical task is being performed that environmental luminances may pose a problem. This is consistent with prior studies of other office tasks where

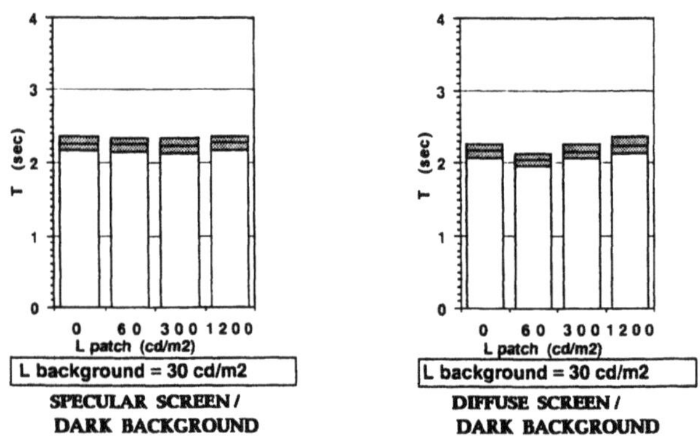

Figure 4. Performance Comparison for Specular vs. Diffuse Screens @ L_b = 30 cd/m2 Dark Background Display (Within Patch)

occcupants were able to perform over a wide range of veiling luminance conditions until they reached a sufficiently low contrast or luminance so as to significantly degrade performance.

Initially, this study suggests that the VDU environment is not as sensitive to lighting conditions as many believe. However, since this study used a short term task, it may also suggest that the effects of environmental luminances on sustained performance with VDU's are important, such as where these luminances may indirectly cause problems where sustained vigilance is required due to decreased contrast. This study also does not address those luminances occupants might prefer for VDU environments, even if changes in luminance do not directly affect performance. This may be especially important where one's preference for certain conditions may lead to enhanced performance and greater satisfaction with working conditions over the long-term, even though an evaluation of short-term performance directly related to the lighted environment would predict otherwise.

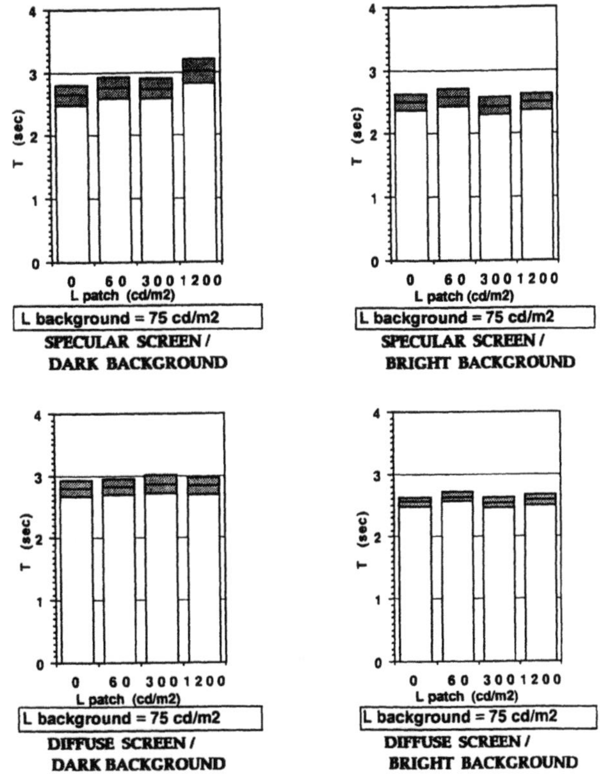

Figure 5. Performance Comparison for Dark vs. Bright Background @ L_b = 75 cd/m2 (Within Patch) All Screen Finishes and Displays

5. References

Adrian, W.K. and Fleming, M.L. (1989). Review of the literature on vision and visual display terminals (VDT) and lighting interactions. New York: Lighting Research Institute.

Sanders, P.A., and Bernecker, C.A. (1990). Uniform veiling luminance and display polarity affect VDU user performance. *Journal of the Illuminating Engineering Society*, 113-123.

PSYCHO-PHYSIOLOGICAL ASPECTS

WORK WITH DISPLAY UNITS 92
H. Luczak, A. Çakir and G. Çakir (Editors)

Precision of convergence of the eyes while viewing a visual display unit

Wolfgang Jaschinski-Kruza

Institut für Arbeitsphysiologie, Ardeystr. 67, D-4600 Dortmund 1, FR Germany

Binocular vision is optimal when a fixated target is imaged onto the center of the fovea in each eye, so that the principle visual directions of both eyes intersect at the fixation point. However, even subjects with normal binocular vision may have a slight deviation from this optimal state. In near-vision, the eyes of many subjects converge behind the fixation point (Fig. 1a). In other cases, they may converge in front of the fixation point (Fig. 1b). These small errors in convergence typically amount to a few minutes of arc and are called exo- and esophoric fixation disparity.

Fixation disparity can be measured psychophysically by presenting two test targets dichoptically, i.e., one to each eye, by means of polarizing filters. The horizontal position of the targets is variable. In case of fixation disparity the targets (shown as open bars in Fig. 1a and b) must have a physical offset in order to coincide with the principle visual directions (shown greatly exaggerated by the dashed lines in Fig. 1), to be imaged onto the center of the fovea and to be perceived in line. From this physical offset, fixation disparity can be calculated. If no fixation disparity is present, the targets must be aligned if they are to appear in line.

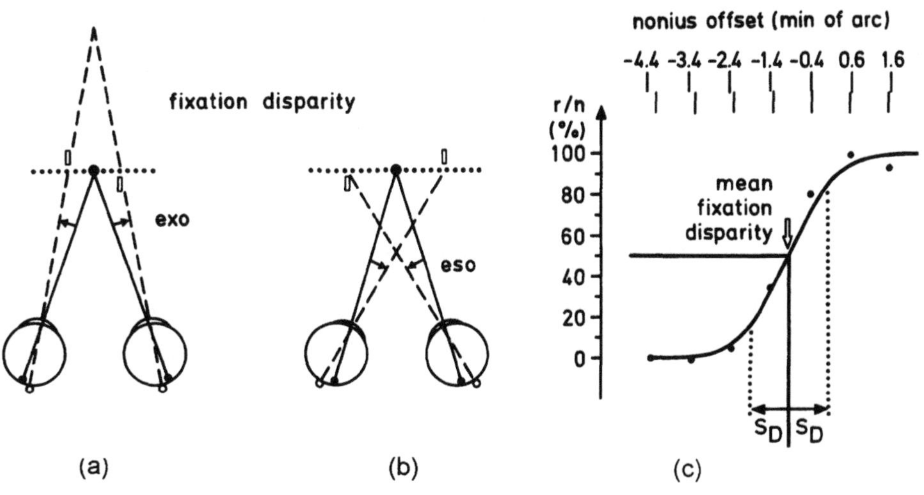

Figure 1. Nonius alignment principle (a and b) and psychometric function (c) for measuring fixation disparity (from [3]).

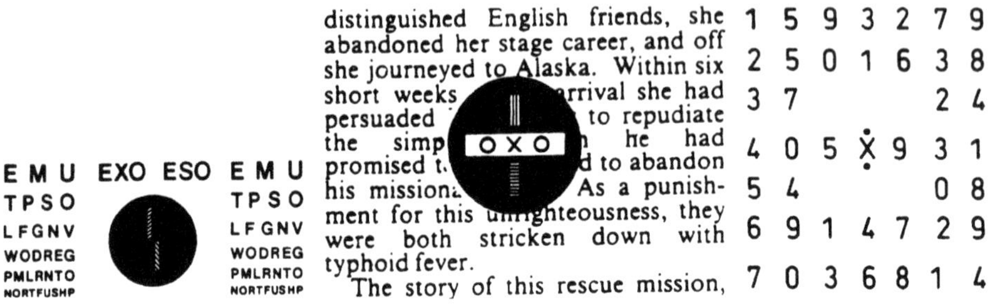

Figure 2: (a) Disparometer (b) Mallett-unit (c) Present test

The nonius alignment principle is used in some clinical tests (Fig. 2). The Disparometer [1] allows the observer to adjust two nonius bars to subjective alignment. Fusion is stimulated by the circular black-white contour; at the fixation point in the middle of the black area no fusion stimulus is presented. When fixation disparity is measured as a function of prism load in front of the eyes, the resulting fixation disparity curves can be useful in the diagnosis convergence problems [1].

In the Mallett-unit [2], the characters OXO are visible with both eyes thus stimulating fusion centrally. Using a modified Mallett-unit it was found that the mean fixation disparity was -1.1' $\pm$ 1.5' exo in subjects with near-vision symptoms and -0.4' $\pm$ 0.7' exo in subjects without symptoms; thus, the symptomatic group had a more exophoric fixation disparity. In other experimental studies [2], visual work induced transient exo-shifts: for example, after several hours of close work, after 30 min reading at low illumination, and after reading at 20 cm viewing distance. The mean effect ranged from 0.5' to 1.5'. After reading at a 40 cm viewing distance no shift was observed. These results refer to mean values in groups and not all subjects fit into this general pattern. Nevertheless, fixation disparity is considered to be a useful parameter for investigating visual fatigue [2].

However, all methods of measuring fixation disparity involve slightly abnormal circumstances which do not coincide with everyday vision [2]. If we think of VDU-work stations we see that the viewing conditions at a cathode ray tube (CRT) terminal are different from those at a test device like the Mallett-unit or the Disparometer. Consequently, it was the aim of the present research to measure fixation disparity in realistic viewing conditions using a visual display unit.

We therefore constructed a special test device [3], in which two dichoptic test targets (points of light made of LEDs) were optically presented above and below the center character "X" on a CRT screen in an array of characters that served as fusion stimulus (Fig. 2c). The nonius targets were presented as a series of short flashes of 100 ms duration. These flashes had different amounts of nonius offset, and after each flash the subject reported whether the upper point appeared to the right or to the left of the lower point.

Fig. 1c shows how frequently a subject reported that the upper target was to the right, as the amount and direction of the offset was varied. By probit analysis a sigmoidal psychometric function is obtained. The 50%-point corresponds to the offset at which the nonius targets were perceived to be vertically aligned and represents the mean fixation disparity. The slope of the function is a measure of the temporal fluctuation of fixation disparity. Stable fixation disparity will lead to a steep psychometric function. When the point of subjective coincidence fluctuates over time, the function will be more flat. Quantitatively, the probability that the instantaneous fixation disparity will be within ± one standard deviation is 68% [3].

RESULTS

1. A display was operated either with a dark background or a bright background at the viewing distance of 50 cm. Five measurements were made on different days, each with 30 nonius target presentations. Thus, each data point is based on 150 responses each for the bright and for the dark background condition. The two polarities produced very similar results. In a group of 16 subjects the correlation between the two display modes was 0.96 for the amount of fixation disparity and 0.86 for the standard deviation of the psychometric function. The group-mean fixation disparity for all observers was about -1.5' exo. The average standard deviation of the psychometric function was 2', which indicates that on average the fixation disparity fluctuated over time in a range of ± 2' with a probability of 68%.

2. The day-to-day variability was tested in 16 subjects. Measurements were made on two days with 180 nonius target flashes in each session. We found a significant test-retest-correlation of 0.9 for the position of fixation disparity. The test-retest correlation of the slope of the psychometric function was about 0.6 ($p < 0.01$). Thus not only fixation disparity but also its temporal fluctuations appear to be an individual characteristic. The correlation between the amount of fixation disparity and the slope (indicating variability) was lower ($r = 0.4$; $p < 0.10$). At least a tendency to smaller slope values (which means a more unstable convergence) was found in those subjects with a stronger exophoric fixation disparity.

3. Fixation disparity (FD) at a 50 cm viewing distance was correlated ($r = 0.52$, $p < 0.025$; $n = 18$) with the vergence state in darkness (DV), which is assumed to be the resting position of vergence [4, 5]. When FD and DV are measured in minarc and meter angle, respectively, the regression line was $FD = -3.0 + 2.1 \cdot DV$.

4. Viewing distances of 85, 47, 31 and 25 cm were compared [6]. The visual angle of the screen characters was 20' in all conditions. 10 subjects performed a search task at the VDU for 30 minutes and measurements were made five times during this period. Fixation disparity remained essentially constant during the half hour period. Fig. 3a shows fixation disparity as a function of viewing distance. Mean fixation disparity increased to stronger exophoria as the display was shifted closer to the eyes ($F(3/27) = 5.21$; $p = 0.005$).

A very similar pattern of results was found in measurements of accommodation which were made concurrently with a laser optometer. No change in accommodation was found during the test period. Fig. 3b shows the accommodative error, that is the lag of accommodation in diopters relative to the optimal accommodation to the actual viewing distance. It appears that the error in accommodation clearly increased when the viewing distance was shortened ($F(3/27) = 18.92$; $p < 0.0001$).

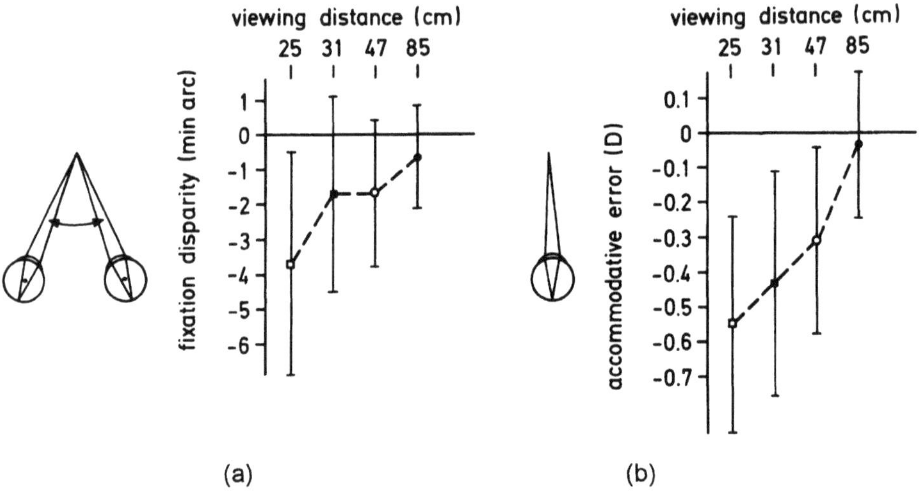

Figure 3. Fixation disparity and accommodation at different distances (from [6]).

Even at the intermediate viewing distance of 47 cm the average oculomotor state was less good than at 85 cm, although the subjects of this study were not presbyopic, and had good visual acuity and stereo vision. The data also showed strong individual differences: in some subjects accommodation or convergence did not change much with viewing distance; in other subjects, fixation disparity and/or accommodative error were clearly increased at shorter viewing distances. The latter subjects can improve their oculomotor state at workplaces by using longer viewing distances which, however, requires larger characters to be easily resolved and larger screens to display a sufficient amount of text [7].

CONCLUSION

The present study shows a technique that is able to measure reliably fixation disparity and its temporal variability while viewing a realistic pattern on a cathode ray tube. The experiments illustrate strong individual differences in different aspects of fixation disparity. No comparison with a hard copy was made. Thus, the present data offer no evidence for differences in oculomotor state when viewing a CRT screen as opposed to viewing a hard copy. These two display modes can differ in several aspects, including spatial resolution and flicker.

Nonius tests as in Fig. 2 measure the error of convergence relative to the principle visual directions which are usually assumed to correspond to the centers of the fovea. This assumption may fail even in normal binocular vision due to sensory anomalies [8]; in such cases the resulting fixation disparity is relative to a center of correspondence that is deviated from the center of the fovea. This adaptation of correspondence may occur in cases of heterophoria and resembles abnormal retinal correspondence in squint, but is different in that it is smaller and is not present in monocular fixation [9]. The Polatest apparatus and procedure [10-15] was designed as a clinical instrument to detect cases of disparate correspondence and to find prisms to compensate both for the motor and the sensory adaptation of heterophoria in order to reduce asthenopic complaints.

Future studies should address the most important question of to what extent fixation disparity is related to visual fatigue while working at a VDU.

REFERENCES

1 J.E. Sheedy and J.J. Saladin. Validity of diagnostic criteria and case analysis in binocular vision disorders. In: Vergence Eye Movements: Basic and Clinical Aspects (eds. C.M. Schor and K.J. Ciuffreda) Butterworths, Boston, USA (1983) 517-540.

2 D. Pickwell. Binocular Vision Anomalies-Investigation and Treatment. Butterworths, London, UK (1989).

3 W. Jaschinski-Kruza and E. Schubert-Alshuth. Variability of fixation disparity and accommodation when viewing a CRT visual display unit. Ophthal. Physiol. Opt. 12 (1992) 411-419.

4 D.A. Owens. Near work, accommodative tonus, and myopia. In: Refractive Anomalies (eds. T. Grosvenor and M. C. Flom). Butterworth-Heinemann, Boston, USA (1991) 318-344.

5 W. Jaschinski-Kruza. Eyestrain in VDU users: Viewing distance and the resting position of ocular muscles. Human Factors 33 (1991) 69-83.

6 W. Jaschinski-Kruza. Fixation disparity at different viewing distances of a visual display unit. Ophthal. Physiol. Opt. 13 (1993) 27-34.

7 M. Bonacker, E. Schubert-Alshuth and W. Jaschinski-Kruza. Ergonomic design of a high-quality VDU monitor with large characters and large screen for full-page mode. In: WWDU'92 Work with Display Units. Abstract book of the 3rd International Scientific Conference on Work with Display Units. Berlin (1992) P-5.

8 B. Wick. Stability of retinal correspondence in normal binocular vision. Optom. Vis. Sci. 68 (1991) 146-158.

9 D. Pickwell. Binocular vision: the Berlin outlook. The Optician 174 (1977) 8-35.

10 H.-J. Haase. Binokulare Korrektion. Willy Schrickel, Düsseldorf, Germany (1980).

11 H. Goersch. Fixationsdisparation erster und zweiter Art, Neues Optikerjournal 11 (1987).

12 D. Methling. Bestimmen von Sehhilfen, Enke Verlag, Stuttgart, Germany (1992).

13 I. Lie and A. Opheim. Long-term acceptance of prisms by heterophorics. J. Am. Optom. Assoc. 56 (1985) 272-278.

14 I. Lie and A. Opheim. Long-term stability of prism correction of heterophorics and heterotropics; a 5 years follow-up. J. Am. Optom. Assoc. 61 (1990) 491-498.

15 R. Brückner. The correction of heterophorias with fixation disparity. Optometrie 2 (1989) 27-42.

WORK WITH DISPLAY UNITS 92
H. Luczak, A. Çakir and G. Çakir (Editors)

Vertical gazing direction and eye movement analysis for a comfortable VDT workstation design

Susumu Saito[1], Midori Sotoyama[1], Toru Suzuki[2], Shin Saito[3] and Sasitorn Taptagaporn[4]

[1]Natl. Institute of Industrial Health, Japan [2]Univ. of Occ. and Env. Health, Japan
[3]Seibo Junior Coll., Japan [4]Min. of Public Health, Thailand

Abstract

Our previous field survey revealed an upward gaze in current VDT operation while other visual works caused downward gaze. According to this results, 2 experiments were conducted on vertical eye movement analysis for a recommendation to a comfortable VDT workstation design. Both experiments on dark vergence and heterophoria ascertained a downward gaze direction to be more comfortable for a visual work than an upward gaze direction. Less fusional effort obtained when working with downward gaze was discussed in the paper.

1. INTRODUCTION

Recently, vertical gazing position has become an interested topic for many researchers in visual ergonomics field. It was revealed to have a relationship with a resting state of the eye as reflected in dark focus and dark vergence. The both are the implication of occulomotor effort and can be useful for understanding and predicting visual fatigue [1]. Then the vertical gazing position may relate to visual fatigue. And since visual complaints are relatively high among VDT (Visual Display Terminal) operators compared to those in other traditional visual tasks, the field survey on vertical eye movements in various visual works was implemented to clarify this situation.

Figure 1 illustrates the results of our study that VDT operation causes upward gaze while other visual works cause downward gaze at work. The mean eye position of VDT operators was revealed to be about 7.5 deg. upward from Frankfurt plane (a line passing through the right tragion and the lowest point of the right orbit), while that of traditional visual workers was about 25 deg. downward

[2]. With upward gaze, eyelid was ascertained to move upwards in physiological synergic action with eyeball, and vice versa for downward gaze [3]. Subsequently, the exposed eyeball surface related to the vertical gazing position was examined to reveal one of the causes of visual strain and eye irritation at VDT work. During VDT operation with upward gaze, the exposed eyeball surface was found to be about twice greater than that with traditional visual tasks [4].

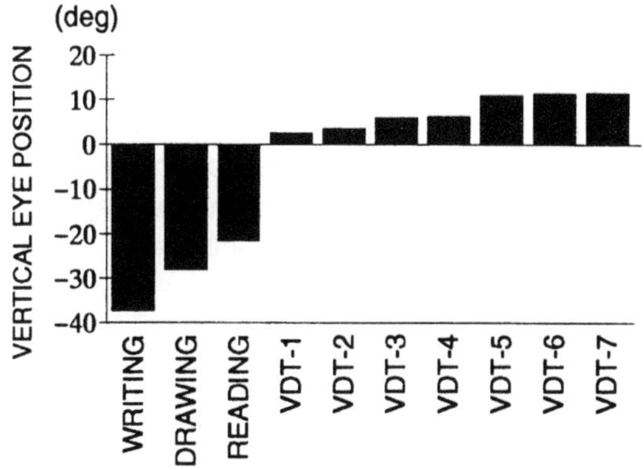

Figure: Difference of vertical eye position among various visual works

In order to give some recommendations to a comfortable VDT workstation design, the analyses of physiological and ophthalmological characteristics of the eye (dark vergence and heterophoria consecutively) related to the vertical gazing position were carried out in two experiments.

2. EXPERIMENT 1: DARK VERGENCE MEASUREMENT

2.1. Method

A TV-type eye camera (NAC-Eye Mark Recorder V) was used to measure dark vergence through binocular eye movement measurement. Fourteen emmetropic subjects (refractive correction included) with an average age of 24.9 yrs. and an age range from 22-31 yrs. were employed in this experiment. They were asked to fix their foreheads and chins at the supporters during the experiment in a darkened room. Firstly, the subjects were trained to incline their eyes upwards and downwards at various vertical eye levels within the limit of the measurement system (45 deg. in vertical direction) without visual stimuli. During the experiment, the subjects were instructed to move their eyes upwards and downwards several times for several levels in darkness. The data of both eye positions in horizontal and vertical planes were recorded in VTR as video signal and decoded into analogue voltage by a video image processor. Then the data were fed to a pen recorder via a DC-amplifier for further analysis. The dark vergence (cm) for each level of vertical eye position were obtained in the analysis.

2.2. Results

The data of each subject on vertical eye position and his/her calculated dark vergence were analyzed by a simple linear regression. A linear regression equation was gained for each subject, and the average of regression equations for all 14 subjects was found to be as followed:

$$Y = 0.63\,X + 46.34 \qquad (n = 14) \tag{1}$$

where X = vertical viewing angle (deg.); Y = dark vergence (cm)

Among all 14 subjects, 9 subjects showed a significant positive correlation between the vertical viewing position and the dark vergence with $r>0.5$ and $p<0.05$. The average regression equation for these 9 subjects became as followed:

$$Y = 1.04\,X + 51.25 \qquad (n = 9) \tag{2}$$

With upward gazing direction, dark vergence was found to shift farther while nearer shift occurred with downward gazing direction. In other words, there was an effect of vertical gazing direction on dark vergence system in 64.3 % of all subjects in this experiment (9 out of 14 subjects).The other 2 subjects showed negative correlation and other 3 subjects showed no relationship ($r<0.5$). The equation (2) can give an estimation of dark vergence (cm) at each vertical eye level for those who express this phenomenon. The dark vergence distance for 0 deg. horizontal eye level was estimated to be about 50 cm from both regression equations.

3. EXPERIMENT 2: HETEROPHORIA MEASUREMENT

3.1. Method

The amount of heterophoria related to vertical eye position was evaluated.

A TV-type eye camera (NAC Eye Mark Recorder V) was again used to measure heterophoria in this experiment. Six subjects without heterotropia (age ranged from 22 to 30 yrs.) were asked to put on the eye camera and to fix their heads and chins at appropriate supporters. The subjects with refractive error more than 1 D (diopter) had full correction during the experiment. The angle of heterophoria was measured by using the alternative cover test while the subject was viewing at each visual target. The visual targets were at 3 vertical gazing levels, namely 15 deg. upward, 0 deg. as a center (primary position), and 15 deg. downward, at the viewing distance of 50 cm. The horizontal eye movement (lateral or medial eye deviation) of the covered eye, which occurred due to heterophoria during the alternative cover test for each vertical gazing position, was detected by the eye camera and fed to a pen recorder for data analysis.

3.2 Results

All 6 subjects showed exophoria (lateral deviation of the covered eye) in the experiment. Table 1 shows the average angle of exophoria measured in 12 eyes with full correction at upward, center and downward gaze. The angle of exophoria at upward gazing direction was found significantly larger than that at the other two vertical gazing levels (by paired *t*-test with $p<0.1$).

Table 1. The amount of exophoria and vertical gazing direction

EXOPHORIA (deg.)	GAZE DIRECTION		
n = 12	15 deg. upward	0 deg. (center)	15 deg. downward
MEAN	3.31	2.71	2.65
S.D.	1.80	1.18	1.13

4. DISCUSSION

Experiment 1 provides the physiological evidence of the influence of vertical gazing direction on vergence system of the eye. The farther shift of dark vergence with upward gaze implies that more fusional effort in the vergence system is needed to fixate a near visual object than with downward gaze. Consequently, there is a higher possibility to get visual fatigue following prolonged near work in upward gazing direction. However, this phenomenon did not occur in all individuals, and the dark vergence distance measured among all subjects revealed a great individual difference. This result necessitates the individual dark vergence data for a recommendation to a comfortable VDT workstation design.

Experiment 2 gives a supportive ophthalmological evidence of greater amount of exophoria occurred in upward gaze than that in horizontal gaze and downward gaze among all subjects. The larger heterophoria with upward gaze implies the more fusional effort in eye movements demanded to keep a binocular vision. This result agrees with the result in experiment 1 that upward gaze probably causes more visual fatigue at work than downward gaze. The preference of vertical gazing direction was also ascertained to be a downward gaze at 23 ± 5 deg. downward from Reid's baseline (a line between the outer canthus and the center of the ear canal) [5].

5. CONCLUSION AND RECOMMENDATION

This paper gives some physiological and ophthalmological evidences of less visual fatigue when working with a downward gaze direction, i.e., nearer dark vergence distance and smaller angle of heterophoria. Visual effort can be reduced by lowering a display height to yield a downward gaze in VDT operation. For a comfortable VDT workstation, it is recommended in the study that the display height should be adjustable for each VDT operator to get a downward gaze, and the viewing distance should be about 50 cm.

6. REFERENCES

1 D. A. Owens, *WWDU'92* (Abstract Book) (1992) B-1.
2 S. Saito, S. Taptagaporn, Sh. Saito, M. Sotoyama and T. Suzuki, *WWDU'92* (Abstract Book) (1992) B-12-13.
3 S. Saito, H. Tada and S. Tsukahara, *Fukushima J. Med. Sci.*, 25, (1978), 101-107
4 M. Sotoyama, Sh. Saito, S. Taptagaporn, T. Suzuki and S. Saito, *Proceedings of the 8th Symposium on Human Interface*, (1992) 517-522.
5 T. Suzuki, S. Taptagaporn, M. Sotoyama, Sh. Saito and S. Saito, *WWDU'92* (Abstract Book) (1992) B-14-15.

WORK WITH DISPLAY UNITS 92
H. Luczak, A. Çakir and G. Çakir (Editors)

Visual work with different gaze inclinations

H. Heuer

Institut für Arbeitsphysiologie an der Universität Dortmund,
Ardeystr. 67, D-4600 Dortmund 1, Germany

Abstract

Subjects with different dark-vergence characteristics worked with a high and a low position of the VDU so that their vertical direction of gaze was about -5° and -35° below the horizontal. Although initially the setup was adjusted for an observation distance of 60 cm, subjects chose a smaller observation distance when the gaze was lower. There was no difference in rated visual and ocular complaints, but the majority of subjects preferred the low VDU position because of a more comfortable direction of gaze and the adjacency of screen and keyboard.

1. INTRODUCTION

One of the reasons for the exploration of different gaze inclinations in visual work is their influence on tonic vergence (or resting vergence). Tonic vergence, operationally defined as the angle of convergence in the dark (dark vergence), has been shown to decline (corresponding to a larger distance) when the gaze is raised and to increase (corresponding to a smaller distance) upon lowering of the gaze. When the head is tilted forward or backward the change of dark vergence is relatively small and uniform across subjects , but larger and different in different subjects when the eyes are raised and depressed [e.g. 1]. Thus with a lower gaze dark vergence corresponds to a smaller distance.

The observation distance in work with VDUs is typically in the range of about 50-80 cm, while the dark-vergence distance with horizontal gaze is mostly larger than 100 cm. Thus, a lower gaze serves to reduce vergence disrepancy, the difference between the angle of convergence during visual work and the dark-vergence angle. There is some evidence that the individual resting vergence and thus - for a constant observation distance - vergence discrepancy is related to rated visual fatigue [2, 3], but this relation has not been found consistently [4]. The present study has been designed to explore the hypothesis that a lower position of the VDU serves to reduce vergence discrepancy and visual fatigue; in addition other potential advantages and disadvantages of different heights of VDUs have been explored.

2. METHOD

The subjects were selected from a sample of 182 subjects - mainly students of the University of Bielefeld - who were screened for certain characteristics of their dark vergence. Dark vergence was measured by means of a subjective procedure that exploits the fact that dichoptic stimuli that are imaged on corresponding points of the two retinae appear in identical visual directions. Details of the apparatus and procedure have been described elsewhere [e.g. 5, 1]. Dark vergence was measured for different combinations of head tilt and eye inclination; the selection of subjects for the experiment proper was based on dark vergence with head tilt or eye depression of -5° and the effect of depressing the eyes by -30° with a forward head tilt of -5°. All subjects who participated in the screening session had normal visual acuity without correction.

The dark-vergence characteristics of the three groups of subjects who were actually selected are shown in Table 1: in group DL dark vergence was small, corresponding to a larger distance, while in group NL and S it was larger; in group DL and NL the effect of eye depression on dark vergence was large, while in group S it was essentially absent; the effect of head tilt was about the same in all three groups. Eight subjects in each group had experience with VDU work, while eight subjects used a VDU for the first time in their life (in group DL two inexperienced subjects were missing because they were hard to find).

Table 1
Dark vergence (in deg) with almost horizontal gaze and the effect of eye inlclination and forward head tilt (-30° in both cases)

head/eye inclination	group DL	NL	S
0 / -5°	1.49	4.64	4.17
-5° / 0	1.42	4.55	4.25
eye inclination	1.44	1.53	0.01
head tilt	0.64	0.84	0.46

After the screening session each subject participated in two sessions which were separated by one week plus/minus one day. The main task during these sessions was proofreading. During each half hour subjects worked on maximally 300 lines of popular scientific text that contained 150 randomly distributed single-letter errors that had to be corrected. The cursor keys were used to move through the text, and for the larger part of the time subjects worked on the bottom line of the sreen.

Visual work was performed with a low and a high position of the VDU. Gaze inclinations relative to the center of the screen were -5° and -35° below the horizontal. The screen was tilted backward by the same angle. Half of the subjects had the high position in the first session and the low position in the second one, while for the other half of the subjects the order was reversed. Initially the observation distance was adjusted to 60 cm. During visual work the head of the subject was unconstrained. By means of video equipment, head tilt and the position of the right eye relative to the initial setting were determined every five minutes during visual work.

Each session started with a warm-up period of 5 minutes that was followed by the first test period. The second test period followed after an additional hour of visual work and the third test period after another half hour. During all three test periods a questionnaire for the assessment of visual fatigue and postural complaints [4] was administered. The questions on visual fatigue were subdivided into "visual complaints" and "ocular complaints". The first were of a more general nature (e.g. "Viewing is difficult for me"), the latter were more specific (e.g. "I have burning eyes"). In the first two test sessions mental fatigue was assessed by means of a questionnaire (BMS II A, [6]) and the critical flicker frequency. In the second test period the subjects assessed some aspects of the conditions of work, and at the end of the last session they indicated their preference for the one or the other VDU position on a bipolar scale and indicated reasons for their preference.

3. RESULTS

The description of the results is limited to some major findings. Although no details of statistical tests are given, differences that are described are statistically significant. In general analysis of variance was used for the postural variables and non-parametric procedures for the questionnaire data.

Overall the direction of gaze relative to the horizontal was -4.2° and -30.5° with the high and low position, respectively. (These were the directions measured relative to the center of the screen; the actual gaze was a few degrees lower because subjects mostly worked on the bottom line of the screen). Of the 26.3° difference between the two conditions only 7.6° resulted from a difference in eye depression, but 18.8° from a difference in head tilt. In the course of visual work the gaze was slightly raised, and the difference in head tilt between conditions was somewhat reduced. Similar to the effect of sustained visual work on the difference between conditions in head tilt, the difference was larger in inexperienced subjects than in experienced ones.

The mean observation distances are shown in Figure 1. For the low VDU position a smaller observation distance was chosen than for the high VDU position. During the first two half-hour periods of visual work the observation distance increased in general; in the last half-hour period this trend continued only in group DL (subjects with a distant dark vergence), and it was limited to the high VDU position. The differences between groups are not reliable; the experienced subjects chose a larger observation distance than the inexperienced subjects (63.4 and 59.7 cm).

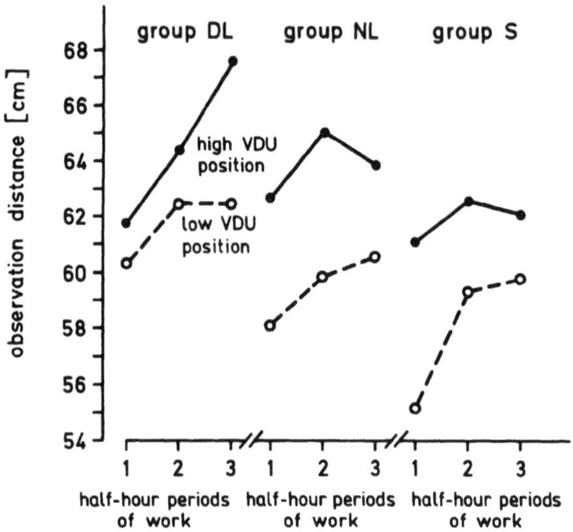

Figure 1. Mean observation distance in the three experimental groups with high and low VDU positions during three half-hour periods of work.

From the screening data on dark vergence and the average head and eye inclinations during visual work average dark vergence was estimated for each half-hour period of work; from the average observation distance and the interpupil distance of each subject the angle of convergence during visual work was estimated. Vergence-discrepancy, the difference of the two estimates, exhibited two major characteristics in addition to its reduction in the course of visual work: (1) in group DL it was larger overall than in groups NL and S because of the difference in dark vergence between groups, (2) in groups DL and NL it was smaller for the low VDU position than for the higher one, but not in group S, because of the difference between groups in the effect of eye depression on dark vergence. Thus, with the lower VDU position the increase of dark vergence as a consequence of a lower gaze was larger than the increase of the angle of convergence as a consequence of the smaller observation distance in groups DL and NL.

In Figure 2 the mean cumulated ratings of "visual complaints" and "ocular complaints" are shown. The ratings increase reliably in the course of work. However, the increase is not stronger in group DL than in group NL and S - this would have indicated a stronger visual fatigue that corresponds to the larger vergence discrepancy in group DL. In addition, the increase of the ratings is not stronger with the high than with the low VDU position - not even in groups DL and NL in which there is a reliable effect of VDU position on vergence discrepancy.

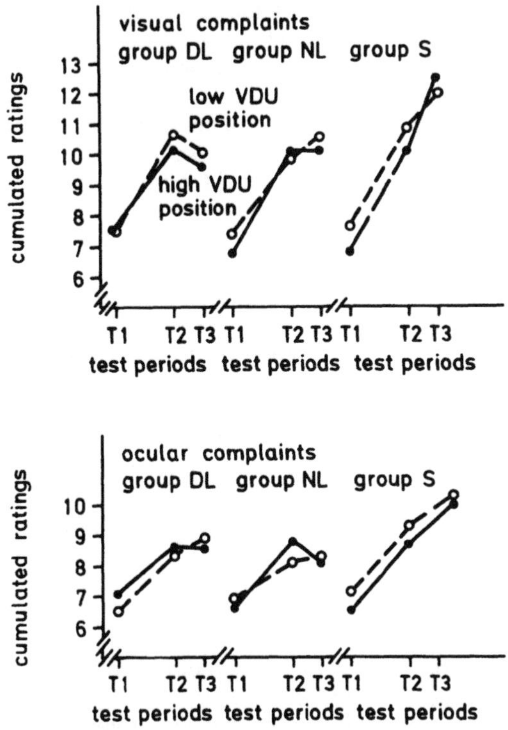

Figure 2. Mean ratings of "visual complaints" and "ocular complaints" in the three experimental groups with high and low VDU positions after 5 minutes (T1), one additional hour (T2) and an additional half hour (T3) of visual work.

Although the low position did not serve to reduce visual fatigue, it was preferred by 28 of the 46 subjects who had experienced both placements; 13 subjects only preferred the low position and 5 were indifferent. In group DL there was a certain balance of preferences; in both groups NL and S the overall preference was for the low VDU position. The reasons that the subjects gave for their choice of the low VDU position were mainly a more comfortable gaze and the adjacency of screen and keyboard.

4. DISCUSSION

The present results on visual fatigue with low and high VDU positions are in conflict with those of Tyrrell and Leibowitz [2, Exp. 2] who reported an advantage of the low VDU position. There may be several reasons for this discrepancy, among them the unnaturally small observations distance of 20 cm in the Tyrrell and Leibowitz study. In addition, to control the effect of different gaze inclinations per se, Tyrrell and Leibowitz used gaze directions of 20° above and below a resting position of about -5° (in the present study such control was implemented by the subjects of group S in whom gaze depression was accompanied only by a negligible change of dark vergence). The use of symmetric gaze inclinations implies that the increase of strain is identical for both directions of deviations from the resting position. This implication may not correspond to reality, and the difference in gaze direction per se may have caused the difference in eye strain instead of the accompanying difference in tonic vergence.

Although this study did not succeed in showing that lower VDU positions are advantageous in terms of visual fatigue, the results on preferences suggest the conclusion that a considerable proportion of VDU users prefer a low position of the VDU that is impossible with most existing furniture. Consistent with the known relation between observation distance and gaze ([7, 8], the subjects chose a smaller observation distance for the lower position of the VDU which could entance the readability of the text presented on the screen. Finally, from an oculomotor perspective there are clear advantages for the low VDU position as described by Suzuki et al., Takeda et al., and Saito et al. (all in this volume).

5. REFERENCES

[1] Heuer, H. & Owens, D.A. Vertical gaze direction and the resting posture of the eyes. Perception, 18, 363-377(1989)

[2] Tyrrell, R.A. & Leibowitz, H.W. The relation of vergence effort to reports of visual fatigue following prolonged near work. Human Factors, 32, 341-357 (1990)

[3] Jaschinski-Kruza, W. Eyestrain in VDU users: Viewing distance and the resting position of ocular muscles. Human Factors, 33, 69-83 (1991)

[4] Heuer, H., Hollendiek, G., Kröger, H. & Römer, T. Die Ruhelage der Augen und ihr Einfluß auf Beobachtungsabstand und visuelle Ermüdung bei Bildschirmarbeit. Zeitschrift für experimentelle und angewandte Psychologie, 36, 538-566 (1989)

[5] Heuer, H. Der Einfluß von Kopf- und Augenneigung auf die Ruhelage des Vergenzsystems. Zeitschrift für experimentelle und angewandte Psychologie, 35, 88-108 (1988)

[6] Plath, E. & Richter, P. Ermüdung - Monotonie - Sättigung -Stress. Berlin: Psychodiagnostisches Zentrum (1984)

[7] Hill, S.G. & Kroemer, K.H.E. Preferred declination of the line of sight. Human_Factors, 28, 127-134 (1986)

[8] Heuer, H., Brüwer, M., Römer, T., Kröger, H. & Knapp, H. Preferred vertical gaze direction and observation distance. Ergonomics, 36, 411-432 (1991)

WORK WITH DISPLAY UNITS 92
H. Luczak, A. Çakir and G. Çakir (Editors)

Psychological and Psychophysiological Effects of Working with Computers: Experimental Evidence

M. Trimmel[a], M. Brand[a], R. Chmelik[a], A. Ewald[b], K.A. Froeschl[c], R. Huber[a], R. Motschnig–Pitrik[c], and M. Haider[a]

[a] Institute of Environmental Hygiene, Department of Psychology, University of Vienna, Kinderspitalgasse 15, A–1095 Vienna, Austria

[b] General Hospital, Centre of Learning, University of Vienna, Währingergürtel 18–22, A–1090 Vienna, Austria

[c] Institute of Computer Science and Statistics, University of Vienna, Universitätsstraße 5, A–1010 Vienna, Austria

Abstract

In 4 experimental studies the impact of working with a computer on some psychological dimensions was investigated. Different groups of users (experts, users, beginners and non–users) were studied by comparing their behaviour, attitudes and performance between groups as well as their short term experimental after–effects.

Data showed group independent experimental after–effects on cognition, motivation, thinking, event–related cortical brain potentials, as well as group dependent after–effects on creativity, memory, and preference of man–to–man communication style. In addition, group differences were also found in the pre task condition for cognition, motivation, communication style, stability of eye preference, thinking, and creativity, indicating long lasting group differences.

Results showed that even man–computer–interaction lasting 30 to 45 minutes leads to after–effects on psychological as well as on psychophysiological dimensions, which are – in part – comparable to detected group differences. This indicates that working with computers leads to short as well as long lasting effects on human performance capabilities, mind and personality.

1. INTRODUCTION

The impact of working with computers on psychological dimensions of the user has often been stated [1,2,3,4,5], however, facts grounded in experimental studies are rare.

In the early 1980s Haider and co–workers [6] started investigations on the impact of working with display units on the visual system. In this time it became apparent that besides 'pure physiological' effects, working with computers is also accompanied by psychological effects. In the following, a group of Viennese researchers started experimental investigations on the impact computer work has on a number of psychological and psychophysiological dimensions. Some main results will be presented in this paper.

Although the data was collected from various experiments, there is a generality in the experimental procedure, which is based on a few hypotheses to be stated in the following. (1) Expected effects of working with computers may be related to the time span as well as the type of work (i.e. word–processing or programming) with computers. Besides immediately appearing well known effects [7,8,9] also (2) short term after–effects as well as (3) long term after–effects were expected. It was also a hypotheses that (4) short term after–effects would be detected by experimental effects, and (5) long term after–effects would be indicated if observed group–effects are similar to detected experimental effects (this also implies that there could be other long term after–effects which are not detected by this approach).

2. EXPERIMENT I

In experiment I the influence of cognitive load as well as paper/pencil vs. computer work on field dependency (a cognitive style), interference tendency (a memory characteristic) and verbal creativity were studied in comparing computer science students and non computer science students.

2.1 Method

2.1.1 Subjects design and task

80 subjects (Ss), 40 students of computer science and 40 students of other faculties took part in a 2 (Groups) x 2 (Low vs. High cognitive load) x 2 (Paper/Pencil vs. Computer work) ANOVA design. The 30–45 min lasting tasks were text editing in the low cognitive load conditions and intelligence items in the high cognitive load conditions, with the exception of the computer work condition of computer science students, who had to do simple programming.

2.1.2. Dependent variables

Field dependency is a characteristic of human information processing (cognitive style). It characterises to what extent someones cognitive processing (especially perception) is influenced by the actual environment (the context). Field dependency was tested with the Embedded Figure Test [10].

Interference tendency describes to what degree elements of memory are influencing each other. It was tested with an advanced German test after Stroop [11].

The dependent variables were evaluated before and after the task. In a pre experiment (with 24 Ss) it had been demonstrated, that the dependent measures were not influenced by the sequence of testing or a preceding pause.

2.2. Results

2.2.1. Field dependency

ANOVA showed statistically significant main effects for Group ($F=8.87$, $df=1$, $p<0.01$), for Pre vs. Post task values ($F=14.9$, $df=1$, $p<0.001$), and also for the experimental condition Paper/Pencil vs. Computer work ($F=4.59$, $df=1$, $p<0.05$).

Mean values for the main effect Paper/Pencil (P/P) vs. Computer tasks (COM) are given in figure 1 and mean values for non computer science students and computer science students in the Pre and Post task condition are given in figure 2.

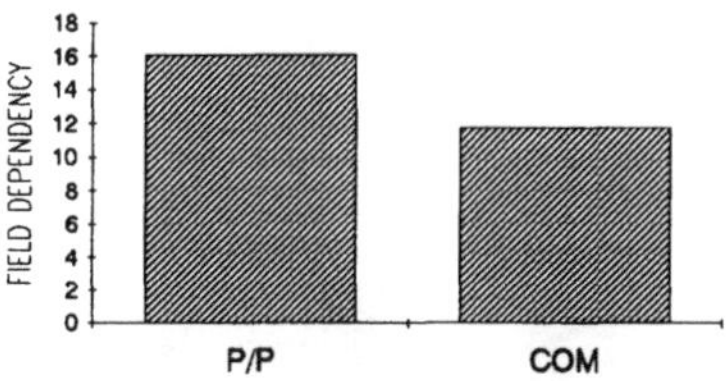

Figure 1.

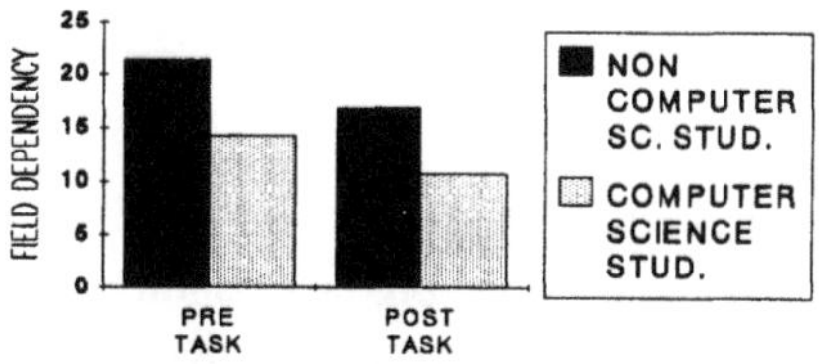

Figure 2.

2.2.2. Interference tendency

Analysis showed an enhanced interference tendency for the non computer science students after computer work (COM). Statistically significant differences ($p<0.05$) were found to pre task values of both groups, to the paper/pencil task in the same group, and to the computer science students after computer work (means are given in figure 3).

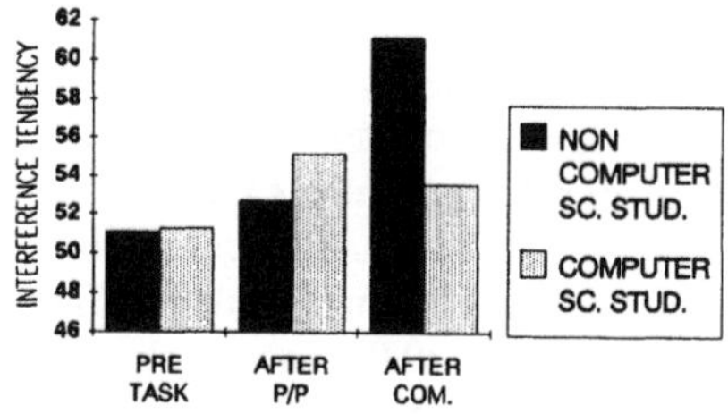

Figure 3.

2.3. Discussion

Results indicate that after a 30–45 min lasting computer task field dependency is more reduced than after a P/P task. Since in the computer science students group, field dependency is smaller than in the control group, it is also indicated that man–computer–interaction leads to short term as well as long term effects on field dependency. A reduced field dependency may be interpreted as a sign of environment–independent human information processing in the sense that motivation and cognitive performance are independent of the actual physical and social situation.

3. EXPERIMENT II

3.1. Method

3.1.1. Subjects, design and task

Subjects, design and task are the same as described in 2.1.1.

3.1.2. Dependent variables

Verbal creativity was tested with the subtest 'Namen erfinden' (find names) of the 'Verbaler Kreativitätstest' (verbal creativity test) [12].

Preferred communication style (verbal vs. non–verbal) was in the pre task condition tested by rating (in the range of 0 to 100) how they would like to explain 9 concepts (e.g. 'Hosenboden') either verbally or non–verbally. In the post task condition Ss had to rate again, but to explain the concept which was actually rated as the most neutral one in reality either verbally or non–verbally (pantomimically).

3.2. Results

3.2.1. Verbal creativity

Whereas in the pre task condition group values differ by statistical tendency (p=0.068) only, in the post task condition non computer science students showed a highly significant (p<0.001) better performance (task independent) in verbal creativity than computer science students (figure 4).

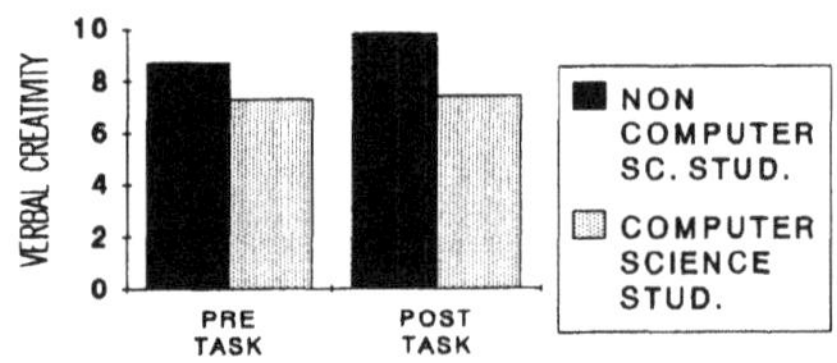

Figure 4. Means of verbal creativity.

3.2.2. Verbal/non–verbal communication preference

Pre task values showed that computer science students rated to prefer a verbal explanation compared to non computer science students. The (F=4.24, df=1, p<0.05) mean values are give in figure 5.

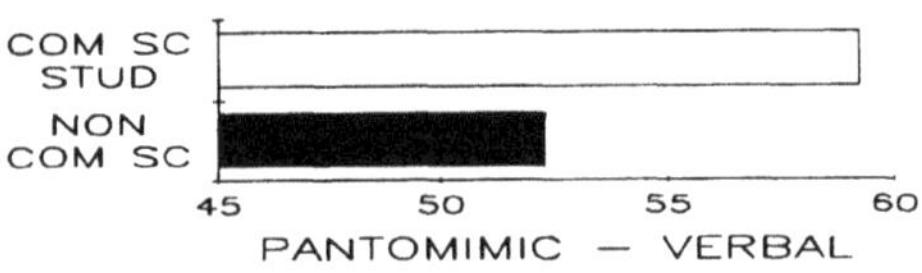

Figure 5. Rated communication preference.

The observed behaviour in the post task condition (for concepts which were immediately before rated as neutral to explain) showed that non computer science Ss preferred a non verbal explanation whereas computer science Ss preferred a verbal explanation (Chi^2=7.45, df=1, p<0.01; see figure 6).

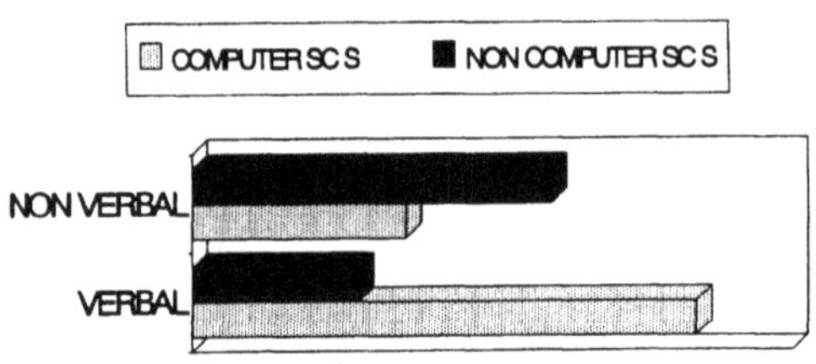

Figure 6. Observed communication.

3.3. Discussion

Results indicate that non computer science students generally have a better performance in verbal creativity than computer science students. This is remarkably pronounced after the task and is independent of the experimental condition.

Computer science students preferred a verbal explanation of concepts compared to non computer science students. Aside of this attitude, computer science students preferred for concepts which were immediately before rated as neutral to explain, a verbal explanation in a real life situation, whereas non computer science students preferred a pantomimic explanation. This results may be interpreted as a sign of a general preference of a verbal as opposed to a non verbal man–to–man–communication in computer science students compared to non computer science students.

4. EXPERIMENT III

4.1. Method

4.1.1. Subjects, design and task

85 Ss (mainly students) participated in a 2 x 2 ANOVA design with the factors Group (User, Programmer) and Condition (Paper/Pencil [P/P], Man–Computer–Interaction [MCI]). To compare pre task values of experimental groups with a control group, data was also collected from 24 computer Non–Users. Experimental tasks for the P/P condition were to describe a sorting algorithm and a description of a graphical presentation of the result. In the MCI condition only Programmers had to program the same task in MODULA and Users had to do their regular work (mainly statistical and word processing applications). The tasks lasted 45–60 min.

4.1.2. Dependent variable

The variable *Locus of Control* (LOC) [13], describes in how far someone attributes certain events either to his own responsibility or to someone or something else.

Pre task LOC (Internally, Externally [I/E]) was evaluated for Stable and Variable (S/V) attribution of Success and Failure (S/F) [14]. Post task LOC (Internally, Chance, Powerful Others) was evaluated for different aspects of life (Work, Social, Mind, Personal, Computer) by an inventory according to [15].

4.2. Results

For the pre task values out of 8 group comparisons (I/E x S/V x S/F) two significant group differences were found, namely for Internally Stable under Success (F=3.44, df=2, $p<0.05$), see figure 7, and for Internally Stable under Failure (F=3.30, df=2, $p<0.05$), see figure 8.

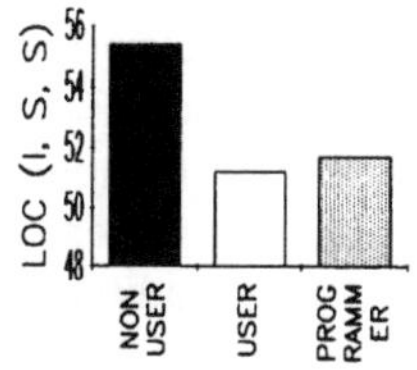

Figure 7.

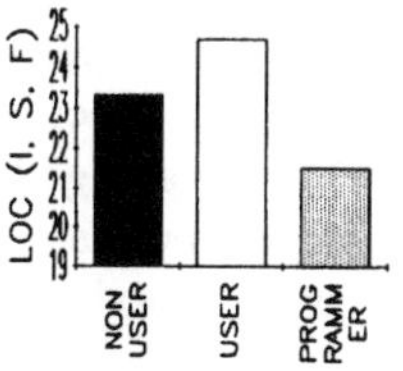

Figure 8.

Two way (Group x Condition) ANOVAs for post task values showed group differences in Internal LOC for Work (p=0.040), in Internal LOC for Computer (p=0.013), in Powerful Others LOC for Computer (p=0.0001) and in Chance LOC for Social (p=0.016), see figure 9.

Group independent experimental effects (P/P vs. MCI) were found for Mind in Intern LOC (p=0.028) and for the Social field in Chance (p=0.081), see figure 10.

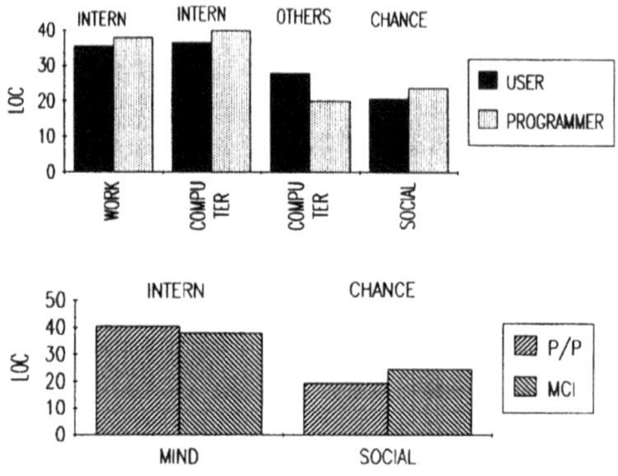

Figure 9 and 10.

4.3. Discussion

Group differences in pre task values indicate, that in general, computer non users feel more personally responsible for conditions which were successfully finished than computer users or programmers. However, for real life conditions (!) which lead to failure, computer users feel more responsible than programmers.

Post task data indicate that programmers – in contrast to users – feel themselves more responsible in the field of Work and Computer whereas in the social field they attribute causality more by chance than users.

Experimental condition effects (P/P vs. MCI) indicate that people feel more responsible for Mind (thinking) after a P/P task than after MCI, and for the field of Social life people attribute after MCI causality more by Chance than after P/P work.

Aside of a number of group differences, the data presented indicates, that MCI influences causality of thinking (a group independent after–effect) and also the perceived causality in social interaction (in the sense of uncontrollability) for which, besides group independent short after–effects, also a comparable group effect was detected.

5. EXPERIMENT IV

5.1. Method

5.1.1. Subjects, design and task

49 Ss (10 programmers, 11 experienced users, 13 beginners, 15 naive non computer users) had to perform 6 tasks each. Each of the 3 computer based tasks (C): text editing (TXT), playing Tetris (TET), computer manipulation (COM) (programmers had to program in Basic, the others had to execute an interactive DOS tutor program); and the 3 paper/pencil (P/P) tasks: text editing (TXT), answering a questionnaire on sensation seeking (QUE), solving an intelligence test (IQT) lasted 15 minutes. The sequence of tasks was balanced across Ss in each group. A 4 (Group) x 2 (P/P vs. COM) x 3 (type

of task: TXT/TXT, TET/QUE, COM/IQT) ANOVA design with repeated measures on the last two factors was used. After each task Ss had to do a 2 minutes lasting acoustical discrimination task, for which cortical information processing was recorded by the electroencephalogram (at F3, F4, Cz, P3, P4 referred to linked mastoids).

5.1.2 Dependent variables

Electrophysiological measures of cortical information processing by means of slow brain potentials [16].

Eye dominance was evaluated immediately after each task by fixing a point in a distance of 5 m trough a whole in a standard paper sheet.

5.2. Results

First results of electrophysiological measures of cortical information processing were presented [17] and showed a significant main effect of P/P vs. C on P300 amplitude. After the computer tasks the P300 amplitude was generally reduced compared to the P/P tasks. Latency of P300 was shortest and also strongly synchronised over the 5 recording locations after the COM task.

No significant effect was found for eye dominance, however, *stability of eye dominance* was different in the 4 groups ($Chi^2=9.19$, df=3, $p<0.05$; see figure 9). Whereas in the control group and in the group of beginners about 50% of Ss showed a variable eye dominance (that means that the same eye was not dominant the 6 times tested), none of the programmers tested showed a variable eye dominance.

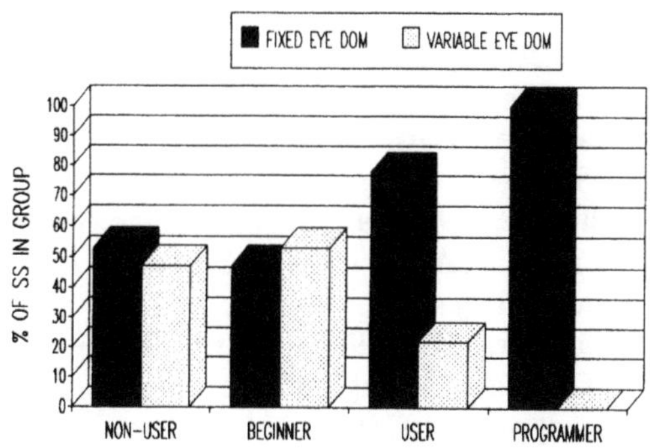

Figure 9. Stability of eye dominance in groups.

5.3. Discussion

Data of event-related cortical information processing showed that after-effects of MCI are different from after-effects of P/P tasks. Analyses indicate generally increased load of computer tasks compared to P/P task and a highly activated and widely synchronised cortical activity under conditions of direct computer manipulation (programming or in the case of beginners learning DOS interactively). This after-effects were found to be independent of the experience of the users (the tested groups) and may therefore reflect short term after-effects.

For stability of eye dominance it was found that programmers showed – in contrast to computer non users and beginners – no variability in eye dominance. This may indicate a rigid behaviour, or one may speculate that eye dominance is related to lateralized hemispheric processing. Under this hypothesis it would be indicated that hemispheric information processing is different in the four groups tested.

6. REFERENCES

1 Frese, M., Ulich, E. & Dzida, W. (Eds.) (1987). *Psychological Issues of Human-Computer Interaction at the Work Place*. Amsterdam: North-Holland.

2 Pflüger, J & Schurz, R.(1989). *Der maschinelle Charakter: Sozialpsychologische Aspekte des Umganges mit Computern*. Opladen: Westdeutscher Verlag.

3 Volpert, W. (1985). *Der Zauberlehrling*. Weinheim: Beltz.

4 Waern, Y. (1989). *Cognitive Aspects of Computer Supported Tasks*. New York: Wiley.

5 Weizenbaum, J. (1978). *Die Macht der Computer und die Ohnmacht der Vernunft*. Frankfurt: Suhrkamp.

6 Haider, M., Kundi, M. & Weißenböck, M. (1980). Worker strain related to VDUs with differently coloured characters. In E. Grandjean & E. Vigliani (Eds.) *Ergonomic Aspects of Visual Display Terminals*. London: Taylor.

7 Boucsein, W., Greif, S. & Wittekamp, J. (1984). Systemresponsezeiten als Belastungsfaktor bei Bildschirm-Dialogtätigkeiten. *Zeitschrift für Arbeitswissenschaft, 38*, 113-122.

8 Çakir, A., Hart, D.J. & Stewart, T.F.M. (1980). *Bildschirmarbeitsplätze*. Berlin: Springer-Verlag.

9 Ulich, E. (1991). *Arbeitspsychologie*. Weinheim: Beltz.

10 Wittkin, H.A. (1971). *The Embedded Figure Test*. Palo Alto: Consulting Psychologist Press.

11 Bäumler, G. (1984). *Farbe-Wort-Interferenztest (FWT) nach J. Stroop*. Göttingen: Verlag für Psychologie.

12 Schoppe, J. (1975). *Verbaler Kreativitätstest*. Göttingen: Hogrefe.

13 Rotter, J.B. (1966). Generalized Expectancies for Internal vs. External Control of Reinforcement. *Psychological Monographs: General and Applied, 80.*

14 Dorrmann, W. & Hirsch, R. (1983). *Manual zur Durchführung und Auswertung des IE-SV-F*. Bamberg: Universität Bamberg.

15 Krampen, G. (1981). *IPC-Fragebogen zu Kontrollüberzeugungen*. Göttingen: Hogrefe.

16 Trimmel, M. (1991). *Experimentelle und Angewandte Neuropsychophysiologie [Experimental and Applied Neuropsychophysiology]*. Berlin: Springer-Verlag.

17 Trimmel, M, Huber, R. & Haider, M. (1992). Mental workload after-effects of paper/pencil vs. computerised tasks indicated by P300. In *Abstracts of the Sixth International Congress of Psychophysiology (IOP)*. Berlin: Bundesanstalt für Arbeitsmedizin.

WORK WITH DISPLAY UNITS 92
H. Luczak, A. Çakir and G. Çakir (Editors)

Reduction of stress by the display of system operations in Human Computer Interaction

H. Holling

Lehrstuhl für Psychologie II, Universität Mannheim, Schloß, 6800 Mannheim, Germany

Abstract

After a short introduction a cognitive stress theory is briefly outlined to provide a theoretical background for the hypothesis that short-term psychophysiological and psychological stress reactions are reduced by the display of system operations in Human Computer Interaction. The results of an experiment support this assumption. Furthermore, type A individuals show higher stress reactions than type B persons.

1. Introduction

It is often shown that system response times (SRT) are a considerable source of stress in Human Computer Interaction. Especially with respect to longer system response times, the question arises whether this stress can be reduced by information about the state of the system during the SRT. There are several possibilities. For example during formatting a disk a system may give no information until the operation is finished or an error occurs. Another possibility is that the visual display unit shows the message "formatting", so that the user knows the system is working. In a further possibility, the computer indicates the amount of SRT elapsed. It may use a numerical format e. g. the display of the percentage of elapsed time or work already done. Often programs demonstrate this graphically by a bar, as the NORTON COMMANDER does when copying a file. Finally, especially if complex operations are performed, such as a compilation of a long source code, more detailed information may be given during the waiting time. This information may be the display of the lines just compiled within a special window.

2. Theoretical background

Does the display of informations cause less stress? Consider the two following situations: (1) formatting a disk and (2) the first compilation of a complex source code. There are several reasons why the display of the state of ongoing operations seems to be more helpful and stress reducing given the second situation. Firstly, when compiling, the subjective probability of an error is higher than during formatting a disk. Secondly, an error in the source code may lead to much more additional work, while an erroneous disk can be changed without great effort. Finally, if there is a program error the programer is more emotionally involved, especially if he attributes this error to his skill.

What can we learn from this example? Stress during SRT is given, if the user expects negative consequences during the system response time, such as additional work or a lower self-esteem due to an error. This statement is a generalization based on a specific example, but we can come to these conclusions by proceeding from cognitive stress theories, especially the stress theory by Lazarus briefly outlined now.

Stress is typically defined as a perceived substantial imbalance between demands and response capabilities, under conditions where failure to meet demands has important perceived consequences. Lazarus (1966) specifies the cognitive processes during stress situations. His main concept refers to cognitive appraisal, defining all those processes used by a person to judge components of a situation according to their relevance for his well-being. These cognitive appraisals include information processing, evaluation and judgement of a situation with respect to the relevance for the person. Lazarus distinguishes three kinds of primary appraisal: irrelevant, benign-positive and stress appraisal. If a situation has no implications for one's own well-being, it will be judged as irrelevant. This situation does not require a personal engagement. None of the personal values or needs are affected. A benign-positive cognitive appraisal will appear, if the outcome of the situation is favorable for a person's well-being. Positive emotions, such as joy and satisfaction are typical reactions. Finally, there is the actual stress appraisal, consisting of three components: challenge, threat and harm/loss. A situation is challenging if a potential profit can be expected. The accompanying feelings could be excitement or encouragement.

If a harm or loss is anticipated as a situational outcome for the person's well-being, an appraisal of the situation as a threat will result. The person involved expects a negative situational outcome and negative consequences of his/her actions and senses that his/her regulation mechanisms will fail. Nevertheless, the goal to cope with the situation and to leave nothing untried will still be pursued. In contrast to the experience of harm or loss, this appraisal of the situation as threatening will enable a person to anticipate coping strategies for the expected impairment. Thus, the experience of threat holds a preventive function. If the situation is ascertained as one leading to harm or loss, personal damage or impairment already occured. Given this situation, the person experiences severe impairment or helplessness.

Holling (1989) has formalized this theory with respect to system response times by means of probability theory. The subjective expected waiting time is specified as a random variable T, the negative consequences are called psychic costs and specified as a real valued measurable function C. Stress intensity (SI) is now defined as the conditional expectation of C, and stress (S) is the integrated stress intensity function. This is a continous measure of stress during the waiting time. Indicators are especially psychophysiological measures. In experiments and field studies, mean stress is often measured over a certain time period, for example by questonnaires.

This mean stress is defined as the expectation of stress. This formalized theory proved as a valuable theoretical basis for investigating stress in many empirical studies.

An important moderator variable, within stress research, is the distinction between type A and type B. Type A individuals are characterized by time urgency, impatience and competitiveness, relatively absent in type B behavior. Type A people tend to work faster than type B even when no time limits are imposed. Forced to slow their pace they feel unsatisfied. In terms of our formalized theory, type A individuals experienced higher costs during waiting times which lead to higher stress.

In most cases negative consequences for the user are reduced by displaying ongoing operations, because: (1) The user knows that the system is working and must not worry, otherwise he has the possibility to stop the program early. (2) The user knows what has already been done, or whether critical points are already passed. Thus, he can better predict possible failures. (3) The user can predict the end of waiting time better and plan the next input at the right time.

3. Hypotheses

We may derive two hypotheses from the above outlined theoretical framework.

Hypothesis 1: If a program displays information about the state of the system a user experiences less stress

Hypothesis 2: Type A individuals experience more stress than type B persons, if no informations about the state of the system are displayed.

4. Experimental design

In an experiment we tested the above hypotheses. 48 subjects from 19 to 33 years of age performed a simulated supervisory control task. They had to correct errors in seven files each consisting of 100 completed forms. Each file contained one or two errors. The subject performed these tasks using two versions of a software program (see figure 1 and 2). One version of the program (see figure 2) gave no information about the state of the task, while the other version always displayed the file and form just checked.

If the program discovered an error it stopped and the user had to correct this error. Figure 3 shows the screen display of the program version with messages about the state of the task if an error occured. The erroneous input here is the 'S' in the displayed line, only numbers were allowed as input. The user had to move the cursor to erroneous sign and type a '0' instead of the letter. In the case of the second program version, no information about the state of task was given during the display of the erroneous line.

Program: STENOX Prototype V2.1 (C) 1988 BeckSoft
Date: 01.09.1992
> Searching for errors. Please wait...   Working on FORM: 12 of 50
Working on FILE: 3 of 7

Figure 1: Screen display of the program version with information about the state of the task, if an error occurred.

Program: STENOX Prototype X.09 (C) 1988 BeckSoft
> Searching for errors. Please wait...

Figure 2: Screen display of the program version without information about the state of the task.

After receiving instructions about the task and performing several training trials, using both program versions, the subjects carried out two experimental trials. 24 randomly selected subjects used the program version with feedback about the state in the first trial and the other version in the second experimental trial, while the other subjects performed these two trials in the opposite order.

During the whole experiment heart rate and electrodermal activity were recorded. Further, anger, anxiety fatigue and activation were measured by a questionnaire after the training trials and after each experimental trial (see Holling, 1989) .

Type A behavior was measured by a German version of the Jenkins Activity Scale (Jenkins, Rosenman & Friedman, 1967). Subjects with values above the median were classified as type A otherwise as type B.

Program: STENOX Prototype V2.1 (C) 1988 BeckSoft
Date: 01.09.1992
> An error occured in the following line 4487113359241738945576845748385834595888473978432935927975 15
> Please move the cursor to the erroneous input by pressing the keys '←' and '→' . Rewrite the incorrect sign with a '0'.
Working on FILE: 3 of 7

Figure 3: Screen display of the program version with information about the state of the task

5. Results

With respect to the psychophysiological measures the mean interbeat interval (IBI) and mean skin conductance level (SCL) were computed for each experimental trial. These averaged values as well as the questionnaire measures represent measures of stress in the sense of our formalized theory. All indicators were scored in such a way that high values indicate high stress.

Table 1 contains the main results. Here we report the standardized differences between the stress measure of both experimental trials $(S_n - S_i) / S_d$, where S_n is the stress measure in the experimental trial without information, S_i the stress measure under the condition with information and S_d the standard deviation of the difference. By this standardization we get an effect measure comparable for all different stress indicators.

The first column of table 1 contains standardized differences between the two experimental trials for all subjects. The statistical significance was computed by t-test for paired samples. These results clearly support the first hypothesis. All stress measures indicate higher stress under the condition without information. The highest differences concerning SCL, anger and activation are signifacant at least at the 5 % - level.

Table 1
Standardized differences of stress measures between the two experimental trials

	All subjects	Type A	Type B
EDA (SCL)	0.61**	0.71**	0.53 **
Heart rate	0.17	0.29	0.05
Anger	0.42**	0.63**	0.22
Activation	0.36**	0.42	0.29
Fatigue	0.19	0.45*	0.05
Anxiety	0.26	0.27	0.26

*:p < 0.05 **: p < 0.01

The standardized differences and the significance computed by paired samples t-test for type A and type B individuals are presented in columns 2 and 3 of table 1. All standardized differences between the conditions without and with information are higher for type A individuals. Additional computed t-test for independent samples (type A vs. type B) yielded significant differences for the variables SCL, anger and fatigue. Thus, even our second hypothesis can be supported empirically by these results.

Summarizing our results we may conclude that computer programs, which display informations about the state of the system reduce the stress of the users. This reduction seems to be larger for type A individuals. Further studies are necessary to strengthen these assumptions.

6. References

Holling, H. (1989). Psychische Beanspruchung durch Wartezeiten bei computergestützten Tätigkeiten. Springer: Heidelberg.

Jenkins, C. D., Rosenman, R. H. & Friedman, M. D. (1967). Development of an objective psychological test for the determination of the coronary-prone behavior pattern in employed men. Journal of Chronic Diseases, 20, 371-379.

Lazarus, R. S. (1966). Psychological stress and the coping process. New York: McGraw-Hill.

WORK WITH DISPLAY UNITS 92
H. Luczak, A. Çakir and G. Çakir (Editors)

Psychophysiology in the Computer Workplace - Goals and Methods

Wolfram Boucsein

Physiological Psychology, University of Wuppertal, Germany

Abstract

A detailed analysis of stress-strain processes at computer workplaces is of major interest for engineers, work psychologists, and physicians. To overcome the current lack of common methodology and theory in this area, a psychophysiological research strategy is presented here. Psychophysiological recording methods are classified with respect to their specific validity for physical, mental, and emotional strain at computer workplaces. As a theoretical background, a neurophysiologicallly-based three arousal model is recommended, and a combined laboratory-field approach is advocated for this kind of research.

1. INTRODUCTION

As a consequence of the ongoing computerization of workplaces, stress resulting from mental challenges came into the focus of attention in stress-strain research. Until recently, *mental stress* during work with display units has been investigated mainly with respect to its impact on performance and subjective well-being. However, this approach is limited, since subjective stress recordings have the disadvantage of being susceptible to faking and require an interruption of work flow. On the other hand, performance measures that are both objective and continuously available can only be regarded as indirect measures of strain.

Physiological recordings have the advantage of being objective measures of strain that can be taken continuously during work. Unfortunately, stress-related physiological changes have been the domain of work medicine so far and were not yet integrated in theory and practice of psychological stress research at visual display units in the field.

Meanwhile, psychophysiological theory and methodology that combine *physiological* methods with *psychological* and *behavioral* approaches have become a standard in laboratory stress research. Applying such a three level approach to the investigation of stress-strain processes at visual display units will integrate the goals and methods of three otherwise separated scientific disciplines, i.e., work medicine, industrial psychology, and engineering. From this deliberate multidisciplinary analysis of stress at computer workplaces, rules for organization of work settings can be developed that will help to reduce physiological and subjective strain, and to avoid stress related performance decrements. As a consequence, psychophysiological stress research can be a useful tool for the identification and prevention of stress related disorders in work with visual display units.

2. PSYCHOPHYSIOLOGICAL RECORDING IN LABORATORY AND FIELD

Various bioelectrical and biochemical parameters have been used in laboratory studies. However, not all of these are easy to obtain at computer workplaces. Their use is limited by recording artifacts caused by body movements or electromagnetic fields, and the restricted number of recording channels in equipment for field studies at real workplaces.

Table 1. Psychophysiological parameters of different categories of strain. The variables are grouped according to their respective physiological systems. "+" means that the values of the parameter in question increase with increasing strain, and "–" that they decrease. More evidence is provided for double plus or minus than for single ones.

Dependent variable	Category of strain: physical	mental	emotional	additional specific indicator functions
EEG beta activity		++		waking state; attention
ERP amplitude		+		stimulus processing, +: vigilance
ERP latency				–: vigilance
Contingent negative variation (CNV)				expectation, response preparation
Heart rate (HR)	++	+	+	–: adaptation, +: effort +: tiredness
Heart rate variability (HRV)		– –	–	concentration, strain
.10 Hz component amplitude		++		
Additional HR		++		
Respiration frequency	+			
Finger pulse volume (FPV)		+	++	
Systolic blood pressure (SBP)	++			
Diastolic blood pressure (DBP)	+	+		
Spontaneous EDA			++	
Electrodermal response amplitude		+		expectation, response preparation
Electrodermal response recovery time		+		resource allocation
Eyeblink frequency	+	+	++	tiredness
Eye movements				level of practice
Pupillary dilatation		+	++	
Electromyogram (EMG)	+	++	+	muscular tension
Tremor	++			tiredness
Core temperature	++			circardian rhythm
Finger temperature			+	
Adrenaline (AD)		++	+	effort
Noradrenaline (NA)	++		+	muscular strain
Cortisol		+	++	
Free fatty acids			++	
Sodium/potassium ratio	+		–	

Since variations of working conditions in the field cannot be realized as controlled as in the laboratory, psychophysiological methods should be tested in simulated computer workplaces before being applied in the field. By such a combined *laboratory-field* approach, hypotheses from field observations can be tested under highly controlled laboratory conditions, and subsequent studies at real computer workplaces may be performed only with psychophysiological variables that have been shown to be relevant measures of strain at simulated computer workplaces. Hypotheses on which physiological variable to use as a marker variable for the specific kind of stress under investigation (e.g., mental stress in computer workplaces) can be gathered from the literature. Most researchers only distinguish between *physical* strain (resulting from muscular work) and mental strain (resulting from cognitive demands of the task). Following a proposal made by Klimmer and Rutenfranz (1983) mental strain should be further divided into *mental* and *emotional* strain (i.e., affective factors). Table 1 provides hypotheses concerning the specific validity of physiological measures, that have been derived from the literature (Luczak, 1987; Boucsein, 1989, 1991).

(1) Parameters of the *central nervous system*. Spontaneous changes in the electroencephalogram (EEG) such as an increasing dominance of the fast, low-amplitude beta waves are observed during mental load. They may also be used to indicate different states of wakefulness or attention. As a more refined measure of stimulus directed central processing capacity, vigilance, or response preparation, event related potentials (ERPs) and stimulus contingent negative variation (CNV) can be taken from the EEG by averaging procedures. However, these procedures require a highly controlled work situation with access to reactions following single stimuli. Furthermore, due to their artifact-proneness, EEG variables have not been much used in field studies.

(2) *Cardiovascular parameters*. One of the most frequently applied parameter in industrial psychology is heart rate (HR), since it figured out to be a robust measure in field studies. It is used as an indicator of physical as well as mental load, but it lacks specific validity. More refined analyses of cardiac activity may use variability measures (HRV) or the power of the .10 Hz component as indicators of mental strain. "Additional HR" can be calculated as the difference of the actual HR to a standard situation such as ergometer performance, and indicates cardiac activity that is not due to metabolic demands of the organism. The recording of respiration without wearing a mask (which may interfere with performance) is enabled by using a thermistor in the nostrils or a strain gauge around the chest. However, these devices do not provide more than mere respiration frequency, which is mainly used to determine the respiratory sinus arrhythmia (a HRV measure), and to control respiratory artifacts in various psychophysiological parameters. Finger pulse volume (FPV) is a very sensitive measure of defensiveness, and therefore mainly indicates emotional strain. Blood pressure (especially systolic BP) is frequently recorded as an indicator of physical strain.

(3) *Biosignals of the skin*. Among these biosignals, electrodermal activity (EDA) can be regarded as the most convenient measure for stress-strain research. Compared to skin humidity and skin temperature, electrodermal activity is easier to record and can be quantified in a more reliable manner. In the present author's laboratory, spontaneous phasic EDA figured out to be a valid indicator of emotional strain that appears during work with display units. Amplitude and recovery of electrodermal responses are valid indicators of certain aspects of information processing, and may therefore be used in a similar manner as ERPs as indicators of mental strain.

(4) Parameters of the *muscular system*. Eyeblink frequency mainly reflects emotional strain but increases also with other kinds of strain. Recording of pupillary dilatation that may be a more sensitive measure of emotional strain requires highly controlled illumination and body movement. Therefore, it is of restricted use in field studies. The electromyogram (EMG) can be used to evaluate the strain of certain muscle groups caused by physical work as well as to evaluate mental or even emotional strain. Especially, EMG may be used in computerized work to quantify specific kinds of strain such as neck muscle tension. Eye movements and muscle tremor are mainly used as specific indicators in this group of variables (see last column of Table 1).

(5) Body *temperature*. Core temperature is frequently used in addition to HR, especially in field studies on night- and shiftwork, since it displays marked circadian variations, and can be recorded easily. Work in accordance with the circadian rhythm is of higher quality so that shift schedules should allow a fast adaptation of the circadian rhythm to the working hours. However, temperature is not suitable for short-term changes. Finger temperature may be used as a slow-changing indicator of emotional strain.

(6) *Endocrine Parameters*. Since blood samples are hardly to obtain during work, an analysis of urine fractions is preferred. However, these cannot indicate effects of short-term stress. Adrenaline (AD) indicates long-lasting mental strain, while noradrenaline (NA) acts as an indicator of physical strain. In addition, corticoids and free fatty acids can be used as indicators of emotional strain at computer workplaces. Cortisol can be recorded with sufficient reliability from saliva probes now. Attempts are made now to use saliva potassium and sodium ions as indicators for different kinds of strain.

Physiological variables may be chosen according to their specific validity as outlined in Table 1. Refined analyses of mental and emotional strain at the computer workplace do not only require tonic measures like heart rate and core temperature, but also *phasic* parameters obtained from evoked responses, or measures that are derived from phasic changes like variability and frequency of these responses. This is necessary to cover both, the effects of long-term and short-term stress.

In addition to the physiological measures outlined in Table 1 subjective and behavioral measures are included in the psychophysiological approach as well. *Subjective* activation, well-being, ratings of bodily symptoms, and other stress related variables may be obtained discontinuously during working pauses, using rating scales of the LIKERT type. As *behavioral* stress indicators, various performance measures (e.g., speed, accuracy, and amount of work) can be continuously obtained from the task itself. In addition, behavior may be videotaped, including mimic and gross body movements. However, their deliberate analysis is time consuming and is therefore not often performed in stress research.

3. RESEARCH STRATEGY AND THEORETICAL BACKGROUND

Unfortunately, research in psychophysiology is often performed without sufficient theoretical background. Refined techniques for recording and data evaluation are available now, but results are frequently interpreted in rather simple theoretical frameworks like one-dimensional arousal concepts. The common theoretical concept of *arousal* refers to shifts in activation whatsoever (i.e., any stressor leads to changes into the same direction in all physiological systems). Beyond simple one-dimensional arousal concepts that still persist in various fields of work and industry research, the last two decades brought more refined multidimensional arousal concepts, which can be connected to brain transmitter systems (cf., Boucsein, 1992, Fig. 48). The advantage of these multidimensional concepts is that they better fit to reality (e.g., to explain why an increase in mental load can be associated with a decrease in HR but with an increase in EDA).

A comprehensive neurophysiologically-based brain model has been provided by Boucsein (1991) to explain the different physiological concomitants of strain at workplaces. The model shows relationships between arousal and *information processing* on the one hand and their dependence on emotional and motivational influences on the other hand. It refers to three arousal systems: arousal system 1 can be referred to as *general arousal* (e.g., level of wakefulness), system 2 as *emotional arousal* (e.g., affective reactions under time pressure) and system 3 as *preparatory* or goal-directed *arousal* (e.g., activation required to work on the task). Arousal systems 1 and 2 are primarily activated by noradrenergic pathways, while arousal system 3 is supported by dopaminergig pathways. The serotonergic pathways on the one hand inhibit general activation (e.g., induce sleep), and on the other hand strengthen the effort component of arousal system 1. This model provides a framework for generating refined hypotheses on the action of different arousal processes on psychophysiological variables. First results from the present author's laboratory are encouraging with respect to its validity for computer workplaces (Kuhmann, Boucsein, Schaefer, & Alexander, 1987).

In *summary*, to enhance the effectiveness of stress-strain research at computer workplaces, a psychophysiological approach is advocated here. As a first step, a deliberate analysis of strain at computer workplaces has to be performed by interdisciplinary cooperation of psychologists with medical and engineering scientists. Furthermore, selection of psychophysiological variables should be made using hypotheses on their specific validity. Refined analyses of mental and emotional strain require not only tonic measures like heart rate and core temperature, but also phasic parameters obtained from evoked responses, or measures that are derived from phasic changes like variability and frequency of these responses. Combined laboratory-field studies leading to an improvement in the design of computer workplaces are recommended as general research strategy. Finally, a neurophysiologically-based modelling of mental and emotional strain during computer work with respect to different arousal systems should be adopted as a common theoretical background.

4. REFERENCES

Boucsein, W. (1989). Psychophysiologische Meßmethoden. In S. Greif, H. Holling, & N. Nicholson (Eds.), *Arbeits- und Organisationpsychologie. Internationales Handbuch in Schlüsselbegriffen* (pp. 389-396). München: Psychologie Verlags Union.

Boucsein, W. (1991). Arbeitspsychologische Beanspruchungsforschung heute - eine Herausforderung an die Psychophysiologie. *Psychologische Rundschau, 42*, 129-144.

Boucsein, W. (1992). *Electrodermal Activity*. New York: Plenum Press.

Klimmer, F., & Rutenfranz, J. (1983). Folgen mentaler und emotionaler Belastung. In W. Rohmert, & J. Rutenfranz (Eds.), *Praktische Arbeitsphysiologie* (pp. 135-141). Stuttgart: Thieme.

Kuhmann, W., Boucsein, W., Schaefer, F., & Alexander, J. (1987). Experimental investigation of psychophysiological stress induced by different system response times in human-computer interaction. *Ergonomics, 30*, 933-943.

Luczak, H. (1987). Psychophysiologische Methoden zur Erfassung psychophysischer Beanspruchungszustände. In U. Kleinbeck, & J. Rutenfranz (Eds.), *Arbeitspsychologie. Enzyklopädie der Psychologie, Serie III. Wirtschafts-, Organisations- und Arbeitspsychologie* (Vol. 1, pp. 185-259). Göttingen: Hogrefe.

INPUT DEVICES
AND
WORKPLACE DESIGN

WORK WITH DISPLAY UNITS 92
H. Luczak, A. Çakir and G. Çakir (Editors)

Character size vs viewing distance on VDTs

P.T. Chang and S. Konz

Department of Industrial Engineering,Kansas State University,Manhattan,KS 66506, USA

Abstract

Two variables that influence visual stress are character height and viewing distance,often combined into one variable, visual angle. Our research,using 9*14 dot and 18*28 dot (double size) characters, shows that, for the same visual angle, larger characters are better. The data confirms (for standard size 9*14 characters) the American National Standard recommendation of 20-22 min of arc. The data also shows the sharp penalties (for standard size 9*14 characters) of characters less than 15 min of arc and the gradual penalties for over 30 min of arc.

1. INTRODUCTION

Viewing distance (in combination with character size) influences the load on the ocular muscles of accommodation and convergence. A closer distance and larger object give greater effort to the ciliary muscle. The force in the extraocular muscles for convergence is linearly related to the angle of rotation of the eyes (1). The closer the distance and larger the object, the greater the convergence strain. Yet if the characters are too small,this also causes strain. What is the best visual angle? And, is visual angle a sufficient description? That is, for specific visual angles, is there any additional effect of character size?

Chang(2) gives 80 references on visual characteristics of the VDT situation; this short paper will only refer to a few of them.

Character structure has an important role in the legibility of VDT displays. Three important variables are character formation, geometric elements of characters, and font design.

Characters can be generated using the dot-matrix method, the raster-written method or the stroke-written method. Most word processing displays use either dot-matrix or raster-written displays. Rasters have visible spacing in the vertical dimension and dot matrix have visible spacing in the vertical and horizontal dimensions. If this spacing is visible, legibility is reduced (3). The spacing is reduced by increasing the number of raster lines (scan lines). Typical scan lines are 525 in the USA and 600 in Europe. High resolution screens can have 729 or 1029 lines.

Size of the dot or line also is important (4),(5).

Geometric elements refer to character height and width,stroke width, inter-character spacing, and inter-line spacing. Evidence for the use of larger characters is given by Fagan et al(6) and Jachinski-Kruza(7).

The general rational for font selection is the ability to avoid confusion among characters.

2. METHOD

2.1 Character design for the experiment

Two different character sizes (9*14 dots and 18*28 dots) were created by the software called *DrHalo*. The fonts are raster-written rather than dot matrix. The 9*14 had 7 horizontal character dots + 1 left spacer dot + 1 right spacer dot (total of 9) and 9 vertical character dots + 2 top leading dots and 2 descender dots + 1 bottom leading dot (total 14). Because the 18*28 font has more dots to work with (especially for "curves" and "slants"), the 18*28 characters are closer to print characters than the 9*14. The font is similar to Times Roman. The height of the capital H was 3.7 mm for 9*14 and 7.4 mm for 18*28. The character width was 54% of character height, stroke width was 14% of character height, distance between characters was 16% of height and space between lines was 70% of height.

The negative display (light characters on a dark background) was monochromatic (amber). The screen had a 12 inch (30.5 cm) diagonal and 60 Hz refresh rate.

2.2 Viewing distance

VDT viewing distance recommendations range from 35 to 70 mm (8), (9), (7). Jachinski-Kruza (10) and Akbari and Konz (11) report that distances over 50 cm were better than 50 cm. Optimum was approximately 65 cm (with a range of 50-80 cm).

2.3 Visual angle

Character height and viewing distance can be combined into visual angle from the formula

$\theta = 3400\ h/d$

where θ = min of arc,h = object height and d = distance of eye to target. Recommended visual angles for VDT characters by Grandjean (12) are 16-25 min of arc and by the American National Standards (13) are over 16 with 20-22 preferred.

2.4 Experimental task

Both the 9*14 and 18*28 characters were viewed at 20,50,80,110,140 and 170 cm. Thus visual angles ranged from 7.4 to 62.9 min of arc for the 9*14 and from 14.8 to 126 for the 18*28.

A total of 12 passages were adopted from the magazine *Business Week* to be proofread by the subjects. Each passage had a total of 1250 words. Reading difficulty (mean of 11 with a range of 10.5 to 11.5) was determined from the Flesch formula GL = .4 (A +P) where GL = Grade level,years, A = Average words per sentence or independent clause, and P = Percent of words with 3 or more syllables. For P, omit (a) capitalized words (except the initial word in a sentence), (b) easy combinations such as screwdriver and guestworker and (c) verbs that reach 3 syllables with the addition of es or ed.

In each passage of 1250 words, there were 50 planned misspellings,with 4 different types, arranged randomly in different lines. There were 13 missing letters (teacher became techer), 12 wrong letter (simple became sjmple),12 reverse letters (higher became higehr) and 13 repeat letter (number became nummber). In all cases the incorrect spelling was designed to be obvious rather than a subtle error.

2.5 Subjects

The 12 engineering students were tested to demonstrate 6/6 vision. Mean age was 27 years (range 20-27). They received extra credit in a course.

2.6 Procedure

The environment was designed to minimize glare by using louvered (egg-crate) ceiling fixtures, an etched screen, and covering the subject chest and worksurfaces with black cloth.

There was a mean of 790 lux in the middle of the visual field

When a subject detected an error, he spoke it aloud and it was recorded on a form by the experimenter. This permitted calculating percent errors detected. In addition, reading time was recorded with a stopwatch. In addition, at the end of each passage the subject rated readability on a 1-9 scale with 1=very bad to 9=very good. For ease of understanding by the reader, this was converted to a 0-100 scale.

3. RESULTS

For each of the three criteria, a 3-way analysis of variance was performed with a least significant difference test.

For all three criteria (subject vote, error detection and time),size,distance and the size*distance interaction was significant. For size, large was better than small for all three criteria. For subject vote, 80,50 and 100 cm were better than 140,170 and 20 cm. For error detection and time, the groupings were more complex but 50 cm was best. Fig. 1,2, and 3 summarize the data. The curves were fitted with a least squares polynomial.

4. DISCUSSION

Fig. 1 shows subject vote vs visual angle. For the conventional size of 9*14, the curve maximum is 20-22 min of arc. If the data for the two sizes is combined, the curve maximum is at 33 min of arc.

Fig. 2 shows proofreading error performance vs visual angle. For the conventional size of 9*14, the curve is quite flat between 25 and 60 min of arc. If the data for the two sizes is combined, the curve maximum is at 38 min of arc--with little difference between 30 and 40 min of arc.

Fig. 3 shows proofreading time vs visual angle. For the conventional size of 9*14, the curve is flat between 15 and 60 min of arc. If the data for the two sizes is combined, the curve minimum is at 35 min of arc with little difference between 30 and 45 min of arc.

The first point to be made is that optimum viewing distance is not solely a function of visual angle. Even at the same visual angle, larger characters,even with the "same" font, are better (probably due to their better shape).

The second point is that, for the conventional character size of 9*14(3.7 mm high on a 30.5 cm diagonal screen), the data confirms the Grandjean (12) recommendations of 16-25 min of arc and the American National Standard (13) recommendations of 20-22 min of arc.

The third point is the severe penalties for small visual angles--especially below 15 min of arc. If designers are to err, it is better to err with large visual angles. Errors and time are not affected much by larger visual angles but subjective opinion begins dropping off (for conventional 9*14 characters) beyond 30 min of arc.

5. REFERENCES

1 Collins,C.,O'Meara,D., and Scott,A. Muscle tension during unrestrained human eye movements. *J. of Physiology* (London),**245**,351-369,1975.

2 Chang,P. Effects of character size vs viewing distance on VDTs. MS Thesis, Kansas State University,Manhattan,KS,USA,1991.

3 Snyder,H. and Maddox,M. Information transfer from computer generated dot matrix displays. *Technical Report HFL-78-3,* Virginia Polytechnic Institute, Virginia,USA,1978.
4 National Research Council, *Video Displays, Work and Vision*, National Academy Press, Washington,DC,1983.
5 Helander,M. Design of visual displays. Chapter 7 in *Handbook of Human Factors*, G. Salvendy (Ed.), Wiley,1987.
6 Fagan,J.,Westgate,T. and Yolton,R. Effects of video display character size, clarity and color in P-300 latency. *American J. of Optometry and Physiological Optics*, **63**,41-51,1986.
7 Jaschinski-Kruza,W. Visual strain during VDT work:the effect of viewing distance and dark focus. *Ergonomics*, **31**,10,1449-1465,1988.
8 Berns,T.(Ed.), *Die ergonomischen Prinzipien der Buroautomation* (Ericsson Information Systems,Bormma,Sweden),1984.
9 Helander,M. and Rupp,B. An overview of standards and guidelines for visual display terminals. *Applied Ergonomics*, **15**,185-195,1984.
10 Jaschinski-Kruza,W. On the preferred viewing distances to screen and document at VDU workplaces. *Ergonomics*, **33**,8,1055-1063,1990.
11 Akbari, M. and Konz, S. Viewing distance for VDT work. *Designing for Everyone*, Y. Queinnec and F. Daniellou,Eds.,Taylor and Francis, 1991.
12 Grandjean,E. *Ergonomics in Computerized Offices*, Taylor and Francis, 1987.
13 *American National Standard for Human Factors Engineering of Visual Display Terminal Workstations*, Santa Monica,CA:The Human Factors Society, ANSI/HFS 100,1988.

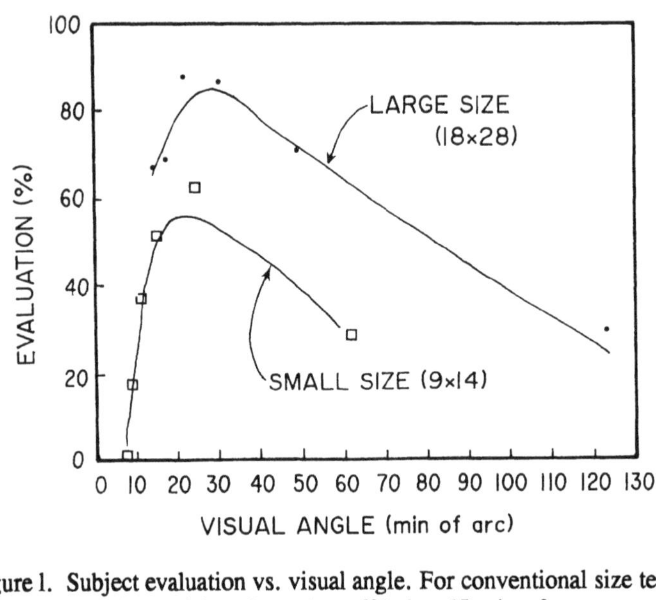

Figure 1. Subject evaluation vs. visual angle. For conventional size text (9*14) the optimum is 20-22 min of arc with a sharp dropoff below 15 min of arc.

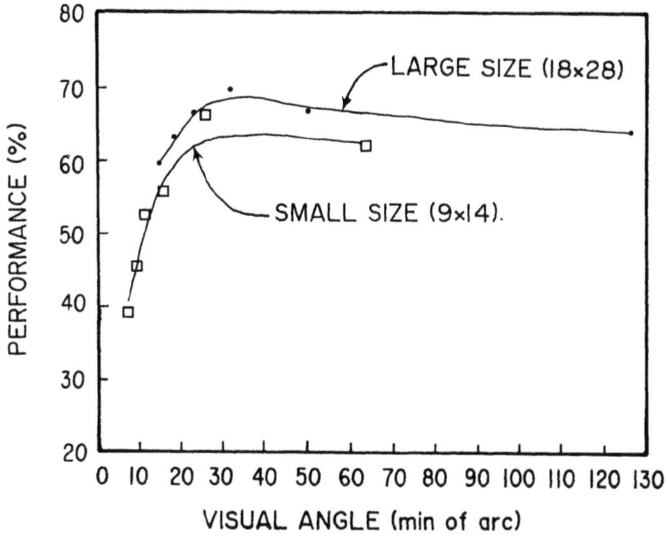

Figure 2. Error detection vs visual angle. For conventional size text (9*14),the curve is quite flat above 25 min of arc.

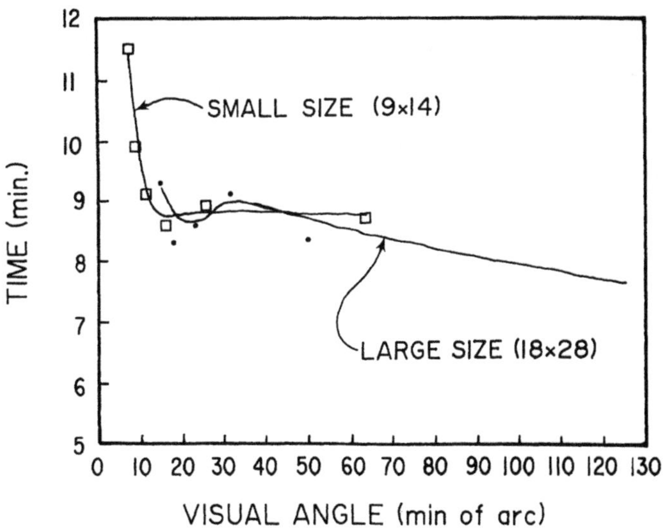

Figure 3. Reading time vs visual angle. For conventional size text (9*14), the curve is quite flat above 15 min of arc.

WORK WITH DISPLAY UNITS 92
H. Luczak, A. Çakir and G. Çakir (Editors)
1993 Elsevier Science Publishers B.V.

Legibility of Visual Display Terminals and an Investigation of Subjective Image Quality Ratings with Respect to Physical Image Quality Measures.

C. B. Edwards and V. J. Demczuk

Human Computer Interaction Laboratory
ERL, DSTOS P.O. Box 1500 Salisbury, South Australia 5108

Legibility of 4 visual display terminals was compared with subjective ratings, and a measure of heart rate variability. Legibility was measured in terms of the confusion that occurred when trying to identify characters in a group of 3 x 3 characters in the centre of each display screen. Displays were placed at different distances from subjects to standardise the character height. The subjects were 15 males aged between 20 and 45 years. Heart pulse intervals were recorded by a pocket sized data logger which measured and stored each pulse period. Photometric measures of the physical characteristics of each display were taken.

Results indicated there was correspondence between reaction time, error rates and subjective ratings of the displays. Error patterns were similar for all displays. There was an interaction between response category (same/different) and the memory and non memory components of this experiment. Each of these components appeared to affect more than one human information processing stage. Display type did not produce any significant effects on heart rate variability. There appeared to be some relationship between the test display session and spectral power but large individual differences swamped any significant effects.

The major objective of this research was to investigate user performance and subjective image quality on VDT's with respect to physical image quality. Modulation transfer Function Area (MTFA) values obtained did not appear to be related to subjective assessment. A Major influence on MTFA values appeared to be the distance between the subject and the display.

1. INTRODUCTION

The goal of this experiment was to investigate user performance and subjective image quality on VDT's with respect to physical image quality using 4 different displays. Display quality is difficult to define and involves a number of factors such as character size, luminance, contrast, resolution, and polarity which combine in some way to produce a display that may be rated as 'good' or 'bad' by subjects. Objective metrics are often related to human performance measures such as legibility which refers to the ease of identification of individual items eg letters and involves detecting and discriminating stimuli. The basic framework of the methodology for our experiment came from several sources. Gorrell (1979) had subjects read 4 x 3 arrays in 5 screen positions. He used alphanumeric characters and symbols taking note of the reading time for arrays, errors made and types of confusions that occurred. Lindgaard (1988) used 6 x 3 alphabetic arrays in 5 screen positions but asked subjects to read only the centre line of the array. She also included subjective ratings. In a study by McNeese and Katz (1987), 3 x 3 arrays of commonly confused alphanumerics were used in the 5 screen positions. These studies formed the basis of deciding to use commonly confused alphanumerics in a 3 x 3 array at the centre of each screen. In our experiment Four displays were used. A Zenith ZCM-1490 Flat VGA display driven by a video Seven VGA graphics adaptor card in a Compaq 386 computer. A Sony Video projector VPH 1030QM driven by a video Seven VGA Graphics adapter card in a Compaq 386 computer which gave a 9 x 14 font. A Private Eye virtual display made by Reflection Technology which is a head mounted display that uses a lens system to present a display and gave a 9 x 11 font. A Genius VHR-400 High resolution monitor by Micro Display Systems and gave a 9 x 14 font.

Displays were placed at different distances from subjects to standardise character height at 12 minutes of subtended visual angle. Brightness levels of the Genius and VGA monitors were set at 50cd/m2, and at 20cd/m2 for the projector. Room lighting was a compromise between normal lighting and dark conditions. The level used was 100 lux which gave a 2:1 contrast for the projector.

Heart pulse intervals were recorded by a pocket-sized data logger which measured and stored each pulse period. Heart rate variablility was calculated using the Rompelman method to determine the 10 second variability (Rompelman, 1982). It has been established that increasing mental load causes a decrease in heart rate variability. Mental load was altered in this experiment by employing 2 tasks, a memory task and a non memory task.

2. METHODOLOGY

Subjects were 15 males aged 20 to 45 years, taken from the staff of DSTOS. All were experienced computer users. Subjects were given an eye test, then fitted with a heart pulse logger and remained seated for 5 minutes in order to obtain a baseline heart rate. The experiment was explained briefly. Displays were presented in random order but the virtual display was never presented first. This was because the virtual display was an unfamiliar device and presenting this first may have had an adverse affect. Characters were presented in a 3x3 array in the centre of each screen. Character combinations were selected from those which produced the highest error rates in a previous experiment (Demczuk & Edwards, 1990). A total of 20 practice trials and 100 arrays were presented on each screen and subjects were instructed to be as fast and as accurate as possible. Subjects were asked to rate each display after each experimental trial. The experimental task was to determine whether all the characters in the array were the same or whether there was one character different in the array. Subjects indicated their response and then identified the characters used. There were two experimental conditions, a memory task which involved remembering the characters used and then identifying them, and a non memory task where the array remained on the screen while the subject identified the characters used. After the experimental trials a baseline heart rate reading was obtained. This concluded the experiment.

3. RESULTS

Objective measures were straightforward with all displays except for the Private Eye display. These results are presented in Table 1. Because of the lens system used to provide the virtual

Table 1.
Summary of the photometric measurements of displays

Display	Character height (mm)	Spot size (mm)	Reflected luminance (cd/m2)	Peak luminance (cd/m2)	Viewing Distance (m)	MTFA
Genius	2.17	0.20	0.3	50	0.62	105
Private Eye	11.7	1.3	0.9	16.5	0.5	3
VGA	4.86	0.45	0.2	50	1.3	186
Projector	30	5.2	10	20	6.5	11

image of the Private Eye, the measurements of spot size were of little value. Further work is required to determine a practical measurement procedure for this type of display. MTFA was calculated using the simplified ANSI algorithm (ANSI/HFS 100-1988). The values obtained do not appear to be related to the subjective assessment. A major influence on MTFA values appears to be the distance from the subject to the display. If the VGA display MTFA is calculated for the same distance as the Genius, then the MTFA value becomes 59, compared to 105 for the Genius. A simple measure like spot size (given minimum brightness and contrast), may be a better predictor of display rating than MTFA.

The pattern of errors was similar for all 4 displays and the projector produced the highest error rates. The 'same' response produced the lower error rates but there was only a small difference between the memory and non memory task for the 'different' responses. Each of the 'different' responses made by subjects were categorised into 'hard' consisting of characters such as 5,S and X,K or 'easy' consisting of characters such as 8,I and U,T. Research from other sources (Ostberg et al, 1989) has demonstrated that 'hard' versus 'easy' character discriminations for 'different' responses would be expected to affect the feature extraction human information processing stage, and the memory versus non memory condition would affect the identification human information processing stage. An analysis of variance was carried out and our results supported these findings. Figure 1. shows the reaction times for the 'different' and 'same' response for memory and non memory components of our experiment. The results indicated that subjects were adopting a different strategy when viewing the projector screen. This change in strategy did not show an increase in reaction time but did show an increase in the proportion of errors. The reaction times for

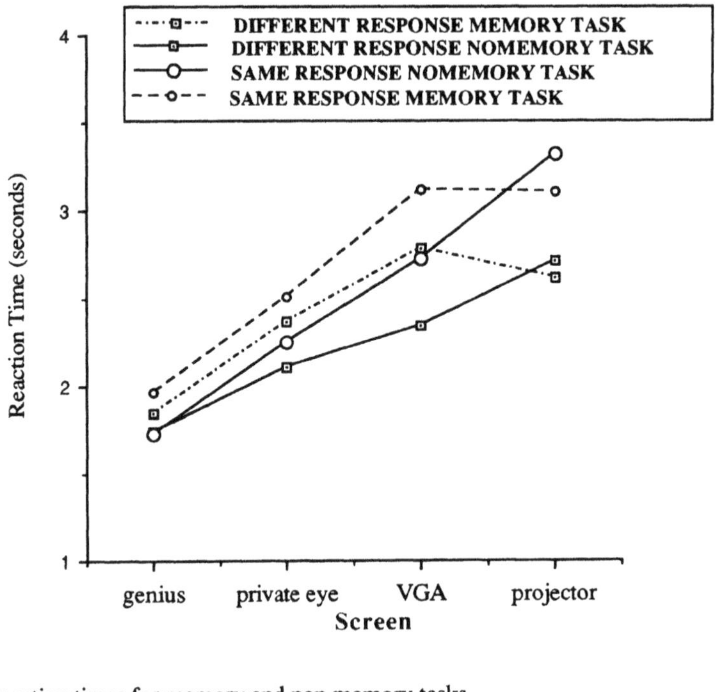

Figure 1. Reaction times for memory and non memory tasks

the memory task were shorter for the projector than the next worst screen, the VGA. Because of the apparent strategy change between the projector and the other 3 screens the projector was eliminated from further analysis. An analysis of variance was carried out and the difference between the 'hard'/'easy' discrimination and the memory component was not significant at the 5% probability level although it was approaching significance. This indicates that there may be an interaction between these components, and that each of these components may be affecting more than one human information processing stage.

The answers to the question "How easy was the display to read?" were rated on a 5 point scale are shown in Figure 2. Subjects rated the Genius as the easiest display to read followed by the Private Eye, the VGA and the projector. Using a t test, significant differences were found between all displays at the 5% probability level with the exception of the Genius display and the Private Eye. Subjects reported visual problems such as difficulty focusing were worst for the projector, then the Private Eye, and VGA with very few problems associated with the the Genius display. Some subjects reported difficulty using the Private Eye head mounted display, but these problems were related to subjects being unfamiliar with this type of device.

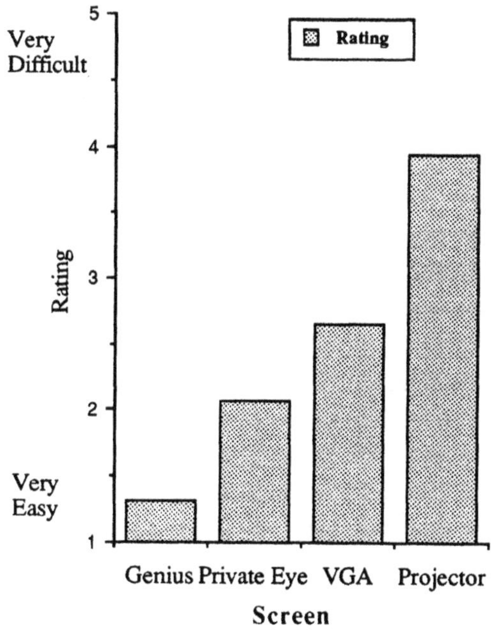

Figure 2. Subjective ratings of display type

No significant difference in heart rate variability was obtained between the rest periods and any of the display periods. Figure 3. shows the heart rate (left axis, upper curve) and 10 second spectral power (right axis, lower curve) profile for one subject. High mental effort is associated with suppression of the spectral power. The peaks correspond to the time each session ended (each test lasted approximately 10 minutes). This suggests that some relationship exists between the test display session and spectral power, but that large individual differences swamped any significant effects.

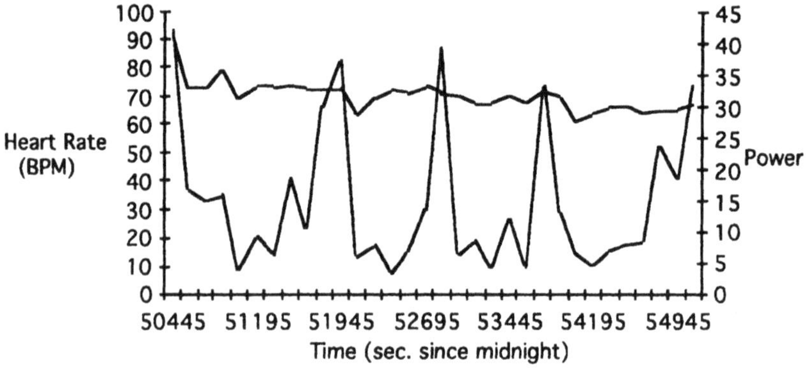

Figure 3. Heart rate in beats per minute and 10 second spectral power

4. CONCLUSIONS

There was good correspondence between reaction time, error rates and subjective rating of the displays. The Private Eye virtual display requires specialized techniques for accurate measurement of spot and character size. The MTFA ratings as calculated by the simplified ANSI method did not appear to correlate with the subjective rating of the displays. Display types do not produce any significant effects on heart rate variability on a recognition task with the methodology used in this experiment.

5. REFERENCES

1. ANSI/HFS 100-1988, American National Standard for Human Factors Engineering of Visual Display Terminal Workstations.
2. Demczuk ,V., Edwards C., Legibility of Visual Display Terminals, Proceedings of the 26th Annual Conference of the Ergonomics Society of Australia (1990).
3. Gorrell, E.L., A Human Engineering Specification for Legibility of Alphanumeric Symbology on Video Monitor Displays, DCIEM, Canada, Tech Report79X01 (1979).
4. Lindgaard, G., Testing for Legibility of Characters on a Screen, Telecom Australia, Branch Paper 152 (1988).
5. Ostberg, O., Shahnavaz, H., Stenberg, R., Legibility Testing of Visual Display Screens, Behaviour and Information Technology, 8(2), 145-153 (1989).
6. Rompelman, O., The Measurement of Heart Rate Variability Spectra with the Help of a Personal Computer, IEEE Transactions on Biomedical Engineering Vol BME-29, No 7, July 1982.

WORK WITH DISPLAY UNITS 92
H. Luczak, A. Çakir and G. Çakir (Editors)

Field Study of a New Type of Computer Screen Technology

Gunnar Ahlström1, Arne Lowden2, Hans Malmkvist3, Bo Schenkman3, Rikard Stöhr1, Rudi Weselka4

1.Telia Research AB, 123 86 Farsta, Sweden
2.The Royal Caroline Institute, Institution for Stress Research, Box 60205, 104 01 Stockholm, Sweden
3.ICL Systems AB, Box 40, 164 93 Kista, Sweden
4.ICL Data AB, Box 40, 164 93, Kista, Sweden

1. Summary

1.1. Background

The aim of the study was to specifically evaluate and compare the different optical ergonomic characteristics of two different types of screen delivered by ICL/Nokia Data in a user environment where screens are used intensively. The study was carried out at Teletjänsten in Sundsvall. A high-quality monochrome CRT screen was compared with an advanced TFT-based flat LCD screen.

1.2. Method

56 telephonists (50 women and 6 men, average age = 36 years) worked for 9 weeks at the LCD screen and 9 weeks at the CRT screen. All the telephonists carried out their normal tasks using the CRT screen. 16 LCD screens were installed and shared by half of the group at the beginning of the experiment. In the middle of the experiment, the LCD screens were replaced by the CRT screens which the other half of the group had used. Three different questionnaires were distributed at different times during the experiment. The questionnaires consisted of questions dealing with various ergonomic aspects, including visual characteristics, flexibility, symptoms of discomfort, health-related anxiety and general sense of well-being when working at a screen. At the end of each 9 week period, the telephonists evaluated their own optical discomfort, fatigue, readability and work load for each shift lasting for over 1 hour and 15 minutes. The shifts were scheduled between 07:00h and 23:00h.

1.3. Results

The result of the questionnaires showed that the LCD screen was considered to be better from the standpoint of readability, and was advantageous in terms of other screen-related characteristics, but that there were still striking similarities between most of the screen-related aspects. The readability of the LCD screen was, above all, better in terms of contrast between text and background, the sharpness of the characters and the brightness of the screen. On the other hand, no difference was found in the design of the characters and the readability of the text. For other screen-related variables, the LCD screen was considered to be better in terms of stability of the display and screen size. On the other hand, no difference was found in flickering and in the occurrence of bothersome reflections. Altogether, the subjects were significantly more satisfied with the LCD screen.

The evaluations relating to an entire day's work showed that readability and symptoms of discomfort were not affected by the kind of screen used. The more shifts worked during the day, the greater the discomfort and the lower the readability. The LCD screen was moved around on the desk to a greater extent than the CRT screen.

2. Background

The equipment used in the experiment comprised Nokia/ICL DU127 colour screens for PC with VGA resolution (640x480 points) and with a 10.5" active screen diagonal which corresponds to a 12-13" screen diagonal for CRT. Monochrome 14" CRT screens (Nokia EWS), which are considered to have good optical ergonomic qualities for this particular type of screen, were used as reference screens. The resolution of these screens is 640x400 dots. It is worth mentioning that these reference screens have better optical ergonomic qualities than any colour CRT screen on the market, intended for similar applications. Both types of screen used in the study displayed black text against a white background. Only text was displayed.

The study was carried out from Week 13 to Week 44, 1991. In the study, the telephonists were engaged in directory enquiry work, - an area of work where the screen is the dominant tool used and an area of work which must be considered to be terminal-intensive and of significance in a field study.

The characteristics studied were specifically, as was mentioned previously, various optical ergonomic characteristics such as brightness, contrast, character sharpness, character design, flickering inter alia.

3. Procedure

The procedure for carrying out the experiment meant that all the telephonists, from the four selected rooms, at the beginning of the experiment, were made to answer a Basic Questionnaire with background questions. The LCD screens were first installed with Group 1 (Rooms 1 + 2). The telephonists in Group 2 (Rooms 3 + 4) kept the CRT screen which was the standard in all rooms. The equipment was checked and replaced if it did not satisfy the optical ergonomic requirements. All the telephonists had about an hour's training in the use of the LCD screen, since there were different function keys on the keyboard compared with the CRT screen. Just over a week after the equipment was installed, all the telephonists received a Screen Questionnaire with questions relating to the screen they were working with at the time. After a further 8 weeks, the same Screen Questionnaire was redistributed to the telephonists. In the second survey it was found that the novelty effect of working with the screens had worn off. From the eighth week a "survey" week was initiated, where each shift of about 1 hour and 15 minutes was followed by a Shift Questionnaire. The subjects filled in the Shift Questionnaires during the next five days. At most, 3 shifts were worked in one day. However, many telephonists did not work full time or alternated work at the screen with other tasks. Consequently they answered the Shift Questionnaires less frequently.

In the middle of the experiment, the screens were exchanged. The CRT screens were returned to the LCD screen users in Group 1 which had been used by Group 2. LCD screens were installed for Group 2. The change of equipment meant that the number of telephonists who tested the LCD screens was doubled at the same time that these subjects could be compared with themselves under two different conditions. The equipment was changed during the summer vacation. In general, the procedure for the second part of the experiment followed the same pattern as the first part. In short, the telephonists worked for 9 weeks at an LCD screen and 9 weeks at a CRT screen.

Three different questionnaires were used in the experiment:

The Basic Questionnaire started off the experiment. The questions dealt with age, sex, experience of work at a screen, eyesight, enjoyment of work and influence over the working situation, as well as work-related stress discomfort.

The Screen Questionnaire was answered a total of 4 times, at the beginning and at the end of each period of 9 experimental weeks. The questions dealt primarily with optical ergonomics, including screen stability, character design, readability, contrast, brightness, flickering, reflections, screen size. The questions also dealt with response times and keyboard as well as well-being when using the screen and the possibility of varying the position of the screen.

The Shift Questionnaire was answered after each shift in the survey week. The questionnaire was shorter and contained questions dealing with fatigue, optical discomfort, readability of the screen, work load and stress during the shift.

4. Results; Basic Questionnaire

There was an even distribution of age, from 19 to 55 years, in the group. The average age was 36 years. The group was dominated by women (50) and a small number of men (6). On average, the subjects had worked at a screen for just over two years, but experience varied considerably within the group. 90% enjoyed their work as telephonists very much/quite a lot. In general, the group felt that they had good eyesight (83%). Optical fatigue, discomfort in the back of the neck and shoulders generally dominated the symptoms of discomfort. In about 20% of the subjects, discomfort was found to occur most of the time/all of the time. The discomfort was generally found to be less prevalent among the subjects than in other groups involved in work at a screen at Televerket. 45% of a group of just over 1600 people reported experiencing optical fatigue on a weekly/daily basis (the Datia project).

5. Results; Screen Questionnaire

5.1 Readability

The results for the optical response to the CRT and LCD screens showed that both screens were considered to be "very good" or "quite good". No differences were found between the screens for the two variables, design of characters and readability of text. On the other hand, the LCD screen was considered to be better in terms of the contrast between the text and the background, and the LCD screen was rated higher in terms of stability of the display and sharpness of the characters.

The two groups differed in their rating of the sharpness of characters. Group 2 felt that sharpness improved with the LCD screen and Group 1 felt that sharpness deteriorated during the nine weeks that they tested the screen.

5.2. Other Screen Characteristics

A clear difference was found for comfort in working with the size of screen provided. In the study, attitudes to the LCD screen were more positive. In addition, the stability of the LCD screen was considered to be better, but the difference is only significant on a 10% level. No differences between the screens were found as regards the response to questions dealing with bothersome flickering and reflections.

6. Discussion

Among the other variables measured, there were subjective symptoms of discomfort (optical discomfort, discomfort in the back of the neck/shoulders, fatigue), work load and ability to perform. It was not possible to link discomfort to the kind of screen used with any of variables. The results of the ratings show that the evaluation of the screen was carried out under comparable levels of discomfort and work load.

The possibility of changing the position of the screen on the desk was important, since there were no fixed workstations. The need for a moveable screen is also shown in the results where the position of the screen was changed before at least every second shift. The CRT screen was considerably more difficult to manoeuvre and also took up more room on the desk which limited mobility. Above all, it was difficult to push the CRT screen further away on the desk for greater reading distance. The LCD screen's advantages in terms of flexibility are indicated by the fact that the LCD screen was moved to a greater extent, in spite of the fact that no specific information on the flexibility of the screen was given before the investigation.

In general, the subjects felt more comfortable working with a screen which was the size of the LCD screen than one the size of the CRT. Since the question dealt with the overall impression, several aspects of the size can be included in the answers. Two aspects are worth noting: the flat format of the screen which affected the amount of space available on the desk and the possibility of moving the screen (see above), as well as the size of the display. The question of the extent to which subjects felt comfortable working with a particular screen size should be followed up by additional questions to determine which aspects of the screen size affected the answers.

Health-related anxiety was more noticeable for the CRT screen. This was probably due to the extensive media coverage on the effects of irradiation and electricity which occurred before the study was initiated.

WORK WITH DISPLAY UNITS 92
H. Luczak, A. Çakir and G. Çakir (Editors)

Method of inputting arbitrary solid shape by hand referring to virtual object in virtual space presented on CRT display

S. Yamada

School of Human Sciences, Waseda University,
2 Mikajima Tokorozawa-shi Saitama pref. 359, Japan

Abstract

A system for inputting arbitrary solid shape by hand referring to virtual object in virtual space was developed and evaluated. The system consists of a presentation system to produce a virtual space between the observer and the large screen, and three-dimensional measurement system to reproduce manually a new shape.

This paper argues some problems for reproduction of the stereoscopic image *in full size*. Those are the ploblem to observe in different conditions of visual system between the virtual object and a hand of the observer, and the ploblem that the hand of the observer sometimes hides the screen presenting virtual space. Since the observational condition in this method is special as mentioned above, there is a possibility that the observer will not perceive the virtual space correctly or continuously. In this paper, the characteristics of human space perception of the virtual space were evaluated.

From the results, continuous perception between the virtual object and his or her hand, and some characteristics of the space perception of the virtual space were investigated.

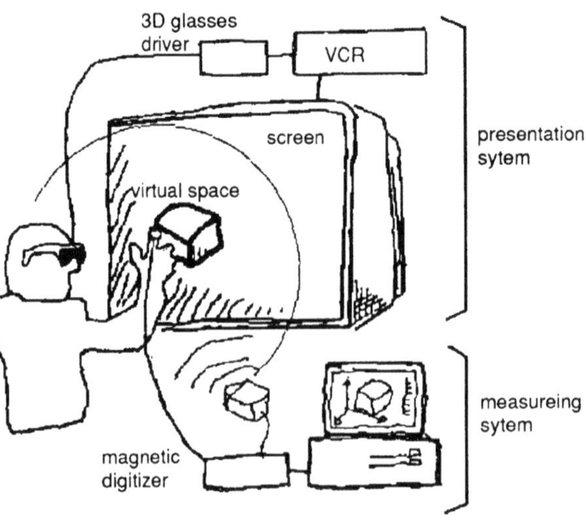

Figre 1 Outline of the system of this method

1. INTRODUCTION

A method is proposed for looking at a virtual object in a virtual reality space (hereinafter referred to as a virtual space), tracing the virtual object by hand, deforming part of the virtual object as required, and manually entering a new three-dimensional shape into a computer by refereeing to the virtual object (Figure 1).

In this system of the method, virtual space is composed of time-shared stereoscopic images displayed on a large CRT screen and three-dimensional digitizer for inputting the position in virtual space directly by our hand. When completed, the technology will allow us to build an operation and visual display system with control per display ratio of 1.

For the accurate formation of three-dimensional image in the virtual space, the subjective position of the object in the virtual space was quantified by the three-dimensional digitizer. The characteristics of human space perception in the system with respect to the virtual space perception investigated accordingly.

1.1. Problems in perceiving the virtual space

The virtual space treated by this study is presented as a binocular stereoscopic image on a screen at a distance from the observer. The observer can directly act on the virtual space by hand. The characteristic of the visual system like convergence and accommodation when the observer looks at the virtual space are different those exhibited when the observer looks at his or her hand (Figure 2). So, there is a possibility that the obsaerver may lose the continuity of observation and perception between the virtual object and the real object or the hand. In addition, when the virtual object is hidden by the hand, the reduction of available space information will be caused.

These points imply the possibility that the space information of the virtual space may not be subjectively perceived as originally intended.

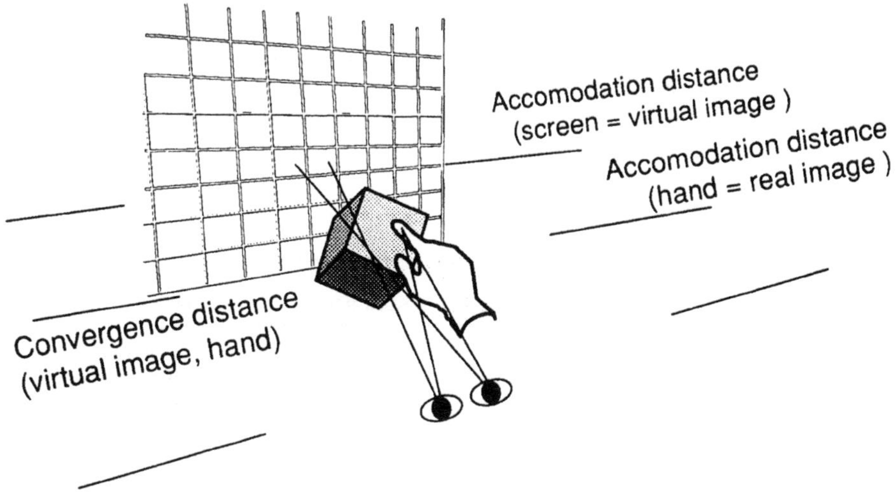

Figre 2 A problem in observing virtual space and hand

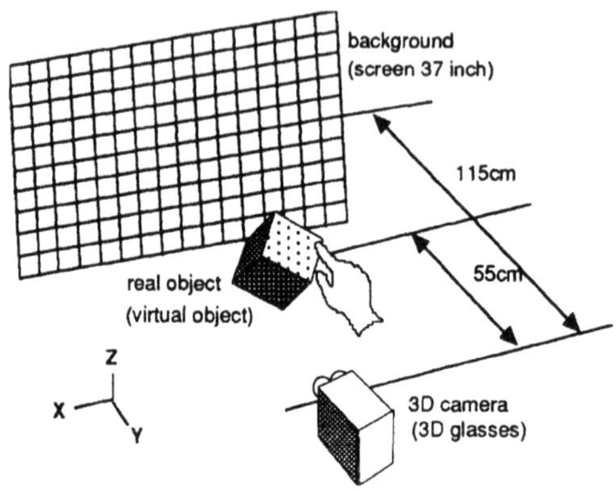

Figure 3 Videotaped (and observed) condition of virtual space

2. METHOD

The virtual space created by the system presents a virtual object *in full size* and allows the observer to reach to virtual object, trace the shape of the virtual object by hand, and enter a new three-dimensional shape into the computer by refereeing to the virtual object.

The proposed system is the combination of a subsystem composing a three-dimensional camera and CRT display screen for constructing a virtual space, and a subsystem for measuring virtual objects with a three-dimensional digitizer (Figure 1).

A cube in the real space was videotaped as time-shared stereoscopic image. The presentation conditions like distance and illumination were controlled so that the videotaped cube could be presented in the virtual space under the same conditions as in the real space (Figure 3). When the cube was videotaped, the vertices of the real cube were entered by the three-dimensional digitizer and used as reference data for comparison (thin wire-frame cubes in Figure 4).

A 37-inch TV monitor (37-CZ1, MITUBISHI) was used for image presentation. The

Table 1
Profiles of the subjects used

Sbj.	age	sex	visual acuity	practice in stereoscopic image
A	24	male	(0.7, 1.0)	practiced
B	40	female	(1.2, 1.2)	not practiced
C	23	female	(1.2, 1.2)	practiced
D	23	male	(0.1, 0.05)	not practiced
E	24	male	(0.7, 1.0)	not practiced
F	25	male	(1.2, 1.2)	not practiced
G	24	male	(1.5, 1.5)	practiced
H	24	male	(0.8, 1.0)	practiced

background (a 5-cm latticed screen) was displayed in full size on the TV monitor. The position of the liquid-crystal shutter glasses (STS-330, UTH) was fixed to limit the apparent motion parallax .

The observation distance was 115-cm and the same as the distance between the three-dimensional camera and background when the cube was videotaped.

The positions of four vertices of each face of a cube (12 cm per side) presented in the virtual space were subjectively perceived and entered with three-dimensional magnetic digitizer (3SPACE, POLHEMUS) by the observer. The observer entered the three-dimensional coordinates of the cube with the probe of digitizer gripped with the right hand. A total of 12 vertices of any three faces of the cube that could be seen from front were entered at random 10 times each or more. Eight subjects, aged 21 to 40 are participated(Table 1).

3. RESULTS

Table 2 lists calculated positions of the center of the cube inputted by each subject. Depth (ΔY) is significantly large in variability and is also large in individual difference between the subjects. And it shows all subjects perceived the cube nearer than the presented virtual cube. In addition the length of the side of the cube inputted was shorter than the presented virtual cube is.

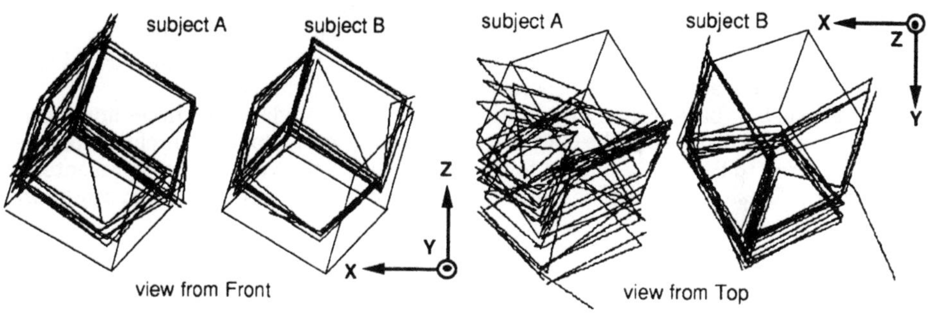

Figure 4 Examples of inputted cube (a cube in the center shows reference position)

Table 2
Shifting of the center of cube inputted (with s.d.) and average length of its side (L)

Sbj.	ΔX	ΔY	ΔZ	n	L
A	-4 ±5.1	10±25.7	27 ±6.6	111	104
B	-1 ±2.4	2 ±6.0	25 ±2.9	95	118
C	-13 ±3.2	2 ±7.2	43 ±4.5	104	118
D	-24 ±4.0	123±17.0	-26 ±4.1	185	80
E	-22 ±3.3	55 ±8.2	3 ±3.7	153	120
F	-20 ±1.9	45 ±8.8	2 ±3.4	177	111
G	14 ±4.1	46±14.5	9 ±5.1	272	119
H	6 ±4.0	86 ±7.6	14 ±5.3	198	119

(unit is [mm], except n)

Figure 4 shows an examples of inputted (perceived subjectively) cube. Though the view from front of the cube inputted by both subject A and B looks the cube was perceived and inputted correctly by both subjects, the view from top shows subject A could not decide the depth of every vertices.

4. DISCUSSION

In this method, the result implies the existence of directional differences in the space perception and individual differences in space accuracy perceived.

Perceived length of the sides of the cube inputted was shorter than the presented cube. And the position of the inputted cube was more closer to the observer. These results probably shows the reduction of the sizes of the perceived space by the observer.

As Iwasaki points out, this phenomenon seems similar to micropsia in ophthalmology (Iwasaki et.al., 1991). Because the visual condition of observation of virtual space is close to the condition how the patients of micropsia see the world.

To avoid the size reduction of the perceived virtual space, further research will be required to make clear of the relation between the special condition of the visual system of this method and perceived size and position.

And From the result, It seems that the occlusion of the screen by observers hand was not a big problem to perceive continuously the positions of the virtual cube. It may be because, before they point the position of the vertices by the three-dimensional digitizer subjects could decide where to point without their hands up.

The virtual space in this method was created only with binocular disparity. Under this condition, the subjects considerably differed in the perception of the virtual space and exhibited low accuracy in the perception in the depth direction.

Factors, such as background information, convergence angle of the three-dimensional camera, size and distance of the CRT display screen, and mental models of the observer, are considered to be closely related to the perception of the virtual space presented on the screen. These factors will be clarified by studying various presentation conditions.

5. CONCLUSIONS

The method to input arbitrary solid shape referring to virtual object was explained as above. The characteristics of human space perception of the virtual space in this method was evaluated. Some problems was pointed out for accurate presentation and perception. The results shows perceived positions of the virtual object varies wide especially in depth, and shows individual differences.

6. REFERENCES

1 Iwasaki, T., Akiya, S., Inoue, T., Noro, K., Position of accommodation to stereoscopic three dimensional images, The Japanese Journal of Ergonomics, Vol. 27, Supplement, pp. 222-223.

2 Yamada, S., Noro, K., Atsumi, H., 1992, Dimensional perception of virtual reality image with real objects, The Japanese Journal of Ergonomics, Vol. 28, Supplement, pp. 366-367.

WORK WITH DISPLAY UNITS 92
H. Luczak, A. Çakir and G. Çakir (Editors)

International Standardization on Colour VDUs

J. Schanda

CIE Central Bureau, Kegelgasse 27, A-1030 Wien, Austria

Abstract

In recent years colour video display units have received general acceptance. With increased addressability of the primary colour channels the number of colours that can be produced on the screen increased to tens of thousands and higher. International standardization became necessary in order to compare the coloured pictures produced with the different VDUs, in order to describe accurately the colours, to find ways to link VDU colours to hard copy colours and specify optimum use of colours in different computer applications.

1. INTRODUCTION

In Europe the *EC Council Directives 89/391/EEC* on '*the introduction of measures to encourage improvements in the safety and health of workers at work*' and *90/270/EEC* on '*the minimum safety and health requirements for work with display screen equipment*' based on *Article 118 a* of the Treaty establishing the European Economic Community directed the interest of display designers and users on the question of establishing international agreement on requirements on VDUs and the working environment of a display terminal, to guarantee a better level of protection of the safety and health of workers.

The EC Directives provide only very general guidance, as e.g.: 'The characters on the screen shall be well-defined and clearly formed, of adequate size and with adequate spacing between the characters and lines. The image on the screen should be stable with no flickering or other forms of instability. The brightness and/or the contrast between the characters and the background shall be easily adjustable by the operator, and also be easily adjustable to ambient conditions. The screen must swivel and tilt easily and freely to suit the needs of the operator. It shall be possible to use a separate base for the screen or an adjustable table. The screen shall be free of reflective glare and reflections liable to cause discomfort to the user.' The detailed measures and the control specifications are the subject of international standards. In the EC this would mean the establishment of CEN and/or CENELEC standards. In world wide harmonization CEN agreed to wait for the global standards developed by ISO, and adopt those for Europe.

2. INTERNATIONAL STANDARDS

ISO 9241: Ergonomic requirements for office work with visual display terminals (VDTs) by *ISO/TC 159/SC4: Ergonomics/Signals and controls* is the fundamental series of standards in this field. The standard consists of 17 parts, it is dealing with: General introduction # Guidance on task requirements # Visual display requirements # Keyboard requirements # Workstation layout and postural requirements # Environmental requirements # Display requirements with reflections # Requirements for displayed colours # Requirements for non-keyboard input devices # Dialogue principles # Usability statements # Presentation of information # User guidance # Menu dialogues # Command dialogues # Direct manipulation dialogues # Form filling dialogues.

From the abovementioned parts several contain information related to the display. The most important of these will be discussed in the following sections.

2.1 ISO 9241-3: 1992 - Visual display requirements

This standard defines the term *image polarity*: Bright image on dark background means negative polarity, dark image on bright background is called positive polarity. Minimum *display luminance* (luminance of radiation emitted and reflected) has to be larger than **35 cd/m²** (character luminance for negative polarity and background luminance for positive polarity).

There are a number of definitions related to contrast, and it is important to use the terms correctly. The following are the most often used terms, their definitions and the required values:

Contrast modulation: $C_M = (L_H - L_L) / (L_H + L_L)$, and $\mathbf{C_M > 0{,}5}$ is required.
Contrast ratio: $CR = (L_H) / (L_L)$, and $\mathbf{CR > 3{:}1}$ is required.
with L_H: higher luminance; L_L: lower luminance:

If luminance is used to code information, then the minimum difference should be: 1,5:1.

2.2 CD 9241 - 8.3 (1992-02-18) Requirements for display colours

(This standard is only in the 'committee draft' stage, thus the following is only preliminary information!) The purpose of the standard is to prescribe basic specifications for colours on VDUs to ensure their optimum visibility, identification and discrimination. The standard summarizes factors affecting colour appearance at the display as originating from the display itself, the image on the display, factors depending on the viewer and on the environment where the display is standing. Table 1 summarizes these factors.

For the colour difference metric to be used in specifying display colour, the 1976 CIE USC Space - CIELUV - has been suggested, although it is mentioned that this space has been specified for colour stimuli subtending approximately 2° at eye level, and in most VDU applications sample sizes are smaller than 2°.

For colour uniformity $\mathbf{\Delta E^*_{uv} \leq 5}$ and $\mathbf{\Delta u'v' \leq 0{,}01}$ is required.

The **misconvergence** (bright line on dark background at 5% level) should be **≤ 20 %**.

Minimum character height is **20'** of arc, the preferred value is between 30' and 45', but for saturated blue the signal area should be larger than 2°.

The standard mentions problems with thin lines if red-orange, red-magenta, blue-purple, or green-cyan pairs are used.

Display	Luminance, spectral distribution & range, type of luminous substance, anti-reflective screen, resolution.
Image	Size. spatial frequency.
Viewer	state of visual adaptation, colour perception ability.
Room	illumination level, illumination colour temperature.

To describe colour differences a metric is recommended, where

ΔL^*: is the metric for brightness difference;

$\Delta u'$: is the metric for red-green difference; and

$\Delta v'$: is the metric for yellow-blue difference.

With such metric one has to keep in mind that ΔL^* overestimates for widely separated targets; $\Delta v'$ overestimates for small targets, compared to $\Delta u'$, by a factor of 5 to 1; and it is difficult to discriminate blue - green due to the small field tritanopia.

Further on it is recommended that for accurate discrimination colour pairs should have a minimum colour difference of $\Delta E^*_{uv} \geq 20$. However it is difficult to give very definite guidance as the permitted colour difference will depend on adjacency and size.

Owing to all these facts and to further complications related to target shape recognition problems the standard recommends the use of luminance contrast metric for colour legibility.

Attention is also drawn to the fact that the simultaneous use of spectrally extreme colours can produce accommodation problems and therefore one should not use blue with $v'<0{,}2$ and red with $u'>0{,}4$ simultaneously. Colours should be used carefully: To avoid background and surrounding image effects, one should use an achromatic background (preferably medium or dark gray) behind chromatic foreground colours; and achromatic foreground on coloured backgrounds (preferably black or white, as gray will tend to appear as complementary colour).

Also the number of colours presented simultaneously should be restricted: If the meaning must be recalled not more than 6 colours should be used, otherwise reference be made accessible; if *search based on colour discrimination* is required **n < 6** and $\Delta E^*_{uv} > 20$.

2.3 Measurement requirements

Colour measurements can be performed by tristimulus or spectral technique, and should be performed at five basic measurement locations (in the middle of the screen and in four corners).

2.4 Further ISO Standards related to VDU colour

2.4.1 Draft Amendment ISO 8613: 1990/DAM2.2

This draft has been developed by ISO/IEC/JTC 1, Information processing - Text and office systems - Office document architecture and interchange format; and deals with colour spaces for the document level architecture.

This document prescribes CIE XYZ as reference colour space and CIELUV as interchange colour space.

2.4.2 Text and Office systems colour architecture (TOSCA)

CIE TC 1-27 'Specification of colour appearance for reflective media and self-luminous display comparisons' is developing recommendations for the specification of colour appearance match between a reflective image and a self-luminous display image.

This Technical Committee acts at the same time as official liaison to ISO/IEC/JTC1/SC18 in the development of colour standards for text and office systems.

2.5 CIE Publ. 60: Vision and the visual display unit workstation (1984)

This publication provides a thorough treatment of all questions related to the visibility of VDUs.

According to this publication the optimum contrast ratio should be in the range $(3:1) < 5:1 < C_R < 10:1 < (15:1)$. The background luminance for office task should be between 3 and 25 cd/m^2 . Experiments have shown that agreeable character luminance range is between 30...125 cd/m^2

The CIE Report suggests the use of not more than six to eight colours. Special attention should be paid if colour deficient observers have to use the computer as well, as many of them might have problems with red colours.

2.6 CIE Publ. 87: Colorimetry of self-luminous displays - A bibliography (1990)

Main chapters of this annotated bibliography, with over 300 entries, are:

- Classical colorimetry as used in colour VDUs;
- Colorimetric measurement and standards of colour on VDUs;
- Colour design and use on VDUs;
- Colour perception.

3. Regional and national standardization

3.1 ECMA - 126: Ergonomics - Requirements for Colour Visual Display Devices, 1987

The European Computer Manufacturers Association developed its own VDU ergonomic standard, where the data differ somewhat from other internationally accepted values: The minimum higher luminance value for white is specified as 45 cd/m^2 and for colour as 35 cd/m^2. The minimum recommended contrast ratio is 3:1 at an ambient illumination of 250 lx.

3.2 European (CEN/TC122/WG5) standards

As mentioned the CEN (European Committee for Standardization) is planning to adopt the 14 Parts of ISO 9241.

In Europe several countries have standards on VDUs (thus e.g.: Austria: *ÖNORM 2630*: Video display work places for digital data and word processing; Great Britain: *BS 7179*: Ergonomics of design and use of visual display terminals (VDTs) in offices; Denmark: *DS nr 100 DS/INF 34-1987:* Workstations with visual display units - Analysis, design , etc. and *DS nr 100 DS/INF 19-1983:* Ergonomic principles in the design of work systems; Germany: *DIN 66 234* Display workstations; the Netherlands: *NEN 3002 Ergonomics* - Ergonomic requirements for the design and use of visual display terminals and their input devices and *NEN 3003 Ergonomics* - Ergonomic principles for the design of office tasks using visual information processing systems, Sweden: *Nat. Sw. Board of Occupational Safety and Health:* Ordinance (AFS 1985:12) concerning work with visual display units (VDUs), *MPR 1990:8 1990-12-01*: Test methods for visual display units - Visual ergonomics; Emission characteristics and *MPR 1990:10 1990-12-31*: User's handbook for evaluating visual display units.

All these standards will have to be withdrawn when the ISO standard adapted by CEN is in force.

3.3 Further national standards

In the USA *ANSI/HFS 100-198 8* American National Standard for Human Factors Engineering of Visual Display Terminal workstations has a number of colour related recommendations - *ANSI IT8 Image Technology Standards* deal with the exchange of colour picture data, line art data, colour proofs and monochrome image data - *ASTM E 1336-91*: Standard Test Method for Obtaining Colorimetric Data from Video Display Unit by Spectroradiometry and *ASTM E-12 on Appearance:* DRC Draft 3, 91.06.19, Proposed standard practice for obtaining colorimetric data from a visual display unit using tristimulus colorimeters are also standards on VDU colorimetry.

The Canadian Standard *CAN/CSA - Z412-M89*: A guidance on office ergonomics, Office equipment: Visual display terminals - screens (monitors) is an other national standard in the field.

4. CONCLUSIONS

As can be seen international standardization helps considerably in unifying VDU coding practice. This will lead to more compatible soft- and hardware constructions, to the easier interfacing of computer systems and unambiguous electronic colour information exchange.

WORK WITH DISPLAY UNITS 92
H. Luczak, A. Çakir and G. Çakir (Editors)

Visual ergonomics of VDUs - testing of the colour characteristics.

Bo Persson, Börje Andrén and Magnus Breidne

Institute of Optical Research (IOF).
100 44 Stockholm, SWEDEN.

Abstract
The major changes of the new revised MPR testing are discribed and explained. A new visual ergonomic control instrument is presented.

1. INTRODUCTION

Visual problems relating to the work with displays are well recognized and established (Knave, B.G. et al 1984 ; Sheedy, J.E. 1992). To solve or to limit these problems, the interdisciplinary research needed should include fields such as image quality, physiology, psychology, lighting, and colour, i.e. fields relevant to the complex nature of the visual problems. The interdisciplinary approach has proven to work well in the visual ergonomic research at IOF.

In this contribution two main results are presented: 1. A new colour display testing method to be included in the MPR-testing. 2. A new visual ergonomic control instrument.

2. THE NEW MPR VISUAL ERGONOMIC TESTING

Two fundamental aspects of the new MPR testing are:

1. The testing should be of interest for practical work with displays.

2. The testing parameters should be tested with, for vision and display ranking, adequately high accuracy.

The short-comings of using stimuli based colour systems in a display testing procedure are well known, and the perceptual Natural Colour System (NCS) was therefore of great interest for the revised MPR-testing. However the NCS-system is developed for surface colours, and even if surface colours can be simulated on a display, luminous colours are the most common type of colours. In reference to this the CIE 1976 (u',v') and CIELUV systems are prescribed in the proposed testing procedure.

Since photopic luminance is not intended to be used as a measure of colour brightness, the colour contrast, field or border contrast can not easily be physically measured. Even if

CIE now supports a number of different types of spectral weighting functions the difference between measurements and actual colour vision is too large. This together with the number of different dot structures used on different displays give the main reasons for not prescribing edge- and line-sharpness testing parameters in the colour testing procedure. Such parameters, based on recent research made at IOF, should however in the near future be added to the testing

3. THE PROPOSED COLOUR TESTING PARAMETERS

The proposed testing parameters are: basic whiteness, colour uniformity, angular dependent characteristics of colour LCDs, straylight and pixel geometry. Basic whiteness tests the basic colour stimulis of the VDU. Colour uniformity, angular dependence, and pixel geometry test well known image quality problems of colour displays.

Straylight is a complex testing parameter relevant to image veils, line sharpness, and the appearance of colours. Five colour CRTs have been tested in accordance to the developed procedure, and the testing parameters have shown a good correlation between visual and photometric data.

4. THE SIGNIFICANT CHANGES IN THE TESTING

The measuring points are subjectively selected by the operator. Furthermore the objects measured are not in the first place letters or other characters that are likely to be dependent on the font and raster frequency.

A notable difference between the ISO 9241-3 testing procedure and the MPR testing is that ISO has defined certain standard points on the screen for testing, while the MPR testing involves a subjective evaluation of the screen for the worst point or points. ISO also prescribes minimum requirements and MPR recommended values.

5. A NEW VISUAL ERGONOMIC CONTROL INSTRUMENT

The work with the new testing parameters showed an urgent need to develop a high quality azimuth, elevation, luminance and radiance scanner for both practical and laboratory visual ergonomic testing. Such an instrument has been developed, and figure 1 shows the luminance distribution of a LCD display with the left active part white, the right part black and with a clear reflex in the right lower corner of the display. Figure 2 shows the luminance distribution of the same display, upper left corner (marked "a"), and a white, and for good visual ergonomics too bright, paper to the right (marked "b") together with the immediate surrounding. This instrument will open new possibilities for high accuracy visual ergonomic testing in the future.

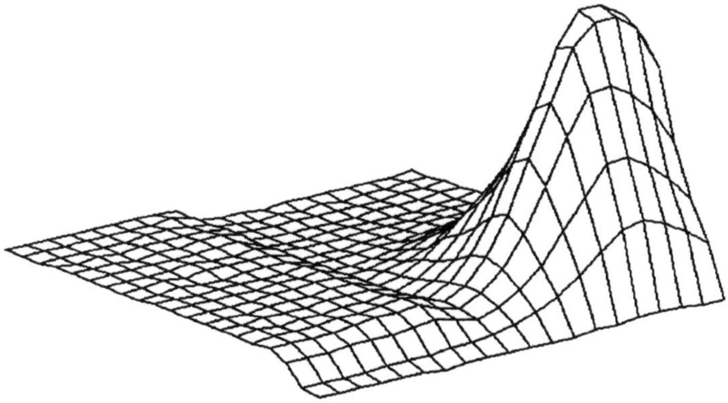

Figure 1. Luminance distribution of an active LCD with a clear reflex.

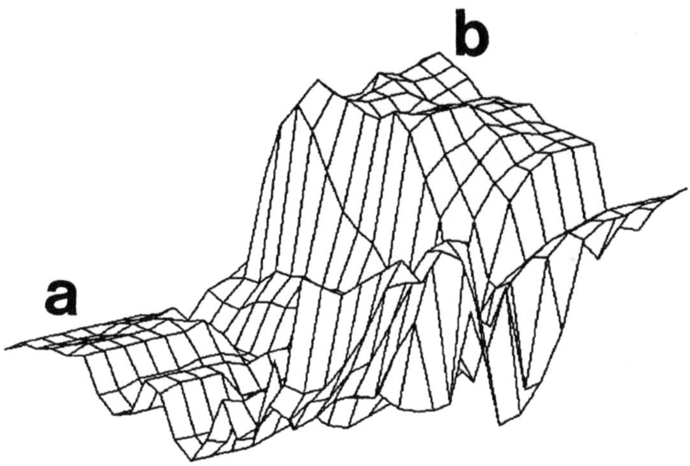

Figure 2. Luminance distribution of a LCD workplace.

6. REFERENCES

Knave, B.G. Wibom, R.I. Voss, M. Hedström, L.D. Bergquist, U.O. (1985) Work at video display terminals among office employees. Subjective symptoms and discomfort. Scan J Work Environment Health 11, 457-466.

Sheedy, J.E. (1992) VDTs and vision complaints: a survey. Information Display 4&5.

WORK WITH DISPLAY UNITS 92
H. Luczak, A. Çakir and G. Çakir (Editors)

The Psychosocial Aspects of Applying Ergonomics to Office Design

M. Joyce[a] and E. Adams[b]

[a]President, The Joyce Institute, 1313 Plaza 600 Building, Seattle, Washington

[b]Ergonomist, The Joyce Institute, 1313 Plaza 600 Building, Seattle, Washington

Abstract

The design of an office environment has extensive psychosocial implications. By involving workers, as well as supervisors and other management personnel in a defined process, an ergonomist can make recommendations addressing the needs of the individual worker in the context of the social culture.

That information contributes to critical recommendations for space planning, workstation configuration, job design, and work organization. In some cases, the information can be used to effectively return injured workers to the workplace.

This paper describes the process used to collect and evaluate data addressing the psychosocial aspects of the office environment and provides case studies of successful implementation of a macro-ergonomics approach to addressing VDT issues in the workplace.

1. INTRODUCTION

The process documented in this paper is grounded on the organizational design and participatory ergonomics literature. The macroergonomics approach, the third generation of ergonomics as defined by Hendrick (1986), means that the technological and physical aspects cannot exist independently of organizational and management consideration (Shipley, 1990). The technical subsystems (equipment, workstation design, environmental characteristics) must be considered in tandem with the social systems (job design, organizational culture, management style, and training.) Given the increasing recognition of the importance of the psychosocial aspects of office ergonomics (Smith, 1986, Bradley, 1989, Sauter, 1985) the process described herein uses a variety of methods for evaluation leading to design conclusion (Wilson, 1990). In particular, the principles of participatory ergonomics are included (Imada, 1991).

The purpose of the process is to enable organizations to make physical and organizational changes to the work and work environment in order to enhance the safety and productivity of the employees.

2. METHOD

There are five steps to the process of considering ergonomics in the design of an office work area. The five steps are: Pre-Planning; Data Collection; Data Evaluation; Recommendations; Implementation/Documentation. Since this is a process that is used in actual work environments, and since the outcome of the process is a set of detailed recommendations addressing the specific problems of an organization, there is a high degree of variability in the application of each step.

2.1 Pre-Planning

The emphasis on psychosocial factors is introduced during the pre-planning sessions. The ergonomist meets with senior management, facilities managers and designers, department managers, safety/health professionals, labor representatives, and human resource professionals to determine concerns and issues, discuss the project in relation to organizational goals, and to identify the specific jobs or work areas to be analyzed. The importance of ensuring that all the parties concerned with implementing the ergonomic solutions understand the project objectives is critical (Joyce, 1989).

2.2 Data-Collection

The data collection process consists of the following: Medical/Safety Records review (as appropriate); Job Analysis; Environmental Analysis. The Job and Environmental Analyses involve interviews with supervisors and employees, videotaping/ photographing of work areas, physical measurement of equipment and work stations and observation and evaluation of environmental aspects of the work area (Adams, 1992).

For the Job Analysis, the ergonomist conducts interviews in a private setting at the job site. The critical questions for attaining psychosocial information address the nature of the job, the demands of the job tasks, interactions with co-workers and personal physical and mental comfort. One series of questions relates to task variety; other questions focus on feedback/ recognition and autonomy/control, since much about a corporate culture is revealed through an organization's approach to these aspects of job design. A final question which provides insight into psychosocial aspects of the job is: "If you could change just one thing about your job or your workspace, what would it be?"

For the Environmental Analysis, both employee interviews and physical measures are included. The analysis encompasses both physical and psychosocial aspects of the work area: the psychosocial aspects include a consideration of densities, traffic patterns and circulation, adjacencies, and work area layouts; the physical aspects include space planning concepts, lighting, noise, air quality and temperature.

2.3 Data Evaluation

The ergonomist integrates the interview responses, correlates the information with the physical observations and measurements and conducts a literature and product search to identify equipment and furnishings and approaches to job/ organizational design that are appropriate to the application.

2.4 Recommendations

The ergonomist then provides recommendations that address both the technical sub-system as well as the social sub-systems. Because of the potentially sensitive nature of the recommendations, particularly those related to supervisory and co-worker issues, the recommendations must be presented in a confidential manner to upper management

2.5 Implementation/Documentation

Implementation is often an iterative process involving the ergonomist and the various members of the organization. The recommendations involving physical changes in the work area design or layout are usually implemented first, but it is often the organizational changes that have the most impact. The Documentation of the changes and tracking over time often provides the basis for an organization's commitment to a macroergonomics approach on a wider basis. In fact, in all the case studies summaries below, the outcome was sincere commitment to ergonomics throughout the facility.

3. CASE STUDY: ADMINISTRATIVE OFFICE IN A MAJOR MANUFACTURING COMPANY

A major manufacturer of durable consumer products provided an ergonomic evaluation for an office employee who had experienced pain and discomfort from a diagnosed upper limb cumulative trauma disorder.

3.1 Issues

The ergonomist, by following the methods described above, identified the following issues:

- Major tasks included composing documents, retrieving file information stored on-line and communicating with outside sources, both in the office and over the phone.
- The workstation was configured and equipped as it had been prior to the introduction of a computer. There was minimal adjustability for the work station equipment and lighting.
- Time pressures negatively influenced perceived work performance. The employee reported "never having enough time to do a proper job". When questioned, management was more than satisfied with the employee's performance, although this was not typically communicated to the employee.

3.2 Recommendations

The recommendations focused first on addressing the physical ergonomics issues, including providing appropriate seating, storage, an adjustable monitor support, a work surface of adequate size and depth and reorganization of the work surface layout. Additional recommendations focused on the modifying the schedule by which computer-related and non-related tasks were performed, improving communication between management and employees, especially regarding performance evaluation, and identifying the need to define job duties to clarify expectations for performance.

3.3 Results

As a result of the implementation of the recommendations, the employee ceased to experience any pain or discomfort related to the cumulative trauma disorder. The ultimate outcome of the improved communication was an internal promotion within one year.

4. CASE STUDY: CLASSIFIED DEPARTMENT OF A MAJOR NEWSPAPER

A major newspaper was experiencing a high incidence of CTD's and a high absenteeism rate in its classified department. The objective of the project was to provide recommendations to reduce these rates.

4.1 Issues

There were four different types of jobs in the department. The disorders primarily occurred in the two positions in which computers were used more than 75% of the day.

All the workstations had serious limitations, primarily related to lack of adjustability. Several areas had high noise levels and visual distractions as a result of an open plan configuration. A new computer system was being installed. The psychosocial issues were as follows:

- certain times of the day and week are perceived as high stress periods
- one group working on an incentive basis felt that some of their tasks interfered with the "important" (income-related) tasks
- two groups were inhibited in their ability to perform well because of inadequate space and/or high noise and traffic levels
- the employees generally felt positive about the value of their work in the organization

4.2 Recommendations

The recommendations focused on the following: space planning to re-configure the workspaces, minimize noise and distraction and provide privacy for area supervisors so they could have conversations with employees; storage requirements to allow for more usable work surfaces; seating and accessories to improve posture and orientation to the equipment; and training of the supervisors and the employees to encourage frequent rest pauses, stretching exercises, and organization of the individual work stations.

4.3 Results

Results of implementation were: eliminated the "paranoia" that workers were expressing about the new system; improved morale since the company was perceived as caring; reduced claims related to cumulative trauma; reduced absenteeism; provided a defense for a pending lawsuit that enabled the organization to clarify the "real issues from the imagined"; convinced management to apply ergonomics and provide training throughout the organization one year later.

5. CASE STUDY: ADMINISTRATIVE OFFICE IN REGIONAL LAW FIRM

A regional law firm provided an ergonomic evaluation for a legal secretary who was diagnosed with tendonitis and was frequently absent.

5.1 Issues

The ergonomist determined that the physical issues were primarily postural and related to the layout of the work area. However, the primary issue was organizational, a "a mismatch between basic personality traits."

5.2 Recommendations

The ergonomist recommended physical changes, including adequate seating and appropriate keying positions and habits, as well as organizational changes relating to reporting relationships.

5.3 Results

Within six months of implementing a change of the attorney/secretary pairing and involving the employee in the selection of the improved seating and accessories, all CTD symptoms have disappeared; and, the employee is motivated and achieving at a high performance level.

6. CONCLUSION

In these and other cases, the relationship between the physical and psychosocial is significant.

7. REFERENCES

Adams, Edie M. (1992). Using Ergonomics to Ensure a Successful Technology-Based Transition. *Proceedings of the International Facilities Management Association*.

Bradley, Gunilla. (1989). *Computers and the Psychosocial Work Environment* (Taylor and Francis).

Hendrick, Hal W. (1986). Macroergonomics: A Conceptual Model for Integrating Human Factors with Organizational Design. In *Human Factors in Organizational Design and Management-II*, edited by O. Brown, Jr. and H.W. Hendrick (North-Holland), pp. 467-477.

Imada, A.S. (1991). The Rationale and Tools of Participatory Ergonomics. In *Participatory Ergonomics,* edited by Kageyu Noro and Andrew Imada (Taylor & Francis), pp. 30-49.

Joyce, Marilyn and Ulrika Wallersteiner (1989). *Ergonomics: Humanizing the Automated Office* (South-Western).

Sauter, Steven L., L. John Chapman and Sheri J. Knutson. (1985). *Improving VDT Work: Causes and Controls of Health Concerns in VDT Use.* Prepared for the Dept. of Administration, State of Wisconsin (The Report Store, Lawrence, Kansas).

Shipley, Pat. (1990). The Analysis of Organizations as a Conceptual Tool for Ergonomics Practitioners. In *Evaluation of Human Work: A Practical Ergonomics Methodology,* edited by John R. Wilson and E. Nigel Corlett (Taylor and Francis).

Smith, Michael J. (1986). Job Stress and VDU's: Is the Technology a Problem?, In *Proceedings of the International Scientific Conference: Work With Display Units* (Swedish Agency for Administrative Development), Part 1, pp. 189-195.

Wilson, John R. (1990). A Framework and a Context for Ergonomics Methodology. In *Evaluation of Human Work: A Practical Ergonomics Methodology*, edited by John R. Wilson and E. Nigel Corlett (Taylor and Francis), pp. 1-29.

WORK WITH DISPLAY UNITS 92
H. Luczak, A. Çakir and G. Çakir (Editors)

User-centred design of an electronic work station for radiologists; the auto-alternator light box metaphor

R. den Buurman

Faculty of Industrial Design Engineering, Delft University of Technology, Jaffalaan 9, 2628 BX Delft, the Netherlands

Abstract

The radiology department of an university hospital is in the process of changing, from using mechanical auto-alternator light boxes for film handling and image analysis, to digital storage of images and electronic workstations. These urgently require experience with a standardised, user orienting, interface for the human computer interaction in the lenghty transition period. This case study discusses the design of such an interface.

The final concept consists of a graphical user interface based on an auto-alternator light box metaphor, with mouse and cursor, pull down menus and icons, suited for direct selection and manipulation. The modular system is divided over four screens to present background information and, related images simultaneously for parallel viewing.

The hardware of the system includes a spacious console with built-in 14 x 14 inch monitors, with a resolution of 1280 x 1280 pixels, that is minimally needed to match perceptually photographic quality.

Preliminary user testing with radiologists using a simplified prototype on a personal computer, is encouraging with respect to ease of use and user acceptance.

1. INTRODUCTION

Radiology departments in hospitals need to handle ever increasing quantities of medical images. Present practice is that every image is recorded on photographic film, even if it is originally obtained in a digital form. For storage and retrieval, communication, diagnostics and economics however, the possibilities of digital techniques combined with electronic presentation of images become increasingly attractive. As a result, all over the world, there are many developments in this field, primarily directed by technological and economic considerations (1).

However, for the people involved, going digital and electronic is very complex and a radical change. Consequently there is an urgent need for user-centred approaches as well. Resulting user-centred information systems should:

- match users' characteristics with tasks requirements
- fit the trajectories of common work practices

- support the management of problems
- provide for communication and consultancy
- have high aesthetic appeal

This paper demonstrates and discusses some of these topics as they relate to a case study on the design of an electronic work station for radiologists at an university hospital in Utrecht, the Netherlands (2). The radiology department there is in the process of changing from using mechanical auto-alternator light boxes for film handling and image analysis, to electronic workstations with possibilities for image manipulation and enhancement and for (picture) communication. These urgently require experience with a standardised, user orienting, interface for the human computer interaction in the, approximately, ten years transition period. The possibilities for the new system are considered to depend largely on immediate understanding, acceptance and adoption by the intended users.

2. ORIENTATION AND ANALYSIS

From literature, observation of present practice and opinions from radiologists and their assistants, the following is concluded. Radiologists are, generally, satisfied with their present procedures around the conventional auto-alternator light box (Figure 1), which they consider highly effective and efficient.

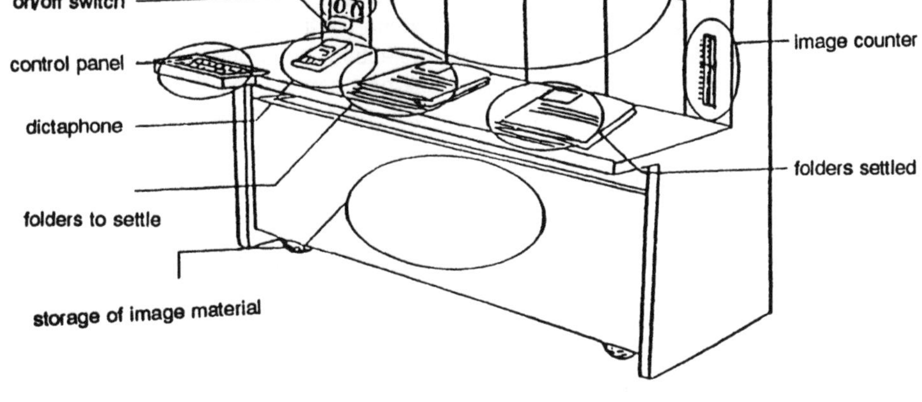

Figure 1. Mechanical auto-alternator light box with light panels, controls, desk area with patient folders and space underneath for storage of image material.

Parallel presentation of several high definition images with facilities for image manipulation and for measuring details and comparing grey levels is an absolute necessity. There is a severe need for having optionally available additional information about the patient's medical history and about the way the images have been generated. Consultation of colleagues and referring physicians should be supported. On the other hand, it became clear that, in between the image sessions, radiologists have a lot of supervisory and administrative tasks. And, for many of them, the system to be designed is their first step towards a totally digital radiology department. They have little experience with computers and are, in general, somewhat conservative, understandably, hesitating to exchange their present familiar and successful procedures and objects for the unknown virtues of the new system. However, radiologists are very sensitive to possible improvements of the quality of their diagnosis and their working speed. In fact, these are the only things they are willing to invest some of their scarce and valuable time in.

After some additional study of existing systems, an assessment of near future technology and an user test to establish the minimally needed image resolutions, it was decided that the interface should:

- support all the radiologists' customary activities, including their research
- maintain familiar procedures and names of objects
- provide at least the same feedback that resulted from working with the physical components on the auto-alternator light box
- simulate the actual presence of high definition photographic material
- provide for a high quality, easy to use, hard copy facility
- make the system act as a flexible and reliable assistant, taking care of all administrative tasks and providing for fast progress of the diagnostic sessions.

3. DESIGN CONCEPT

The final concept consists of a window driven user interface based on an auto-alternator light box metaphor, with a single mouse (or tracking ball) and cursor, pull down menus and icons and suited for direct selection, annotation and manipulation. The modular system is divided over one desk-part screen and three light box-part screens to present background information and related images simultaneously for parallel viewing.

Programmed system intelligence facilitates layout, manipulation and enhancement of images. In the images alphanumeric and graphic information on parameters relevant to image generation and diagnostics can be included. The desk-part screen (Figure 2) contains a menu bar, some icons acting as buttons and three permanent windows.

- a *patient window*, containing name, age, sex and registration number
- a *contents window*, indicating the available photographic material, at choice in a pictorial or in an alphanumeric form, and
- a *report window*, connected to the hospital information system and providing information on the patient's medical status, laboratory data and the requests of the referring physician.

There is also an optional *system window* giving feedback on time and session progress.

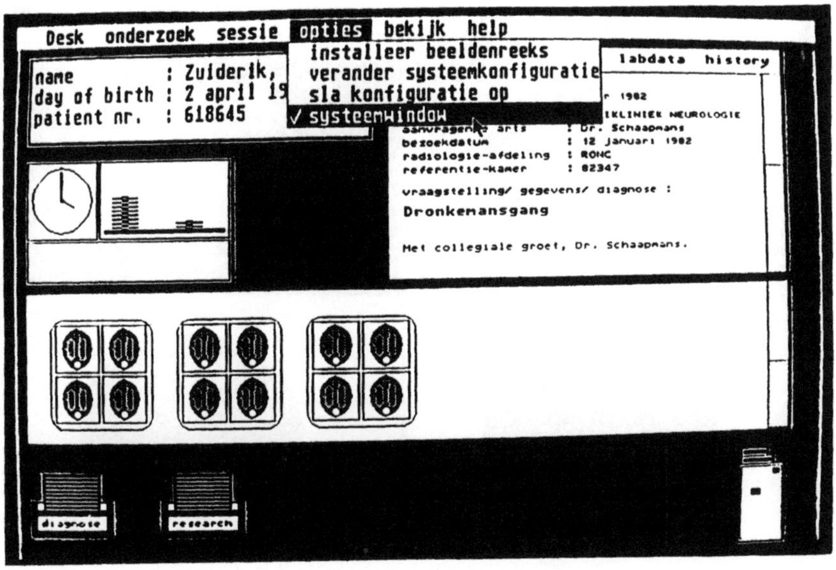

Figure 2. Desk-part screen with the three permanent windows and, upon request, the additional system window giving feedback on time and progress.

The three light box-part screens include a menu bar and resizeable image windows - one, four, or sixteen on a screen - with their buttons and, upon request, alphanumeric data on image generation and tools facilitating measuring and judging of image details. An example is shown in Figure 3.

The user interface is designed to accommodate busy radiologists and their assistants inexperienced in computer use, working with complex systems in the time limited transition period.

The hardware of the system consists of a spacious console with four built-in 14 x 14 inch monitors, with a resolution of 1280 x 1280 pixels, that appears minimally needed to match perceptually photographic quality (3). In addition, the console, accommodating several people at the same time for training and consultation purposes, offers a large desk area. The hardware set up is designed according to anthropometric guidelines with respect to seating posture, reach and lines of sight. The design is facilitated and tested with the help of ADAPS, a computer programme for the assessment of anthropometric design.

Preliminary user testing with radiologists using a simplified prototype of the new system on a personal computer is encouraging with respect to user acceptance and ease of use.

Due to technical, financial and organizational difficulties however, the real system still has not been implemented.

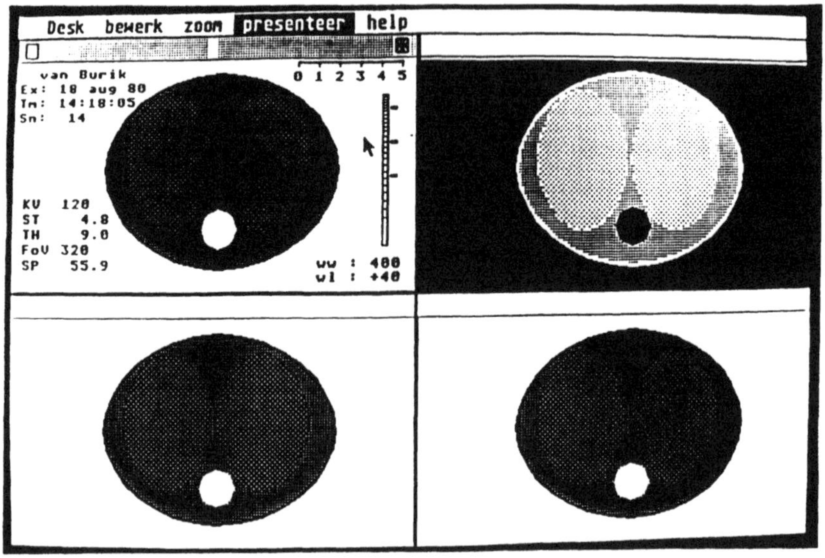

Figure 3. Light box-part screen containing four images. One of the images has been inverted and another one supplemented with alphanumeric data and grey and centimeter scales.

Acknowledgement

The author is indebted to J.H.W. Schuttenbeld, M.Sc. in Industrial Design Engineering for his major contribution to this project in the framework of his study.

4.REFERENCES

1 Dutch PACS Project, Phase-1 (1986-1989), Management summary, Sinteur, Leiden, 1990

2 Schuttenbeld, J.H.W. and B.M. ter Haar Romeny, Design of an user interface for a PACS viewing station, Proc. SPIE Conference on Medical Imaging. R.H. Schneider and S.J. Dwyer (eds.). SPIE, Vol. 767, 1987.

3 Seeley G.W. et al. The use of psychophysics as a system design aid: comparison of filmscreen to an electronic review console, Proc. SPIE Conference on Medical Imaging. R.H. Schneider and S.J. Dwyer (eds.). SPIE, Vol. 767, 1987.

WORK WITH DISPLAY UNITS 92
H. Luczak, A. Çakir and G. Çakir (Editors)

The Design of Control and Communication Centres with Multiple Displays

John Wood

Communications Complex Design (CCD) Limited

76, Church Street, Weybridge, Surrey, England

Abstract
Control rooms pose some special challenges to the ergonomist designing for VDU environments. When compared to other VDU workstations, say in offices, the control room designer needs to take account of such special factors as 24 hour operation, high concentrations of equipment, equipment sharing, diurnal rhythms and safety critical operations.

A summary of some of the key ergonomic considerations in control room design are presented together with a resume of some of the work currently under way on developing standards for these environments.

1 WHY ARE CONTROL ROOMS SPECIAL?

There is an enormous range of different types of control room - from multi-operator centres handling air-traffic control to single position controls dealing with the security of a prison. Whilst the equipment and operating practices may differ from one centre to another some common features can be found which, collectively, can distinguish control rooms from other working environments [1].

Most control rooms operate continuously 24 hours a day, seven days a week, for anything between 5 to 15 years. During this period many will need to accommodate equipment upgrades, changes in working practices and increasing workloads all without serious disruption to their primary control function. Essential maintenance of control room equipment has also to be undertaken while the room is operational and it is for the ergonomist to ensure that the conflicting demands of the maintainer and operator can both be met without any unnecessary disruption to either. Shift working is likely to result in each workstation being used by up to 5 different operators over a short period whereas in an office most workstations are dedicated to an individual.

Many control tasks are, by their nature, paced by external events and the control room operator may have little choice in the timing of their response. It is when such paced decision making is combined with safety critical systems that the ergonomist is faced with some of his most demanding challenges. A final feature which distinguishes many control environments from others is the density of equipment associated with any work position - most of us will have seen the pictures of the NASA Mission Control room.

2 ARCHITECTURAL AND BUILDING DESIGN CONSIDERATIONS

It is unlikely that the control room will exist as an entity on its own and the control will often associated with a number of other functional spaces which need to be considered at the same time. In the early planning for a new control centre we have found it useful to define the set of other spaces closely associated with the control room itself and to plot out their operational links with it. Such ancillary rooms, or spaces, may have supporting functions to do with equipment, staff welfare or the security of the centre itself. The figure below illustrates the concept of the 'control complex' of which the control room is but one component.

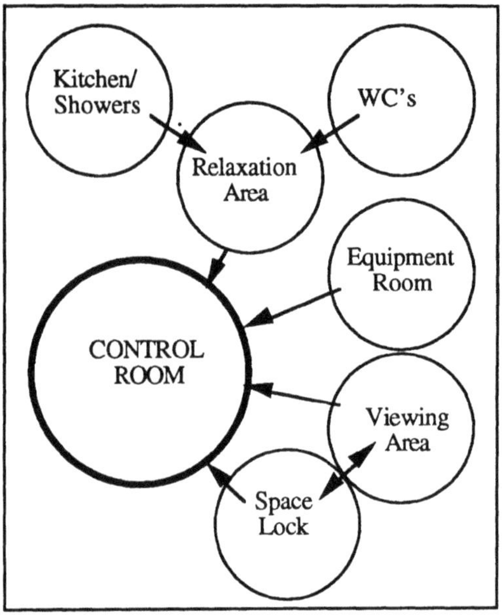

Fig. 1: Concept of a 'Control Complex'

In order to translate a list of functions into possible space layouts we have found it useful to prepare 'interrelationship' charts. These charts plot-out the various links between the functional areas - whether they are visual, circulation, cabling or message passing. Such a matrix then allows for the preparation of a 'bubble diagrams', in which the relationship between the control area and its associated supporting functions are schematically drawn up. When subsequently developing control complex layouts the bubble diagrams and interrelationship matrices provide an operational framework to assess alternative options.

Many control room design projects are unnecessarily hampered by the choice of space in which to house them. Rooms which are square tend to offer the greatest flexibility as far as control room layout options are concerned whereas long rectangular rooms, or those with a dog-leg should be avoided. Structural pillars, service duct access and doorways all reduce the actual usable space in a control room and it is a wise precaution to scrutinize potential control sites with this in mind before finally selecting an area.

The vertical dimensions need also to be carefully considered when looking at possible locations In our experience restricted floor to ceiling heights and control rooms with split ceiling heights can both give rise to problems, Fig. 2. Split ceiling heights create potential difficulties in balancing the lighting and thermal environments in the different areas - a common complaint is that whilst the temperature is too cool in the area with the lower ceiling height it is considered too hot and stuffy where the ceiling is lower.

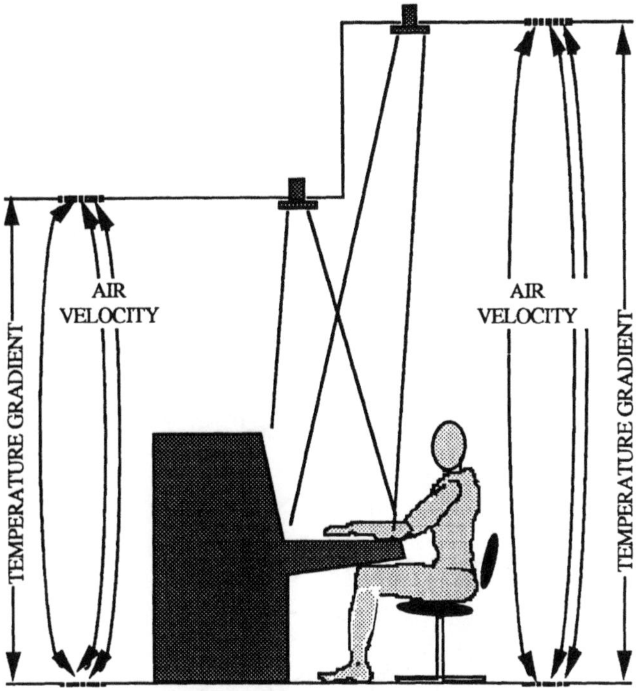

Fig. 2: Problems Created by Split Ceiling Heights

The lighting of control rooms has always been a difficult problem and many of the early attempts at carefully controlled downlights failed to adequately resolve the inherent conflict between the levels of illumination required on the worksurface and those on the screen. Indirect lighting has offered the possibility of using higher levels of ambient lighting which can meet the requirements of the desktop whilst avoiding veiling reflections on the screen.

Observations in a number of control rooms, supported by light measurements, has shown a common phenomenon with artificial lighting levels varying during a 24 hour cycle - even in windowless rooms! This observation underlines the need to design for high levels of flexibility in a lighting scheme.

3 GROUP AND TEAM WORKING

Team working is a common feature of control rooms involving both equipment sharing, pooling of information and joint decision making. In any particular control environment the way in which individuals interact with each other will depend on such factors as the time of day, levels of workload and the nature of the control tasks being undertaken. The ergonomist, in his planning, needs to adequately predict these formal and informal interactions. By using an interrelationship matrix, in which all the possible links between staff are plotted, the operational links which the control will need to accommodate can be documented and agreed. Such an interrelationship matrix should include visual links, auditory links, paper-passing requirements and 'social' links which become more important during quieter periods.

When examining the physical arrangement of staff, particularly when equipment is shared, reach and viewing requirements should be tempered by a proper consideration of *proxemics* [2] which concerns itself with man's perception of social and personal space. Proxemics identifies a series of zones around any individual starting with an "intimate zone" which is entered by, say, only a doctor through "personal". "social" and "public" zones at ever increasing distances from the individual. We have identified problems when shared tasks require operators to encroach each others' intimate zones. A workstation layout should aim to achieve an arrangement of equipment which keeps operators outside each others "intimate zones", Fig. 3:

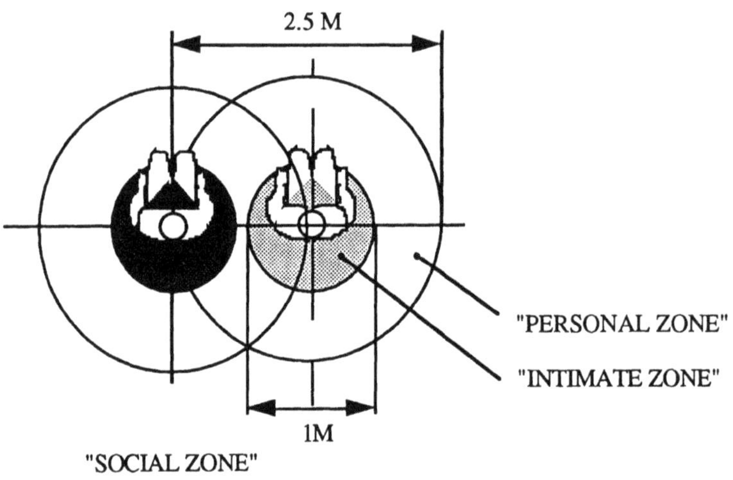

Fig. 3: 'Proxemics' - Personal, Social & Intimate Zones

STANDARDISATION

The European Directives concerning the use of display screen equipment [3] have been a welcome development since they have drawn the attention of a wider audience to the problems of working with VDU's and provided legislative muscle to the implementation of minimum standards. The impetus for these new laws can be traced back to the introduction of VDU's in the office environment.

Many control room characteristics are entirely different to those in offices with higher densities of equipment, 24 hour operation, safety critical tasks and team working. A new standard is being prepared which specifically addresses the ergonomics of control room design and operation. This multi-part, international standard on the Ergonomic Design of Control Rooms [4]is being written in 8 parts: a summary of the proposed structure and content is presented below:

- **Part 1 - Principles for the Design of Control Centres** presenting a step by step procedure for the ergonomic design and specification of a control centre
- **Part 2 - Control Complex Layout** - architectural considerations including space allocation, functional interrelationships and security.
- **Part 3 - Control Room Layout** - covering such aspects as console arrangement , location of secondary workstations, storage, maintenance access, circulation routes, windows and preferred locations for wall displays.
- **Part 4 - Workstation Layout & Dimensions** - plan layout principles for single and multiple workstations, vertical dimensioning for sit / stand operator positions, secondary workstation layout, maintenance design, panel and equipment layout principles.
- **Part 5 - Displays & Controls** - encompassing such aspects as man-machine interface design, information structuring, input devices, output devices including overview displays and CCTV.
- **Part 6 - Environmental Requirements** - a distillation of good practice on , for example, artificial lighting, heating, acoustics, interior design, finishes and the control of natural light.
- **Part 7 - Principles for Evaluation** - presenting evaluation techniques and how they can be applied at various stages of the design programme.
- **Part 8 - " Applications"** - will address specific types of control environment.

By 'decoupling' the general principles from 'applications' it is intended that the individual applications can be updated independently from the more stable background principles.

REFERENCES

1	Wood, J	Control Room Design Standards, Proceedings of the Ergonomics Society, Taylor & Francis, 1990
2	Hall, E	The Hidden Dimension, The Bodley Head Ltd, 1966
3	90/270/EEC	Council Directive on the Minimum Safety and Health Requirements for Work With Display Screen Equipment 29 May 1990
4	ISO 11064	Ergonomic Design of Control Centres - (8 Part Standard currently under preparation)

WORK WITH DISPLAY UNITS 92
H. Luczak, A. Çakir and G. Çakir (Editors)

Video Display Units for Safety Relevant Tasks in NPP Control Rooms? - Steps to pass the licensing procedure in the FRG

G. Becker, P. Sommer, TÜV Rheinland, FRG

Introduction

The state of the art of VDUs and the supporting computers allow sophisticated forms of information presentation and adequate control of power plants. Positive experiences with such technologies are reported for conventional plants. The possibility of preprocessing of information allows the visualisation of process interactions and an indication of the limits of operation. History and trends of process variables may be presented.

In a VDU control room the variety of components installed is very limited. Thus they are much cheaper than conventional control rooms.

These advantages are the reasons for dealing with the new development, especially in view of possible further improvements in nuclear safety. This aspect is important in Germany as the dynamic improvement of safety which corresponds to the state of science and technology is required by law.

Development trends

The German NPP manufacturers are designing a new generation of video display control rooms /1/ on the basis of computer aided process information systems /2/. Several other countries, e.g. France /3/, Canada /4/ and Japan /5/, are developing similar control room layouts using modern computer technology. The general principles of these designs are similar. There are work places for each of the 2 - 4 operators, there is some kind of overview panel and there is some kind of panel or workplace especially dedicated to safety relevant tasks. The French design uses conventional instruments for its safety panel, while German manufacturers intends to base the safety panel on computers /11/.

The operators use touch screens for most of their actions and additional conventional buttons for controlling the VDUs and special safety functions. In the German design the touch sensitive screens are separated from the information displays.

General Safety Requirements

For several years computers have been used in control rooms as additional tools. The automation of operator tasks and safety relevant actions has a long tradition in German plants even if the impact of advanced technology and the balancing of automation and human action is still under discussion /6/, /7/. The replacement of conventional hard wired control systems and the introduction of VDU based digital information processing is nevertheless more a revolution than a stage of development.

The change to new technology in the NPP control room therefore has to be prepared very carefully in order to benefit from new technology but - more importantly - to avoid the disadvantages. It is therefore necessary to remember the basic requirements laid down in the safety criteria:

- from the control room, the power plant must be controlled safely during operation *) and maintained in a safe condition in the event of an accident
- in the event of function loss of the control room it must be possible to survey and maintain safe conditions from outside the control room
- an adequate survey of the state of the plant under all conditions of operation must be possible at all times
- the control room and the tasks of the shift personnel must be designed under ergonomic aspects in such a way that they offer the conditions required for an optimal behaviour of the employees with respect to safety.

On the basis of these general safety requirement detailed criteria and technical standards have been developed over the years. These standards are focussed on conventional hard wired instrumentation and controls. They cannot be applied to VDU-Display design and software driven actuators. Thus some utilities, who have developed their own VDU-pictures, complain about the unsolved licensing problems.

With respect to the new technology the general criteria need some interpretation. The third requirement for example appears quite weak, as it calls for a "adequate survey of the state of the plant". This must be seen against the background of the court decision which requires "dynamic protection of the Base Law on Health". In this light - and this is our interpretation - the improvements in safety as compared with the conventional control room must be shown; only this will be "adequate". There should be no doubt on this due to poor evaluation methods.

New control room technology and licensing

The licensing procedure in Germany includes strict requirements with respect to the technical equipment to be installed in nuclear power plants. The successful operation of components over long periods has to be proven or the equipment has

---

*) the German term is "Bestimmungsgemäßer Betrieb" which includes normal operation, incidents not terminating the plant operation, and operation after shut down.

to be "qualified". The new information processing system is based to a large extent on software which has to be qualified. Thus the qualification of the software is one problem to be solved.

The other problem is the qualification of the interface and work design for the new control room.

Up to now, conventional control rooms were based on a steady development. Interface changes between the subsequent power plant generations were small. The evaluation of the adequacy of the operator tasks and the control room design was based to a large extent on previous experience. Mock ups of panels and the whole control room were sufficient for evaluating the improvements for new plants.

The replacement of conventional displays and controls with VDU displays requires different methods to make sure that problems relating to the human factor are solved correctly. Therefore an iterative design process using a dynamic simulation of tasks is necessary. The software generated pictures on the screens have to be qualified as already stated by the German Reactor Safety Commission.

The software qualification process

The problem of software qualification is not the focus of this paper but as the manufacturer intends to replace all types of conventional instrumentation, some comments are necessary.

In conventional control rooms the instrumentation is already divided in several classes with respect to safety. Correspondingly the qualification requirements for e.g. operational instrumentation are different to safety relevant instruments because the latter backs up the former.

The manufacturer therefore proposes different requirement-levels for different types of software. Furthermore in their opinion the safety relevant computers shall be redundant /11/.

With the state of the art of software qualification only very small software programs can be proven to be free of faults. For larger programs only the probability of perfectness may be assessed. We doubt that this obstacle may be overcome in the near future. Therefore we propose to design the accident instrumentation in the control room as well as the emergency control room on the basis of conventional I&C technology. This would simplify the licensing procedure for the new control room devices considerably.

Furthermore we do not believe that redundancy of safety relevant computers may be shown to be the state of the art. In safety relevant applications redundant computers as well as the software should be produced by diverse manufacturers as is usual in the aircraft industry.

The design of all other panels including the support of safety relevant tasks with preprocessed information may be based on digital information processing provided the questions of interface design are solved according to the IEC-procedure (see below).

Human factors questions

This section deals with some of the ergonomic questions, which are to be solved within the design process. The current state of the planning of German manufacturers is reflected as far as possible.

Functional analysis and function assignment

Information presentation for the operators will be based on pictures integrating several process variables. The preprocessing means a shift of more functions towards the machine. This could probably increase the likelihood of design errors hidden in the technique (latent errors) perhaps complicating the problem solving task of the operator. This means that the adequacy of this new function assignment must be assessed. The positive experience with traditional function assignment to man and machine may not be sufficient as assumed in /11/.

Serial presentation of information

The panel layout of conventional control rooms virtually represents a "world map" of the process, where system positions include relevant meanings for the operators. Thus the design of separate work places for each operator must be supplemented with additional survey panels compensating for the more serial presentation of information. The necessity of such survey panels is one of the findings of simulator experiments /3/. All new design proposals now include such survey panels.

But the separation of the operators whereby each has his own work place has other implications. The operator work is team work especially during disturbances. The influence of the operator separation on the effectiveness of the "network of heads" during problem solving seems to us to be an unsolved question.

Integration of information

The presentation of highly integrated information implies several questions with respect to operator task and the licensing process e.g.

- how may the operator check that the input signals of a picture are correct? Operators in conventional control rooms always check if a sensor defect may be the cause of the new signal by comparing it with other related displays.
- how is it possible to check that unexpected situations at the plant, not previously considered, may be identified?
- how to convince operators to trust the system if there are (unavoidable?) bugs in it?
- what are the consequences for the training of the operators? Considerable knowledge and skills are required for the handling of the information system (e.g. knowledge of (all?) pictures, which picture for which task?, skill/knowledge to find the right picture)

These are some of the several problems which must be solved in order to show that the new technology has advantages over the old conventional displays.

How to solve the HF-problems

The procedure of the qualification of the control room interface in principle is well known. For new control room equipment according to the German standard KTA 3904 /8/ an iterative design process based on thorough task analysis is required. Meanwhile the international standard IEC 964 /9/ proposes a comparable procedure of iterative steps:

1 Functional Analysis
2 Function assigment to man or machine
3 Verify, if the assigment corresponds to the capabilities of man and machine (revise if necessary)
4 Job analysis
5 Control room detailed design
6 Verify detailed design (revise if necessary)
7 Integrate control room design
8 Verify control room system (revise if necessary)

Thus the general methods are available. As the technology changes are of a general nature discussions between the authors as safety consultants and the manufacturer have been initiated on the basis of the existing cooperation in a standardization commitee. The consultants proposed runing a special licensing process (Vorbescheidsverfahren) regarding the more general control room features independent of specific plants.

Conditions for solving the problems

As one may imagine the task of showing the superiority of the VDU based control room will be a difficult one. A possible way of solving the problems would be the application of the iterative design procedure based on the IEC 964 flowgraph.

The main focus of this procedure will be the job analysis. We think it might be possible to select a number of typical tasks from the huge number of conceivable work situations of operators on the basis of a careful analysis. For this selected number of tasks detailed studies with experienced shift personnel have to be executed. A necessary prerequisite of such studies is a simulator covering all features of the selected tasks /3/,/10/. If no other sophisticated measurements are available at least pair comparison of the same jobs performed with old and new technology may show which solution is preferable.

The method of showing the advantage of the new design on the basis of a sample of tasks will necessarily end up only with a probability that the design is superior but not with certainty. Thus there is a need to have back up systems with convincing features. Such back up systems in German plants are the accident I&C and the emergency control panel.

As we have shown above the licensing problems of safety relevant computer based I&C are not sufficiently solved. Therefore it is necessary to design the above mentioned back up systems in conventional hard wired technology. There is no other way to pass the licensing procedure.

References

/1/ Hinz, W.; Kollmannsberger, J.: Screen based control rooms: a vision of the future. In: Nuclear Engineering, Dec. 1991

/2/ Hofmann, H.; Fisch, H.D.; Lochner, K.-H.; Mertens, U.: Microprocessor-based Information and Control Systems for Safety and Non-Safety-Applications in the Nuclear Power Plants of the Nineties, Transaction on the ENS/ANS-Foratome Conference, Lyon (France) 1990, Sept 23-28, 1820-1890

/3/ Paziaud, A., 1991: Simulater Based Verification for 1400 MW PWR Main Control Room. In: Jahrestagung Kerntechnik '91, Deutsches Atomforum, Bonn, 1991.

/4/ Olmstead, R.A., 1992: Control Room Systems and I&C Systems for Canadian CANDU Nuclear Stations. In: IAEA AGM-Report on Guidelines for Control Room Design. Wien, 1992.

/5/ Iwaki, K.; Shirakawa, T., 1992: Development of the ABWR Type Control Room Panels. In: OECD/NEA-IAEA Int. Symp. Nuclear Power Instrumentation & Control, Tokio, 18.-21.5.1992.

/6/ IAEA: Impact of advanced Technologies on Reactor System. Proceedings of a Technical Commitee Meeting/Workshop in Vienna, 6-8 Nov. 1989

/7/ IAEA: Balancing Automation and Human Action in Nuclear Power Plants. Symposium 9-13 July 1990. Vienna: IAEA, 1991

/8/ KTA 3904: Warte, Notsteuerstelle und örtliche Leitstände in Kernkraftwerken. Fassung 9/88

/9/ IEC 964: Design for control rooms of nuclear power plants. International standard, 1989

/10/ Becker, G.: Simulator experiments as method giving feedback to improve the man-machine interaction in Nuclear Power Plants. In: Proceedings of the IAEA Specialists' Meeting on the Human Factor Information Feedback in Nuclear Power. Riso, Denmark, 1987

/11/ Kollmannsberger, J.; Heßler, C.: Gestaltung moderner Bildschirmwarten. DAtF-Herbsttagung, 14.-15. September 1992, Königswinter

WORK WITH DISPLAY UNITS 92
H. Luczak, A. Çakir and G. Çakir (Editors)

ERGONOMICS AND COMPUTER SYSTEMS - VIDEO IN TWO PARTS

J. De Meyer[a], H. D'Hertefelt[b], J. Gaussin[c], R. Leonard[d], R. Patesson[e] and E. Wendelen[f].

[a]Occupational Health Physician, Ergonomist, Service Médical Interentreprises M.S.R.

[b]Sociologist NOVA-INRCT

[c]Professor, Work and Organisational Psychology Unit, U.C.L.

[d]Scientific Manager Ergoconsult

[e]Professor, Computers and Human Sciences Section U.L.B.

[f]Industrial Psychologist INRCT-NOVA

These videos are a joint production of three Belgian Institutions :

* the National Institute for research on Working Conditions (INRCT-NOVA)
* the Service Médical Interentreprises "MSR"
* the Service Médical Interentreprises "Santé et Travail".

It was made by GSARA with support from the Commission of the European Communities (Executive Producer : Paul Lhoir).

The two videos (each about 26 minutes long) deal with two different worlds : one about work in industry and the other about office work. A common part of both videos covers the European directive of May 29, 1990 (90-270-CEE). This directive stipulates that "Member States shall bring into force the laws, regulations and administrative provisions necessary to comply with this Directive by 31 December 1992". The most important provisions are the following :

* Employers shall be obliged to perform an analysis of workstations in order to evaluate the safety and health conditions to which they give rise for their workers, particularly as regards possible risks to eyesight, physical problems and problems of mental stress.
* Workers shall receive information on all aspects of safety and health relating to their workstation.
* Every worker shall also receive training in using the workstation before commencing this type of work and whenever the organization of the workstation is substantially modified.
* The employer must plan the worker's activities in such a way that daily work on a display screen is periodically inter-

rupted by breaks or changes of activity reducing the workload at the display screen.

* Workers shall be entitled to an appropriate eye and eyesight test carried out by a person with the necessary capabilities :
  - before commencing display screen work,
  - at regular intervals thereafter, and
  - if they experience visual difficulties which may be due to display screen work.
* Workers shall be entitled to an ophtalmological examination if the results of the test referred to above show that this is necessary.
* If the results of the test or of the examination referred to above show that it is necessary and if normal corrective appliances cannot be used, workers must be provided with special corrective appliances appropriate for the work concerned.

There is no chronological or hierarchical order in either videos on "Ergonomics and Computer Systems". Each video deals with distinct professional fields and can be looked at separately. However, the two of them have one and the same goal : to admit the idea that ergonomics requires a "multi disciplinary approach" involving each of the social participants, from employer to user.

Through a series of concrete cases, the aim of the ergonomic approach is emphasized : that of adapting work to man and not vice-versa.

FOR INSTANCE, DESCRIPTIONS OF SOME SEQUENCES OF THE TWO FILMS:

FILM 1 : WORK IN INDUSTRY

- A ship en route to England
  Points covered : information technology is used in the most wideranging places. The computer is a tool like any other. Its ability to integrate information provides undeniable advantages, but it has to be adapted to every stage of the work done by humans.
- Industrial design office.
  Here, engineers draft blueprints for ready-to-use "turnkey" factories. Points covered : a high-performance tool - CAD : computer-aided design - side-by-side with traditional drawing boards. Computers here are still simply an aid; they don't regulate everything. For various reasons, designers sometimes prefer to return to the drawing board, where they can obtain a better overview of the whole project and get a clearer idea of what they are aiming at.
- An electricity generating station, on an evening when it is due to be started up again.
  Points covered : the computer controls most of the commands and simplifies operations. Unfortunately, not every command can be computerised (mainly for cost reasons), and some

mistakes were made when the room was built. In emergency situations, the mental input of the operators therefore gains considerably in importance.

- A water purification plant.
  Although, from a technical point of view, this workspace appears to be an excellent example of the integration of information technology (well-lit, well-ventilated control room, a large number of information points allowing cross-checking...), some of the day-to-day realities were not taken into account at the design stage. Important point : systems designers are hardly ever the users. Consequently, they are not aware of actual user-requirements. A preliminary ergonomic study often enables omissions to be detected and rectified.
- A large chemical concern.
  Points covered : personnel training is a short-term investment. A large number of errors and ommissions can be avoided in this way. Article 6 of the EC Directive of June 1990 now requires that all VDU operators be given basic training and continued guidance.
- Contribution by Mrs Annie Drouin, ergonomist at "Electricité de France".
- EC Directives, June 1990.
  Regarding : eye tests, an alysis of the work post in order to evaluate safety and health conditions, and the taking of regular breaks or changing acitivities in order to avoid becoming overstrained.
- A large glass-making factory.
  Point covered : what factors indicate that this control room is well-designed ? The furniture, physical factors, the placement of screens, the way commands are handled, the fact that all the data-carriers work in synergy?... In other words, the fact that the user has been kept in mind at all times. Proof before your eyes!
- After-sales service dispatching unit.
  Making changes to the workspace, adjusting working hours, adapting equipment : these are all welcome improvements. But they are not alway enough. Point covered : once information technology has been adapted to simplify worker's tasks, the software also needs to be adapted to serve the same end. Badly-adapted software can create more problems than it solves!
- Contribution by Mrs Annie Drouin.
  Essential point : ergonomics acts as an "interface" between the operator, who is confronted each day with specific requirements, and the designer, who is not always fully aware of these requirements.
- Car production line.
  Here, the computer monitors the tests carried out on each vehicle at the end of the production line. The use of computer systems establishes a reliability factor and guarantees the overall quality of the finished product. As such, the task of the operator is optimised, but his scope

for initiative is virtually non-existent. The underlying question is : what part does the worker play in the finished product? Reducing the intellectual content of the job does not necessarily increase the worker's involvement...

- Coffee roasting factory.
  The computer does not always have all the information needed at its disposal, particularly as a large proportion of this information is subjective and can only be assessed by people, e.g. taste, colours, shapes, etc. Point covered : ergonomics cuts across the observations of a wide variety of disciplines and each case is different.

FILM 2 : OFFICE WORK

- Inside a government office.
  Point covered : the introduction of information technology, a rearrangement of the workspace or the installation of a new workspace are ideal occasions to launch a detailed ergonomic study. The picture shows us a "before and afer" situation : the particular focus of this analysis. There is praise for certain software manufacturers who have realised that the ergonomic aspect of their products are a major advantage ... not least from a commercial point of view!
- Contribution by Mrs Annie Drouin, ergonomist at the EDF.
  Essential point : ergonomics acts as an "interface" between the operator, who is confronted each day with specific requirements, and the designer, who is not always fully aware of these requirements.
- Inside a bank.
  Another resounding success : this bank has perfected (by changes to software, screens and workspaces, among others) a "made-to-measure" training, allowing each of its employees to benefit from training designed to suit them. Other point covered : the importance of being able to carry out the same task using various different procedures : the idea of cross-checking information, tailoring the work to the workers.
- Inside a telephone exchange.
  A new computerised switchboard for dealing with telephone enquiries : 10,000 calls a day. Highly successful from the point of view of the arrangement of the physical working environment, the lay-out of the workspace, etc. In 95% of cases, the computer has replaced the traditional phone book... even so, 5% of calls still cannot be categorised. Point covered : the software has still to be adapted to the new system, in the first place so that it corresponds to actual working methods, but above all so that it corresponds to the way in which customers formulate their enquiries.
- Contribution by Mrs Annie Drouin.
  Point : one of the aims of ergonomics is to make sure

people no longer feel they are controlled by computers, but are themselves in control...

- The trading room of a financial institution.
  Every day, foreign exchange dealers carry out financial transactions involving hundreds of millions of francs... Point covered : improved systems of communication, the increasing range of information sources available and the ability of the computer to integrate information make it possible to reduce both uncertainties and the mental input of the operator. Even so, it is up to the dealer to make the right decision at the right time. The user still remains the centre of the system.
- Public transport system.
  An operational support service was established serveral years ago on a number of bus routes in a European capital. The aim of this system is to help cope with the growing density of urban traffic and to provide real-time management of the routes. Point covered : the fact that the system is interactive not only increases the participation of drivers in the management of their route - while reducing the uncertainties of their job - but il also enables all the other users to benefit.
- In an architect's office.
  There are now programmes for "plan processing" (drafting complete architectural plans on computer) as opposed to the more usual "word processing" found elsewhere. This involves numerous advantages both for the architects and his clients. Point covered : the attractiveness of software developed and manufactured with transparency and userfriendliness in mind. Conlusion of EC Directives requiring that "...the software must conform to the task it is being used for, must be simple to use and able to be adapted to the level of knowledge or experience of the user".

TO SUM UP :

The aim of ergonomics is to match working conditions - and tools - to people, and not the other way around. Means : studying, analysing each case in detail from all angles. Result : people are no longer controlled by computers, but are themselves (once more) in control.

(Distributed by DISC, rue du Marteau 26, B-1040 Brussels - Tel. 2/218.58.85. - Fax 2/217.29.02.)

WORK WITH DISPLAY UNITS 92
H. Luczak, A. Çakir and G. Çakir (Editors)

ACCESS TO COMPUTERS WITH GRAPHIC USER-INTERFACES FOR THE BLIND:

J. Frank, FRANK AUDIODATA, P.O.Box 1161, D-68790 Oberhausen, GERMANY

A progress report on a seemingly paradoxical Project

ABSTRACT: A description of "classical" methods to make PCs accessible for the blind is followed by details about our "TASO" or "AudioScreen", allowing them for the first time to work efficiently with 2-dimensional structures like spread-sheets. The problem with new "GUI-type" software and our current efforts to solve it, the "VISA-project", is portrayed.

1. Who are we? - A brief introduction

FRANK AUDIODATA, a company with today 65 employees, develops, produces and sells PC-based workstations for the blind and partially sighted. Founded in 1981, the first PC-systems were installed in the autumn of 1984. We have by now installed about 2.000 computers for the visually impaired in Germany, the UK, BeNeLux, Scandinavia, Switzerland, the USA and many other countries. The founder and sole owner, H.-Joachim Frank, has himself been blind during early childhood and today he is partially sighted. Additionally, 7 employees are visually impaired. This has naturally lead to very pragmatic and relevant concepts. One of our main aims is integration, which we ourselves daily practise at work.

2. Computer access for the blind, applications and users

A typical configuration is a standard PC connected to a speech-synthesiser or Braille-display with special adaptive software. As PCs become ever more available, for desk- or lap-top usage, and as they can easily be interfaced to almost all host computers by means of "emulations", they are the de-facto standard. The users constitute a wide variety: students, typists, telephone operators, programmers, lawyers, judges as well as highly qualified office-workers, physiotherapists (they have office-work too!), scientists and administrators...

3. Classic computer access methods: the screen-reader program

Leaving aside specialised software for the blind, it becomes necessary to make a PC-screen accessible with synthetic speech in a common manner for all "normal" application-programs that are in "text-mode" (i.e. no graphics!). The most often realised way to do this is a "screen-reader-program" that puts - on user-command - the screen-text or certain parts of it out to a speech-synthesiser including text-to-speech conversion. The screen-reader runs "in the background" (i.e. quasi-parallel) to the application (e.g. a word-processor) and has no screen-output of its own, but just monitors the screen-content of the application-program.

This seems to be a simple and elegant solution, but it has at least one severe drawback: one needs an extreme capability of abstraction and good short- as well as long-term memory to work it successfully. Commands that are implemented are of the following type: where am I? (line/column), where is the cursor? read a line, move up/down one line, move left/right one word, spell current word, mark current column for later reference (tables!) and so on... It is difficult to imagine the problems of navigating around "in the dark" on a computer-screen with a few keystrokes, especially when the same keyboard is used for this as well as the application-program (switching from "operating" to "listening-mode" is necessary!). This makes acceptance very low for many potential users. We therefore undertook the task of finding a better solution in 1982, after having started with "special software" and later implementing and testing an early "screen-reader".

4. The breakthrough: TASO and AudioScreen

In 1983 we were granted patents on our TASO-principle (T_actile A_coustic S_creen O_rientation). Briefly described, it combines spatial representation with orientation-tones and directly controlled synthetic speech. The most visible elements of this are two sliding keys, one vertically oriented and to the left of the computer-keyboard, the other slider running horizontally below the SPACE-bar of the keyboard.

These two sliders, the vertical "Line-Slider" and the horizontal "Column-Slider" give a direct access with absolute X/Y-positions to the (typically) 25 lines and 80 columns of the computer-screen. When moved, the line-slider seems to "generate" one tone for every line it is passing over, and the user can immediately distinguish empty lines (=high beeps) from lines containing information (=lower tones). Also, the cursor-line is clearly discernible by a specific "buzz", and the frequency of the tones for full lines are in groups repeated every 5 lines. The column-slider "gives out" tones when moved horizontally. Here also, a high beep denotes "empty here" (i.e. a SPACE), and there are specific tones for capitals / small letters / digits / other symbols like punctuation and the cursor. All this is hard to imagine, but it sure is easy in practice right from the start! The orientation is learned nearly subliminally, and the tones - as they correlate with movements of the hand - are acquired by unexperienced users very quickly. Large tone-intervals ensure that a "musical ear" is really not needed.

Thus far we have only described the orientation. The control is straight-forward: pressing the line-slider will start the readout of the selected line, stopping when the sliding key is released. If the column-slider is positioned on a SPACE, pressing it will start speaking the rest of the line (to the right of the selected column), or the word "in which" the column-slider is positioned will be spelled out.

All this gives an excellent direct screen-access, and even working with typically 2-dimensional structures (e.g. tables) and indented text is very easy with the TASO. That gave us the idea to name the whole hardware/software-system connected with it the "AudioScreen", because for blind people it is a true substitution for a video screen.

It is impossible to describe here all the details of operation that we have added during our years of experience. It should, however, be noted briefly that we often employ two other media complementary to audio, also under TASO-control: Braille-displays for the blind and "large print", a screen-magnification for people with residual eyesight.

5. The big new problem: GUI-software

All techniques mentioned above require that THE COMPUTER HAS TO WORK IN "TEXT-MODE"! Up to 1991, this has been the most widely used so far as real work (i.e. no games) was involved, of course with the exception of typical graphic applications like CAD, which are not relevant for the visually impaired anyway. Today, no access exists for the visually impaired to new GUI-software, greatly endangering their integration at work! GUIs ("Graphic User Interfaces", meaning e.g. windows, icons, menus and pointing devices) make it much easier to use computers without having to learn complex commands, as everything is presented in a very obvious manner -OBVIOUS TO THE SIGHTED! It is no understatement to argue that there is a real danger of a rapid "de-integration" of blind and partially sighted computer users and users of devices with computer-equivalent output that will abound in the future as long as "THE GUI-PROBLEM" is not solved. THE VISUALLY IMPAIRED STAND NOT ONLY TO STAGNATE, BUT TO LOOSE GROUND IN THE MODERN WORK- AND ALSO EVERYDAY-ENVIRONMENT !

Since 1984 (the first "MAC"), we became aware of this GUI-access problem and went to great length keeping in touch with top research, reviewing our ideas and recently starting experiments with our TASO in a GUI-context. We achieved positive results in this preliminary phase and thus started our European R&D-activities:

6. VISA - An EEC-funded project to get GUI-access for the blind

The VISA (=Video-Interface & -Signal Analysis)-project aims at a general solution for this problem as defined in the EEC-TIDE work plan (TIDE=Technology for the Integration of Disabled and Elderly persons). VISA uses a subset of robotic vision for smart screen translation plus a modification of our TASO / AudioScreen. VISA uses a high-throughput processor and intelligent image-and structure processing to analyse the screen and extract the relevant information for the blind user. The human eye-brain-system and its perception, analysis and processing of screen-information as well as intuitive and established rules used in GUI- programming can help to create an interactive man / machine model.

7. Proposed approaches to date: design of specific "bridge-software"

A simple way to get around most of the problems seems to be a program to intercept the interaction between the user program -e.g. a word processor or spreadsheet package- and the GUI. Here is an example: A currently widely used GUI is "WINDOWS 3.1" by

Microsoft. Any programmer wishing to create applications running under Windows 3.1 can acquire a special software-"Tool Kit". This specifies all the functions, sub-programs and necessary pointers to interact in a correct way with WINDOWS 3.1. By the same token, using the same definitions, it should be possible to write a "bridge-software" to give the necessary (text-type) information e.g. to speech-synthesisers, Braille displays etc., creating a quick and relatively low-cost solutions for a limited range of applications. It may work for certain "nicely-programmed" packages, but this surely is a miscalculation. The situation gets clearer from the negative side: there would be the necessity for a multitude of packages and versions, not functioning with many application programs, a need for frequent updates. To stay with our example: assumed the bridge-software is a solution for some useful applications under WINDOWS 3.1... What about X-Windows (UNIX), Presentation Manager (OS/2) and all those other GUI-interfaces coming along in the future? What about other systems like the MAC or Workstations? What about programs using WINDOWS 3.1 but not confirming to the "Tool Kit"-standards (like Microsoft's own EXCEL, programmed "non-standard" to make it run faster...)? What even about a small change - let us say to WINDOWS X.Y probably "not quite compatible"? This is an endless task!

8. A better solution: an interface using the video signal - "VISA"

After reviewing the situation over and over again since 1984, we concluded that only a radical approach could help here: an intelligent "robot" to look at the video screen, describe the possible inputs or choices to the visually impaired user, and also relieve them of the task of "mouse-navigation"... Cameras are not needed, because every computer has some form of video-outlet, even small Notebooks are able to connect to an external monitor. This situation will probably stay the same for the next 15 to 20 years, even if there will be ever higher resolutions. Manipulators are also not needed with the VISA-"robot", because a mouse does not have to be moved physically, but can be simulated through an RS-232-connection from the VISAcomp to the host.

The elementary questions of user access were - in our opinion - very often wrongly put: WHAT should be the right USER-INTERFACE ? All sorts of multi modal-, 2D- and 3D- interfaces have been written about without ever seeing the real need: getting the information out of the application- or host-system without having to mess with the software inside it and then converting it into a manageable form for the visually impaired.

The most complex part of this chain between the applications computer and the user is the VISAcomp (=VISA computer) with it's OCR- and pattern recognition software and fast data-reducing hardware. Besides or in addition to the AudioScreen (TASO), other adaptations like Braille displays can of course also be connected to VISAcomp.

9. TASO, AUDIOSCREEN and the GUI-environment

It is now clear that the TASO or AudioScreen could provide excellent results in a GUI-context, the reasons being:

1. the two sliders allow a sort of "active eye movement" very well suited to the exploration of unknown screen-layouts. Of course, this is mainly useful in tutorial situations or when the user is not yet well acquainted with the structure of the program he works with. In a "Fast Interaction-Mode", the window opening up e.g. in a corner of the screen has to produce direct speech (or braille) output, without recourse to the sliders, but whenever track is lost or unusual situations occur, even for the expert user the TASO is a great help.
2. the sliders can be and already are used in certain applications to select items, effectively "clicking on a position with the mouse", which is a great part of current GUI-interaction.
3. the tonal feedback from the TASO allows very fast, 2-dimensional search for "priority areas" (the attribute of "priority" or "importance" is of course a matter to be decided by the analytical and interpretative work of the VISAcomp in translating the GUI-type screen into a readable format for a visually impaired person. An example for this would be a blue window on a generally red screen, and within the window there is a yellow menu-bar. Here "priority" would be given first to the menu-bar, then to the window and last to the rest of the screen.
4. there is a very convenient way of distinguishing "real text " and "meta-text" on the TASO-driven AudioScreen. If VISAcomp has been given the word "delete" to denote an icon resembling a waste bin, that word will be represented simply as one point on the screen with a very different "icon-beep" discriminating it from "real text" on the screen.

10. The VISAcomp software: modelling the "screen-eye-brain chain"

First, the video data stream is considerably reduced by a so-called VISAboard. It is granted that not every screen of the 60 to 100 per second does need evaluation, but still, with all it's OCR- and pattern-recognizing capabilities, the VISA-software is a real challenge. The VISAcomp-software does and can not provide first-time interpretation of icons. It has to be trained, i.e. words are attached to icons when they first appear. Of course, a user of VISA will get the "collective experience" from several different GUI-environments in the system, and the amount of icon-knowledge will grow with use and also by updates. In any case, a user who is partially sighted can get an enlarged image of an unknown icon and "name it" himself, a blind user must ask a sighted person for help if a totally new icon is encountered.

11. Conclusion:

We think that the chance to develop an intelligent screen-interpreter for the blind and partially sighted is now here, and the splitting of the task into the VISAboard (data reduction), the VISAcomp (screen analysis) and the TASO / AudioScreen (interface to the blind user) is the right way to go about it. Detection of priorities and context-dependent interaction is now realisable, and we are doing just that now.

WORK WITH DISPLAY UNITS 92
H. Luczak, A. Çakir and G. Çakir (Editors)

Computer-assisted Rehabilitation (CURE)

Yvonne Bosilj and Alexander Trubetzkoy

Siemens Nixdorf Informationssysteme AG, Project "Computers help curing", Dreizehnmorgen-weg 46, 5300 Bonn 2, Germany

Abstract
The project "Computers help curing" deals with the computer-assisted rehabilitation after cranial-cerebral traumas; which is a range of applications to benefit the motorial handicapped. Due to cranial-cerebral traumas after injuries caused by accidents in the household, during road traffic or at sports activities, many individuals are taken out of their professional life. In most cases the way to a professional reintegration may be long and difficult.
The subject of the following pages will be the description of this way as well as the supporting possibilities by means during the rehabilitation and the professional integration.

1. Application of Computers in the Medical sector

Computers have been made use of in medical science for quite some time already; in the somatic sector, e.g. for the computer tomography, and in the psychological-neurological sector for the examination of psychological and neurological malfunctions. A further and relatively new means of applying computers at the therapeutical as well as post-therapeutical phase in connection with the rehabilitation of cognitive functional disturbances or disorders.

2. Functional Disorders and disturbances

These disorders mainly involve effects of a cranial or cerebral trauma after injuries due to accidents in the household, road traffic or during sports as well as cerebral tumors, apoplexies or infections.

The project "Computers help curing" focuses on the rehabilitation of functional breakdowns having been triggered by a cranial-cerebral trauma. In this connection, the following functional disorders may occur:

- Aphasia (disturbances of the speech functions in the widest sense and in various degrees of severity)

- Dyslexia (reading and writing disturbances)
- Dysmnesia (verbal and/or visual, short-term memory, long-term memory)
- Disorders of the attention and concentration
- Perception disturbances (visual, auditive and tactile)
- Impairment of the spatial orientation
- Impairment of reaction and reaction readiness
- Disorders related to the interaction of various functions (visual-motoric co-ordination, considering, planning, acting etc.)
- Loss of cultural skills and technologies (school knowledge; skills having been obtained by training and education)
- Disorders of large parts of motoricity

3. Diagnostics

There will be no uniform diagnostical pattern in the case of a cranial-cerebral trauma. The breakdowns depend on the type and severity of the area affected and arise individually extremely seldom only. There is much more frequently to be assumed, a combined breakdown of the various neuro-psychological function areas.

The first diagnostic step consists of the detection of the involved disorders or disturbances by means of test based psychological logopedic and pedagogic examinations, ergotherapeutical and professional stress tests. The target is the initiation of a specific and concerted training process concerning the breakdowns detected.
In the early phase, the therapeutic approach cannot yet cover the treatment of individual performance disturbances, but must preferably treat the complex breakdowns existing at that time.

4. Therapy

The therapeutic approach in this phase includes the motivation of the patient to render possible access to the memory of the past still existing , i. e. to the memory of past events. Functional exercises, approaches to speaking, communication and behaviourism training are carried out parallel therewith.

Although an astonishing number of successful results has been achieved with the methods described, specific problems arise in some cases, particularly in connection with patients who, due to their distinct motoric disorders, are not in a position to carry out reasonable complicated movements with their extremities so that they can only be therapeutically treated to a rather insufficient degree.

A further problem consists of the illness-related low motivation of the patients. An intensification of the restricted motivation takes place by the rather children-like arrangement and make-up of the working media. The training tasks of the early rehabilitation period are mostly derived from the special school paedagogics and are conceived and made up of correspondingly. However this make-up can be hindrance for the rehabilitation of adults.

5. Application of Computers in the Rehabilitation Sector

At the suggestion of Mrs. Hannelore Kohl, the president of the "KURATORIUM ZNS für Unfallverletzte mit Schäden des zentralen Nervensystems" (CURATORY ZNS for Accidentally Injured with damage to the Central Nervous System/CNS), which has set itself the task as a non-profit and charitable organisation, the rehabilitation promotion of accident victims with cranial-cerebral injuries and which was founded in 1983, there was established the project "Computers help curing" in co-operation with the neurological hospital Hessisch Oldendorf of the Association of German Cerebrally Injured and the company Nixdorf Computers (now Siemens Nixdorf Informationssysteme AG). It is their target to solve the problems, having arisen during the execution of the therapeutic rehabilitation, by means of specially developed and manufactured hardware and software.

In the first phase, special keyboards were developed which render possible quick access to the cognitive cerebral performance training for the patients in spite of the severe motoric restrictions which do not allow them to command and control the usual training means (positioning trainer, paper and pencil tasks). For example large-panel keyboards for patients with essential motorial disorders, keyboards which can be operated with head or mouth bars, foot-operated keyboards, split type two-panel keyboards to be fastened to both sides of a wheelchair in order to compensate an essentially restricted field of movement. With a total of 15 special keyboards and various accessories such as stroke deceleration, distance plates, stands and tripods etc., most restrictions and limitations can be compensated. The special keyboards allow the training in an early phase already where writing or drawing tasks are impossible to fulfill due to the distinct disturbances.

Computer training programms suitable for the cognitive therapy were developed at the same time. Various programms allow the training of cognitive functions such as perception, memory, concentration, logic etc. A notable motivation increase has been achieved by the adultoriented design of the programms. The existing breakdowns can be better compensated, because both the patient and the therapist can choose and determine the learning rate. Each type of task can be further individualized by the determination of various parameters so as to adapt the learning velocity to the specific requirements. As compared with printed learning means and material, the possibility of differentiated learning aids and specific acknowledgements of the results yields an essential enlargement of the spectrum.

Patients with severe concentration, perception or memory disturbances are able to process a larger scope of tasks, as would be possible in the therapy without computer assistance. The computer-assisted therapy enables a quick change of methods and media in the course of one treatment unit so that the quickly arising fatigue and the low mental stressing capability of patients with cranial-cerebral injuries can be improved.

The most handicapped patient enjoys a substantial experience of success an account of his training on the computer which would have been denied him in part, in the event of other task settings.

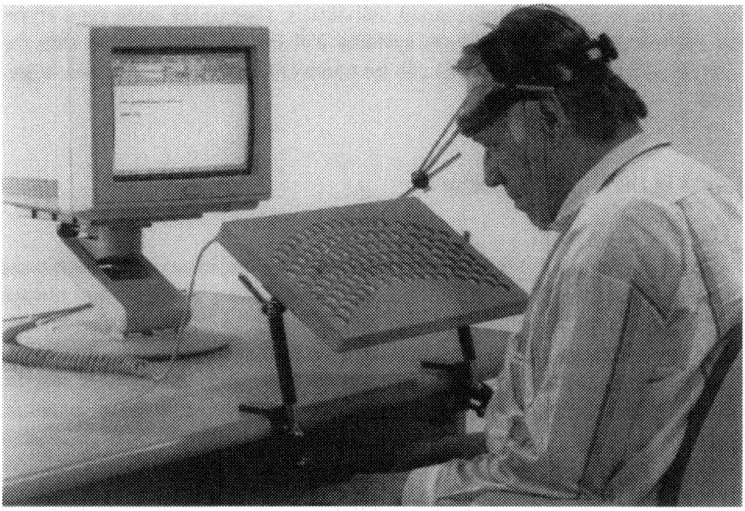

6. Preparation of the Professional Integration

Subsequent to the early rehabilitation, there will take place the preparation for the professional reintegration. The relevant computer programms must be designed in form of an accurately matched concept. Apart from the training of individual neuro-psychological functions that are now possible, one focus concentrates on the cultural techniques (mathematics, German, general knowledge, geography, specialized knowledge and proficiency).
Also helpful is the installation of a model office at the clinic or hospital where the workflow of a real enterprise can be simulated. Here, the patients can learn and train in such subjects as invoicing, placing of orders, handling and execution, bookkeeping etc., with the aid and under the supervision of the therapist.
The cognitive training takes place along with the handycraft training (joinery, metal working etc.).

7. Professional Integration

In spite of all therapeutic measures, the motoric disturbances of the patients frequently cannot be fully eliminated. This aggravates the professional integration in post-therapeutic phase. Irrespective of remaining motoric disabilities, the application of special keyboards, particularly designed and matched to such disabilities, in combination with suitable retraining methods renders possible a professional reintegration at a computer workplace (e.g. in the commercial sector, as an employee in charge of defined matters, as a programmer).
As most office workplaces are equipped with computers, there will be numerous possibilities of establishing workplaces for motorially handicapped individuals. Due to the open-type architecture of the special keyboards, special computer systems will not be necessary so that the existing equipment can be utilized. The keyboards can be connected to PCs, UNIX and large-scale computer systems.

8. Computer Assistance in the Domestic Sector

Apart from the professional integration, life in the domestic or household environment places requirements for the handicapped with a restricted motoric coordination which cannot always fully be met in spite of a handicapped-compatible living space. The computers can also be reasonably made use of in this sector by taking over multifold control and monitoring functions. With the environmental control system MULTIKOM, up to 256 electrical devices can be controlled and monitored via the computer (electrical door openers, electrical window openers, rouleau control, operation of the lighting system etc.). Particulary in the case of restricted movability, it is of advantage when the major part of the required electrical in-house functions can be operated from a central workplace.

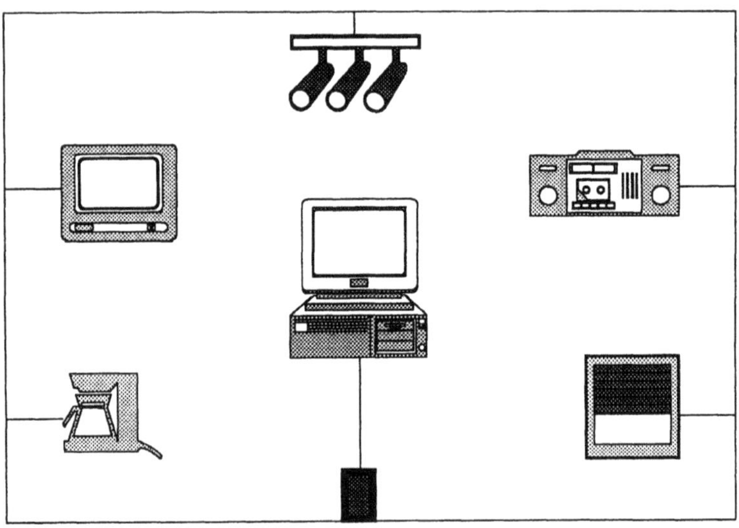

9. Prospects

The experience having been gathered since the beginning of the project "Computers help curing" five years ago shows that the assistance by computers for handicapped people presents an appropriate and necessary enlargement of the existing measures both in the rehabilitation phase and in the post-rehabilitative sector. The possibilities of application presented within the framework of this paper are only a beginning of the assistance. In the future, too, the co-operation of the KURATORIUM ZNS with the rehabilitation hospitals and the company Siemens Nixdorf Informationssysteme AG will provide new application possibilities of computers for the compensation of disabilities.

For further informations, please contact:
Siemens Nixdorf Informationssysteme AG
Projekt "Computer helfen heilen"
Dreizehnmorgenweg 46
D-5300 Bonn 2
Telephone: (0228) 303-0

WORK WITH DISPLAY UNITS 92
H. Luczak, A. Çakir and G. Çakir (Editors)

The Effects of System Response Time on Directory Assistance Operator Worktime

Jody E. McCain

Bellcore, 435 South Street, Room 1A345, Morristown, New Jersey 07960 USA
(author now at: Bell Atlantic NSI, 1310 N. Courthouse Rd, 4th Fl., Arlington, VA 22201)

Abstract

Directory assistance operators provide telephone numbers to customers who supply the names of businesses or individuals. In this study operators answered simulated requests for directory assistance under varied levels of system response time. System response time was defined as the interval between the subject's depression of the database search key to the beginning of the painting of the computer screen. System response time was varied from .1 to 3.7 seconds, in intervals of .4 second. Average worktime per call was the dependent measure of the operator's performance. Average worktime increased by .4 second with each .4 second increase in response time. There was no effect of system response time on operator accuracy.

1. INTRODUCTION

An important consideration in the design and evaluation of computer systems is the effect of system response time on the users' productivity. System response time is defined as the time interval between when the user requests an action of the computer to when the computer responds with the requested feedback. Several laboratory and field experiments have manipulated system response time with varied results (Butler, 1984; Dannenbring, 1984; Martin & Corl, 1986; Thadhani, 1984). One commonly-held explanation for the variation in results is that system response time effects depend upon the nature of the task.

Directory assistance operators respond to requests from customers for information regarding telephone listings. An operator must obtain the appropriate information from the customer, type it into the retrieval system, scan the listings that are returned from the directory assistance database, and select an appropriate telephone number. The task of a directory assistance operator is repetitive with a short cycle time. The system response time of the database query request of the telephone operator can be as much as 15% of the total cycle time. Based on both the lack of a clear predictive theory for system response time and the need for generic requirements for new telephone operator systems, it was important to determine the effect of system response time on the task of the directory assistance operator.

This experiment was designed to determine, "how system response time effects a directory assistance operator's efficiency." System response time was defined as the time from which the operator depressed the search key (business or residence) until the listings began to paint the screen. Productivity was defined as the total worktime necessary for the directory assistance operator to listen to the customer request, key in the appropriate information, scan the database listings on the screen and choose the corresponding target listing if it is present or key appropriately if it is absent.

A secondary objective of the study was to verify a previous study (Springer, 1987) which found that directory assistance operators take longer to scan the screen and to find the target listing, with more information displayed on the screen. It was desirable to confirm this finding for two reasons. First, confirmation of this finding would add validity to the recommendation that operators key more to narrow down the amount of listings the database returns to the operator's screen. Second, the ability to verify the finding would add validity to the simulated directory assistance task and the experimental procedure used in this study.

2. METHOD

2.1. Subjects

Ten Directory Assistance operators from the New York Telephone Madison Directory Assistance Bureau participated. They were chosen by their management under the following criteria: each operator had at least one year's service and was rated as a satisfactory performer at the time of the study.

2.2. Apparatus

The experiment ran on the Operator Services Laboratory Simulator (OWLS), an IBM PS2-based directory assistance simulator. The PS2 emulated an IBM directory assistance system in both the input screen format and the listing screen format. Actual listing screens from the IBM Indianapolis, Indiana database were collected and used in the simulator. The IBM PS2 QWERTY keyboard, equipped with custom IBM directory assistance keycaps, was used to input data into the simulator. Both statistical and timing data was gathered by the IBM PS2. The particular target selected was also collected as a measure of accuracy.

Customer recordings were made from scripts read by volunteers, following the format of actual customer requests. A variety of voices, accents and background were used for to produce a realistic sound. The recordings were stored on an optical disk to enable the subject to work an entire shift of 1000 calls. They were able to request additional replays of the customer recording if they wished. Customer requests were divided into two basic types; business and residence. The percentage of calls by call type was empirically derived. Subjects wore monaural headsets and were allowed to manipulate the audio level of the voice playback within three preset levels.

The screens were of three different lengths: quarter, half or full. Additionally, the target appeared either in the top quarter, the second quarter or the bottom half of the screen. A random number generator was used to determine the target placement for each of the screens within the appropriate condition. These conditions of screen size and target placement were counterbalanced across the 1000 calls and system response time conditions described in Section 3.2. There also were a specified number of calls that did not have the customer requested listing present. These calls are known as *no finds*. The percentage of *no finds* used in this study was 18%. The *no finds* were also counterbalanced across call type and screen size.

The calls and screens were arranged into 10 blocks of 100 calls each. The assignment of calls to a particular block was random within the constraints of call type, screen size and target placement. The screen "painting" of listings appeared instantaneous. The time between each call was specified as .10 seconds.

3. PROCEDURE

3.1. Experimental task and training

Each subject was told that they would be performing the directory assistance job with a simulator. Subjects were told that the purpose of the experiment was to test the operation of the simulator and how they, as operators, interacted with the simulator. The subject's task was to listen to the customer's request, decide what to key to obtain the listing, key what they had decided, choose whether it was a business or residence listing, scan the screen for the customer request and choose the target if it was present. It was necessary to key only four letters of the requested information: the first four letters of the last name of a residence listing and the first four letters of the first major word in a business listing. Following the keying of the four letters, the operator depressed either the business or residence key. If a listing was not obtained on the first search, it was considered a *no find*. The subjects were asked to work as fast as they could while keeping errors to a minimum.

Subjects were instructed on the use of the simulator, including hardware, keying procedures and format of the listing screens. Following the verbal training period, subjects took practice calls until they were comfortable with the system and the keying procedures. This training period lasted about 15 minutes. The experimenter was available to the subject during the entire experiment, and the subject was told that they could ask questions at anytime during the experiment.

3.2. Experimental Variables

There were two within-subject variables manipulated in this experiment. The first variable was system response time. All subjects experienced the 10 levels of system response time which were .1, .5, .9, 1.3, 1.7, 2.1, 2.5, 2.9, 3.3, and 3.7 seconds.

The second within-subject variable was a combination of the two screen-formatting factors. The first was the amount of information on the screen and the second was the position of the target on the screen. The six levels of this combination variable were as follows: 1. quarter screen (5 lines) with the target listing appearing within lines 1-5; 2. half screen (10 lines) with the target appearing within lines 1-5; 3. half screen with the target appearing within lines 6-10; 4. full screen (20 lines) with the target appearing within lines 1-5; 5. full screen with the target appearing within lines 6-10; and 6. full screen with the target appearing within lines 11-20.

A Graeco-Latin 10 x 10 square design was used to counterbalance the order effects of both system response times and the blocks of screen listings with the purpose of minimizing practice and fatigue effects.

3.3. Working Conditions

Subjects worked within their normal office conditions at a separate desk with the simulation equipment. They worked their customary hours and took their standard breaks, a half-hour lunch and two 15-minute breaks (before and after lunch).

4. RESULTS

Statistical analyses were performed on each operator's average worktime. These average worktimes, shown in Table 1, were analyzed in a two-way repeated measure (10 x 6) analysis of variance (ANOVA). The average worktime means do not include data from the *no finds* condition nor the error data. These data were analyzed separately. A statistically reliable main effect of system response time was found, F (9, 540) = 12.11, p < .01, such that average worktime clearly increased as system response time increased. A second significant effect was found for the screen format variable, F (5, 540) = 11.89, p < .01. Planned comparisons revealed that average worktime increased as the amount of information on the screen increased and as the target position moved down the screen. It is also true that when the target remained constant (whether it was in the top quarter or the middle of the screen), adding more listings beyond the target also increased average worktime. The interaction did not reach statistical significance.

A trend analysis was performed on the system response time variable to see to what extent a linear expression accounted for the data. It was found that a linear expression accounted for 96% of the variance in the data.

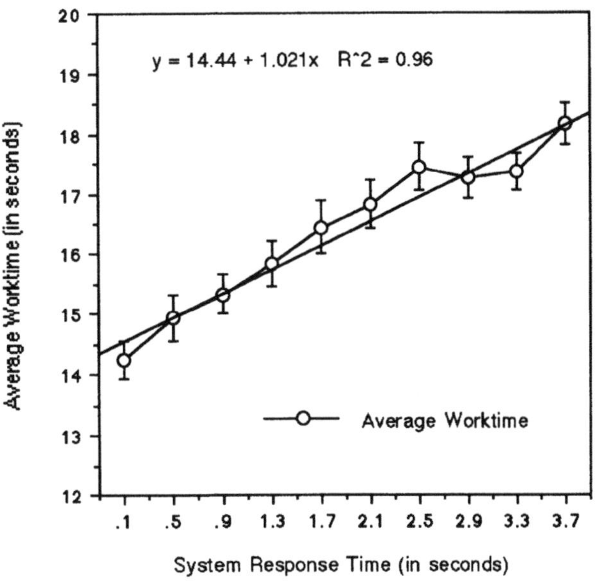

Figure 1. Average worktime as a function of system response time.

A separate 2-way ANOVA was performed on the 18% of the calls that were defined as *no finds*. Again the system response time was a within-subject variable. Since there was no target present, the second variable was solely the amount of information on the screen; quarter, half or full. The results of the *no find* analysis followed the same pattern as those reported above. A significant main effect of system response time was found, F (9, 239) = 2.31, p < .01. Once again, average worktime increased as system response time increased. Screen size was also statistically significant, F (2, 239) = 38.75, p < .01, such that average worktimes increased as the amount of information on the screen increased. The interaction did not reach statistical significance. The trend analysis revealed that 67% of the variance in the *no find* data could be accounted for by a linear expression. Error rates were examined separately across all of the levels of system response time. No statistically significant differences were found.

At the end of each session the operator was asked to give feedback on the simulator. Two out of the ten subjects commented on the slow system response times and compared the speed of the simulator unfavorably to the speed of their current system.

5. DISCUSSION

The results reveal that discrete system response times have a linear relationship with average worktime in a directory assistance task, such that as the system response time increases or decreases so does average worktime. This finding has significant implications for the design of systems for use in Directory Assistance. An increase or decrease in system response time, brought about by design changes, can be expected to raise or lower operator productivity a similar amount, provided no other significant changes are made.

The significant finding in the size/target combination variable is not surprising. Previous Directory Assistance studies corroborate that the more listings present on the screen the longer it takes the directory assistance operator to find the correct listing. This is most apparent when the target is in the middle or the bottom of a full screen. An average increase in average worktime of approximately 2.5 seconds occurs from when the target is in the first five lines of a quarter screen to when it appears in the middle or bottom of a full screen. This finding along with the more surprising finding that, even when that target is in the top quarter of the screen, additional listings on the screen increase average worktime, highlights the importance of "keying more to see less."

It is important to note, however, that in this experiment system response time was manipulated at discrete levels. In other words, there was no variability in the system response time. Variability refers to the variance associated with the mean delay. For example, the mean delay with a variance of .1 second or 1.0 second. Theory behind the effects of variability of system response time on performance suggests possible detrimental effects because of the unpredictable nature of the system response, although research in other disciplines has failed to support or reject this finding conclusively. A second study has been conducted to answer the question: "What effect does varying the system response time in wide and narrow ranges around several levels of system response time have on average worktime?"

6. REFERENCES

Butler, T.W., (1984). *Computer response time and user performance during data entry.* AT&T Bell Laboratories Technical Journal. 63, 1007-1017.

Dannenbring, G.L., (1984). *System response time and user performance.* IEEE Transactions on Systems, Man, and Cybernetics. SMC-14, 473-478.

Martin, G. L., & Corl, K. G. (1986). *System response time effects on user productivity.* Behavior and Information Technology, 5(1), 3-13.

Springer, C. J. (1987) *Directory assistance screen formats: impact on operators' scanning times.* Bellcore Letter # IL-87/-09/047.

Thadhani, A. J., (1981) *Interactive user productivity.* IBM Systems Journal. 20, 407-423.

FATIGUE
AND
HEALTH HAZARDS

WORK WITH DISPLAY UNITS 92
H. Luczak, A. Çakir and G. Çakir (Editors)

PREVENTION OF VDU-RELATED MUSCULOSKELETAL PROBLEMS; A SHIFT FROM A SPECIALIST'S TO A PARTICIPATORY APPROACH

Ilkka Kuorinka

Institut de Recherche en Santé et en Sécurité du Travail du Québec, 505 boul. de Maisonneuve Ouest, Montréal, Qué., H3A 3C2, Canada

Abstract
The musculoskeletal problems related to VDU work are considered to be commonplace. Their nature as clinically vaguely-defined disorders and the variety of signs and symptoms require new approaches in prevention. The elements of a participatory approach along with the ergonomic improvements of the workplace in the prevention of musculoskeletal problems are presented.

1. MUSCULOSKELETAL PROBLEMS

Work-related musculoskeletal disorders (in the text the acronym WRMD is used for work-related musculoskeletal disorders) are a controversial problem. Some specialists bluntly deny its existence (Hadler, 1990 1), some opinions see it as a socially induced, ephemeral phenomenon (Cleland, 1987 2), whereas others feel that it will be the most important safety and health related problem of working life in the 90's (Fine, 1989 3). A growing consensus is that work-related musculoskeletal problems at work are important and that their prevention is feasible and cost-effective.

VDU-related musculoskeletal problems are less convincing and less clear than those in industry. A consensus seems to exist that neck-shoulder and hand-wrist are the main anatomical locations of VDU-related musculoskeletal problems and that problems can be in some cases serious. The agreement ends here. Some studies have shown a correlation between the strain from working with VDU screens and/or the intensive use of the hands in keying (Guggenbuhl and Krueger, 1989 4), but in other cases such an association has not been found (Fahrbach and Chapman, 1990 5, Bergqvist et al., 1989 6). The Scandinavian researchers have pointed out that the observed association or lack of it may depend on the differences in work load, willingness to take corrective actions when early symptoms appear, work organization, etc.

Several features of the musculoskeletal problems influence the prevention strategy:
- we are dealing with a phenomenon which has a variety of symptoms and which probably has several causal factors (although the repetitive or static load are common immediate causes),
- we are dealing with a problem where the reaction and attitudes of the sufferers modulate the outcome. The classical medical model does not explain these diseases well.

It seems that we have to reject the one-cause-one-outcome model and adopt a risk-factor and/or system model. The risk-factor approach applies well when our understanding of the mechanisms is still limited. The system model helps us to understand the interrelations and dynamics of causal factors when sufficient information on causal factors is available. It seems that we are currently able to understand the situation mainly from the risk-factor point of view, except possibly for hand-wrist repetitive traumas where even quantitative information is beginning to be available.

2. PREVENTION

The model of prevention of WRMDs is usually inspired by the classical medical model: causal factors trigger a pathological process, which eventually reaches a state of an apparent disorder: the host of pathological processes becomes an ill person. The mechanical stresses, forces and repetitive movements are usually considered as necessary and sufficient causes of disorder (Armstrong et al, 1993 7). The preventive actions are mostly inspired by the above models and follow three lines: ergonomic improvement of work stations, improvement of the organizational work factors (job redesign, breaks, time limits for VDU work periods, etc.) and physical activation of workers (increasing physical activity, fitness programs, etc.) (Shephard, 1992 8). All these have been shown to have beneficial effects at least on subjective morbidity.

These usual modes and targets of prevention tend to rely on specialists: ergonomists, safety agents and medical professionals.

While waiting for more solid information on the causal factors of WRMDs and by taking into account the nature of the WRMDs and in the light of the meagre results of prevention in general, a parallel strategy to using specialists only may be appropriate: a participatory approach to prevention. A participatory approach is also a step towards a system model of understanding the WRMDs.

It is interesting to note the results of a Finnish study (Lindstrom, 1991 9) on the implementation of information technology in the banking and insurance fields. The employees were asked about the usefulness of various resource groups for them during the implementation process. A majority of respondents (70%) felt that computer specialists were very important in ensuring good work practices and well-being at work. The corresponding percentage for supervisors was 54%, and for occupational safety and health specialists, 27%.

However, 74% of the respondents felt that they themselves were most important in the implementation of information technology. A cautious interpretation of the results points to the significance of participatory approaches: there seems to be the self-confidence, willingness and capacity to participate in designing one's own work and workplace.

3. PARTICIPATORY ERGONOMICS

In primary prevention, that is, prevention of causes, attention has been paid increasingly to psychosocial factors (i.e., length of task cycles, boredom, low control, poor content of tasks, etc.) and participation as well in its subset, participatory ergonomics. A hypothesis has been proposed that psychosocial factors through various mechanisms, such as stress (Smith, 1987 10) also cause WRMD. In the prevention of WRMDs, participatory ergonomics can be seen as an effective means for achieving psychosocial goals in improving job content, combined with the physical improvements of workplaces.

Reports on participatory approaches in the prevention of WRMDs are not numerous compared to those in an industrial context (Noro and Imada, 1991 11). Most of the reports which deal with VDU's and participation describe representative participation, the activities of safety committees, etc. Only rarely is the focus on the actor, the worker, employee him/herself at work, work organization and the workplace.

4. ELEMENTS OF A PARTICIPATORY ERGONOMIC PROJECT

There are many ways of carrying out participatory ergonomic projects in VDU environment. Each case is unique and different from the others, and also produces different outcomes as shown for participatory projects in general by Cotton et al (1988 12).

There seem to be some elements that increase the probability of success in a participatory project. They can be outlined by two proven procedures.

Sen (1987 13) underlines the need for adapting the approach to the target group. He in fact proposes the use of different approaches for different target groups: quantitative for the technically oriented, strategic for management, and qualitative for workers.

Kogi (1991 14) proposes a six-step procedure to implement changes in workplaces (building on local practice, focus on achievements, linking working conditions and management goals, learning-by-doing, exchange of experience, and promoting worker involvement). Although developed for developing countries, this approach seems to be fully valid in industrialized countries also.

5. CONCLUSION

The participatory approach seems to be a promising way to tackle work-related musculoskeletal problems either to correct an existing situation or to prevent problems at the source. The higher initial costs from training and from implementing a project are usually largely compensated by shorter run-in periods and by more effective use of production tools and better control of work-related musculoskeletal disorders.

1. N.M. Hadler, J.Occup.Med. 32(1990):1,38-41.

2. L.G. Cleland, Med.J.Austr., (1987):147, 236-239.

3. L.J. Fine, NIOSH testimony on repetitive trauma disorders, June 6 (1989).

4. U. Guggenbuhl, H. Krueger, in: Work with Display Units '89, (1989), 121-128.

5. P.A. Fahrbach, L.J. Chapman, J.Am.Ass.Occup.Health, 38(1990):1, 32-36.

6. U. Bergqvist, B. Nilsson, M. Voss, R. Wibom, E. Wolgast, in: Work with Display Units '89, (1989), 1-11.

7. T. Armstrong, P. Buckle, M. Hagberg, L. Fine, B. Jonsson, A. Kilbom, I. Kuorinka, G. Sjogaard, B. Silverstein, E. Viikari-Juntura, Scand.J.Work Environ. Health, (1993), in press.

8. R.J. Shephard, Medicine and Science in Sports and Exercise, 24(1992):3,354-370.

9. K. Lindstrom, Int. J. Human-Computer Interaction 3(1991):4,339-361.

10. M.J. Smith, Behaviour and Information Technology, 6(1987):3, 243-255.

11. K. Noro, A.S. Imada, Participatory Ergonomics (eds.), Taylor et Francis, London, (1991).

12. J.L. Cotton, D.A. Vollrath, K.L. Froggatt, M.L. Lengnick-Hall, K.R. Jennings, Academy of Management Review 13(1988):1, 8-22.

13. T.K. Sen, in: Handbook of Human Factors, G. Salvendy, ed., John Wiley and Sons, (1987), pp. 453-469.

14. K. Kogi, in: K. Noro, A.S. Imada (eds) Participatory Ergonomics, Taylor et Francis, London, 1991, pp. 73-80.

WORK WITH DISPLAY UNITS 92
H. Luczak, A. Çakir and G. Çakir (Editors)

Musculo-skeletal disorder, visual fatigue and psychological stress of working with display units: Current issues and research needs

Choon-Nam Ong

Departmant of Community Medicine, National University of Singapore, Kent Ridge, Singapore 0511, SINGAPORE

Abstract

This paper reviews some of the recent literature concerning musculokeletal disorders, visual and psychological stress of VDU operators. Although the prevalence of musculoskeletal disorder is rising in various countries, the aetiology is still not clear. Debate on this problem usually centres on task related and socio-psychological factors. The problem of visual fatigue tends to link to musculoskeletal complaints and work stress. There is however, no evidence that VDU work would lead to permanent eye damage. VDU workstress is usually arised from either the task itself or owing to socio-psyschological predisposing factors. These issues suggest that multi-disciplinary approach is required to provide more precise and objective methods for evaluating VDU workload. An international collaborative project has been initiated recently to investigate the problems of Musculo-skeletal, visual and strees of VDU operators (MEPS) in various countries. It is hoped that with a multi-disciplinary approach using a more comprehensive approach will systematically identify and address some of these problems so that preventive measures can be taken.

1. INTRODUCTION

Visual display units (VDUs) have now become a common feature in offices, banks, industry and even at home. Today, in many large organizations, such as airlines and banks, the operation of computer terminals has become a full-time job for many workers. They were first used at control panels and display systems in industry, research and military activities. Now the personal computer has brought VDUs into offices and homes. It is the scale of expansion that is new, not VDUs (Lee, 1985).

The development of VDUs and their incorporation into the work environment has been so rapid that it has raised aprehension among the users. How to fit the technology to the work environment thus becomes an important function for many who are concerned with the health of VDU operators.

Numerous studies have suggested that a poorly designed workplace incorporating a VDU can cause a variety of physical and psycho-social problems, including visual fatigue, musculoskeletal problems and stress. This paper summarises some of the current knowledge related to these issues and attempts to suggest some preventive strategies.

2. Musculoskeletal problems and the use of VDUs

Occupational disorders of the musculo-skeletal system are not new. In his published "Treatise on the Diseases of Workers" in 1780, Ramazzini, an Italian physician made reference to workers experience from "certain violent and irregular motions and unnatural postures of the body". The 1893 edition of Gray's Anatomy described a "sausage-shaped swelling" of the hand that it characterised as "washer woman's sprain". Today the names may be different, but the pain/disorder is the same.

From the ergonomics point of view the introduction of VDUs in offices leads to an integration of employees in a man-machine system associated with workloads due to constrained posture, eye strain and psychological problems.

The first report of musculoskeletal discomfort of VDU operators came from Hultgren and Knave (1974). It was found that VDU users, who remained sitting in the same position for long periods of time and paid attention to a specific task were more prone to feelings of tiredness. Many recent studies have also suggested that VDU operators have more health complaints than conventional office workers (WHO, 1986). The symptoms reported were of various types, e.g. pain, stiffness, fatigue, cramps, numbness and tremors. Quite often they would occur in specific parts of the body; with neck, shoulders and arms being some of the more common sites. The symptoms also occurred with varying frequency; daily, occasionally or never (Huntling et al 1981).

The aetiology of these musculoskeletal problems is not clear. Debate on the relationship between musculoskeletal complaints and VDU activity usually centres around the following aspects:

1. Task related factors; the main causes are due to constrained and insufficient posture, frequency of repetitive movement, poor workstation and equipment design, bad task design and increased muscle tension associated with mental load.

2. Non-task related factors; The complaints may be related to bio-demographical elements such as age, previous musculoskeletal injuries, emotional stress family burden or environmental factors.

3. Psycho-social factors; depends on social practices, psyscho-social perception, prevailing imagery about the complaints and others (Jeyaratnam 1992).

It has been shown that the highest incidence of localized musculoskeletal problems is found in jobs involving repetitive keyboard work. The lowest figures are reported among typists engaged in traditional clerical work (Figure 1).

There have been very few studies on chronic muscular disorders among VDU users. In 1980's there was a significant increase in the number of reported RSI cases seen in Australia and is commonly referred to as repetitive strain injuries (RSI). However, musculo-skeletal disorder of this nature has long been a subject of debate. Recent reports from the United States also indicate that there is an increase incidence of strain injuries in users of visual display units. Comprehensive survey cited keyboard operators in occupations related to information and data processing as having the highest risk of injuries. Among some display unit users, the conditions of the musculo-skeletal disorders were so severe that clinical treatment were required, including surgical intervention. The true prevalence of musculo-skeletal disorder among VDU operators is unknown. Prevalence rates from 1% to more than 50% have been quoted in various studies (Silverstein et al 1986).

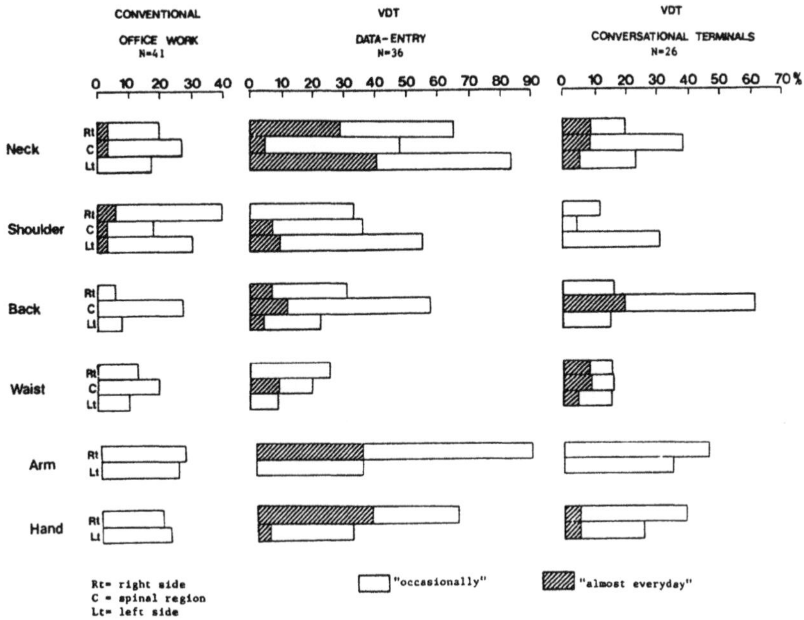

Figure 1. Prevalence of musculo-skeletal complaints among conventional office workers using electronic typewriers, word processing operators and data entry operators using keyboards.

The US Bureau of Labour Statistics has recently showed that claims for repetitive motion disorders or repetitive motion trauma (RMT) suffered by intensive computer keyboard operator has increased remarkably (Table 1). The 1989 figures indicated that RMT is now accounted for more than half of all the job related illnesses. The disorders led to lost in productivity and higher workmen compensations, as well as law suits against computer vendors. This reflects that technological changes could lead to loss in productivity and higher health costs.

In contreast, RSI is relatively unknown outside Australia or US. It could be that the problems are known but there is no epidemic of RSI.

The patho-physiological mechanism underlying musculo-skeletal problems and how it leads to RSI, tenosynovitis and carpal tunnel syndrome are in a large extend still unclear. It is however important to note that perceptions and interpretations of the nature of RSI depend on processes of social negotiation. What is considered an illness is not given solely by nature but is also tied up with current medical practice, prevalent theoretical frameworks, the social system, prevailing imagery about health and disease and so forth (Bammer and Martin, 1988).

Table 1. Number of reported illness in US, 1988 and 1989.

Illness	1988	1989
Total occupational illness	240,000	284,000
Repetitive motion disorders	115,000	147,000

Source: U.S. Bureau of Labour Statistics

The predominant causes of musculo-skeletal disorder or RSI lie in the nature of the work. There are numerous ergonomic factors and others due to unsatisfactory work pattern with too little variation and too high a work rate for too long a time, this is particularly so when workers are on piece work rates. Certainly, it is a matter that warrants urgent attention since far too many computer users are having to suffer pain and inconveniences which should be avoided.

3. Effect of VDU work on the eyes and vision

VDU operators have been shown to have higher prevalence of subjective visual symptoms or distress. Reported prevalences varied, levels between 40-92% for occasional problem to 10-40% for daily complaints. The prevalence varied considerably due to a number of factors related both to the study design and work situation.

The individual eye symptoms noted differ between different studies, but can be separated into two categories: 1) eye being painful, irritated, burning, red, tingling - related to ocular asthenopia symptoms, and 2) vision being blurred, double or flicker - visual symptoms. In most studies, the ocular symptoms were more common than the visual. Higher prevalences were also noted among conversational terminal users than data entry operators. This is because the former need to have their visual attention turned more towards the screen. Most of the recent findings have suggested that work duration, in particular, the total time looking at the screen, may be a primary factor in determining the visual problem. Problems were also noted to be more prominent among workers who had less workplace control, higher work pressure and high job dissatisfaction. Glass wearing VDU operators also tend to report more visual problem than those without lenses (Horgan, 1992). It is possible that incorrect glasses and non-corrected astigmatism may be related to these observations. In older people a correlation was noted between decreased visual acuity and increased visual complaints.

The possibility of permanent eye damage, due to VDU work has been suggested. Considerable debate has been focused at the question of pathological changes of the eyes, acquired myopia has also been figured in recent discussion.

4. Psyschosocial stress of VDU work

There is at present no conclusive evidence that working for long hours with VDUs can cause damage to physical health, but there are indications that prolonged use of VDUs has frequently been associated with complaints of tiredness and other symptoms of stress at work.

4.1 Work Related Factors

Studies have shown that even if all environment and work stations are at their optimum conditions, we still find VDU operators with visual and muscular complaints. Job demands, both physical and psychological could influence the severity, frequency of VDU operators health complaints. It is however, logical to consider that psychological demands can produce physical as well as emotional complaints. Some support for this view is suggested by several major studies on VDU operators (Smith et al, 1987; See also review by Ong et al ,1988). In contrast, the amount of time working at the VDU was not very predictive of the frequency of visual or muscular complaints. While the types VDU work activity was with the more mundane, boring, repetitive VDU jobs showing higher levels of both visual and muscular problem.

The evidence as to whether VDU operators have greater job demands than other occupations is mixed. In most cases, the evidence is confounded by other ergonomic factors, as well as the lack of adequate study designs. Ostberg and Hogberg (1990) found that when VDU operators had little control over job tasks, 72% complained of monotony, while with greater control, only 10% complained of monotony. NIOSH evaluations indicated that clerical VDU operators reported less work involvement, job autonomy, self esteem, supervisor support and peer cohesion with greater work pressure than professional VDU operators (1985). These findings suggest that lower social economic group may feel a higher job stress. The results also showed that job stress factors were highly predictive of health complaints. It appears that job design factors, primarily high paced work, lack of control, and pressures severe as deadlines are more prevalent in VDU works. The recent findings of NIOSH (Sauter et al, 1992) have added new horizon to the growing body of information on the importance of work organization and psychological factors in the etiology of musculo-skeletal problems in VDU work on heavy cognitive or information processing demands. The studies showed that the job risk factors among the VDU operators include heavy work pressure and surges in workload, concers over job security, lack of social support and amount of daily VDU work. Additionally, routine work and heavy information processing demands were common predictors on musculo-skeletal disorders.

4.2 Psychosocial and demographical factors

Two recent studies (Jeyaratnam et al 1989; Ong et al 1991) have taken into consideration that bio-demographics or psychosocial factors may affect the health complaints of VDU operators. Their results demonstrated that working mothers were more pronounced in health problems. The authors believed that the prenatal and perinatal stress may have an effect on their working health, too. These findings revealed that psychosocial factors do play a part in the development of health problem, such indications should be treated with great circumspection.

It was also observed that a significant difference in complaints about musculoskeletal problems was seen among different ethnic groups in Singapore,

(Jeyaratnam, 1992). These differences are likely to reflect the different level of pain perception among different races.

Clearly, occupational and social-psychological factors play an important part in the pathogenesis of the resulting syndrome.

4. Research needs and Preventive strategies

Visual problem and musculo-skeletal disorder are the two most common health complaints among VDU operators. These two problems, which arise from a number of specific factors, can be eliminated or prevented. However, methods of preventing VDU workstress will require an integrated approach involving improved workstation design, a well-scheduled work-rest regime, job design and employee education. One must be awared that this kind of multi-displinary approach will require the use of sound principle; a fundamental change in management philosophy and employees co-operation.

To date, ergonomic intervention strategies which have focused on addressing the risk factors for musculo-skeletal system have met with varying degrees of success (Aaras, 1990;Ong, 1990 and Thomson, 1990). Worker selection and education have been attempted with a small degree of success and effective only to some extent. It can be said that a considerable amount of investigations performed hitherto have failed to provide practical solution towards solving the problem. More attention should be given to the design of the input device (keyboard) to reduce the human effort (musculo-skeletal strain). More care should also be taken to see that workers carrying out repetitive work have a proper work schedule with adequate pauses. The functional components of the task, which is an important feature in man-machine relationship, also need to be carefully researched.

A more objective mean of measuring the muscle load would contribute significantly to assist keyboard manufacturers in better digned input device. The use of portable EMG machine was found to be a reliable and accurate tool for evaluating muscle load (Aaras, 1990), more research are needed to focus on the physiological load and how it affects the performance and well-being of operators are obviously required.

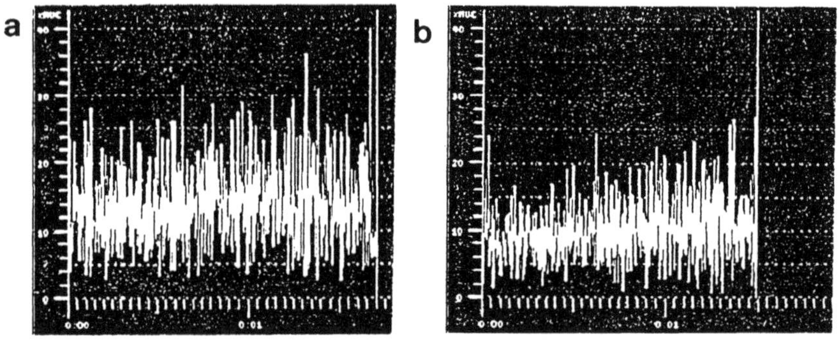

Figure 2. Electromyogram of right tipeza muscle of an operator using a) an electronic type writter and b) an electronic keyboard. Significant differences were noted for the muscle load. (Unpublished data of K.C. Tan and C. N. Ong).

A literature search on musculoskeletal problems related VDU task has indicated that most of the studies were focused on the physical aspect of workplace design and external work load. These elements no doubt are important, but a more comprehensive approach to this problem also requires a better insight on activities within the human components of the man-machine system. It is important to mention that the predominant cause of workstress problems lies in the nature of the work. Thus studies to examine this problem should include determination of excessive muscle activity due to unnecessary tension or poor keyboard design (Figure 2) and bad working posture (Ong et al, 1989). The assessment of musculoskeletal load and its effects would provide worthwhile values of long-term prevention of the problems. What should be the acceptable load on the muscle during prolonged periods? Is there a threshold level for various parts of the muscle involved with keyboard task? Could there be different thresholds for operators of different age? Certainly, study on the causal factors is warranted.

A participative, interventive multidisciplinary team approach that incorporates work design analysis, environmental and equipment modifications to cater for specific local conditions and realities are essential (Dainoff and Cohen, 1992). This approach is expected to improve well-being of the workers and effectiveness of the work.

An international project to investigate the musculo-skeletal, eye and psychological stress (MEPS) was initiated recently to compare health complaints among different VDU work groups in different countries. This multi-country study hopes to investigate the performance and well-being of the VDU operators under an optium working condition through ergonomic intervention (Shahnavaz and Johansson, 1992). This is an important step forward. It is heartening to learn that several countries in Europe, Asia and America will be participated in this research programme. A multi-disciplinary approach with professional skill is what we all need to suceed. Further work is obviously required to delinate the precise musculo-skeletal and visual conditions in relation to keyboard work so that preventive measures may be taken by both the equipment designers and the users.

REFERENCES

Aaras, A. Load related musculoskeletal illness:Is ergonomic workplace design a sufficient remedy? In:Work Design in Practice, ed. by C.M. Haselegrave, J.R. Wilson, E.N. Corletts and I. Manenica, Taylor & Francis. London.(1990)

Bammer G. Review of current Knowledge-Muscouloskeletal problems. Work with Display Units 89. In: Berlinguet L. and Berthelette D.(eds) Elsevier. p.113.(1990)

Bammer G and Martin B . The agruments about RSI: An examination. Commu. Hth. Studies 12(1988):348-352.

Dainoff M. and Cohen B. A participative approach to ergonomic intervention:Egronomic as total quality. Abstract Book, WWDU'92. Berlin (1992)

Horgan G. Optometric Methods for MEPS-VDU Berlin study. Abstract Book, WWDU'92, (1992).

Hultgren G.V. and Knave B. Discomfort glare and disturbances from light reflections in an office with CRT display terminals. Appl. Ergo. 5 (1974):2-8

Huntling G. et. al. Postural and visual loads at VDT workplace. Ergonomics, 24 (1981):917-923.

Jeyaratnam J. Musculoskeletal problem: Asian perspective. Abstract Book, WWDU'92. Berlin, (1992).

Jeyaratnam J. et al (1989). Musculoskeletal Symptoms among VDU operators In:Work with computers. Ed. M.J. Smith and G.Salvendy. Elsevier, pp.330.
Lee, W.R. Working with visual display units. Brit. Med. J. 291(1985):989-991.
Ong C.N. Ergonomic intervention for better health and productivity. In Promoting Health and Productivity in the Computerised Office Ed. Sauters. et al, Taylor & Franics (1990)
Ong C. N. et al. Anthropometrics and display station preferences of VDU operators. Egronomics 31 (1988) :337-341.
Ong C. N. et al. Technological change and work related musculoskeletal disorder: A study of VDU operators. In: Toward Human Work. (Eds) Kumashiro M and Megaw E. Taylor and Francis (1991).
Ostberg O, Hogberg G. Perspectives on ergonomic issue in a VDT Office. InIn Promoting Health and Productivity in the Computerised Office Ed. Sauters. et al, Taylor & Franics (1990)
Sauter S and N.G. Swanson. The effect of frequent rest breaks on preformance and well-being in repetitive VDT work. Abstract Book, WWDU'92, Berlin.(1992)
Shahnavaz H, and Johannson A (1992) Instruments for ergonomics investigation of VDU work:MEPS project. Abstract Book, WWDU'92. Berlin.
Silverstein B et al. Carpal tunnel syndrome: Causes and a preventive strategies. Seminars in Occ. Med. 1 (1986):213-219.
Smith M.J. et al An investigation of health complaints and job stress in video display operations. Human Factors, 23(1987): 387-400.
Thomson D. Effect of exercise breaks on musculoskeletal strain among data-entry operators:a case study. In Promoting Health and Productivity in the Computerised Office Ed. Sauters. et al , Taylor & Franics (1990).
World Health Organization. Working document on the use of video display terminals. WHO, geneve (1986).

WORK WITH DISPLAY UNITS 92
H. Luczak, A. Çakir and G. Çakir (Editors)
1993 Elsevier Science Publishers B.V.

Summary of Two NIOSH Field Studies of Musculoskeletal Disorders and VDT Work among Telecommunications and Newspaper Workers

S. Sauter, T. Hales, B. Bernard, L. Fine, M. Petersen, V. Putz-Anderson, L. Schleifer and T. Ochs[1]

National Institute for Occupational Safety and Health, 4676 Columbia Parkway, Cincinnati, OH 45226, USA

Abstract

The potential health effects of work with video display terminals (VDTs) have been a subject of study at the National Institute for Occupational Safety and Health (NIOSH) for over a decade [1]. The present report provides a synopsis of two recent NIOSH epidemiologic studies of musculoskeletal disorders among VDT operators. Together, these studies represent the most ambitious effort by NIOSH to investigate the scope of musculoskeletal disorders and associated risk factors in the VDT workplace. Distinctive aspects of these studies include the broad range of potential risk factors investigated (both the physical and psychosocial work environment), and the use of physical examinations of workers to define musculoskeletal outcomes. Of special importance, investigation of the psychosocial environment included factors such as cognitive (i.e., information processing) demands, which have received little attention in prior investigations of VDT work, as well as emerging concerns such as exposure to electronic monitoring of work performance.

The results of these studies show both psychosocial and physical workload stressors to be predictive of musculoskeletal strain, although the magnitude of effects was often modest. These findings are supportive of recent research highlighting the role of psychosocial factors in the etiology of occupational musculoskeletal disorders [2-3], as well as earlier NIOSH investigations indicating similar effects [4-5]. An important common tie between the present studies is the significance of variables denoting workload demands (e.g., work pressure in the telecommunications study, and time working "under deadlines" in the newspaper study) as predictors of musculoskeletal disorders.

Reports providing a more complete description of study methods and a broader delineation and interpretation of findings are in preparation by NIOSH [6-7].

1. TELECOMMUNICATIONS STUDY (T. Hales, Principal Investigator)

In 1989, NIOSH received a joint request from the Communications Workers of America and US West Communications to evaluate the effects of VDT work on musculoskeletal disorders among Directory Assistance Operators (DAOs). To address this concern, a cross-sectional study of 533 telecommunications workers (including DAOs and workers from four additional job classifications) from three different metropolitan areas in the U.S. was conducted.

The study focused on the upper extremity (UE) musculoskeletal system, which was assessed using a symptom questionnaire and also via physical examinations. Data on worker demographics, individual factors (extant medical conditions and non-work activities), work practices, work organization and psychosocial aspects of work, including electronic monitoring of performance, were obtained from all participants by questionnaire. For one group of DAOs, the total number of keystrokes per day was generated from company computer records. The physical workstation was assessed by the NIOSH study team using direct measurement and checklists of workstation configuration, and work postures were assessed while employees operated their VDTs.

Two types of musculoskeletal outcomes were defined for analysis:

1) Potential work-related UE musculoskeletal disorders (UE *disorders*) defined by physical examination and by questionnaire (based on self-reports of frequency, duration and intensity of symptoms, and absence of prior injury), and 2) UE musculoskeletal symptoms (UE *symptoms*) defined by (the same) questionnaire alone (based on a cumulative score of symptom frequency, duration and intensity). The expression "potential work-related disorders" is used because self-report (i.e., questionnaire) data were used to define the work-relatedness of symptoms.

Relationships between workplace factors and UE *disorders* were assessed by multiple logistic regression models generated for each of four UE areas (neck, shoulder, elbow, hand/wrists). Associations between workplace factors and degree of UE *symptoms* were assessed by multiple linear regression models generated for each of the same four UE areas.

Over ninety percent of 573 selected employees participated in the study. Fifteen employees were excluded from the analyses because they were employed at their current job less than 6 months. The mean age of the remaining participants was 38 years, and the mean seniority on the current job was six years. Seventy-eight percent of participants were female, and 74% described themselves as "white."

Twenty-two percent of participants met the case definition for potential work-related UE *disorders*. Probable tendon-related *disorders* were the most common (15% of cases). Probable nerve entrapment syndromes represented less than five percent of cases. The hand/wrist was the UE area most affected (12% of participants), followed by the neck area (9%), the elbow area (7%), and the shoulder area (6%).

Pre-existing injury data from U.S. West Communications suggested that the DAOs would have the highest prevalence of *disorders*. This expectation was not supported by current findings. Although 22% of DAOs had musculoskeletal *disorders* that were potentially work-related, this prevalence was lower than rates for two of the four comparison jobs in this study.

Numerous individual and job variables were predictive of the two musculoskeletal outcome measures in the final regression models. However, most of the significant predictors had only modest elevations in odds ratios, or explained only modest proportions of the variance in outcome measures. Regarding demographic and individual characteristics, female gender was among the factors associated with increased UE *symptoms*. Also, type of eye glasses used was predictive of both UE *disorders* and *symptoms*. Notably, recreational activities were not associated with any *disorders* or *symptoms*.

Several variables denoting intensified workload (e.g., increasing work pressure, high information processing demands, and surges in workload) were associated with increased UE *disorders*. All three of these variables were also associated with increased UE *symptoms*. (Alternately, self-reports of overtime work and increasing hours of VDT work were associated with reduced UE *symptoms*.) UE *symptoms* were also found to be buffered by increased social support from coworkers and supervisors.

Of special interest, five of eleven variables assessing workers' perceptions of the effects of electronic performance monitoring were associated with increased UE *symptoms*. (However, no effects were seen for UE *disorders*.) UE *symptoms* were most common among workers who perceived the monitoring system to adversely affect social and supervisory relationships, and to cause increased workload and reduced work motivation.

Information to estimate the total keystrokes per day was available for 174 (71%) DAOs. Increasing total keystrokes per day was not associated with UE *disorders* or *symptoms* in the final models. However, the low number of keystrokes performed per day by DAOs (mean=15,950) limits the ability to generalize these results to other VDT workers such as data entry operators who may perform many times this number of keystrokes per day.

Reliable analyses of postural and workstation design factors were precluded by methodological limitations, including high correlations among predictor variables, low variation in several predictor variables, and the fact that DAOs were not assigned to specific workstations (thereby reducing reliability of exposure measurements).

2. NEWSPAPER STUDY (B. Bernard, Principal Investigator)

Also in 1989, NIOSH received a request from the Los Angeles Times for assistance in evaluating UE musculoskeletal disorders among employees using VDTs at two of its facilities. Editorial staff speculated that the introduction of VDTs and a keyboard specially designed for use in the Editorial department may have been responsible for an increase in musculoskeletal disorders at the newspaper. To assess the nature and distribution of employee UE symptoms, and possible causal factors, four departments (Circulation, Classified Advertising, Accounting and Finance, and Editorial) were selected for study.

2.1 Phase I

In Phase I of the study, UE symptoms were evaluated by use of a self-administered questionnaire, and cases of UE disorders were defined by questionnaire alone (unlike the telecommunications study). However, the questionnaire criteria for definition of cases was similar to the questionnaire criteria used for *disorders* in the telecommunications study (i.e., frequency, duration, and intensity of symptoms in the affected area, and absence of previous injury). The questionnaire was also used to obtain information on worker demographics and individual factors, job history, job tasks, and work organization and psychosocial aspects of the work environment. Physical ergonomic aspects of the workstation and workplace were also assessed but, similar to the situation in the telecommunications study, circumstances (e.g., ongoing redesign of workstations and of the physical work environment) precluded the reliable evaluation of these variables as risk factors for UE disorders.

Over ninety percent of 1050 eligible employees participated in Phase I. The mean age of the participants was 39 years, and the mean seniority on the current job was 11 years. Fifty-six percent of the participants were female. Forty-one percent of participants reported symptoms meeting the case definition for at least one UE disorder. Neck symptoms (26%) were the most frequently reported, followed by hand/wrist symptoms (22%), shoulder symptoms (17%), and elbow symptoms (10%). Employees in the Editorial Department had the lowest prevalence of UE disorders (38%) of the four departments studied.

Multiple logistic regression analyses were performed on the Phase I data to determine important risk factors for UE disorders in the neck, shoulder, and hand/wrist separately. As in the telecommunications study, variables corresponding to increased workload demands (e.g., increased time working under deadline; increased job pressure) were associated with increased neck, shoulder, or hand/wrist disorders. But contrary to the telecommunications study, greater time working at the VDT keyboard was also associated with increased disorders. Again, these effects were buffered by higher levels of supervisory support.

Women were more likely to report symptoms in several upper extremity areas, but this may reflect the concentration of women in jobs involving more risk factors.

2.2 Phase II

In Phase II of the investigation, a case-control study using selected participants from Phase I was conducted to determine whether Phase I risk factors would be confirmed using a more restrictive hand/wrist case definition. Randomly selected cases who fulfilled the criteria for a hand/wrist UE disorder on the Phase I questionnaire were compared to controls with respect to results of an UE physical examination (focusing on the hand and wrist) and nerve conduction velocity (NCV) testing.

One-hundred-thirty participants were randomly selected from the hand/wrist cases identified in Phase I, and 99 controls were randomly selected from the Phase I participants reporting no UE symptoms. On physical examination, 53% of cases and 12% of controls had one or more positive hand/wrist findings. As in the telecommunications study, tendon-related cases were the most common (over 30% of cases).

Multiple logistic regression analyses were performed to identify risk factors associated with the more restrictive hand/wrist case definition, which involved both positive physical findings and the questionnaire criteria (i.e., similar to the telecommunications study). The results were consistent with Phase I findings; e.g., female gender and increased time spent typing at the VDT were among the important predictors of disorders.

NCV testing was performed on randomly selected Phase II participants (61 cases and 35 controls). Initial analysis of nerve conduction data showed no important differences between the cases and controls, although the direction of differences tended to be consistent with greater impairment of nerve function among cases.

In a final step, the case definition was restricted further, requiring symptoms and physical findings in the median nerve distribution of the hand, and NCV differences between cases and controls were reassessed. More pronounced differences in several NCV measures resulted, but the magnitude of these differences were still quite small and may not reflect any clinically significant impairment of nerve function.

3. CONCLUSIONS

The results of these studies add to the growing body of evidence that psychosocial factors contribute to the development of musculoskeletal disorders among office workers who use VDTs. Variables denoting increased work pressure seem especially salient in the present studies.

The mechanisms linking the psychosocial environment at work and musculoskeletal disorders in VDT work are poorly understood and warrant further investigation. Among the many possibilities are stress-related increases in muscle tension and consequent biomechanical strain. Or an impoverished psychosocial environment and physically demanding work may simply go hand-in-hand.

Several sources of potential bias, including study design limitations, disease misclassification, and exposure misclassification could have influenced the results and interpretation of the present studies. Regarding the latter source, it is possible that many of the workplace factors associated with UE *disorders* and *symptoms* in the telecommunications study are surrogates for the job titles investigated, since there was considerable variation in the prevalence of disorders across job titles. Further, in both studies, the cross-sectional study design cannot determine whether self-reported working conditions were causally related to musculoskeletal outcomes, nor the direction of causation. Also, neither study fully addresses the possible impact of non-work-related stress factors, or their possible associations with work-related musculoskeletal disorders. Our results are based on the assumption that non-work stressors are probably similar between symptomatic and non-symptomatic workers, and do not confound or modify the results to a large degree. Finally, the possibility for statistically significant associations due to chance alone (i.e., Type I error), must be considered, given the large number of analyses completed.

4. FOOTNOTES

[1]Since the completion of this research, L. Schleifer has joined the U.S. Internal Revenue Service, Washington, DC, and T. Ochs has joined the General Electric Corporation, Cincinnati, OH.

5. REFERENCES

1. NIOSH Publications on Video Display Terminals (REVISED). NIOSH, DTMD, Cincinnati, 1991.
2. P. Leino, J. Epi. and Community Health, 43 (1989) 293.
3. S. Linton and K. Kamwendo, J. Occup. Med., 31 (1989) 609.
4. M. Smith et al., Hum. Factors, 23 (1981) 387.
5. S. Sauter et al., Comm. Assoc. Comput. Machinery, 26 (1982) 284.
6. Health Hazard Evaluation Report 89-299-2230, NIOSH, DTMD, Cincinnati, 1992.
7. Health Hazard Evaluation Report 90-013-2277, NIOSH, DTMD, Cincinnati,1993.

WORK WITH DISPLAY UNITS 92
H. Luczak, A. Çakir and G. Çakir (Editors)

An image analyzing approach to working postures for screen and keyboard use of Visual Display Units

M. Nakaseko[a], K. Morimoto[b], K. Nishiyama[c] and H. Tainaka[d]

[a]Department of Hygiene, Kansai Medical University, Fumizonocho 1, Moriguchi, Osaka 617, Japan

[b]Faculty of Engineering and Design, Kyoto Institute of Technology, Matugasaki, Sakyo, Kyoto 606, Japan

[c]Department of Preventive Medicine, Shiga University of Medical Science, Seta-tsukinowacho, Ohtsu 520-02, Japan

[d]Ergonomic Laboratory, Osaka Prefectural Institute of Public Health, Nakamichi, Higashinari, Osaka 537 , Japan

Abstract

An image analyzing method was designed to quantify the postural elements associated with static muscle tension in the neck, trunk and arms of Visual Display Units (VDU) operators. Postural measurements were made by videotaping the VDU operators using the keyboard and the display screen to determine the neck and trunk postures. An ergonomic evaluation of 199 operators found the trunk to be bent at each level of the thoracic and lumbar regions. Tilt of the neck was associated with an increasing degree of forward bending of the thoracic region. Finally, Extended arms and Raised elbows were found to be related to use of the poorly designed VDU workstations.

1. INTRODUCTION

Many studies describe the occurrence of muscular skeletal disorders like occupational cervicobrachial disorder (OCD) as being linked to repetitive motion and static tension problems among VDU operators [1, 2]. Grandjean reported that constrained postures are certainly the most frequent form of static muscular work and the main causes of constrained posture are carrying the trunk, head or limbs in unnatural positions [3]. Postural characterization of VDU work helps to identify which of the postural elements pose the health risk for muscular skeletal disorder. Ergonomic evaluation using an image analyzing method provides a quantitative measure to evaluate the postural stress at various anatomical sites of the muscular-skeletal system which contribute to OCD. In this study the image analyzing method was designed to describe quantitatively postures associated with static muscle tension in operators working with VDUs. Other independent ergonomic evaluation measures included reach and height of the workstation components.

2. SUBJECTS AND METHOD

Two ergonomic evaluations were used to identify several postural characteristics associated with static postures during VDU work: (i) The ergonomic evaluation of static postures at anatomical sites consisted of videotaping the VDU operators at work. The video sources included left or right side view of the 199 VDU operators of covered postures during keyboard or screen display use at 72 VDT workstations of the console type. The images studied were obtained from the averaged image of 10 to 30 frames, which were derived from the video source by a framegrabber from 3 - 4 minute segments of the usual VDU task. The measurements on the computer display included angle of tilt of the neck and the angles at 5 selected points along the vertebral line. (ii) Other independent ergonomic evaluation of static postures at the VDU workstation measured reach and height of the workstation components.

One hundred and ninety-nine VDU operators (men: N=125 and women: N=74) participated in a field study. Their age (mean+SD) was 34+11 years for the men and 42+12 years for the women (range from 18 - 63 years). The average body height was 169+8cm for the men and 156+6cm for the women.

3. RESULTS AND DISCUSSION

3.1. Descriptions of VDU tasks and workstations

The workstations studied consisted of a VDU with a fixed keyboard and chair capable of small adjustments. The keyboard had several differences in key layout and arrangement from the QWERTY type of alphanumeric keyboard. The height of the keyboard from the floor was 71cm. The distance between the middle row of keys and the front edge of the table was 15cm. The workstation also included a narrow table 15cm deep and 70cm high. The operators, therefore, were able to use it as source document holder or support their hands. However, this layout required the operators to extend the upper extremities when using the keyboard. The VDU operators tasks mainly fell into two categories; one was a data entry task, the other was an information inquiring task. In the result of 10 operators studied, keyboard use accounted to 7 - 47% of the regular working hours. The operators sat for 75% of their working day, including VDU and other office work.

3.2. Inclination of the neck in VDU work

Fig. 1 shows the distribution of the neck angle of 179 VDU operators while performing their usual daily jobs.

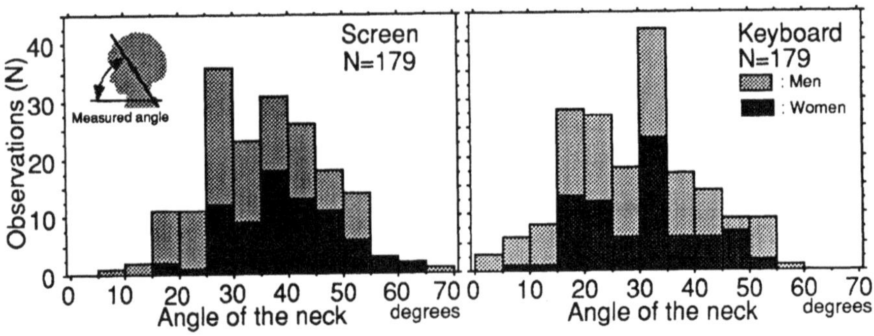

Figure 1. Distributions of the neck angle of 179 VDU operators during their usual daily jobs.

The neck angle was assessed as the angle of a line between the seventh cervical vertebra (C_7) and the earhole to horizontal.The results reveal that the use of keyboard was associated with a marked tilt in neck position with a mean angle of 28.6±11.6 degrees. The tilt was 35.6±11.0 degrees while looking at the screen display and 58 - 61 degrees when looking forward with the head in an upright position. The significant inclination of the neck suggests a link not only to the use of an unfamiliar keyboard but also poor design of unadjustable and fixed workstation components. These ergonomic disadvantages tend to produce a lot of tension and constant repetitive motion of the neck.

3.3. Trunk posture during VDU work

Table 1 shows the mean and standard deviation of the observed angles at five points up the spine during VDU work. There was a statistically significant difference in the neck angle and the angle of the forward bent of the trunk at C_7 between keyboard and screen display use. However there were no differences at other levels of the spine.

Table 1. Mean and standard deviation of angles at various points along spine during keyboard and screen display use.

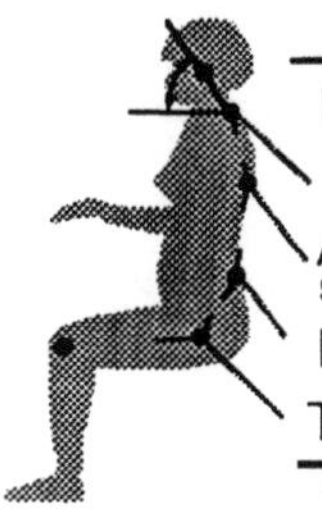

level of measured points	Keyboard use N=199 Mean (SD)	Display use N=199 Mean (SD)
Neck angle**	28.7 (11.6)	35.5 (11.0)
C_7	157.0 (10.5)	163.7 (9.7)
Angulus inferior scapula	140.5 (8.8)	140.7 (8.5)
Iliocristale	134.1 (13.3)	133.6 (13.2)
Trochanter	146.4 (12.1)	146.6 (12.7)

** P<0.01 Degrees

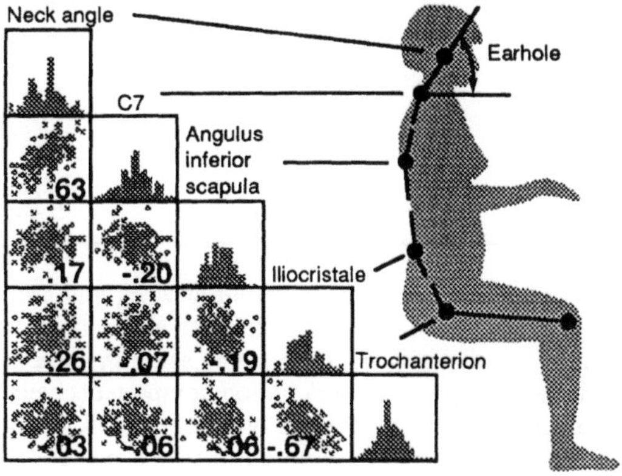

Figure 2. Scattergrams for the forward bent of the trunk during keyboard use for five height levels along spine.

As shown in table 1, the averaged postures had the trunk forward bent and the neck strongly tilted with the trunk moving very seldom. The neck tended to change to a more tilted angle during keyboard use. Fig. 2 shows the matrix of scattergrams for the forward bent of the trunk during keyboard operation for five height levels along spine. The figures in each scattergram show the correlation coefficients for each combination of the scattergram matrix. The results show that the forward bend of the trunk posture at the level of the thoracic vertebra was positively related to an increase in the neck angle, whereas at the lumbar level trunk posture was associated with leg posture, dependent on an inclination of the overall trunk posture. Only one postural difference was found between the keyboard operation and screen display use, the angle between a line running from the earhole to C_7 and the angulus inferior scapula level of the spine. This posture leads to a strong tendency for constant head movement between the keyboard and the screen display without any movement of the trunk. It can thus be said that postural settings are obviously determined by two movable regions of the spine, which are associated with an inclination of the angle of the neck.

3.4. Constrained posture in the upper extremities at VDU workstations

As shown in Table 2, for the postural element measured, there were statistically significant differences in eye level and shoulder height between men and women but there were no significant differences in elbow, wrist and seat height. It discloses that the eye and shoulder heights are mainly in relation to difference of the body height which is likely to associate with the forward bend of the trunk posture but the posture in the upper extremities strongly depends on the fixed height of workstation compornents.

Table 2. Mean and standard deviation of postural measurements obtained from 199 VDT operators while working at VDT.

cm

Height from floor	Men (N=125) Mean (SD)	Women (N=74) Mean (SD)
Eye level	113.5 (4.7)	110.6 (4.2)
Shoulder	99.1 (4.1)	97.2 (3.8)
Elbow	71.8 (3.7)	72.4 (3.4)
Wrist	72.7 (2.1)	73.1 (2.1)
Seat	45.9 (2.5)	45.5 (2.2)

Fig. 3 shows the plots of elbow height, seat height at work and arm length against body height for 179 VDU operators. The result shows that the elbow height was nearly the same level as keyboard height, and that seat height was the same in spite of differences in body height. This means that the unadjustable workstation components cause the VDU operators to hold constrained postures that are associated with a high risk of the neck-shoulder-arm pain. The taller operators, especially, are required to take a posture with their arms rather extended, with the elbows raised and with a marked forward bend in the trunk, in order to operate the keyboard.

It seems that this constrained posture is likely to cause serious static muscle tensions, physical discomfort and less efficient movements in the neck- shoulder - arm-hand area.

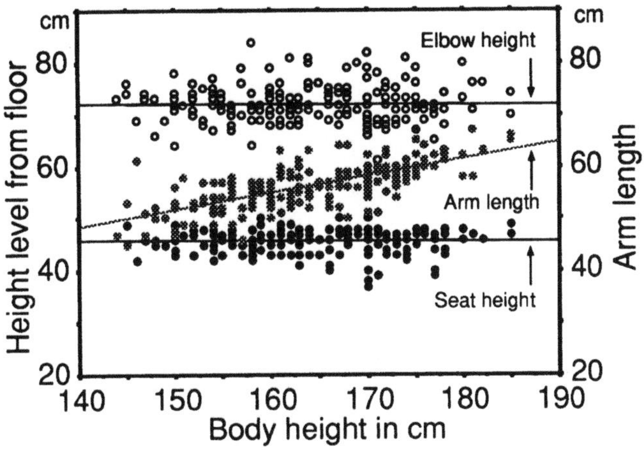

Figure. 3. Relation of seat height, elbow height and arm length to body height in 179 VDT operators.

4. Conclusions

From an image analyzing approch to assess quantitavely postural elements associated with muscular tension of the neck, trunk and shoulders. It is revealed that VDT operators took postures with the neck tilted as well as the trunk forward bent at the height level of the thoracic and lumbar region. The angle of tilt was more acute in keyboard operating work than in screen display work. Moreover the angle of the tilt of the neck was associated with an increased degree of bending of the trunk at a thoracic level of the spine. The trunk posture was associated with movements of lumbar and hip regions. An increase in movement in the hip region was likely to cause forward bending of the trunk. Finally the position of the upper extremities was found to be linked to poor designed VDU workstation.

Recent studies show that there are several evidences to suggest that a properly designed workstation can reduce a muscle tension of neck-shoulder area for the operators working with VDTs [4]. Grandjean [3] pointed out that regardless of the body height, the great majority of the VDT operators preferred to leaning back posture. It is great important to introduce adjustable workstation components to provide leaning back posture, which relates to reduce an inclination of the neck as well as to permit a natural position of the trunk.. It is noted that inexperienced VDT operators are more likely to take forward bent posture because of looking a position of the key on the keyboard. Keyboard design with a special key layout and arrangement is obviously related to an unnatural posture.

References

1. W. Hunting, T. Laubli and E. Grandjean, Postural and visual loads at VDT workplaces, Part 1: Constrained postures, Ergonomics, 24 (1981) 917.
2. K. Nishiyama, M. Nakaseko and Uehata, Health aspects of VDT operators in the newspaper industry, E. Grandjean (ed), Ergonomics and Health in modern offices, Taylar & Francis, London, (1984) 113.
3. E. Grandjean, Ergonomics in computerized offices, Taylar & Francis, London, 1987.
4. M. Nakaseko, H. Tainaka and M. Itoh, An ergonomically designed VDT workstation for reducing postural stress in the shoulder-arm-hand area, WWD'89 Abstracts (1982) 150.

WORK WITH DISPLAY UNITS 92
H. Luczak, A. Çakir and G. Çakir (Editors)

VDT Repetitive Motion Health Concerns in the U.S. Telecommunications Industry

D. E. LeGrande, M.A., Director

Occupational Safety and Health Department, Communications Workers of America, AFL-CIO, CLC, 501 Third Street, N.W., Washington, D.C. 20001

Abstract

The CWA has identified visual display terminal (VDT) safety and health issues as a top priority of the union's members.

As a result of the union's activity, musculoskeletal repetitive motion health complaints have been identified on an ever increasing basis. To determine the degree and severity of member health problems, in January, 1989, CWA's Occupational Safety and Health Office developed and distributed a VDT repetitive motion survey to identified CWA officers.

Some 8,000 CWA members from 108 locals representing telecommunications employees completed and returned the VDT repetitive motion questionnaire. Analysis was performed for four different occupations: operators, service representatives, clerical VDT operators, and maintenance administrators.

Collected data revealed that represented telecommunications employers were not providing ergonomic VDT working conditions. In turn, a catastrophic number of respondents reported experiencing a variety of health symptoms and disorders ranging from hand and wrist pain to medically-diagnosed carpal tunnel syndrome.

In turn, analyzed data and reports were used to negotiate improved VDT work environments.

To determine the degree to which VDT repetitive motion illnesses continued to occur and in preparation for 1992 collective bargaining with the same represented telecommunications companies, in June, 1991, CWA's Occupational Safety and Health Office distributed its VDT repetitive motion survey to identified CWA officers.

This paper presents individual and comparative data from both 1989 and 1992 surveillance efforts.

Paper

The Communications Workers of America (CWA) represents 600,000 workers in the U.S. and Canada. Of these, 500,000 are employed within the U.S. telecommunications industry and 450,000 of represented telecommunications workers use VDTs to perform their jobs. The introduction of VDTs into represented telecommunications workplaces began during the mid to latter 1970's. In the future, it is anticipated that VDT use will continue to increase.

Since 1979, the CWA has identified visual display terminal (VDT) occupational safety and health issues as a top priority of the union's members. In turn, such recognition has been translated by CWA's Occupational Safety and Health Office into the development of educational materials and training, the provision of technical assistance to the union's leaders and members, and the sponsoring/conducting of survey and scientific research.

In part, during the early 1980's this work led to the identification of an increasing rate of member musculoskeletal VDT repetitive motion health complaints. Initially, limited to the occurrence of upper extremity musculoskeletal health symptoms, by 1984, repetitive motion illnesses or cumulative trauma disorders began to be reported. By 1988, CWA had identified many catastrophic occurrences of VDT repetitive motion illnesses.

The most noteworthy case involved 500 workers employed as directory assistance operators by U.S. West in Denver, Colorado. These employees utilized VDTs throughout their work shift to perform their jobs. During the latter part of 1985, a variety of upper extremity musculoskeletal symptoms were reported to the local union by some 40 directory assistance operators. By 1986 and 1987, increased numbers of members reported repetitive motion health symptoms as well as disorders. During 1987, the company agreed to enter into meaningful negotiations with CWA to resolve workplace ergonomic concerns. By the end of 1987, supported by a comprehensive settlement on VDT workplace ergonomics from the U.S. Occupational Safety and Health Administration, the union and the company had reached agreement on all physical ergonomic factors. By 1988, nearly half of the 500 directory assistance operators had reported some form of diagnosed repetitive motion illness, with nearly 100 of the cases being carpal tunnel syndrome.

During 1988 and 1989, with the implementation of VDT workplace physical equipment largely underway and, in some cases, completed, labor and management began to develop and introduce amendments to work organization factors. In particular, topics such as training, increased rest breaks, VDT exercises, and alternate work were addressed.

The Denver, Colorado case was matched by similar incidents throughout the U.S. in cities such as Sacramento, California; Phoenix, Arizona; Dallas, Texas; Orlando and West Palm Beach, Florida; Madison and Milwaukee, Wisconsin, Cleveland, Ohio,

Lexington and Paducah, Kentucky, Annapolis, Maryland, and Syracuse, New York.

To assist in and hopefully ensure the early identification and treatment of VDT repetitive motion symptoms and illnesses, CWA's Occupational Safety and Health Office worked with Local unions to educate members about VDT workplace ergonomics and, through the use of survey tools, identify repetitive motion health problems associated with poorly designed physical and work organization ergonomic factors. In turn, treatment and prevention strategies were introduced.

Given that the majority of the union's activities take place within the collective bargaining environment, CWA attempted to work cooperatively with represented telecommunications employers to identify and resolve member repetitive motion health symptoms and disorders as well as poorly designed VDT workplace environments. Unfortunately, until 1989, when CWA and U.S. West reached their landmark agreement to fully cooperate in the resolution of VDT workplace ergonomic-related health problems and the provision of properly designed VDT working conditions, except for isolated cases, no other represented telecommunications company agreed to fully cooperate in the resolution of VDT workplace ergonomics. (In fact, this is still the state of affairs between CWA and most represented telecommunications employers.)

1989 CWA VDT Repetitive Motion Illness Survey

As a result of this lack of cooperation between CWA and most telecommunications employers as well as the companies' insistence that member repetitive motion health symptoms and disorders were not work-related, the union's Occupational Safety and Health Department developed and initiated its 1989 "CWA VDT Repetitive Motion Illness Survey."

The survey process was intended to, in part, better identify the degree and severity of member repetitive motion health problems and how represented employers were responding to union and member concerns.

Questionnaires were distributed to CWA District Vice Presidents and local union presidents with instructions to target intensive VDT users, i.e., those workers who used VDTs more than 50% of their work day to perform their jobs. Some 8,000 CWA members from 108 local unions representing all major represented U.S. telecommunications employers and CWA regional offices completed and returned the VDT repetitive motion questionnaires.

This surprisingly high response rate was an indication of how serious the VDT repetitive motion problem was perceived by the union's members. However, the number of responses was believed to constitute only a small percentage of the total number of CWA members who use VDTs to perform their jobs who had developed repetitive motion health problems. Reasons for not responding to the union's request for information included a lack of awareness of the relationship between musculoskeletal repetitive motion health problems and VDT work, fear of employer reprisal for complaining of VDT workplace health and design problems, and fear of losing job security.

It was anticipated that members employed in intensive VDT work would experience the greatest number and most severe types of repetitive motion illnesses. The basis for this opinion was factored upon both physical and psychological ergonomics or workplace design. In workplaces where there was a lack of adherence to physical design factors (e.g., VDTs, chairs, tables, and illumination), one would anticipate finding a high number of visual (e.g., eye irritation, burning, itching, soreness) and musculoskeletal (e.g., hand and wrist, arm and shoulder, neck and back, and leg pain) health complaints.

Compounding poor physical working conditions with poor work design factors (e.g., work pace, workload, monitoring, lack of worker input into how work is designed), one would expect to find a number of psychological and psychosocial related health problems (e.g., headaches, nausea, muscle tension, irregular menstrual periods, and chest pain), as well as a greater occurrence of physical symptoms.

Since physical ergonomic factors lend themselves to this type of survey investigation, the union's survey focused only upon physical variables.

Analysis was performed for four different occupations: directory assistance operators, service representatives, clerical VDT operators, and maintenance administrators. Workers in each of these jobs utilized the VDT intensively to perform their jobs. A significant number of employees in each of these occupational classifications responded to the survey.

For example, completed questionnaires were received from:

- 2,031 directory assistance operators;
- 2,722 service representatives;
- 1,216 clerical VDT operators;
- 513 maintenance administrators.

Although additional surveys were returned from members in other occupations, insufficient quantities within each occupation were received to merit analysis.

Collected data from all four occupations indicated catastrophic findings. For example, a majority of directory assistance operators reported experiencing the following health symptoms: hand and wrist pain (63%), numbness or tingling of fingers (50%), arm or shoulder pain (72%), neck or back pain (84%), and leg pain (51%).

Of particular concern, the following repetitive motion illnesses were reported: cysts on hands or wrists (13%), diagnosed tendonitis (14%), and medically-diagnosed carpal tunnel syndrome (6%). Thus, collected data suggested that 33% of directory assistance respondents had a repetitive motion disorder.

Information received from service representatives indicated similar results. Following were reported occurrences of health symptoms: hand and wrist pain (45%), numbness or tingling of fingers (38%), arm and shoulder pain (70%), neck or back pain (85%), and leg pain (45%).

Reported data was even more alarming for repetitive motion disorders: cysts on hand or wrists (9%), diagnosed tendonitis (15%), and medically-diagnosed carpal tunnel syndrome (4%). Therefore, survey results indicated that 28% of responding service representatives had a repetitive motion disorder.

Similarly, large numbers of responding clerical VDT operators reported repetitive motion health symptoms: hand and wrist pain (45%), numbness or tingling of fingers (34%), arm and shoulder pain (65%), neck or back pain (76%), and leg pain (37%).

Collected data specific to repetitive motion illnesses indicated: cysts on hands or wrists (9%), diagnosed tendonitis (16%), and medically-diagnosed carpal tunnel syndrome (5%). Thus, 30% of responding clerical VDT operators indicated suffering repetitive motion disorders.

Responding maintenance administrators reported the following health symptoms: hand and wrist pain (36%), numbness or tingling of fingers (35%), arm or shoulder pain (65%), neck or back pain (76%), and leg pain (38%).

Of particular concern were the reported occurrences of repetitive motion health disorders: cysts on hands or wrists (12%), diagnosed tendonitis (18%), and medically-diagnosed carpal tunnel syndrome (5%). Therefore, 35% of responding maintenance administrators indicated having repetitive motion disorders.

Clearly, reported data indicated CWA members employed in the noted occupations were experiencing catastrophic rates of repetitive motion illnesses.

1992 CWA VDT Repetitive Motion Illness Survey

As a result of continued reports of member repetitive motion health symptoms and illnesses and represented telecommunications employers' reluctance/refusal to deal with the union in a meaningful fashion specific to the identification, treatment, and prevention of VDT member repetitive motion symptoms and illnesses, in 1991, CWA's Occupational Safety and Health Office re-initiated its "CWA VDT Repetitive Motion Illness Survey."

Completed during early 1992, the research effort was intended to assess represented telecommunications employers' progress in implementing ergonomic VDT workplaces and success in reducing worker repetitive motion health symptoms and disorders. Also, survey data would allow the union to better determine the degree and severity of musculoskeletal health symptoms among CWA-represented VDT workers. Finally, collected information would allow for the comparing and contrasting of health symptoms and disorders and working conditions data from the 1989 and 1992 surveys.

The 1992 survey was disseminated using the same methods as the 1989 effort, i.e., to regional Vice Presidents and local union presidents. In turn, directions were provided to target members in telecommunications jobs in which VDTs were used intensively to perform their work. Completed surveys were returned to the CWA Occupational Safety and Health Office for analysis.

Some 8,000 members from 83 locals representing five of the union's seven districts and a majority of represented telecommunications employers completed and returned the VDT repetitive motion illness survey.

The large response rate was an indication of the seriousness with which CWA members viewed the VDT repetitive motion issue. As was the case in 1989, the number of responses was believed to constitute only a minimal percentage of the total number of union members who use VDTs intensively to perform their work who have developed repetitive motion health symptoms and disorders.

Analysis was performed for four different occupations: directory assistance operators, service representatives, clerical VDT operators, and technicians. Workers in each of these jobs were involved in intensive VDT use.

Completed questionnaires were received from 2,876 directory assistance operators, 3,988 service representatives, 1,503 clerical VDT operators, and 760 technicians.

Although additional surveys were returned by members in other jobs, within each occupation insufficient numbers were received to merit analysis.

Data received from directory assistance operators indicated catastrophic occurrences of VDT repetitive motion health symptoms and disorders. Symptom data indicated the following: hand and wrist pain (73%), numbness or tingling of fingers (59%), arm and shoulder pain (78%), neck or back pain (86%), and leg pain (53%).

Of particular concern, very large numbers of directory assistance operators reported suffering repetitive motion illnesses. For example, 14% indicated having cysts on their hands or wrist, 17% said they had been diagnosed with tendonitis in their arms or wrists, and 9% reported having medically-diagnosed carpal tunnel syndrome. Thus, 40% of the directory assistance operators reported having a repetitive motion illness.

Findings from service representatives depicted similar concerns. Of respondents, 61% indicated experiencing hand or wrist pain, 47% said they had numbness or tingling of fingers, 71% said they experienced arm or shoulder pain, 85% reported neck or back pain, and 42% indicated experiencing leg pain.

More significantly, 11% of service representatives indicated having developed cysts on their hands or wrists, 16% said they had been diagnosed as having tendonitis in their arms or wrists, and 8% reported being medically-diagnosed with carpal tunnel syndrome. Therefore, 35% of responding service representatives indicated having VDT repetitive motion illnesses.

Clerical VDT operators reported high rates of health symptoms and disorders. 55% indicated having hand and wrist pain, 46% said they had numbness or tingling of finger, 67%

reported arm and shoulder pain, 78% indicated having neck or back pain, and 39% said they experienced leg pain.

Of more concern, the following percentages of respondents reported suffering repetitive motion disorders: 11% cysts on hands or wrists, 18% diagnosed tendonitis, and 9% medically-diagnosed carpal tunnel syndrome. This data shows that 38% of responding clerical VDT operators indicated having repetitive motion illnesses.

Collected data from the union's 1992 national survey included significant numbers of completed questionnaires from technicians. Receipt of such large numbers of surveys from this occupational grouping may, in part, be an indication of increased technological change within the telecommunications industry, i.e., greater numbers of technicians used VDTs to perform their jobs as opposed to hand tools and other less sophisticated work methods.

Technicians reported the following health symptoms: hand and wrist pain (48%), numbness or tingling of fingers (39%), arm and shoulder pain (62%), neck or back pain (71%), and leg pain (34%).

Of particular concern, 9% of responding technicians reported cysts on their hands or wrists, 15% said they had diagnosed tendonitis, and 9% indicated having medically-diagnosed carpal tunnel syndrome. Thus, 33% of responding technicians said they had developed repetitive motion illnesses.

Comparison of 1989 and 1992 Data

1989 was a landmark year for CWA in its continued efforts to successfully identify, recommend treatment for, and prevent member VDT workplace repetitive motion health symptoms and disorders and, in turn, have represented employers provide ergonomic VDT working conditions. The negotiated agreement with U.S. West to fully and jointly cooperate in the resolution of VDT workplace design concerns as well as the occurrence of identified worker repetitive motion symptoms and disorders throughout the U.S. telecommunications industry convinced other CWA-represented telecommunications companies to begin to introduce well-designed physical ergonomic equipment into VDT workplaces. Even though, in most cases, these companies were acting unilaterally with no involvement from CWA, the union believed their efforts to provide physical ergonomic VDT working conditions would lessen the occurrence of member repetitive motion illnesses.

However, data from the union's 1992 VDT Repetitive Motion Illness Survey suggests that, in and of itself, provision of improved physical ergonomics does not significantly reduce or eliminate worker repetitive motion health symptoms and disorders.

When comparing the union's 1989 and 1992 survey results for directory assistance operators, service representatives, and clerical VDT operators, two particular findings are noted. First, represented employers provided improved physical VDT working conditions. Second, increased numbers of worker health symptoms and disorders were reported. This is particularly true for illness data where cases reported in 1992 exceeded those reported in 1989 by as much as 100%.

Directory assistance operators indicated the greatest improvements in physical VDT working conditions. The 1992 survey results indicated 94% as compared to 91% in 1989 of respondents reported they were provided adjustable chairs; 71% as compared to 53% in 1989 said they were provided angularly adjustable VDTs; 60% as compared to 43% in 1989 indicated being provided height adjustable tables or work surfaces; 70% as compared to 63% in 1989 reported they were provided thin, well-designed keyboards; 62% as compared to 66% in 1989 said VDT work area illumination levels were too bright causing glare and making screen characters difficult to read.

Responding service representatives reported improvements in physical VDT working conditions, but not to the same degree as directory assistance operators. For example, 81% as compared to 80% in 1989 said they were provided adjustable chairs; 87% compared to 79% indicated they were provided angularly adjustable VDTs, and 57% compared to 67% in 1989 reported VDT workplace illumination was too bright causing glare and making screen characters hard to read.

Similarly, clerical VDT operators responding to the 1992 survey indicated improved VDT working conditions. For example, 83% as compared to 81% in 1989 indicated they were provided adjustable chairs, 82% as compared to 79% said VDTs were not equipped with screen angle adjustability, and 49% as compared to 57% reported VDT work area illumination was too bright causing glare and making screen characters hard to read.

Collected data as well as various scientific studies suggests that attention to both physical and psychological or psychosocial ergonomic factors are necessary to prevent VDT workplace repetitive motion health symptoms and illnesses. Future research efforts should emphasize both physical and psychosocial ergonomic factors and their interrelationships. Failure to adhere to the "balance theory" will result in the occurrence of repetitive motion health problems.

Of concern to those involved in U.S. industrial or labor-management relations is the degree to which management interests are reluctant to accept the "balance theory" and supportive scientific data and adopt a comprehensive approach to identifying, treating, and preventing, VDT workplace repetitive motion illnesses. Rather than work towards the common good -- including labor, management, and public policy -- these opponents of industrial, social and political progress are preventing U.S. workers from realizing their potential and real worth and keeping the U.S. economic and political systems from realizing their full potential.

WORK WITH DISPLAY UNITS 92
H. Luczak, A. Çakir and G. Çakir (Editors)

MUSCULOSKELETAL DISORDERS AMONG DATA ENTRY WORKERS

Robert DeMatteo, Ontario Public Service Employees Union, Toronto, Ontario, CANADA
Margaret Denton, McMaster University, Hamilton, Ontario, CANADA
Lynda Hayward, Guelph University, Guelph, Ontario, CANADA

INTRODUCTION

Data Entry operators performing repetitive, one-dimensional tasks under computer monitored quota systems may be at increased risk of developing musculoskeletal (MS) disorders. Given the nature of this intensive VDT work, this risk may not be completely offset by conventional interventions such as regularly scheduled rest breaks and work station design modifications.

STUDY OBJECTIVES

The objectives of this study are to: 1) determine the prevalence of upper extremity (UE) disorders among data entry clerks; 2) compare the prevalence of disorders in data entry clerks to that in general clerical workers; 3) determine whether these disorders are associated with various biomechanical and work organization factors with a view to developing appropriate intervention strategies.

METHODOLOGY

Study Design: This is a cross-sectional prevalence study of data entry clerks and general office and clerical employees. It was designed to identify prevalence and contributing factors at one point in time.

Sample and Research Setting: This study included two groups of office workers: The large majority of subjects are data entry clerks from data entry operations in Ontario's Public Service. They use VDTs solely to input data. Key stroke rates are electronically monitored and recorded. They work under a norm of 11,400 stroke/hour. Rates are reviewed weekly, and comparisons are made for the same worker and the relative standing of the individual to the whole group. On average they spend more than 6 hours a day on VDT work..

For the purposes of comparison a group of clerical employees from a community college and Ontario's Legislative Assembly were included. These workers are not monitored and do not work under a quota system. They perform a variety of VDT tasks and other office duties. On average they spend less than 6 hours per day on VDT work.

Research Instrument and Measures: A self-reporting survey questionnaire was developed to elicit responses to questions designed as measures of health outcomes and working conditions exposures. For health outcomes, respondents were asked to indicate whether they: 1) were medically diagnosed as having MS disorders of the UE from a list provided in the questionnaire; 2) experienced any muscular pain, numbness, tingling, swelling, weakness of the UE (once a monthe to almost daily); 3) experienced psychosomatic symptoms such as exhaustion, loss of appetite, irritability, sleeplessness, dizziness, headaches, and nausea (once a month to almost daily).

For work exposure measures, questions were asked to ascertain: 1) biomechanical factors such as repetitiveness (keystroke rates) , awkward postures, static loading, and workstation design features; 2) work organization factors such as monitoring, quota systems, work load, work pressure, work hours, and rest break schedules.

Analytical Methods: Responses to the questionnaire were numerically coded, and the data entered into an IBM AT computer for analysis using SPSSPC+, a statistical package specifically designed for the social sciences. The analytical procedures used included univariate analysis to obtain frequencies for descriptive purposes, as well as bivariate and multivariate methods such as cross tabulation and multiple linear regression analysis to examine association between variables.

RESULTS

The questionnaire was administered at 13 office worksites to 382 subjects. 292 respondents completed the questionnaire for a response rate of 76.4 percent. Approximately 78 percent were data entry operators and the remaining 22 percent included secretaries and other clerical occupations.

The incidence of diagnosed musculoskeletal injury occurred in 26 percent of the population, with cervical strain (10 percent) most commonly reported. The overall incidence of one or more MS symptoms experienced from once a week to almost daily was approximately 67 percent over the past six months. Thirty-five percent of those experiencing MS symptoms visited a doctor in the last three months, and 89 percent reported using some form of treatment.

Over 80 percent of respondents reported one or more psychosomatic complaints once a week to almost daily. The most commonly reported complaints were exhaustion and fatigue (54 percent), neck and shoulder tension (43 percent), headaches (43 percent), irritability (33 percent) and sleeplessness (32 percent). Approximately 50 percent of these visited a doctor in the last six months for these symptoms.

Comparison of Prevalence

The prevalence of ill health was highest among data entry operators on every health outcome parameter. As can be seen in Table 1, the average number of diagnosed injuries was almost three times higher for data entry operators compared to other office workers (.72 vs .24). Similarly, the average number of musculoskeletal symptoms occuring almost daily was over two times higher for data clerks (3.3 vs 1.2) and the average number of psychosomatic complaints was one and one/half times higher (5.2 vs 3.3) for data entry clerks.

Table 1 **Health Outcomes by Occupation: Mean Values**

	Diagnosed Injury	MS Symptoms	StressSymptoms
Data Entry	**0.72**	**3.27**	**5.26**
General Office	**0.24**	**1.24**	**3.27**
P values	<.05	<.0000	<.004

This trend is also apparent in the extent to which individuals experience multiple symptoms. Twenty-seven percent of data entry operators reported six or more MS symptoms compared to 7.3 percent of other office workers. Similarly, 35 percent of data entry operators reported seven or more psychosomatic symptoms while only 12.2 percent of other office workers reported this number of symptoms. As well, data clerks were four times more likely to have visited a doctor about these problems (25% vs 6%). These differences were significant at the .05 level or better.

Working Conditions:

Work regimes differed substantially between data entry operators and general office staff. 71 percent of data clerks reported working 7 or more hours a day on a VDT compared to 11 percent of general office workers. Similarly, 40 percent of data entry operators reported working six to ten hours overtime per week compared to 6 percent of general office staff.

On the other hand, only 9 percent of data clerks reported working more than 1 and one half hours without a break compared to 39 percent of general office workers. Similarly, 84 percent of data clerks reported taking a break every hour compared to 27 percent of general office staff. And only 13 percent of data clerks reported missing a rest breaks almost daily compared to 36 percent of general office staff.

At the same time, only 5 percent of data clerks indicated that they could moderately to frequently walk around compared to 42 percent of general office staff. Similarly, only 15 percent of data clerks could vary their hand or arm positions moderately to frequently compared to 65 percent of general office staff.

Data entry procedures also involve significantly more twisting of the wrist with 74 percent of operators reporting that their work involved constant twisting of the wrist compared to 26 percent of general office workers. As well, 60 percent of data clerks complained that the thickness of the key board caused them to bend their hands awkwardly compared to 33 percent of general office workers.

Relationship Between Health Outcomes and Working Conditions:

To examine the relationship between working conditions and health outcomes correlations were analyzed through zero order regression analysis, as a first step, to evaluate whether an association was present and the strength of that association, if it existed.

To this end, summary measures of health outcomes were created by pooling the number of symptoms reported by respondents for musculoskeletal injuries and symptoms and psychosomatic complaints. The resulting scale for musculoskeletal symptoms ranged from a low of 0, those with no symptoms, to a high of six or more symptoms. Similarly, the scale for psychosomatic complaints ranged from a low of 0 to a high of seven or more symptoms.

The results of the zero order regression analysis show that stress is most strongly related to musculoskeletal symptoms ($R=.64$) followed by work station design problems ($R=.45$), computer monitoring ($R=.37$), postural mobility ($R=.34/.29$), hours spent on a VDT($R=.32$) and years of experience($R=.19$). These relationships were significant at a .03 value or better. However, the analysis could find no significant association between key stroke rates and musculoskeletal symptoms ($p<.4103$). Moreover, the relationship between the longest time spent keying without a break was negatively related to musculoskeletal symptoms ($p<.005$).

While the analysis shows a strong and significant relationship between levels of stress and musculoskeletal symptoms, the levels of stress were strongly influenced by a number of work environment factors that seem to act as significant stressors. Among these, work station design problems (R=.30) followed by computer monitoring (R=.27) and inability to walk around (R=.27) were the most strongly related to levels of stress at a significance level of $p<.001$.

In the next step of the analysis the data were analyzed using standard multiple linear regression analysis which allowed an assessment of the relative contribution of factors while controlling for the affect of all other factors.

Table 2 **Multiple Regression Analysis: MS Symptoms**

		Regression Coefficients	
Design Problems		**.158***	
Stress Levels		**.382***	
*p<.01	R=.704		R^2 =.476

Table 2 shows that when all other associated factors are controlled and analyzed simultaneously, stress, followed by work station design problems produce the most pronounced and significant effect on musculoskeletal disorders, and can explain approximately 48 percent of the variations in musculoskeletal disorders. However, as can be seen in Table 3, the results of multiple linear regression analysis of stress as a dependent variable, the levels of stress, are in turn, more strongly influenced by lack of postural mobility, followed by work station design problems.

Table 3 **Multiple Regression Analysis: Stress Levels**

		Regression Coefficients	
Design Problems		**.413***	
Postural Mobility		**.651****	
** P<.04	*P<.0002	R=.393	R^2=.119

DISCUSSION

On the basis of the data presented here, data entry operators have a significantly higher incidence of musculoskeletal injury and experience higher levels of musculoskeletal symptoms and psychosomatic disorders than general office workers. The analysis suggests that the interaction of several factors contribute to the higher prevalence of MS disorders among data entry clerks independent of key stroke rates.

On the one hand, the lack of postural mobility and the consequent maintenance of constrained awkward postures due to work station design problems contribute directly to disorders. Indeed, the lack of postural mobility obviate the potential ameliorative effects of routine rest break regimes. The analysis showed that, despite the fact that data entry clerks worked shorter periods without a break, they reported a higher incidence of musculoskeletal disorders than general office workers who had a greater opportunity frequently change posture. It seems that autonomy over mobility is much more important as an ameliorative measure than just having scheduled rest breaks.

On the other hand, computer monitoring in single task VDT work appears to contribute indirectly to musculoskeletal disorders. Computer monitored quota system is a psychosocial stressor that operates to restrict autonomy of decision and movement, and creates pressure to constantly push ones self. In this regard, the present study is consistent with the findings of previous studies linking psychosocial factors with MS disorders (2,3,6), and in particular, the role that computer monitoring plays in this context (7). Although the mechanism for this is not clearly understood, this study suggests that monitoring leads to constrained postures by reducing autonomy over postural mobility, a well established contributing factor for the development of MS disorders (1,4,5). As well, monitoring creates a pressurized work environment that increases muscular tension and thus the propensity for injury.

This suggests that musculoskeletal disorders are not so much a result of the keying demands of data entry work, but more likely a result of the work organization demands. Computer monitoring and low task variety restricts postural mobility and creates high levels of psychosocial stress and muscular tension. These act together with poor work station design to produce musculoskeletal overload and consequent pain, fatigue and injury.

Intervention strategies must consider the influence of work organization on biomechanical factors and the need to change work organization in addition to contemplated changes in the physical features of the work environment.

REFERENCES

1. Hunting, W., Laubli, T., Grandjean, E. (1981) Postural and visual loads at VDT workplaces: Constrained postures. Ergonomics 24: 917-931.
2. Leino, P. (1989) Symptoms job stress predict musculoskeletal disorders. J. Epidemiol. Community Health 43: 293-300.
3. Linton, S.J., Kamwendo, K. (1989) Risk factors in the psychosocial work environment for neck and shoulder pain in secretaries. J. Occup. Med. 31 (no. 7) : 609-613.
4. Maeda, K., Hunting, W., Grandjean, E. (1982) Factor analysis of localized fatigue complaints of accounting-machine operators. J. of Human Ergology 11: 37-43.
5. Sauter, S.L., Schleifer, L.M. (1991) Work posture, workstation design and musculoskeletal discomfort in a VDT data entry task. Human Factors 33(2) : 151-167.
6. Sievers, K., Makela, M., Klauka, T. (1989) Work stress and musculoskeletal disease (English summary). In Kalimo, E., Kallio, V. (Eds.) Juhlakirja Jaakko Pajula II. Helsinki: Kansanelakelaitos 425-440.
7. Smith, M.J., Caragon, P., Sanders,K.J., Lim, S.Y., LeGrande, D. (1992) Employee stress in jobs with and without electronic performance monitoring. Applied Ergonomics. 23(1): 17-28.

WORK WITH DISPLAY UNITS 92
H. Luczak, A. Çakir and G. Çakir (Editors)

Changes in the Visual System Resulting from Radar Screen Work

V. Koitcheva, V. Stantchev

Institute of Hygiene, Sofia

Abstract

Visual function of air-traffic controllers is studied in real work conditions, after two hours work on radar screen and two hours rest. Result indicates there are changes in dark focus, nearest point of accommodation and the threshold of electric sensitivity. Two hours of rest are not sufficiently effective for complete overcoming of the changes in vision.

Introduction

During the last several years a large number of investigations is devoted to the work with VDUs. Different types of activity are studied in a number of professions. (Bauer, H.C. et al 1989; Koitcheva,V., Zlateva,V. 1986). One of these professions is this of traffic controllers, which requires near point fixation of a screen that is characterized by an unusual contrast pattern, often by annoying reflections. The peculiarities of the visual fatigue in this profession are comparatively poorly studied (Östberg, O. 1980). Even more scanty are the investigations, which trace the rehabilitation processes in the visual system after work on radar screen and the optimal work rest schedules.

The primary focus of this research was to examine the changes in some basic visual parameters of air traffic controllers as a result of the work on radar screen. The secondary focus of this research was to evaluate the effectiveness of the existing work and rest schedules.

Method and subjects

Examinations were carried out on 26 air traffic controllers, men, at the age of 27 to 41. To obtain a representative sample, no specific criteria limited subject selection. All wore their normal refractive correction if any, so subjects had a visual acuity of 1 minute of arc. All subjects had a normal stereoscopic vision. Subjects were not encouraged to maximize their efficiency but were told to work at an individual comfortable speed.

The following methods were used: measurement of the nearest point of accommodation (PP), defining the electric sensitivity of the eye by determining the threshold of electric stimulation, leading to the appearance of phosphene, timing observations, measuring the eye-screen distance, evaluating the lighting conditions of different parts of the work place, subjective estimation of visual strain which included ocular and visual symptoms and the evaluation of the work load by the administration of a questionnaire. The dark accommodation was measured with a hand optometer (Jaschinski-Kruza, 1988), based on the polarized Vernier principle. Dark accommodation was measured in both eyes and averaged. The subjects received preliminary information on all methods used for the investigation. All tests were performed by the same operator at the same time of the day in order to avoid eventual effect on the results from the day-night rhythm of the visual functions. The visual task presented a predominantly static load of the oculomotor system because subjects looked at the VDUs during the work at a viewing distance about 50 cm.

The time schema of the study was the follow:

1. Assessment of the ophtalmologic status.
2. Measurement of visual parameters: threshold of the electric sensitivity, dark focus, nearest point of accommodation.
3. Two hours of real work on radar screen.
4. Measurement of the visual parameters.
5. Questionnaire.
6. Two hours rest period.
7. Measurement of the visual parameters.

The periods of work and rest in real conditions were organized in such a way, that after 2 hours of work on the screen follows 2 hours rest period or shift to another activity, where the vision is not the leading one.

"T"-tests for paired observations were calculated for all measured variables.

Results and discussion

The traffic controllers observe the radar screen on which are given graphics, figures and letters in type of information. The background of the screen is dark brown, the up signs are amber coloured. The gaze of the operator is directed not only to the radar screen but also to the board of meteorological information, to the written documents etc.

The time observations show that for 1 hour the traffic controller shifts his gaze to the different parts of the visual field 300 to 400 times, looks at the screen for 54 to 75 % of the 2 hours working period. The radar screen is irregularly illuminated by the running ray. The images of the airplanes appear for a short period of time and disappear to the following cycle of the radar. For this short interval the traffic controller has to appraise where exactly is the airplane and in supreme moments he has to assess the interdisposition of the airplanes, the direction of the flights and velocity. During the day shift for an hour 10 to 18 flights are controlled.

The evaluation of the lighting conditions in the workplace shows an irregular distribution of the brightness in the visual area of staff. The illumination of the screen is between 10 and 20 lx, and on the desk the local lighting is up to 100 lx. In the limits of the visual areas fall in light spots of illumination up to 200 lx.

Those observations point out that the work of the traffic controllers is characterized by an uninterrupted occupation of the sight in conditions of irregular distribution of the brightness in the visual field at a mean eye screen distance 53 cm.

The results show clearly the expected changes statistically significant in the visual parameters after 2 hours uninterrupted work on radar screen: bringing further away the nearest point of accommodation, increase of the threshold electric sensitivity and shifting the dark focus in myopic direction (fig. 1, 2, 3). We have found statistically significant difference between initial - 53 cm and final - 59 cm mean eye-screen distance.

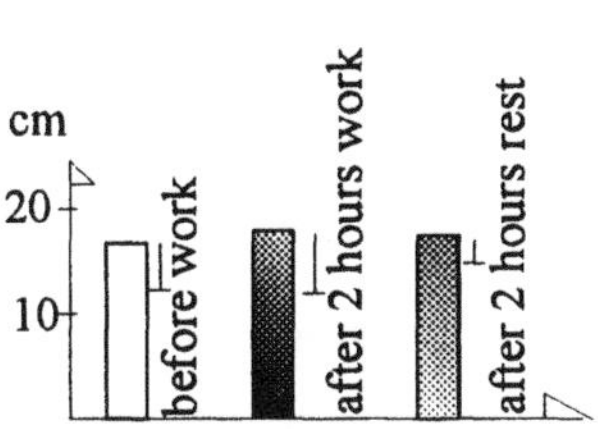

PP
Fig.1

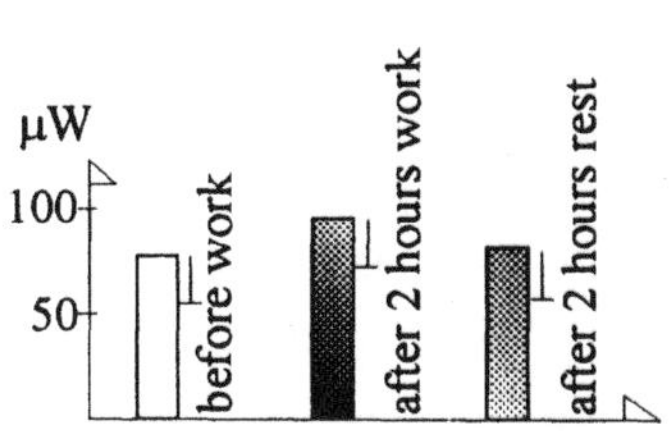

threshold of electric sensitivity
Fig.2

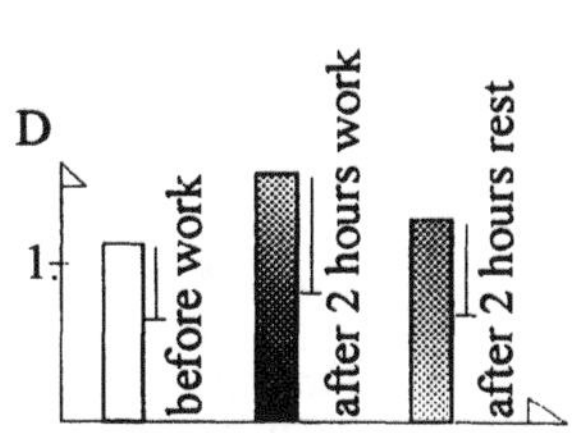

tonic accommodation
Fig.3

The inquiry performed on the existing complaints concerning vision shows that from 26 examined persons 23 have the classic symptoms of visual fatigue - photophobia, burning eyes, tearfulness, reddening of the eyes, headache, tired eyes. Most of the examined subjects classified the subjective feeling of visual fatigue after 2 hours work on the radar screen as strongly manifested and pointed out the presence of 2-3 subjective symptoms of visual fatigue at the same time.

Both literature data (Jaschinski-Kruza, 1988) and our studies in laboratory conditions show the dependance of the changes in the dark focus from the individual state of the tonic accommodation and the distance eye-object of observation. The results received from this study also support this affirmation. At the viewing distance 53 cm more significant changes are found in the group of persons with far dark focus (fig.4).

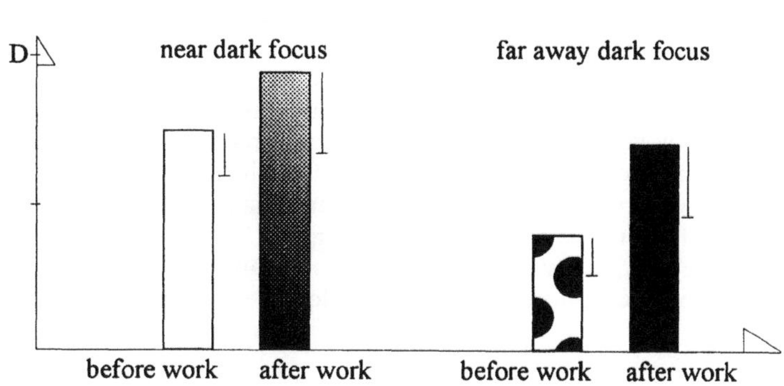

Fig. 4. Changes in the tonic accommodation

For the group with far dark focus the values increase from 0.8+0.2 to 1.3+0.5 D (t=3.92, n=14) and for the group with near dark focus from 1.5+0.3 to 1.9+0.5 D (t=2.94, n = 12). This results show that the persons who have initial state of tonic accommodation responding relatively to a further distance of sight than the visual task and therefore load more the accommodation, have more significant changes in the dark focus at the end of 2 hours work period on radar screen.

In the group of far dark focus we observe subjective symptoms of visual fatigue more strongly expressed as given on table 1.

Table 1
Subjective symptoms of visual fatigue in persons with different type focus

	Far dark focus - to 1.3 n=14		Near focus - above 1.3 n=12	
	Number of complaintes			
	strong	weak	strong	weak
burning	8	2	3	2
tearfulness	3	1	1	1
readening	5	1	3	1
photophobia	1	-	1	-
headache	1	3	1	1

A possible reason for this differences could be find in the hypothesis that the visual fatigue is influenced by initial dark focus, since subjects with a more distant position of accommodation in darkness tend to report stronger visual fatigue.

In the both groups of subjects we find significant moving away of the nearest point of accommodation more expressed in the group with the far dark focus - from 16.6+3.8 to 19.4+4.0 cm (n=14, t=2.3) and from 14.7+3.2 to 16.5+3.9 cm (n=12, t=5.0) in the group with near dark focus. This date needs a more detailed study of the interrelation between the tonic accommodation shifts and the position of the nearest point of accommodation.

One of the most important problems, related to the work with VDUs is that for the duration of the work periods and the rest between. Literature data give different proposals for the work-rest schedules defined empirically or on the assessment of the subjective discomfort in models of work on screen in laboratory conditions.

The air traffic controllers left their workplaces after 2 hours period of work on radar screen and passed the following 2 hours engaged in an other activity, excluding near to the eyes work.When measuring the visual parameters after the 2 hours rest, it was established that the changes in the threshold of electric sensitivity, in the tonic accommodation and in the nearest point of accommodation decrease, but they don't reach the initial values, measured before work (fig. 1, 2, 3). It means that the rehabilitation processes in the visual system are not complete and the traffic controllers start their next period of work on radar screen with lower functional possibilities of the visual system, which is prerequisite for occurrence of more expressed visual fatigue during the following work period. The results show also that 2 hours of rest is a means decreasing the visual fatigue in traffic controllers, but it is not sufficiently effective for the complete overcoming of the changes in vision at work on the radar screen. Possible reason for this is the way of getting along during rest, a well as the psychophysiological stress effects of the work.

References

1. H. G. Bauer et al. Conference "Work With Display Units", Montreal, 1989.
2. V. Koitcheva and V. Zlateva. Conference "Work With Display Units", Stockholm, 1986.
3. W. Jaschinski-Kruza. Vision Research, 28, 1271-1275, 1988.
4. O. Östberg. In Ergonomics Aspects of VDU. Ed. by E. Grandjean, E. Vigliani. Taylor and Francis Ltd., London, 1989.

WORK WITH DISPLAY UNITS 92
H. Luczak, A. Çakir and G. Çakir (Editors)

How to Eliminate Vision Symptoms - Treat the Eyes and Fix the Environment: A Report from the VDT Eye Clinic

James E. Sheedy, University of California, School of Optometry, Berkeley, CA 94720

ABSTRACT

Visually related symptoms at video display terminals (VDTs) occur when the visual demands of the task exceed the visual skills of the individual. At the VDT Eye Clinic we have been successful at relieving symptoms by diagnosing and treating vision disorders and by analyzing and improving environmental factors. This paper presents the results of recent studies and the clinical methods of resolving visual problems.

INTRODUCTION - VISUAL PROBLEMS

Eye and vision problems are by far the most frequent health related problems reported by video display terminal workers. Most studies into health related symptoms of VDT workers show that eye-related problems are the most frequent, but there is a wide variation in the percentages of VDT workers who experience eye-related problems[1-3]. The primary reasons for this wide variation include differences in the study populations and in the study methodologies. Worker groups with poorer eye care, poorer VDT equipment, poorer office ergonomics, and with older workers will have more eye problems.

In order to assess the extent of the visual problems in a different manner, I surveyed 5,686 randomly selected U.S. optometrists (25.3% responded) with a mail questionnaire concerning VDT patients in their practice[4]. On the average, 14.25% of their patients are obtaining the examination because of "symptoms primarily related to using a video display terminal". This means that approximately 10 million of the 70 million general eye examinations given annually in the US are due to problems at the VDT. There are approximately 60 million VDTs in use in the US. The following symptoms were reported to occur in the following order of frequency by the optometrists:

1. Eyestrain	5. Neck / back aches
2. Headaches	6. Photophobia
3. Blurred vision	7. Double vision
4. Dry or irritated eyes	8. After-images

Most of these symptoms have long been recognized as associated with demanding visual work - especially demanding near visual work. Secretaries, accountants, bookkeepers, draftsmen and others with demanding near visual jobs have commonly experienced these symptoms. However, in the survey of optometrists 680 said (549 said not) that their VDT patients have symptoms that other near point workers do not have[4]. The VDT task is an example of a task which can be particularly visually demanding and therefore will cause symptoms in a greater percentage of workers than will a less visually demanding task. The optometrists also were unable to confidently arrive at a diagnosis and treatment (health care practitioners are not always 100% certain of their treatment) more frequently for VDT patients (20.87%) compared to non-VDT patients (14.05%). The individual responses were tested with a paired t test, and the difference is statistically significant with $p < 10^{-13}$, d.f. 1105. This is a clear indication that the visual problems of VDT patients are more difficult to resolve than for other patients. This may be due to the visual environmental factors which are largely outside of the control of the optometrist.

Whether or not a particular individual will experience symptoms associated with near visual work depends upon the match between the visual skills of the individual and the visual demands of the task. Many individuals have marginal visual disorders which do not cause symptoms when the individual performs less demanding visual work, but will cause symptoms when the individual performs a more demanding visual task. Since each persons visual system and capabilities are different, and every (VDT) work environment is different, individual assessment is required to solve any given patients symptoms.

VDT EYE CLINIC

The VDT eye clinic is one of the specialty eye clinics of the School of Optometry at the University of California at Berkeley. Treatment at the VDT Eye Clinic relieves the symptoms of VDT users by diagnosis and treatment of vision disorders, provision of ergonomically designed spectacles, and analysis of the patients' work station environment through an in-office simulation and making suggestions for improvements. Patients with visual complaints or symptoms associated with work at a VDT are scheduled for their primary eye examination in this clinic. Prior to being examined, patients are mailed a questionnaire which asks them to make numerous observations and measurements of their work environment. Patients receive a complete general eye examination which includes in-depth assessment of the functioning of the eyes at near viewing distances. After most of the visual functions have been measured, but before the eyes have been dilated for the internal examination, the patient is seated at a VDT workstation which can be adjusted to match the measurements which the patient has made on their own work environment. The goal is to simulate, within limitations, the patients own work environment within our clinic. This allows for visual ergonomic analysis and proper prescription and spectacle design. Detailed descriptions of the clinical techniques and procedures are published elsewhere[5-8].

VISUAL DISORDERS AND TREATMENTS

Based upon the survey of optometrists[4] and upon our reported findings in the VDT Eye Clinic[7-8], the primary visual conditions which are causative of symptoms and which require correction are discussed below. Specific details about the clinical diagnoses and treatments have been reported previously[5,9].

Presbyopia. This is the condition in which the normal age-related loss of accommodation (ability to change the focus of the eye for near viewing distances) results in an inability to comfortably maintain focus on near objects. As a result of presbyopia, most people need to wear reading glasses or bifocal lenses in their early forties. The power of the proper corrective lens depends upon the remaining accommodative ability of the individual and the working distance.

Very frequently the prescription which the presbyope uses for other near tasks such as reading is not effective at the VDT. The "usual" bifocal correction is designed for a "normal" viewing distance of 40 cm and the bifocal segment is located in the lens for a downward gaze angle of about 25 degrees. The VDT is usually at a viewing distance which is somewhat greater (50-60 cm) and the viewing angle is only 10-15 degrees downward. A presbyope who tries to wear their "usual" bifocal correction at the VDT will either not see the VDT clearly or will need to assume an awkward posture - resulting in neck and back strain. Most VDT workers have other viewing needs such as reference materials. The particular prescription and spectacle design depends upon the remaining accommodative abilities and the viewing distances and angles which are required to perform the tasks. In most cases, this requires a separate pair of spectacles.

Nearly all VDT workers who require bifocals for normal visual tasks will require a separate pair of spectacles for their VDT work. It is very important that these workers measure the distance from their eyes to the VDT screen and to the reference documents, and also note the height of these tasks relative to their eyes. This information should be brought with them to their eye examination since it will influence the prescription which is given.

Accommodation. Normal pre-presbyopic patients have adequate accommodative abilities to function comfortably at near working distances. However, many workers have a reduced amplitude of accommodation for their age or accommodative infacility (inability to quickly and responsively change the level of accommodation). We have diagnosed 33% of our pre-presbyopic patients with accommodative disorders[8], nearly identical with the 34.6% accommodative disorder frequency rate indicated by the survey of optometrists[4]. These conditions result in blur at near working distances and/or discomfort. They also can result in post-VDT distance blur due to spasm of the accommodative mechanism. It is possible that poorer resolution on some VDT screens exacerbates accommodative problems because of the poorer accommodative stimulus.

Patients with accommodative disorders can generally be treated with spectacles which relieve the accommodative effort required to see clearly at near working distances. Some conditions can be treated with vision training exercises.

Eye Coordination. Even though most people keep their eyes aligned when viewing an object, many patients have difficulty maintaining this ocular alignment and experience symptoms such as fatigue, headaches, blur, double vision, and general ocular discomfort. Visual sensory feedback is utilized to keep the eyes aligned and to avoid double vision. Without this sensory feedback the eyes would assume their "position of rest" with respect to one another. If the position of rest is outward or diverged, the patient has exophoria. If it is inward or converged, the condition is esophoria. Small amounts of esophoria or exophoria are not usually clinically significant. The magnitude of the deviation and the ability of the patient to expend the necessary neuromuscular effort to overcome the deviation are factors in determining whether the condition causes symptoms.

Eye alignment at near viewing distances is more complex than at distance because of the ocular convergence required to view near objects and because of the interaction between the ocular convergence and accommodative mechanisms. It is possible that poor resolution of some VDT screens exacerbates ocular coordination problems because of the reduced quality of the sensory fusion stimulus. Treatment of these conditions can include spectacle refractive or prismatic correction, or vision training exercises.

Refractive Errors. Many patients simply need an accurate correction of refractive error (myopia, hyperopia, astigmatism). Patients with hyperopia must exert more accommodative effort to see clearly at near distances than non-hyperopes. Therefore many hyperopic VDT patients require refractive correction whereas they may not require it for a less visually demanding job.

Dry, Irritated Eyes and Contact Lens Problems. VDT work results in a higher gaze angle than other common near work. This also results in an approximate doubling of the exposed ocular surface area. Since the amount of tear evaporation is directly related to the exposed area of the tears, the higher gaze angles associated with VDT work result in greater tear evaporation. It has also been shown that VDT work significantly reduces the blink rate[10]. In many cases the office environment is low in humidity and can contain toxic matter, further contributing to dry or irritated eyes. Many individuals have a borderline dry eye condition which is exacerbated in a VDT working environment.

The solutions to these problems can include alterations in the work station arrangement, improvement of air quality, discontinuance of contact lens wear, artificial tears, or punctal occlusion

VISUAL ENVIRONMENTAL ISSUES

There are several aspects of the VDT task which make it especially visually demanding and/or contribute directly to symptoms. Mitigation of these problems can often directly eliminate symptoms or reduce the demands of the task so that symptoms don't result from marginal visual disorders. In our clinical experience, the most important visual environmental factors are as follows. A more complete discussion of these factors appears elsewhere[6].

Lighting. Improper lighting is likely the largest environmental factor contributing to visual discomfort. The most important principle of good lighting is: eliminate bright sources of light from the field of view and strive to obtain a relatively even distribution of luminances (brightnesses) in the field of view.

Bright sources of light in the field of view create discomfort glare. This can be demonstrated to most individuals by having them look straight ahead in a room with overhead fluorescent lights, and then shielding their eyes with a visor (or their hand) and noting the immediate improvement in comfort. This has become a particular problem for VDT users because they view more horizontally in the room than do workers who view materials on a desk. This results in the bright overhead lights and windows being more centrally located in the field of view. This is further exacerbated by the use of dark background VDT screens in which the luminance disparity between the screen and the other objects in the room is worsened. Methods of fixing this problem include: turning off selected luminaires, reducing the light levels, use of window blinds or drapes, parabolic louvers on the fluorescent luminaires, wearing visors, changing the workstation orientation, eliminating auxiliary workstation lighting, changing to a light background display, and changing wall treatment among others. Indirect lighting systems often provide good quality lighting.

Reflections. Room illumination will cause light to come back off the VDT screen because of the reflective glass surface and the underlying phosphor. This additional light coming off the VDT interferes with the image on the VDT and reduces visibility. This is a greater problem with dark background displays. Anti-reflection screens of glass construction are preferred over those made of mesh because they don't cause a decrease in resolution. Hoods can also be used to shield the VDT from incident room illumination.

Workstation Arrangement. The workstation should be arranged so that most of the visual work is located in front of the worker and so that the various visual tasks are located relatively close to one another. Document holders help to locate reference materials close to the screen so that excessive eye and body movement is not required to look back and forth. The screen should be located so the worker views 10-15 degrees downward. If the screen is higher it usually results in neck ache due to tilting the head backwards. It also results in the eyelids being open wider and less frequent blinking. This can cause dry eye, contact lens discomfort, and greater exposure to airborne toxicants which can cause eye irritation.

Design of Visual Display. Good resolution is important for proper visual function. Extended viewing of poor resolution images can be particularly taxing on the accommodative and ocular alignment systems. In a recent study[11] a group of 15 subjects read 17% more lines ($p<0.05$) in a 30 minute reading session on a higher resolution monitor compared to a VGA monitor. The subjects were also significantly more comfortable after reading on the higher resolution monitor.

White background displays have several advantages over black background displays: better brightness relationship with the surrounding room (they should be adjusted in brightness to match the immediate surrounds), less affected by reflections, and performance has been measured to be better[12].

There is some evidence that suprathreshold flicker rates are detected by the retina and cause discomfort. It may be desirable to use refresh rates higher than the common 60 cps, especially for white background displays where the size of the flickering image is considerably larger than for black background displays. The color of the display is probably not of great significance to visual comfort or performance, so long as the contrast between the letter and background is good.

SUMMARY

The visual symptoms and symptoms of discomfort experienced by VDT workers result from a visually demanding work environment which overtaxes the visual abilities of many workers. Proper visual diagnosis and treatment along with proper ergonomic design can resolve most of the problems.

REFERENCES

1. Smith MJ, Cohen BGF, Stammerjohn LW. An investigation of health complaints and job stress in video display operations. Human Factors, 23(4), 387-400, 1981.

2. Dain SJ, McCarthy AK, Chan-Ling T. Symptoms in VDU operators. Am J Optom Physiol Optics 65, 162-167, 1988.

3. Collins MJ, Brown B, Bowman KJ. Visual discomfort and VDTs. Centre for Eye Research, Department of Optometry, Queensland Institute of Technology, 1-37, 1988.

4. Sheedy JE. VDTs and vision complaints: A survey. Information Display 8(4&5), 20-23, 1992.

5. Sheedy JE. Video display terminals - solving the vision problems. Chapter in: Problems in Optometry - Environmental Optics, Sheedy JE, editor, 2(1), 1-16,1990.

6. Sheedy JE. Video display terminals - solving the environmental problems. Chapter in: Problems in Optometry - Environmental Optics, Sheedy JE, editor, 2(1), 17-31,1990.

7. Sheedy JE, Parsons SP. Vision and the video display terminal - clinical findings. In: Promoting Health and Productivity in the Computerized Office: Models of Successful Ergonomic Intervention, edited by Sauter S, Dainoff M, Smith M. Taylor and Francis Ltd, London, 1990.

8. Sheedy JE, Parsons SP. The video display terminal eye clinic: clinical report. Optometry and Vision Science, 67(8), 622-626, 1990.

9. Sheedy, JE. Six no-nonsense ways to help computer users. Optometric Management, Cover story, June, 1992.

10. Patel S. Henderson R, Bradley L, Galloway B, Hunter L. Effect of visual display unit use on blink rate and tear stability. Optometry & Vision Science 68(11), 888-892, 1991.

11. Sheedy JE. Reading performance and visual comfort on a high resolution monitor compared to a VGA monitor. Journal of Electronic Imaging, accepted for publication, 1993.

12. Sheedy JE, Bailey IL, Fong D, Ostermeier M, Stanton S. Task performance and contrast polarity on hard copy and video displays. Proceedings of SPIE/SPSE symposium on electronic imaging science and technology. Society of Photo-Optical Instrumentation Engineers, Bellingham, Washington, February, 1990.

WORK WITH DISPLAY UNITS 92
H. Luczak, A. Çakir and G. Çakir (Editors)

SIGNIFICANCE AND ROLE OF WORKING CONDITION ANALYSIS IN ERGOPHTHALMOLOGICAL SURVEILLANCE OF VIDEO DISPLAY UNIT OPERATORS

Piccoli B.,D'Orso M.,Troiano P.*,Ferrario M.,Carabelli I.*,Pierini F., Grieco A.,Miglior M.*

Inst. of Occupational Health,Univ. of Milan,V. S.Barnaba 8 ,20122 Milan.

*Inst. of Ophthalmology (1st),Univ. of Milan,V. F. Sforza 35,20122 Milan.

Introduction

From reviewing the literature it is clear that the high prevalence of asthenopic disturbances in VDU operators has a multifactorial origin (1,3,4,5,7,8).

This has important consequences in Occupational Medicine and in Ergophthalmology,not only from a research point of view but also for preventive aspects,with specific enphasis on health surveillance and design of work stations.Indeed, it seems more than ever true that if each aspect of the problem is analysed separately (visual function,lighting,chemical pollution etc.) ergophthalmological studies, even though vast and accurate, have little hope of interpreting aethiologically the asthenopia of VDU operators.(2)

For these reasons we have tried to set up a global methodology to analyse and study the relationships between VDU work and visual disturbances.

This methodology has been developed and perfected by trial and error during investigations carried out in work places by our Division of Ergophthalmology from 1988 to 1991;35 firms were examined involving 1216 operators.Particular care has been used in calculating data concerning the analysis of the exposure which has been described with some imprecision in previous published studies.

Usually exposed groups are classified either by using data obtained by self-administered questionnaires (which, according to our experience, are not very reliable) or by information based only on a general description of the work done ("data entry", "word processing", "programming,"etc.) and on the duration of the work. Sometimes even just in terms of dichotomic exposure levels such as "VDU user" or "VDU non user".

Assuming that exposed and non-exposed categories have the same probability of being misclassified,the expected effect would be a reduction of the association between exposure and asthenopia.It is quite possible therefore that in many investigation the reported absence of correlations between the prevalence of asthenopic disturbances and categories of operators is due to these deficiencies.

In fact imprecise evaluation of the " visual load ", i.e. observation distance per observation time (the equivalent of the "dose" in toxicology), can remarkably affect the final result.

Materials and methods

A total of 169 VDU operators from three firms were included in the study. The investigation consisted of three subsequent steps.
The first step was to gather some basic data from the firms such as planimetries of the offices indicating VDUs workstations, technical characteristics of the heating and cooling system, main technical characteristics of VDUs in use, personal and job-related data of the working population.
This information was analysed in terms of reliability and consistency.
With this data in hand,all the specific work stations were inspected to further verify the previously gathered data and to closer examine the type and the conditions of the exposure.
During these visits the required visual effort and the lay-out in relation to the natural and artificial light source were particularly observed. The presence of either microclimatic conditions capable of causing ergophthalmological discomfort or of air-borne substances having an irritative effect on the ocular surface were also carefully checked.
The second step of the investigation consisted in the collection of subjective data by interviewing each operator, at the work place.
These included questions about lifestyle, family history, general and ocular history, task description, opinion of the work environment and lastly asthenopic symptomathology occurring in relation to work.
Interviews took approximately half an hour per subject.
The third and final step was the evaluation of the visual function (including:case history,clinical ocular examination,refraction,orthoptic examination, simultaneous perception by synoptophore,fusion at far and at near by prisms,stereopsis at far by synoptophore and at near by Titmus Stereo-test,lateral and vertical phoria at far and at near by cover test,divergence and convergence at far and at near by prisms/cover test,proximal point of convergence and near point of accomodation).
Among the 169 subjects considered exposed according to the information provided by the firms, following the previously illustrated checks, 46 were unsuitable either because they were assigned only occasionally to VDU work or because their duties did not require VDU work at all.
In the remaining 123 subjects (57 males av.age 42.5, 66 females av.age 35.3)the work with VDUs mainly consisted in "data entry", and "data acquisition" tasks, more or less equally distributed;all VDUs had CRT display with negative presentation and white or green or amber phosphors.
Finally, to better correlate the exposure data with the asthenopic symptomatology, an experimental multifactorial "score" was elaborated by using an unweighted sum of scores of the principal exposure factors (table 1) reported in the literature to be correlated with asthenopia.
The score which varies from a minimum of 7 points (worst conditions) to a maximum of 21 points (best conditions),has been applied to each work station.
Concerning the symptomatology, subjects were considered asthenopic when they suffered from two or more occasional symptoms (e.g. at least once a week), or of one frequent symptom (two or more times per week).

Results

Examination of ocular refraction and motility revealed a high prevalence of alteration in the evaluated parameters (table 2 and 3).
There were only 13 subjects with no abnormalities.
The subjects were divided into four groups according to their refractive alterations and motility disturbances.Prevalence of asthenopia did not show statistically significant differences among these groups (table 4).
On the other hand the mean values of the multifactorial score showed a statistically significant difference in refraction and motility impairment categories.Moreover disaggregating these data according to the presence or absence of symptoms,symptomatic subjects reported lower scores in every abnormal category but a higher difference was found in the group of subjects who did not suffer from any ocular impairment (table 5).As shown in figure 1, the number of referred symptoms is statistically significant related to the score according to a linear function. A high prevalence of symptoms seems to be predicted by a low score.
An univariate analysis (data not presented) of the parameters considered in the score has shown that the duration of exposure is statistically significant in relation to asthenopia ($p<0.01$).

Conclusions

Our data confirm the high prevalence of asthenopia in VDT/PC operators.
Prevalence of asthenopia does not seem to be related to the different alterations of ocular refraction and motility probably because the former are mostly well corrected while among the latter there were only a few subjects with "unstable functional compensation".
The application of the "score" has shown on the contrary a high correlation with the symptomatology in the whole sample.Moreover among subjects without ocular impairments the score seems to better discriminate between symptomatic and asymptomatic subjects.
The exposure time (last parameter of the score,see table 1) is confirmed as significantly correlated to the symptomatology.
These results confirm that a correct and precise assessment of exposure is of basic importance to make detailed associations between asthenopia and its occupational causes.
Further confirmation of the validity of this index could be reached by additional studies,involving many other populations.
The accuracy of the collection of the environmental and working exposure parameters could be improved by the use of more objective evaluation and quantification of type and duration of work as well as more detailed investigations about all chemical and physical factors potentially causing ocular disturbances.

References

1) Bergqvist U.
Possible effects of working with V.D.U.:Brit.J.Ind.Med.,46,217,1989.
2)Grieco A.,Piccoli B.
Nota 1:metodo per la valutazione del carico di lavoro visivo e delle condizioni illuminotecniche dei posti di lavoro:Med Lav,5,496,1982.

3) Knave B.,Wibom R.,Voss M.,Hedstrom L.,Bergqvist U.
Work with V.D.T. among office employees.Subjective symptoms and discomfort.:Scand. J.of Work and Environment Health,11,457-466,1985.
4) Molhave L.
The Sick Building Syndrome caused by V.O.C.s:Proceedings of the Indoor air quality International Symposium,St. Louis Missouri,U.S.A.,May 1989.
5) Molhave L.
The influence of V.O.C.s on indoor air quality:Symposium on indoor air quality and health,Perugia,October 1991.
6) Piccoli B.,Maltoni R.,Zambelli P.L.,Grieco A.
Lo studio delle luminanze al posto di lavoro:metodo e risultanze di una ricerca sul campo:A.I.D.I.I.,VIII Congresso Nazionale,1988.
7)W.H.O.
V.D.T. and workers health:Publication n.99,Geneve,1987.
8)W.H.O.
Update on V.D.T. and workers health:3,october 1990.

Table 1:Parameters of the score for the evaluation of each work station.

Parameter	3 Points	2 Points	1 Point
Video position	Facing	< 45	>45
Work surface	Opaque-dark	Opaque-light shiny-dark	Shiny-light
Protection from natural light	No natural light or venetians	Other protection	No protection
Sheilding from artificial light	Grille	Screen	Absent
Luminance ratio (*)	Slight	Moderate	Intense
Air conditioning	Centralized	Localized	Absent
Average exp. time	< 3 hrs/day	3-5 hrs/day	> 5 hrs/day

(*)inside of the "occupational visual field" (6).

Table 2: Ocular refraction. (*)

	Emmetropia		Myopia		Ipermetropia		Astigmatisms		Tot.	
Frequency	62	50.4%	17	13.8%	12	9.8%	32	26.0%	123	100%

(*) 29 subjects were presbiopic.

Table 3: Ocular motility.

	Ortophoria		Exophoria		Esophoria		Other impairments		Tot.	
Frequency	74	60.2%	14	11.4%	25	20.3%	10	8.1%	123	100%

Table 4: Asthenopia prevalence by refraction and/or motility impairment.

Pathology	No symptoms		Symptoms		Tot.	
None	4	30.8%	9	69.2%	13	11.5%
Motility impairm.	5	55.6%	4	44.4%	9	8.0%
Refraction impairm.	31	50.8%	30	49.2%	61	54.0%
Both	9	30.0%	21	70.0%	30	26.5%
Tot.	49	43.4%	64	56.6%	(*)113	100.0%

(*) subjects with tropias excluded
Chi-squared test (3 d.f.) n.s.

Table 5: Mean environmental score by ocular pathologies and presence of asthenopia.

	No symptoms	Symptoms	Total (*)
Pathology			
None	17.75 (sd.0.96)	11.00 (sd.2.50)	13.07 (sd.3.86)
Motility imp.	14.20 (sd.1.79)	14.00 (sd.3.55)	14.11 (sd.2.52)
Refraction imp.	16.06 (sd.1.36)	14.60 (sd.3.06)	15.34 (sd.2.45)
Both	15.89 (sd.1.26)	14.66 (sd.2.22)	15.03 (sd.2.04)

(*) One way ANOVA :p<0.05

Figure 1: Association between symptoms sum and exposure score value.

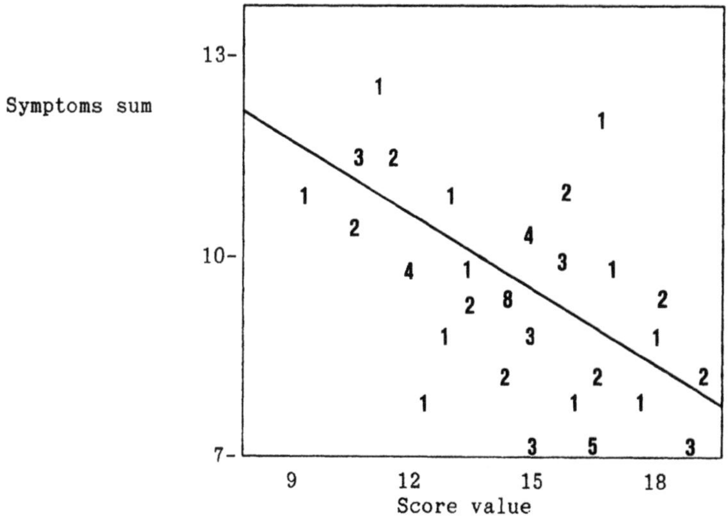

r= -0.48 (p<0.01), R-squared = 0.23, y= 15.48 -0.401x

WORK WITH DISPLAY UNITS 92
H. Luczak, A. Çakir and G. Çakir (Editors)

Subjective symptoms and ophthalmological findings in VDU employees

G. Cornelio[a], S. Da Pozzo[b], R. Ferri[a], P. Perissutti[b], L. Petronio[a]

[a]Occupational Medicine Service, P.le Canestrini 2, 34100 Trieste, Italy

[b]Ophthalmology Department, Children Hospital, via dell'Istria 65/1, 34100 Trieste, Italy

In recent years, several studies have focused worldwide on the high incidence of eye discomfort among VDU operators. Various hypotheses have been put forward to underline and support the role played by various factors, such like work environment, lighting conditions, different job tasks on VDU, quality of VDU image and the predisposing effect of some ocular disorders like refractive errors, use of spectacles, reduced visual acuity and oculomotor impairment.
The purpose of this paper is to give a contribution to shed light into this research field and provide some recommendations not only to VDU operators, but also to labour organizations, offices and companies in order to prevent as much as possible the occurrence of visual and ocular complaints.

1. METHODS

This study involved 610 operators (336 females, 274 males) working at VDU with three different tasks (software industry, postal office, newspaper); all subjects were first interviewed and then examined by the same researcher. The interview was performed by means of a questionnaire including items on time spent at VDU (daily worktime, VDU length of service, glance time), environmental data (illumination conditions, indoor climate, noise), VDU characteristics (colours, readability of characters, screen position, annoyance by flicker and reflections), frequency of ocular and visual complaints, Mc Collough effect and headache.
According to the AOA suggestions, the ophthalmological examination was performed evaluating best visual acuity (corrected or not), refraction, oculomotor and sensorial situation, intraocular pressure, colors discrimination and fundus ophthalmoscopy. The statistical evaluation was performed on all available data by means of the chi-square test, in order to find significant correlation between symptoms on one side and environmental data and/or ophthalmologic findings on the other.

2. RESULTS

Table 1 summarizes age and sex distribution and mean values of VDU exposure in the population.

Table 1
Distribution of subjects by age, sex, working time with VDU

	MALES	FEMALES	ALL
No. subjects	274	336	610
Mean age (yrs)	36	33	34
Mean work with VDU (yrs)	5.6	3.3	4.3
> 10 yrs (%)	18.7	6.2	11.8
Hours/day at VDU(mean)	4.0	4.5	4.3
> 4 hours/day (%)	60.2	74.0	67.8
Glance time at VDU ("long"%)	16.5	22.0	19.6

Table 2 shows the distribution (total and separated for sex) of asthenopic symptoms, divided into ocular and visual. In the same Table the prevalence of headache and the incidence of Mc Collough effect are shown.

Table 2
Prevalence of reported complaints

Ocular symptoms	Total %	Males %	Females %
Eye heaviness	68	64.2	71.1
Eye burning	57.2	54	59.8
Eyes red and tearing	49.2	50.4	48.2
Photophobia	48.2	36.1	58
Visual symptoms			
Myopization	46.1	46.7	45.5
Trouble in focusing	55.9	56.9	55.1
Double vision	27.4	26.6	28
Headache	32.8	25.3	39
McCollough effect	10.3	11.3	9.5

Table 3 shows the effect of daily worktime and prolonged glance time on symptoms occurrence.

In Table 4 the correlations between complaints and VDU characteristics are shown.

Table 3
Correlation between symptoms and daily worktime and glance time

	Daily worktime (> 4 hrs.)	Long glance time
Eye tired and heavy	$p < .0001$ (T), $< .001$ (M)	$p < .0001$ (T), $< .001$ (F), $< .01$ (M)
Eye burning	$p < .001$ (T) $p < .01$ (M)	$p < .001$ (T - F)
Myopization	$p < .01$ (T - M)	
Trouble in focusing	$p < .01$ (T - M)	
Headache	$p < .01$ (T - F)	$p < .001$ (T - F)

T = Total population M = Males F = Females

Table 4
Correlation between screen characteristics and symptoms

	Ocular discomfort	Visual fatigue
Reflections on screen	$p < .0001$	n.s.
Characters/background colors (if different from black-white)	$p < .0001$	$p < .001$
Short eye-screen distance	n.s.	$p < .0001$
Flicker annoyance	$p < .01$	$p < .01$
Bad characters readability	$p < .01$	$p < .01$
Bad characters resolution	$p < .01$	$p < .001$

The correlation between lighting conditions, environmental characteristics and eye complaints are shown in Table 5.

Table 5
Effect of lighting conditions, microclimate and noise on eyestrain

	Ocular discomfort	Visual fatigue	Headache
Bad illumination	$p < .0001$	$p < .01$	$p < .01$
Noisy workroom	$p < .001$	n.s.	$p < .001$
Bad microclimate	$p < .001$	n.s.	n.s.

The prevalence of corrected and uncorrected refractive errors is shown in Table 6,

Table 6
Population profile according to proper or improper correction of refractive errors

Glasses users	296 (48.5)	* Proper glasses	173 (28.4)	* Improper glasses	123 (20.1)
No glasses	314 (51.5)	* Emmetropes	227 (37.2)	* Uncorrected ametropes	87 (14.3)

In Table 7 are summarized the factors that resulted significant for the occurrence of visual fatigue, ocular symptoms and headache.

Table 7
Summary of significative factors in eyestrain and headache onset

Visual fatigue	Ocular discomfort	Headache
Daily worktime > 4 hrs (in males only)	Sex	Sex
Uncorrected/partially corrected small refractive errors	Long glance time (in females only)	High-rythm job
Use of spectacles	Daily worktime > 4 hrs. (in males only)	Noisy environment
Decompensating heterophorias	Length of service > 3 yrs. and < 10 yrs.	
Convergence insufficiency	Reflections	
	Bad lighting conditions	
	Bad microclimate	
	High-rythm job	

3. DISCUSSION

From the literature on VDU complaints, it is well known that females report more eyestrain than males. In our population, on average, females are younger than males, report a shorter length of service at VDU, but their daily worktime (specially when shifts > 4 hours a day are considered) and their percentage of prolonged glance time of VDU are clearly higher than in males (Table 1). This could be the first key to understand why they report more eyestrain than males; in fact, ocular discomfort is more frequent in females (p =.001), while the prevalence of visual fatigue is almost the same in the two sexes (Table 2). The percentage of those who report no ocular discomfort is 11.5%, while the correspondent percentage for visual fatigue is 16.2%.
Significant correlation has been pointed out between daily work at VDU and glance time on one side and asthenopia on the other; the threshold of four hours a day is the starting point for a significant increase of complaints (Table 3) and the "longlasting" glance time is a real factor, when compared to an "average" glance time. Surprisingly, a by-sex-analysis makes evident that a significant correlation for daily work at VDU appears quite only in males, while for the glance time it appears quite only in females.
All VDU characteristics, except reflections, reported on the questionnaire as "average" or "bad" resulted to be significantly related to both ocular and visual complaints (Table 4); reflections on VDU screen were strongly correlated to ocular discomfort only. Furthermore it became evident that positive-polarity screens are well accepted by operators, specially black/white screen colours. Workroom lighting conditions perceived as unsatisfactory (i.e. both excessive/insufficient illumination) resulted to be strongly related to ocular discomfort, but only weakly to visual fatigue (Table 5).
In Table 6 it can be noted that 210 operators (34.4% of the population) work at VDU with uncorrected or partially corrected refractive errors and among them visual fatigue is significantly higher (p=.011). Both in spectacle wearers and in

non-wearers small uncorrected or partially corrected refractive errors reducing visual acuity at levels ranging from 7 to 9/10 are related to higher levels of visual fatigue, while subjects with visual acuities lower than 7/10 appear to be more "protected" from fatigue onset. This fact confirms that, differently from the small visual defects, the great ones are not related to high levels of complaints.
Exophoria at near was found in (18.5% of all subjects); in this group eyestrain was more common than among ortophoric subjects, but the difference was not statistically significant. Instead, in 29 subjects latent exodeviation had the tendency to decompensate into manifest deviation; among these subjects double vision was significantly more frequent than in ortophoric ones (p=.006). The same trend was observed among operators with convergence insufficiency (p=.018), thus suggesting that work at VDU represents a critical task for operators with latent diplopia.

4. CONCLUSIONS

The main goal of research on eyestrain affecting VDU operators is the identification of ocular and environmental predisposing factors and then the accomplishment of a prevention campaign to all labour organizations, companies and offices. The present research underlines the pathogenetic role played by some environmental, work-related and ophthalmological factors and suggests that in VDU operators eyestrain can be really reduced working on three main aspects (Table 7): i) improve the work environment and the workstation design and characteristics as much as possible; ii) introduce a new working style that includes periodical visual breaks into the working shift and a shorter glance time at VDU; iii) perform periodical ergophthalmological examination to recognize eye conditions that can lead to high levels of eyestrain. A correct and full approach to the problem with this wide-oriented protocol well borne in mind would surely guarantee better working conditions to all VDU operators.

5. REFERENCES

1 U.O.V. Bergqvist: Video display terminals and health: a technical and medical appraisal of the state of the art. Scand. J. Work. Env. Health., 10 (supp2) (1984) 1
2 S. Diamond: Headache from video display terminals. Postgr. Med., 82 (1987) 184
3 K.G. Nyman, B.G. Knave, M. Voss: Work with video display terminals among office employees. IV: Refraction, accommodation, convergence and binocular vision. Scand J Work Environ Health 11 (1985) 483
4 L. Rose: Workplace video display terminals and visual fatigue. J Occup Med 29 (1987) 321.

WORK WITH DISPLAY UNITS 92
H. Luczak, A. Çakir and G. Çakir (Editors)

Eye screening and basic medical examination of employees at visual work places in Germany

K. Behling, AG 1.9 Ausschuß Arbeitsmedizin des Hauptverbandes der gewerblichen Berufsgenossenschaften, Verwaltungs-Berufsgenossenschaft, Mönckebergstr.7, W-2000 Hamburg 1, Germany.

1. Abstract

The special german principle of examination in occupational health "Visual display work places" (G 37) will be discussed.

2. Introduction

In Germany the "Commitee for Occupational Health" (Ausschuß Arbeitsmedizin) had published 44 different "Principles of Special Preventive Examination in Occupational Health" (Berufsgenossenschaftliche Grundsätze für Arbeitsmedizinische Vorsorgeuntersuchungen). According to these principles in 1991 about 12000 physicians examined employees in over 2 million medical check-ups (2,389,617).

In 1982 a group of physicians, i.e. works doctors, physicians of health insurances and ophthalmologists, chosen by the Commitee for Occupational Health, published the first examination principles for vision tests, the G 37.

About 4000 of the above-mentioned over 10,000 physicians have the license to test eyes and eyesight of the employees who spend a great deal of each working day at visual display units (VDU) for various purposes. In 1991 300,000 check-ups were carried out with these visual tests. 1600 special eye physicians have the license for ophthalmologic examinations if the results of the check-ups make them necessary.

In 1992, ten years later, roughly the same group, chosen by the Commitee for Occupational Health, published a revised G 37 "VDU-Work-places" (Bildschirm-Arbeitsplätze), taking in consideration the new council directive of the European Communities on the minimum safty on health requirements for work with display screen equipment (90/270/EEC) and the experience of the vision examinations done from 1982 til 1991 by the physicians.

3. Criteria

In october 1991 the Commitee for Occupational Health published the criteria for selection if an employee using VDU has to be examined or not examined. The so called ZH 1/600.37 says that any worker who habitually uses display screen equipment as a significant part of his normal work shall be entitled to the test G 37 carried out by a physician with a special license. Every worker not older than 40 years shall be checked every 5 years and older than 40 years shall be checked every 3 years. A vision test must also be provided if an employee reports discomfort or visual difficulties which may be connected with the visiual requirements of his work.

4. Document

The health and vision examination can be documented on a green paper edited by the above mentioned group G 37 "VDU-Work-Places".

After the health and vision test a green certificate is given to the employer and the employee.

5. General Health

The physician has only to state if there are any objections regarding health for starting or continuing work at the VDU-workplace or if there are no objections. In 1991 872 times "objections regarding health" were documented for VDU-work-places, that are 0.3 percent.

During the health and vision tests several questions are to be answered. Are there complaints such as asthenopic symptoms, i.e. ocular discomfort, eye fatigue, eye strain or visual discomfort at VDU-work place or even during normal reading. Which kind of glasses or lenses are worn? Are there any ophthalmologic diseases. Are there musculo-skeletal problems regarding the back, neck and shoulder, legs and arms? What about headache, dizziness, epilepsis or other neurological symptoms? Are there diseases like diabetes, concerning the thyroid or other endocrine glands? What about the heart and vascular system like high pressure, what about medication?

After the history of illness is reported the description of the work place is next important. Which kind of work does the employee carry out at his VDU-work-place. How many hours does the person work using a VDU. Had he received training at VDU-workstation before commencing this type of work. If there are any indications for diseases of the musculo-skeletal system or pains in the neck, shoulder, back and extremities, a physical examination has to be carried out. It is important to know, that many slender asthenic individuals and some obese middle aged individuals have discomfort in the back. Their backs ache much of the time and the pain interferes with effectiv work. The physical examination is positive for slack musculatur and poor posture. Pain in the neck and between the shoulder blades is a common complaint among thin, tense and active women and seems to be related to tout muscles. To decide if the complaints are due to the equipment of the workplace the physician, i.e. the works-doctor, has to inspect the arrangement of display-unit, keyboard, work desk and chair. The environment has to be inspected, too, like space requirements, lighting, noise, heat and humidity. All the abnormalities of the physical examination are to be recorded by using the green paper. But normally it is hard to decide if there are any relations between the mentioned risk factors of the individuals, the individual muskulo-skeletal problems and the special factors of the workstation.

6. Vision Test

Then the vision test is performed. It is important to know, that persons in late childhood and adolescence have increasing difficulty in focusing the eyes and in seeing clearly, i.e. the abnormalities usually can be traced to myopia. Later in life cataracts, glaucoma, retinal hemorrhages and detachments are the most frequent causes of visiual disturbances. In the vision test it is recommended that the acuity is examined at a viewing distance of 33 cm, of 55 cm and at long distance, because it is impossible to avoid differing viewing distances while working with VDU. The accomodation, i.e. the switch to see from various distances is a particular problem for the presbyopia. The older employees have presbyopia, i.e. a restricted accommodation ability. In the measurement of visual acuity the Landolt rings are prescribed, that are black rings with a small gap on the top, bottom, on the right or the left side or between top and right side and so on. It is recommended that the visual acuity should be better than 10/12, i.e. the 1.2 minutes of arc big gap of a 12 minutes of arc big Landolt ring is definitely recognized in the right position. Rows of diminishing size of these Landolt rings are to be regognized til a row with at least three out of five signs is correctly recognized. A patient with a refractive error should wear eyeglasses for the test.

In figure 1 the flow chart of the preventive medical examination G 37 is shown. If there is a visual acuity less than 10/12, the patient has to go to an ophtalmologist of his own choice, has to get new eyeglasses if necessary, and has to repeat his vision test within the next three months. An employee is to be supplied with special glasses tested for his work, if a vision test shows that these are needed and ordinary spectacles cannot be used. Since 1990 in Germany the costs of the special VDU-glasses, which are needed only at the VDU-work-places, have to be paid by the health insurance.

After the acuity vision test has been done the occupational physician has to examine the quality of central vision, colour vision, oculomotor coordination, phoria and stereopsis.

The quality of central vision is examined by a standard Amsler-chart, i.e. a square with dark lines on a white background in which horizontal and vertical parallel lines make up a perfectly squared surface. In the centre there is a black spot which serves as a fixation point. Keeping the gaze fixed upon the spot you have to see the four corners of the square and an intact network with quite straight and parallel lines, in other words all lines are perfectly regular.

The colour vision test is performed by comparing pairs of special colours in a vision instrument or by reading coloured numbers on a special coloured background.

The strabismus or phoria is an eye-muscle imbalance that results in improper alignment of the two eyes. Once binocular fusion is established, any type of ocular muscle balance causes diplopia, i.e. images then fall on different and noncorresponding parts of the retinas in the 2 eyes. After some time, however, patients learn to supress the image of one eye. If this happens at an early age, i.e. there is a commitant strabismus of congenital nature, the person may later have a diminished visual acuity in that eye. The test will be performed with a test equipment where the fusion is broken up by regarding two quite different figures with each eye.

During the stereopsis test the patient has to distinguish stereoscopic demonstrated figures at diminishing stereo angles. He has to distinguish if a special stereoscopic figure is in front or behind of a reference plane til a stereo angle of 2 minutes of arc is reached.

7. Special Vision Test

If the special vision tests show abnormalities or the acuity is less than 10/12 and there are eye-complaints by VDU-work you have to send the employee to an ophthalmologist with the special license. This special eye-physician has to examine the patient and has to write an ophthalmological certificate. The occupational physician, i.e. the works-doctor, has to decide if there are any objections regarding health for working at the VDU-workplace.

Strabismus and diplopia, ocular pain, photophobia, inability to read or recognize objects can but do not have to be factors for the medical certificate. The question is: Do these abnormalities interfere with his personal well-being while working at VDU-workplaces. If there are severe complaints, the works doctor cannot recommend to the employer that the person should work at VDU-workplaces. The works doctor has to give the medical certificate "Unlimited Objections regarding to Health". In this connection it is important to say, that one-eyed persons are not excluded from working at VDU-workplaces.

8. Costs

In Germany the employer has to pay about 70 DM according to the medical tarif for the preventive medical examination in occupational health regarding to VDU-workplaces, i.e. for the G 37, if there is no works doctor in his company, who normally carries out the G 37.

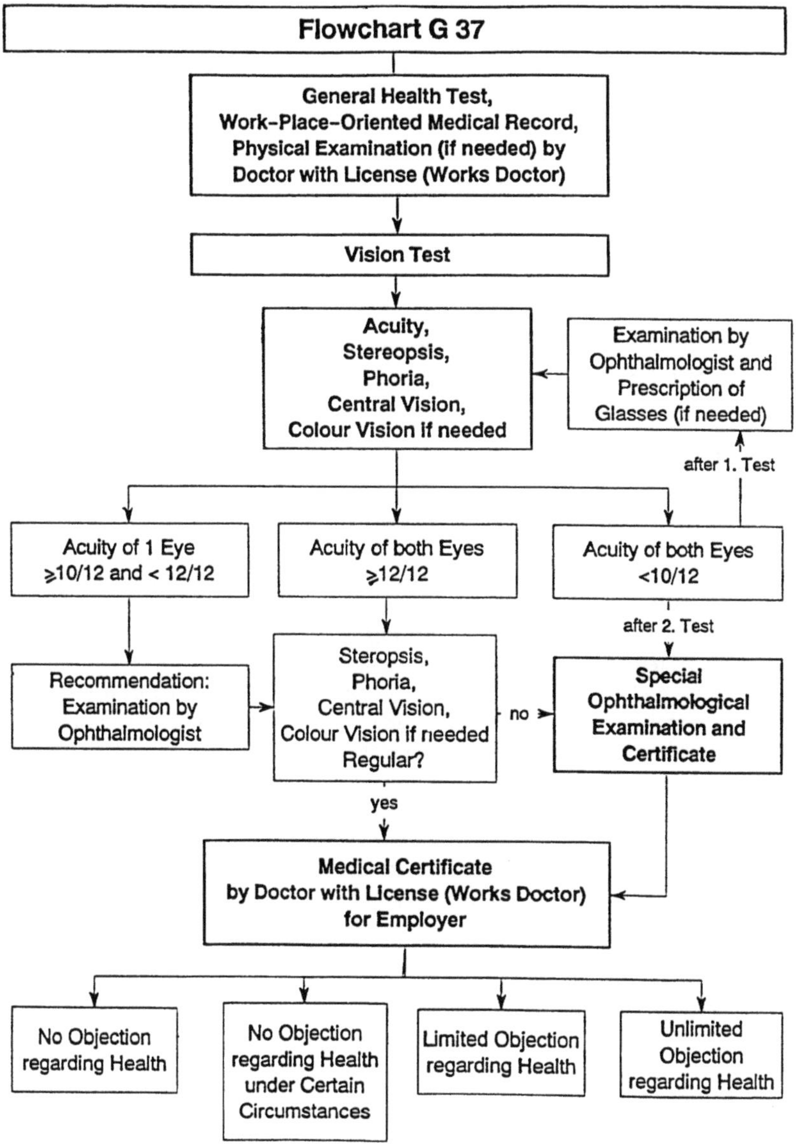
Flowchart G 37
General Health Test,
Work-Place-Oriented Medical Record,
Physical Examination (if needed) by
Doctor with License (Works Doctor)
Vision Test
Acuity,
Stereopsis,
Phoria,
Central Vision,
Colour Vision if needed
Examination by
Ophthalmologist and
Prescription of
Glasses (if needed)
after 1. Test
Acuity of 1 Eye
≥10/12 and < 12/12
Acuity of both Eyes
≥12/12
Acuity of both Eyes
<10/12
after 2. Test
Recommendation:
Examination by
Ophthalmologist
Steropsis,
Phoria,
Central Vision,
Colour Vision if needed
Regular?
no
Special
Ophthalmological
Examination and
Certificate
yes
Medical Certificate
by Doctor with License (Works Doctor)
for Employer
No Objection
regarding Health
No Objection
regarding Health
under Certain
Circumstances
Limited Objection
regarding Health
Unlimited
Objection
regarding Health

Figure 1

WORK WITH DISPLAY UNITS 92
H. Luczak, A. Çakir and G. Çakir (Editors)
1993 Elsevier Science Publishers B.V.

Visual comfort and performance measures of VDUs tested in comparative multi-display experiments

M.C. Boschman and J.A.J. Roufs

Institute for Perception Research (IPO), Eindhoven University of Technology, P.O.Box 513, 5600 MB Eindhoven, The Netherlands

1. INTRODUCTION

In order to obtain optimum visual comfort during prolonged, intensive visual tasks, the parameters of VDUs have to be tuned to the human visual system. Criteria for these parameters have to be found in measures which are directly related to the ease with which information can be extracted from a display. Measures based upon visual comfort and performance have been introduced by Roufs et al. [1] and Roufs and Boschman [2]. The measures used included objective variables - *search velocity* and *eye movement variables* registered in a letter search task in pseudo-text - and a subjective variable - *judgement of visual comfort* using a 10-point scale - which were measured simultaneously. They also introduced printed stimuli to serve as references when results of different experimental sessions need to be compared. In the medium-quality range all measures were shown to be closely correlated. However, in the high-quality range visual comfort may increase while all other measures level off (Boschman and Roufs, [3]). Taking both the complexity and effectiveness of measurement into account, search velocity was found to be the most suitable objective measure and delivers at least as much information as the eye movement parameters. Hence, the only quality measures studied in this paper are comfort judgement and search velocity.

The main purpose of the experiments to be described in this paper is to check whether the aforementioned methodology resolves the relatively small display-quality variations that exist between the different commercially available terminal displays used in these experiments.

2. APPARATUS

A multi-display panel was set up to evaluate eight terminal displays and printed references under well-defined physical conditions. The equipment was divided into two sections.

In the first part the eight different terminal displays were placed on two tables. The terminals were connected to a μVAX computer via addressed RS-232-C lines. Room illumination consisted of fluorescent strip-lighting that was concealed, so that direct reflections were prevented. In order to provide diffuse illumination, the test-room walls were covered with white sheets. This resulted in a vertical illumination E_v of 340 lx on all terminals.

Printed references [2] were presented to the subjects in the second part of the apparatus. The contrast and background luminance of these stimuli were controlled via a combination of direct and mirrored light sources that were driven by the μVAX computer.

Head-chin supports restricted the subject's viewing distance to 53 cm in front of the terminals and 100 cm in front of the print references. At each table a button case was available to register the subjects' responses.

3. EXPERIMENTS

3.1. Experiment 1

In this experiment the effects of contrast polarity and near-vision correction were also investigated. The stimulus set contained eight different VDUs and two print references that were driven in both contrast polarities. The peak luminance of the VDUs was set to 70 cd/m^2.

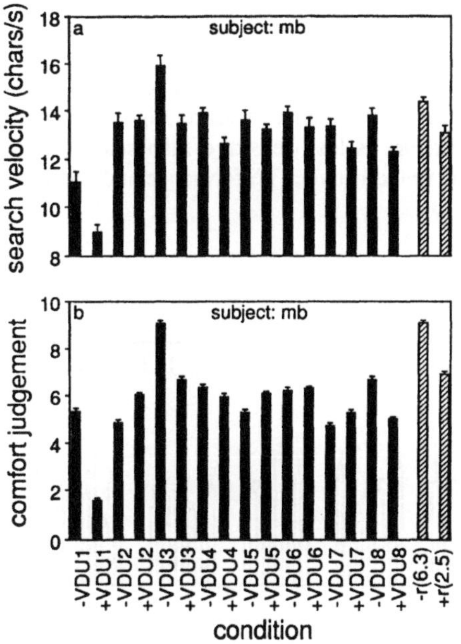

Figure 1. The results of experiment 1 for subject mb. The two bars on the extreme right of each plot represent the results of the print references. Fig 1a shows the performance results and Fig 1b the scaling results for mb. See the text for a description of the labels.

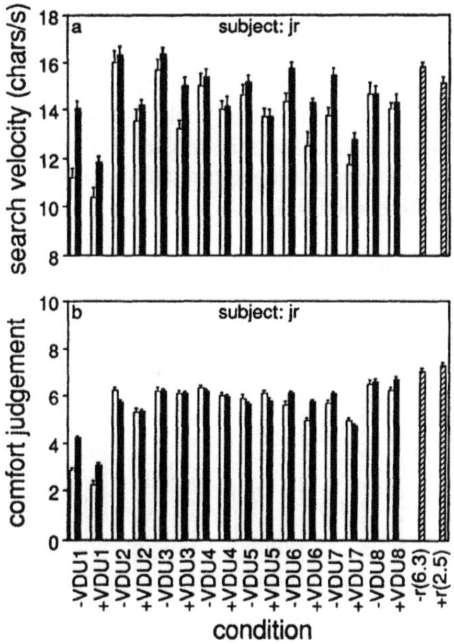

Figure 2. The results of experiment 1 for subject jr. For each VDU stimulus the results are plotted for both the corrected (black bars) and uncorrected (white bars) visual conditions.

Two subjects with a considerable age difference, mb (age 35) and jr (62), participated. The older subject performed the experiment twice: with and without his reading glasses (refracted for 33 cm). The subjects' task was to count the target letter 'A' in pseudo-texts and to give their impression of visual comfort on a ten-point scale afterwards. They then moved in front of another display. The experiment consisted of five 40-minute sessions, in which every condition was presented twice. Prior to the first session a test sequence of 18 stimuli containing all conditions was presented as a trial.

The results of experiment 1 are shown in Figures 1 and 2. The search velocity (Figs 1a, 2a) was corrected for session trends by normalizing the data per session to the average results of the print reference stimuli. Afterwards, the mean normalized search velocity was scaled back to the proper range. In Figures 1b and 2b the scaling results are plotted. The comfort scale is constructed according to Thurstone's law of categorical judgement condition D [4]. The terminal stimuli are labeled 'VDU', followed by integer numbers; r(*C*) indicates the print references with contrast ratio *C*. The sign in front of the labels corresponds to contrast polarity (+ means bright characters on a dark background)

The results for subject mb are shown in Figure 1. Significant performance differences are found between different displays (Fig. 1a). It is also clear that in most cases this subject performed significantly better with decremental contrast polarity. The subjective measure (Fig. 1b) shows similar results. The correlation between scaled comfort and search velocity was found to be considerable ($r = 0.87, p < 0.001$).

The results for subject jr are plotted in Figure 2. Besides the effect of image polarity, we see that the effect of visual acuity is also reflected in the performance measure. Figure 2b, however, suggests that for this subject the comfort measure is less sensitive than search velocity. Nevertheless, a high correlation coefficient was found between performance and comfort ($r = 0.79, p < 0.001$).

3.2. Experiment 2

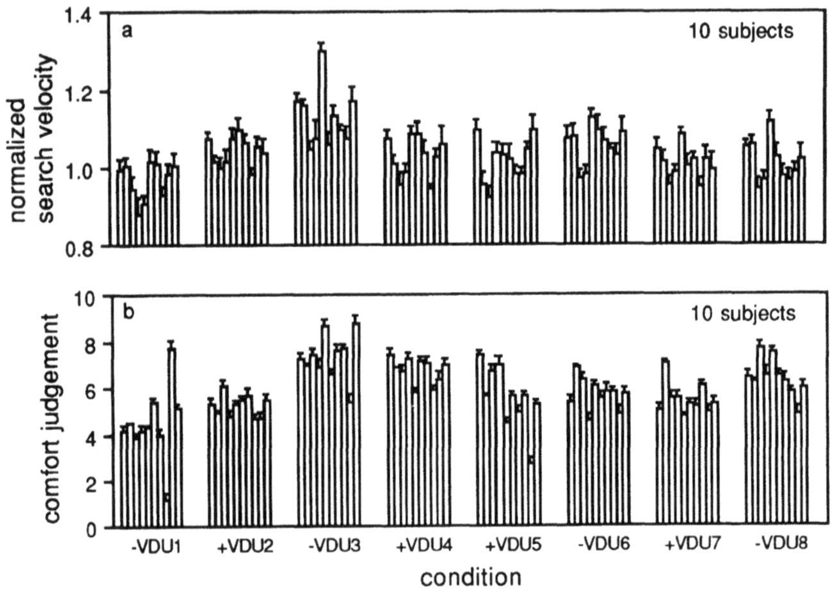

Figure 3. Combined results of experiment 2 for 10 subjects. In Fig 3a the normalized search velocity and in Fig 3b the Thurstone scale values for judged visual comfort are plotted.

In experiment 1 the peak luminance was arbitrarily set to a constant value for all displays. However, this is probably not the optimal setting for each display in both polarities. For experiment 2 we first selected one polarity per VDU. Prior to the main experiment we asked ten subjects to adjust the brightness setting of the displays to their personal optimum. Eventually, we set the display brightness settings to the averages over all subjects. In order to obtain a better frame of reference, some print reference stimuli with varying contrast were added to the set.

The subjects who varied in age from 24 to 62 all had normal or corrected-to-normal near visual acuity. The same experimental procedure was followed as in experiment 1, except for the last session, during which the subjects were asked to comment orally upon positive or negative effects of display properties on their comfort judgement. They were free to say whatever came into their minds about various display characteristics. Every subject participated in three 45-minute sessions, in which each condition was presented three times. The results of experiment 2 are plotted in Figures 3 and 4. Figure 3a shows the performance results concerning the VDU stimuli for all subjects. In order to make the results comparable for different subjects, we calculated the normalized search velocity: i.e. the search velocity divided by the average search velocity over the print conditions. Due to the presence of low contrast conditions in the print reference set, the average performance level for these conditions (refer to value=1 in Fig. 3a) is in most cases found to be lower than the level of performance for the VDU conditions. In Figure 3b the comfort judgement results are plotted for all subjects. It is clear that both measures are sufficiently sensitive to the relatively small quality variations over different VDUs.

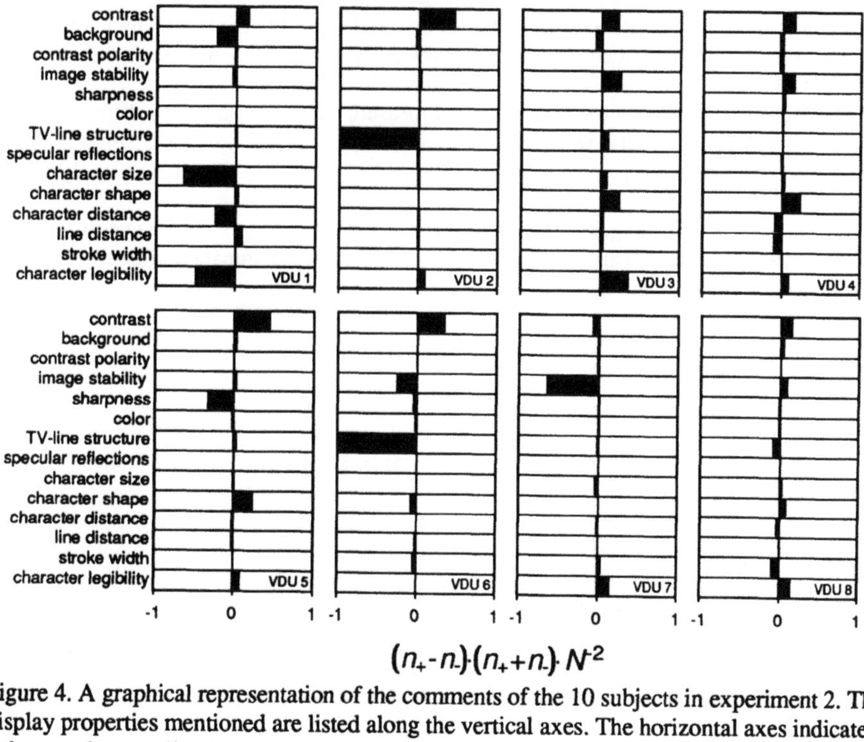

Figure 4. A graphical representation of the comments of the 10 subjects in experiment 2. The display properties mentioned are listed along the vertical axes. The horizontal axes indicate a balance of normalized weighted differences between the number of subjects that made positive and negative comments about these properties. See text for a full description.

It is also obvious that there are some significant comfort and performance differences between subjects. Looking at the individual results of the subjects, the degree of correlation between the subjective and the objective measure is found to be strongly subject-dependent: the correlation ranged from $r = -0.49$ ($p = 0.22$) to $r = +0.98$ ($p = 0.004$).

In Figure 4 an attempt has been made to make a graphical representation of the comments of all subjects for each VDU. The subjects made comments about various display properties, which can be found along the vertical axes. The horizontal axes indicate the differences between the number of subjects that made positive (n_+) and negative (n_-) comments about various properties. This difference is weighted by the number of subjects that made a comment on this property, and normalized to values between -1 and +1. (N = total number of subjects, i.e.10).

4. CONCLUSIONS

- Both visual comfort and search velocity vary significantly over the different display terminals. This shows that these measures are sufficiently sensitive to discriminate between displays of different manufacturers. However, the strength of their correlation is subject-dependent.
- In general, at a constant peak luminance setting, subjects performed significantly better with dark characters on a bright background than with white characters on a dark background. This is probably not exclusively an effect of image polarity.
- Significant effects of near-vision correction are reflected by the performance measure. The effects are the largest when characters are small. The subjective measure is less sensitive to acuity changes.
- Visual comfort must be a multi-dimensional measure which is spanned by different attributes. Its value depends on the weights that subjects apply to the various display properties. Differences between subjects may be explained by the fact that subjects apply different weights.
- The present study suggests that subjective comfort might be less sensitive than the performance measure. This may however be attributed to a summation of opposite effects of different display properties.

REFERENCES

1 Roufs, J.A.J., Leermakers, M.A.M. & Boschman, M.C. (1987) Criteria for the subjective quality of visual display units. In: B. Knave and P.-G. Widebäck (Eds):Work With Display Units '86.Amsterdam: North Holland, 412-417.

2 Roufs, J.A.J. & Boschman, M.C. (1991) Visual comfort and performance. In: J.R. Cronly-Dillon (Gen.Ed.): Vision and Visual Dysfunction, Vol. 15: J.A.J. Roufs (Ed.): The Man-Machine Interface. London: The Macmillan Press, Chapter 3, 24-40.

3 Boschman, M.C.& Roufs, J.A.J. (1990) Comparison of methods for the evaluation of VDUs: II. The effect of bandwidth. In: J. Morreale (Ed.): SID International Symposium, Las Vegas, Digest of Technical Papers. Playa del Rey, CA: SID, 17-20.

4 Torgerson, W.S. (1958) Theory and Methods of Scaling. NY:John Wiley and Sons Inc.

WORK WITH DISPLAY UNITS 92
H. Luczak, A. Çakir and G. Çakir (Editors)

Do VDUs harm the eyes? A report of a six year study of VDU operators

B. L. Cole[a], J. D. Maddocks[a] and K Sharpe[b]

[a]Department of Optometry and [b]Department of Statistics, University of Melbourne, Parkville, Australia

Abstract
The vision and ocular health of 642 persons who used a VDU at work was assessed annually for six years and compared to a control group of persons who did not use a VDU at work. The VDU group had a slightly higher prevalence of some symptoms of visual discomfort than the control group but the need for glasses or for a change of glasses was a more important factor in determining the probability of occurrence of symptoms. On average the VDU group was slightly more myopic than the control group but this difference did not increase in the course of the study There were no differences of note in the prevalence of external eye disease between the groups. The VDU group had a higher prevalence of abnormal signs on ophthalmoscopy than the control group on entry to the study, but in the succeeding 6 years more control subjects exhibited new signs of retinal abnormality. The control group had more lens opacities on entry to the study and although more members (11) of the VDU group developed cataract in the course of the study than did members of the control group (2), the difference was not statistically significant. Moreover, it was the members of the control group who had lens opacities who more often suffered significant loss of visual acuity.

1. INTRODUCTION

The introduction of VDUs to the work place over the last two decades has given rise to a number of concerns about health and safety that have been the subject of numerous investigations, a great deal of discussion and much controversy. It has been claimed that VDU work can give rise to excessive symptoms of visual discomfort, can cause cataract, myopia and other visual disorders. Although some of the heat has gone from the debate, there is still not a clear picture on whether or not VDU cause visual problems and if they do, the magnitude of the problem.

The first question is whether or not VDU work cause more visual symptoms than non VDU office work?

A number of surveys of visual symptoms of VDU operators have provided data to support the contention that VDU work commonly gives rise to symptoms of visual discomfort. However, not all the studies used a control group so they were simply reports of the prevalence of visual symptoms and could say nothing about whether or not VDU work was more likely to cause symptoms than conventional office work. Moreover, not all studies support the view that VDU work cause visual symptoms substantially more often than non VDU office work[1,2,3,4].

The next question is whether VDUs can harm the eyes. It has been suggested that VDUs may harm the eyes because they may emit UV, X radiation or radio frequency radiation. Dr Zaret[5] has been the principal and most vigorous advocate of this controversial view and although there is no convincing evidence the concern persists. Indeed it seems that VDUs do not emit biologically harmful radiation in sufficient quantity to have any effect on the eyes and vision[6,7] Nor is there convincing epidemiological evidence that VDU work is associated with a risk of ocular damage[8,9] However, these surveys have their deficiencies and none surveys VDU operators over a period of time.

2. METHOD

We assessed the vision and ocular health of a large group of VDU operators and of a control group over a period of six years. The sample was 642 VDU operators comprising all the VDU operators employed in a large metropolitan utility who used a VDU for at least one hour a day, and 673 employees of the same organisation who did not use a VDU at work. The gender and age of the VDU and control groups were as closely matched as practical. The subjects were given a comprehensive eye examination in the first year which was repeated annually over the succeeding five years for all subjects who remained in the employ of the utility. The eye examination was to a standard protocol and was conducted in the same consulting room throughout the period of the study. It included a questionnaire of symptoms administered by a clerk, standardised measurement of visual acuity, both unaided and with present glasses, refraction, corrected visual acuity, external eye examination, ophthalmoscopy, biomicroscopy and assessment of binocular and accommodative functions. Examiner bias was eliminated by making sure that the optometrists carrying out the examination did not know who were VDU operators and who were not.

The objective of the study was to ascertain whether or not the VDU group showed a higher prevalence of visual and ocular disorders than the control group on entry to the study and whether over a six year period the VDU group showed a higher incidence of visual disorders.

3. RESULTS

Symptoms In the first year of the study, the VDU group reported certain visual symptoms significantly more often than the control group, namely sensitivity to glare, aching sore eyes, blurred vision and ocular fatigue, but not other symptoms such as headache, burning or gritty eyes and watery eyes. Although the differences between the VDU and control group are statistically significant they are not large.

Moreover, in the case of the symptoms of blurred vision and ocular fatigue, the need for glasses was a very much more important factor than whether or not a VDU was used. A regression analysis on age, gender and the need for glasses or a change of glasses showed that while VDU use is still a significant factor in the occurrence of the symptoms it is marginal in relation to the need for glasses or the need for a change of glasses.

Visual acuity and refraction The VDU group had significantly lower unaided visual acuity and was significantly more myopic than the control group. The difference in mean refractive error was 0.35 D which is consistent with the difference in mean unaided visual acuity of LogMAR 0.04.

If VDU use is a factor in causing myopia it would be expected that the myopia of the VDU group would increase more rapidly than that of the control group. The VDU group did not show a more rapid increase of myopia than the control group. We conclude that the myopia of the VDU group is a chance result or due to self selection.

In any event, in a regression for refractive error on age, sex and group (VDU/Control), group accounts for less than 4% of the variability in refractive error. Forty three percent of the subjects wore glasses on entry into the study and there was no significant difference between the groups. Glasses were prescribed for the first time for 6.2% and existing glasses were changed for 11.4%. Prescribing rates were slightly higher for the VDU group but the difference was not significant. The lack of clear differences between the control and VDU groups in the proportions wearing glasses, needing glasses for the first time or needing a change of existing glasses, does not support the proposition that myopia or other kinds of refractive error are more prevalent or progress more rapidly among VDU workers.

Ocular disease Corrected visual acuity is a measure of loss of visual function due to disease. There was no difference in the corrected VA of the two groups.

There was no significant difference between the two groups in the prevalence of external eye disease except that the VDU group had a higher prevalence of ptosis, a difference that is too bizarre to attribute to VDU exposure.

The VDU group exhibited ophthalmoscopically visible abnormal signs more often than the control group (10.3% cf 7.8% of subjects) on entry to the study and showed a significantly higher prevalence of abnormal ophthalmoscopic signs of actual or potential significance. However, in the ensuing 6 years, more members of the control group (1%) exhibited new ophthalmoscopic signs of actual or potential significance than the VDU group (0.4%).

It has been said that VDUs may cause cataract of the lens of the eye. In fact the control group was found to have significantly greater prevalence of lens opacities at the time of entry to the study. However, many lens opacities are insignificant developmental anomalies and are not cataract in the clinical sense. If cataract is defined as a concurrence of lens opacity and corrected VA reduced below 6/6, there were 11 (1.7%) control and 9 (1.3%) VDU subjects with cataract on entry to the study.

In the course of the next 6 years, 11 VDU workers and 2 non-users developed cataract. This difference is suggestive but is not statistically significant when analysed in relation to the number of annual assessments. Moreover, of the 16 subjects who had cataract and whose visual acuity continued to decline through the course of the study, only four subjects had their visual acuity reduced below 6/12 and all were members of the control group.

We classified lens opacities of those subjects who had reduced visual acuity (<6/6) or who had declining visual acuity as a result of a lens opacity into those that had a form that might conceivably be characteristic of radiation damage and those that had a form quite different from that usually ascribed to radiation cataract and found that 1.8% of VDU subjects and 1.4% of control subjects had lens opacities of a form that might conceivably be attributable to radiation damage, a difference that is not significant.

4. CONCLUSIONS

VDU workers may experience some symptoms of visual discomfort more often than non VDU workers but the differences are not great. Need for glasses to correct refractive errors and presbyopia is a more important cause of visual discomfort than whether or not a person uses a VDU.

Even though our VDU workers were on average more myopic than the control group, it is unlikely that VDU work is associated with myopia since the myopia of the VDU group did not progress at a greater rate than the control subjects.

The data does not support the view that VDU work will cause cataract or other eye disease.

5. REFERENCES

1. Coe , JB, Cuttle, K, McCellan, WC, Warden, NJ and Turner, PJ *Visual Display Units* Report W1/80 Wellington. New Zealand Dept Health. 1980

2. Starr, SJ, Thompson, CR and Shute, SJ Effects of video display terminals on telephone operators *Human Factors* 24, 699 - 711, 1982

3. Smith, AB, Tanuka, S, Halperin, W and Richards, RD Correlates of ocular and somatic symptoms among video display terminal users *Human Factors* 26, 143 - 156, 1984

4. Sauter, S, Gottleib, MS, Jones, KC, Dodson, VN and Rohrer, KM *Job and Health Implications of VDT Use. Initial Results of the Wisconsin-NIOSH Study.* Communications of the ACM, 26, 284 - 294, 1983

5. Zaret, MM Cataracts and visual display units *in* Pearce, BG (Ed) *Health Hazards of VDTs?* Chichester. John Wiley 1980

6. Moss, CE, Murray, WE, Parr, WE, Messite, J and Karches, GJ *A Report on Electro-magnetic Radiation Surveys of Video Display Terminals* Ohio. National Institute for Occupational Safety and Health, Division of Biomedical and Behavioural Science. 1977

7. Elliott, G, Gies, P, Joyner, KH and Roy, CR Electromagnetic radiation emissions from video display terminals (VDTs) *Clin & Exp Optom* 69, 53 - 61, 1986

8. Bergqvist, UO Video display terminals and health *Scand J Work, Environ and Health* 10, Supl 2, 1984

9. Nat Res Council *Video Displays, Work and Vision.* Washington DC. National Academy Press 1983

WORK WITH DISPLAY UNITS 92
H. Luczak, A. Çakir and G. Çakir (Editors)
1993 Elsevier Science Publishers B.V.

The Effects of Exercise on the Health and Performance of Data Entry Operators

Naomi G. Swanson and Steven L. Sauter

National Institute for Occupational Safety and Health
4676 Columbia Parkway, Cincinnati, Ohio 45226 USA

1. INTRODUCTION

A recent study at the National Institute for Occupational Safety and Health (NIOSH) has demonstrated the efficacy of frequent restbreaks in reducing psychological and musculoskeletal strain, and increasing productivity, among video display terminal (VDT) workers (Sauter and Swanson, 1991). Nevertheless, subjects in this study exhibited increasing discomfort and declining productivity over the course of the workday (i.e., the increased restbreaks greatly reduced, but did not eliminate, the stresses associated with VDT work). These performance and comfort decrements may be due to the static loads and constrained postures inherent in VDT work which are only partially counteracted by increased restbreaks. As an alternative to passive rest, physical activity has been recommended as an effective means of counteracting these stresses (Winkel, 1987), and a number of exercise programs designed for VDT users have been promoted as having health and productivity benefits (e.g., Austin, 1984; Krames Communications, 1986). The purpose of the present study was to determine whether physical exercises, inserted into a frequent restbreak schedule, would further reduce, or eliminate, daily comfort and productivity decrements in a repetitive VDT task.

2. METHOD

2.1 Subjects

The subjects were 37 experienced (female) data entry operators (ages 18 to 38), recruited from a local temporary employment agency. All subjects were in good health, as established by a pre-employment medical examination. Subjects also met a minimum performance requirement of 6000 keystrokes/hour of numeric data entry (i.e., slow to medium data entry rate).

2.2 Design and Procedure

Subjects performed a right-handed data entry task, using the number pad of an IBM 3163 PC. Data were entered from United States IRS 1040-EZ tax forms, stacked on a document holder placed in front of the VDT screen. Ergonomic chairs and tables were adjusted according to each subject's preferences before testing.

All subjects underwent a 400-minute workday of baseline testing with only one break of 45 minutes for lunch. They were then randomly assigned in blocks of 1-4 subjects to either a passive rest break or an exercise break condition for experimental testing during two, subsequent, 400-minute workdays. In addition to the 45-minute lunchbreak, both groups received the following rest break schedule: Ten-minute breaks were provided after 100 minutes of data entry in the morning and afternoon; 3-minute minibreaks were provided at 50-minute intervals in the morning and after 30, 65 and 150 minutes of work in the afternoon; and, 30-second microbreaks were administered every 10 minutes during the morning and afternoon.

Subjects in the passive break condition sat passively during the 3-minute and 30-second breaks, while subjects in the exercise break condition performed simple, inconspicuous, exercises during these breaks. The exercises targeted the neck, shoulders, back and extremities, and could, with the exception of a "walking-in-place" exercise, be performed while the subjects were seated at their workstations. Exercise names appeared as prompts on each subject's VDT screen during the performance of the exercises.

2.3 Measures

The results of two health measures (i.e., musculoskeletal discomfort and mood state) and one productivity measure are reported in this paper. The musculoskeletal discomfort items assessed musculoskeletal discomfort in the legs, back, neck, buttocks and left and right arms. The mood scale items measured fatigue, boredom and workload dissatisfaction. Both the musculoskeletal discomfort and the mood state items were assessed eight times during each of the two test days: At the beginning and end of the day, and before and after the midmorning, lunch and mid-afternoon restbreaks. The productivity measure, keystrokes/hour, was measured continuously throughout each worksession.

2.4 Analyses

The health and performance data were aggregated over the 100-minute worksessions in the morning, and the 105-minute and 95-minute worksessions in the afternoon, for a total of four worksessions per day. A mixed design analysis of variance (ANOVA) was used to assess the effects of exercise breaks vs passive restbreaks on performance and comfort, as well as changes in these outcomes across the workday.

3. RESULTS

3.1 Musculoskeletal Discomfort and Mood State

There were no differences between the two break conditions in musculoskeletal discomfort or mood state. Both break conditions showed increases in musculoskeletal discomfort across the workday, with the greatest increases in discomfort reported for the right upper arm, right forearm/wrist/hand, back and neck. Additionally, in both conditions, subjects reported increasing boredom, less energy and greater dissatisfaction with workload and workpace across the workday.

3.2 Keystroke Productivity

With regard to productivity outcomes, there were no differences between the two break conditions in baseline performance, or in overall daily keystroke production levels. However, the analyses did indicate different patterns of performance decline over the sessions for the two break conditions on the two test days. Post hoc analyses, comparing the session means for each restbreak group, showed a significant decline in keystroke production over the last half of each workday for the passive restbreak condition. The exercise break condition, on the other hand, showed no significant decline in keystroke production until the final worksession of the second test day.

4. DISCUSSION

The present results indicated that breaks containing simple, inconspicuous, stretching/flexing exercises provided no health (i.e., comfort and mood state) benefits beyond those obtained with frequent, passive, restbreaks. Exercise did not eliminate the increases in discomfort, or the decrement in mood state, across the workday. However, the decline in keystroke production across the workday was less pronounced for the exercise break group than the passive restbreak group. This suggests that exercise breaks may act to stabilize performance over the course of a workday.

5. REFERENCES

Austin, D. (1984) Tone Up at the Terminals. Verbatim Corporation.

Krames Communications. (1986) Fitness at the Terminal: Comfort Tips for Computer Users. Daly City, CA: Krames Communications.

Sauter, S.L. and Swanson, N.G. (1991) Increased Restbreaks Yield Increased Productivity in Repetitive VDT Work. Paper presented at the 35th Annual Meeting of the Human Factors Society, San Francisco, CA, September 2-6.

Winkel, J. (1987) On the significance of physical activity in sedentary work. In B. Knave and P,-G. Wideback (Eds.) Work With Display Units 86, Amsterdam: Elsevier Science Publishers B.V.

WORK WITH DISPLAY UNITS 92
H. Luczak, A. Çakir and G. Çakir (Editors)

Frequent, Short Breaks During Computer Work: The Effects on Productivity and Well-Being in a Field Study

Robert A. Henning, Sabina M. Alteras-Webb, Pierre Jacques,
George V. Kissel, & Anne B. Sullivan

Industrial/Organizational Division, Department of Psychology,
University of Connecticut, Storrs, Connecticut 06269-1020, USA

Abstract

A field study was conducted to validate the use of frequent short breaks from computer work as a means to improve operator productivity and well-being. The 20 VDT operators performing claims processing at a large insurance company were given frequent short breaks from computer work (with or without stretching exercises designed to reduce musculoskeletal discomfort) in addition to their conventional mid-morning and mid-afternoon rest breaks. The break schedule was similar to the one tested in laboratory studies conducted by NIOSH. Mood state and musculoskeletal discomfort (at the start of the workday, at mid-day, and at the end of the work day) was assessed throughout a nine-week period; 3 weeks of baseline (no added breaks), 3 weeks of breaks only, and 3 weeks of breaks & exercises. Productivity measures for each worker were obtained from company records. Results indicated that eye comfort improved under the break & exercises condition, and that productivity increased. The results provide evidence from a real-world setting that frequent short breaks from computer work can benefit both operator well-being and productivity.

1. Introduction

VDT operators performing repetitive tasks are known to experience fatigue and musculoskeletal discomfort that is not completely offset by conventional rest breaks. Results from laboratory studies at the National Institute for Occupational Safety and Health (NIOSH, USA) reported at this meeting (Sauter & Swanson, 1992; Swanson & Sauter, 1992) suggest that worker productivity and well-being can improve when workers take frequent, short rest pauses while remaining at their workstations. In the NIOSH studies, scheduled microbreaks lasting 30 seconds after 10 minutes of work, and 3 minutes after about 50 minutes of work, with or without simple stretching exercises, occurred in addition to conventional rest breaks.

The present study was a validation effort to determine if the positive effects of frequent breaks from computer work, with or without stretching exercises, could be replicated in a real-world setting. Two field studies were conducted at separate claims processing divisions of a large insurance company. The results from the smaller study site are reported here.

2. Methods

2.1. Subjects

20 VDT operators performing claims processing tasks at a large local insurance company participated on a voluntary basis. Operators worked a minimum of 7.5 hrs per day over a 5-day work week. A flex-time policy allowed workers to work between the hours of 6 AM and 6 PM.

2.2. Rest Break Administration System

Small indicator lights (LEDs) mounted on the video display and document holder of each workstation were used to signal operators to take a short break from computer work. The LEDs were controlled by a dedicated microcomputer.

2.3. Procedure

Participants participated in a repeated-measures design over a nine-week period. During the initial three-week baseline period, no additional computer breaks were administered.

During the second three-week period, participants were instructed to take four short "computer breaks" each hour (three 30-sec breaks and one 3-min break) in addition to their conventional 15-min mid-morning and mid-afternoon rest breaks. When the LED indicator lights signalled a 30-sec computer break, operators were instructed to cease computer operations, sit back in their chairs, and relax for the duration of the break. During the 3-min computer breaks, however, operators were asked to perform alternative forms of work; that is, to perform anything but computer work (e.g., return processed claims to a central depository).

At the start of the final three weeks of the study, an exercise specialist trained operators to perform a set of stretching exercises that were developed to reduce the musculoskeletal discomfort associated with prolonged periods of uninterrupted VDT use. Operators were asked to perform at least one of these exercises during the 30-sec computer breaks, and a set of two complementary exercises during the 3-min computer breaks in addition to performing alternative forms of work.

Operators were asked to complete surveys of their mood state and musculoskeletal discomfort three times each day throughout the 9-week study; at the start of the workday, at mid-day before lunch, and at the end of the work day. Operator ratings of mood items (e.g., "I feel tense") were combined into mood scales for fatigue, tension, and vigor. Operators rated the extent of musculoskeletal discomfort of separate regions of their body; eyes, back, legs and feet, hands and arms, and neck and shoulders.

Productivity for each VDT operator was obtained from company records. Productivity was calculated on a weekly basis as the operator's work output (number of claims processed) per the time available for claims processing. The time available for claims processing did not always equal the total hours worked per week because it was not possible to process claims during periods of computer system failure or group meetings.

2.4. Analysis

Due to attrition and other factors over the extended study period, the number of participants dropped from 20 to 13 for the mood and discomfort measures, and from 20 to 10 for the productivity measures.

Repeated-measures ANOVA was used to test for within-subject differences across the three conditions (baseline, breaks only, breaks & exercises). Tests were considered statistically significant at the .05 level. Tests at the .10 level were reported as trends. Greenhouse-Geisser epsilon was used in all repeated-measures ANOVA analyses to adjust the degrees of freedom in the **F**-tests for within-subjects effects.

2.5. Results

No significant changes in mood state were found across the three conditions.

Eye comfort was found to varied significantly across conditions ($\underline{p}$ = .041). Eye comfort increased above baseline levels in the breaks-only condition and also in the breaks & exercises condition, with the greatest increase above baseline occurring in the breaks & exercises condition.

Leg comfort also varied across conditions, but only at the level of a trend ($\underline{p}$ = .105). Leg comfort showed an increase above baseline levels, but only in the breaks & exercises condition.

Finally, productivity varied significantly across conditions ($\underline{p}$ = .018). Productivity showed an increase in both the breaks-only condition and the breaks & exercises condition, with the greatest increase occurring in the breaks & exercise condition.

3. Discussion

The results of this field study provide evidence that VDT operators can benefit from a work regime that includes frequent short breaks from computer work. The results replicate many of the same beneficial effects of added rest breaks in the laboratory studies conducted by NIOSH.

A reliable experimental effect was found for eye comfort, where eye comfort improved with the addition of computer breaks, and improved further when exercises were added to the break schedule. This finding of improved eye comfort is consistent with earlier related research that was reported by Sundelin et al. (1986) at the WWDU conference in Stockholm.

A less reliable effect was detected for a second body comfort measure, leg comfort. Leg comfort tended to improve at the level of a trend, but only in the breaks & exercise condition. This increase in leg comfort may be explained by one of the stretching exercises that required the operator to briefly stand next to their workstation while performing the exercise. This activity may have improved leg comfort by increasing blood circulation in the legs.

A reliable experimental effect was also found for operator performance, performance improved during both computer break conditions. The lack of a performance decrement when frequent rest breaks are administered is not unexpected. Short rest breaks capitalize on the rapid rate of recovery that occurs early in a rest break period, helping prevent the accumulation of fatigue over the workspell (Rohmert, 1973). The time lost to work during the short break periods is usually compensated for by an increase in productivity during the subsequent work periods.

An important finding in the present study is that frequent, short computer breaks can benefit both operator well-being and productivity. This result has practical implications for those who are considering testing new rest break schedules in their workplace. It appears unlikely that the addition of added computer breaks will compromise the productivity of VDT operators. Since stretching exercises during short breaks from computer work are likely to provide other benefits as well, such as reducing the risk of repetitive strain injuries, the positive impact on operator productivity reported here makes further tests of new rest break schedules even more desirable.

The results of this study must be viewed with some caution due to the inherent limitations of the pseudo-experimental design that was employed. It cannot be ruled-out that the positive effects of the computer break program reported here were due to confounding factors external to the study. However, for the experimental effects to be detected in such a limited sample suggests that the beneficial effects are relatively robust.

4. Conclusions

The present study provides empirical evidence that frequent short breaks from computer work can benefit the well-being of VDT operators and improve their productivity.

5. References

Rohmert, W., 1973. Problems of determination of rest allowances, Part 2: Determining rest allowances in different human tasks. Applied Ergonomics, 4, 3, 158-162.

Sauter, S.L., & Swanson, N.G. (1992). The effects of frequent rest breaks on performance and well-being in repetitive computer work. WWDU '92, Berlin.

Sundelin, G., Hagberg, M., & Hammarstrom, U., 1986, The effects of pauses on muscular load and perceived discomfort when working at a VDT word processor. Proceedings of the International Scientific Conference: Work with Display Units, Part 1, pp. 501-502, Stockholm.

Swanson, N.G., & Sauter, S.L. (1992). The effects of exercise on the health and performance of data entry operators. WWDU '92, Berlin.

USER INTERFACES

WORK WITH DISPLAY UNITS 92
H. Luczak, A. Çakir and G. Çakir (Editors)

Window design and location for messages in interactive systems

P. J. Haubner

Ergonomics Department, Siemens Research - Centre, Paul Gossen - Straße 100, 8520 Erlangen, Germany

Abstract

How the information, contained in messages, can be identified and exploited by users of human-computer systems depends on the structuring of the content as well as on the formal design of message areas or windows. For this reason investigations have been carried out with the objective of empirically clarifying important human factors aspects of message display.The results demonstrate that task performance and user acceptance are influenced by temporal and spatial factors of presentation. Some practical guidelines could be deduced.

1. THEORETICAL PRELIMINARIES

Dialogue systems are, from the user`s point of view, tools incorporating external knowledge memory. While performing tasks, the following questions play a dominating role for the user in this context:

1. Which knowledge is externally stored and is available to the user for solving his problem ?
2. How can this knowledge be accessed and retrieved ?
3. How is external knowledge functionally related to problem solving and how can this knowledge be exploited ?

The "orientation problem " and the "access problem" are mainly cocerned with the design requirement of "transparency of the dialogue" and the "application problem" relates to "task adequacy" and "application comfort".

Messages are usually displayed in computer initiated windows. Therefore, the "application problem" is to be addressed, primarily. The information has to be detected, identified and matched to the task context. In general, messages are represented for interactive dialogue systems using different techniques (command, mask, direct manipulation) in computer initiated windows.Their appearance on the screen can be either permanent or temporary at a fixed place or at a variable location.

With a fixed message area the window containing the message, can be axcised in a permanent or in a temporary frame.Resulting variants of these produce arguments both for and against from an ergonomics viewpoint, and lead to system designers` attitudes which have evolved historically.

The following questions, which arose during design walkthroughs and which could not be resolved on theorethical grounds nor by experience, formed the basis for the hypotheses tested:

1. How to place messages at either fixed or variable locations ?
2. How to display windows for messages, permanently or temporarily ?
3. How to choose distances between windows and their instigating events on the screen ?

The theoretical framework for these questions can be related to three aspects, which play the primar role for perceptive and cognitive processing of messages:

- Stimulus detection, and recognition of the class of information (e.g. "Message")
- Identification of the meaning of the message (e.g. "Warning")
- Association with other objects displayed on the screen (e.g. spatial location relative to an item initiating the message)

The appearance at the same position, usually at the upper or lower screen edge supports allocation of information class, since this indicated position can be related to other information in the semantic network of the user (Mahling 1985).

However, class allocation prerequires previous detection of the message , which can be hindered if the user`s attention is not concentrated near such screen areas, or even more serious if the field of view becomes restricted due to strain (Voss 1982).

In addition, it can be expected, the more distant the window is from it`s instigating element on the screen,the more this association deminishes (Metzger1975).

Clarification does not thereby appear possible on a theoretical basis.Therefore, several window configurations were tested empirically in the context of a series of experiments on information access in direct manipulation interfaces using an end user sample of 30 observers (Haubner 1992).

2. EMPIRICAL INVESTIGATION

The following configurations of windows or rather message boxes, schematically represented in figure 1, were tested in our "Interface Lab" using an experimental setup to simulate a realistic office environment. Lighting, room layout, workplace design and arrangement etc. were optimized according to established ergonomics principles.

The message box was surrounded by a frame. It`s positon on the screen could be fixed or variable. It could be diplayed permanently or temporarily.

This resulted in the configurations as shown in figure 1, which we term window (box) type.The distance of the window (box) from an element on the screen which instigates the message could be close, middle or further apart.

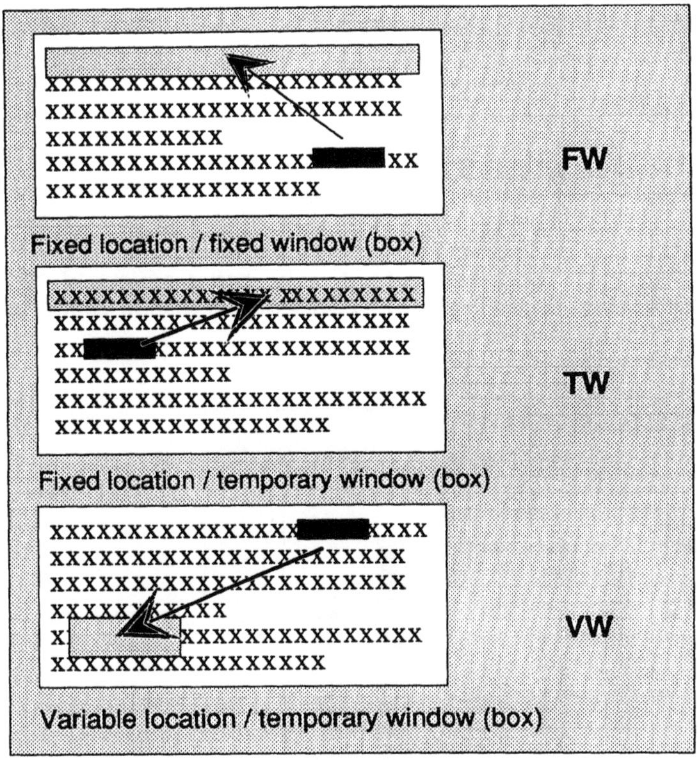

Figure 1. Test situation and schematic screen layout

The experimental design was such that the following parameters could be treated as fixed or random factors in a multidimensional analysis for related samples:

Fixed factors: Location,
Window Type,
Distance (from related item)

Random factor: End users

As dependent indicator variables "Objective Performance", operationalized by detection time and detection rate, and "Subjective Responses" such as experienced strain and preference, measured by psychometric scaling, were used.

The responses were scaled by means of the "constant sum" version of magnitude estimation (Torgerson 1962). Additionally, we applied a questionaire of items on experienced job performance. The items had to be assessed on a five point rating scale. The experimental data were treated by a multidimensional analysis of variance for related samples.

3. EXPERIMENTAL RESULTS

The results of the statistical analysis exhibited that human performance as well as the users` attitudes are signifcantly influenced by each of the three factors (location, window (box) type, distance) above a type I error of $\varepsilon = 0.01$. Interactions of first and higher order were insignificant or could be explaint by means of control variables.

In general, variable windows (boxes) turned out to be better performed and accepted than the fixed windows configurations. As an example, this is shown in figure 2.

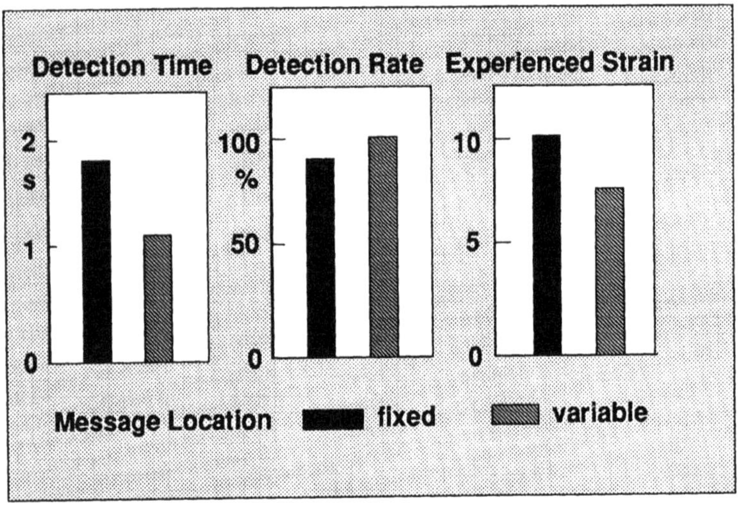

Figure 2. Influence of message location on task performance and response scaling

Compared with fixed locations, detection time for variable location is about 40%less. The plot in figure 3 exhibits the same relationship for fixed andvariablelocation parameters in the case of distance between the instigating event and the window. Since we also calculated distance in terms of visual angle, we could conclude that the best performance and user acceptance resulted in the parafovea, followed by foveal and peripheral distances.

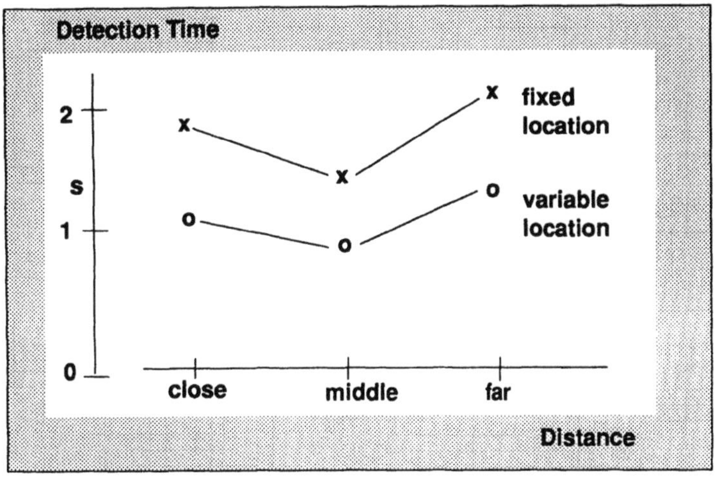

Figure 3. Influence of distance on performance (detection time)

Similiar results have been obtained for the dependency of the observers' responses on the distance and on the location stimuli.

From the outcome of the experiments several practical conclusions can be drawn with respect to ergonomics guiding principles on the design of message windows for interactive systems, e.g. present messages in variable windows, prefer parafoveal locations and avoid permanently displayed fields, if a fixed area becomes unavoidable.

4. REFERENCES

Haubner, P.J. Design of Dialogues for Human-Computer Interaction, in, Methods and Tools in User-Centred Design for Information Technology (Galer, Harker, Ziegler,Eds.), North Holland, Amsterdam-London-NewYork-Tokyo, 1992, 203-236

Mahling, D. Vergleich verschiedener Dialogsysteme in Fenstertechnik, Diplomarbeit TU Braunschweig / Siemens AG, ZT FWO 2, 1985

Metzger, W. Gesetze des Sehens, Verlag W.Kramer, Frankfurt, 1975

Voss, M. Aufnahme und Verarbeitung von Information unter dem Aspekt der Beanspruchung, Dissertation, Universität(TU) Karlsruhe, 1982

WORK WITH DISPLAY UNITS 92
H. Luczak, A. Çakir and G. Çakir (Editors)

What do system designers know about software ergonomics and how to improve their knowledge?

J. Hüttner and H. Wandke

Department of Psychology, Humboldt University Berlin,
Oranienburger Straße 18, O - 1020 Berlin

Abstract
Software designers were asked about their actual knowledge in software ergonomics and their expectations for support in designing ergonomic user interfaces. In a first inquiry with (n=82) software designers it was shown that there is little or medium knowledge in ergonomics. In a second inquiry (n=44) designers wished mainly advice-giving support of traditional and computer-based type.

1. Ergonomic design of user interfaces

While the ergonomic design of hardware components is acknowledged as a domain of human factors specialists ergonomic software design is often considered to be a matter of experience and common sense. Since software development is frequently performed in small "venture enterprises", programmers have not only to take care of the functional layout of the programs but also of the ergonomic design of the user interface. An European survey showed that most of the 13.000 firms working in software development are such small enterprises. They have no special departments with human factors experts accompanying the products.
It is said such "normal" programmers don't know so much about ergonomical software. Is that an old prejudice or a current fact? Some recent investigations support the last opinion (Maaß, Rosson & Kellogg, 1987; Aschersleben & Zang-Scheucher, 1989; Molich & Nielsen, 1990).

2. Empirical analyses - what designers know

In an empirical study using questionnaires it was analysed how much software designers know about ergonomic design of user interfaces and where the deficits are. A similar study showed what kind of supporting tools they wish to improve the ergonomic quality of software products.
In the first study 50 software firms and 82 system designers took part. There was a high percentage of young firms (58% are not older than three years) with a small number of employees (54% have no more than 2). The firms put their main emphasis on developing very

specialised software for specific customers. In that domain they work often with DOS-PC's (78% use DOS only).
They responded to an announcement published in three German computer journals. Sofar, it can be assumed that these firms and their designers are highly interested in software ergonomics. This conclusion is supported by data: 46% of them declared to use modern developing techniques.
They were asked for their knowledge of the state of the art in the scientific landscape of software ergonomics. 63% reported to know ergonomic literature, but this is not entirely scientific material from our point of view. Among other things they refered to software manuals or technical articles in computer journals. There could also be the same misunderstanding in interpreting the high percentage of the knowledge of institutions. Designers mentioned often their former universities and academic teachers in computer science, although no research in software ergonomics has been carried out there.

Table 1
Knowledge of the scientific landscape

literature	63%
key scientists	25%
institutions	48%
conference series	16%

The notice of scientific discussions and further information is obviously lower than we supposed.
Another special indicator of knowledge about software ergonomics might be the distribution and application of ergonomic standards and guidelines shown at the following table.

Table 2
Ergonomic standards and guidelines known and applied by the 82 participants of the study. Multiple answers were possible.

standard or guideline	known (%)	applied (%)
DIN 66234	22	11
ISO 9241	1	-
IBM SAA/CUA	55	31
Apple Guidelines	15	7
other guidelines and in-house standards	20	6
no standard or guideline	10	26

The most important norm in Germany DIN 66234 is known by 22% of the subjects. One person knew the forthcoming ISO standard. Only the complex of SAA and CUA by IBM was better known and applied. More than the half stated to know this standard but only 31% of the whole sample used it in daily work. The Apple Guidelines were known by 15% and only 7% took them for programming software. The last line is remarkable: 26% used nothing at all.

In the last part of the first questionnaire we went into technical terms and abbreviations of software ergonomics. We asked for 54 terms and only 6 of them were known by more than 75%. However, we found 4 terms known by less than 15%.
The next table shows the terms and their spreading. The last column shows obviously that programmers mean something different than we assumed with the term "literature on software ergonomics", since e.g. the acronym HCI is found in nearly all articles and books on software ergonomics.

Table 3
Knowledge of software ergonomic terms and abbreviations (examples)

known by > 75%	known by ≅ 50%	known by > 15%
default	functionality	UIMS
pull-down menu	consistency	(user interface
prompt	self-descriptiveness	management systems)
icon	error tolerance	CSCW
WYSIWYG	context-dependent help	(computer supported
pop-up menu	pictogram	co-operative work)
	system response time	HCI
	mouse sensitive area	(human computer
	dialogue control	interaction)
	user friendliness	UIT
	learnability	(user interface tool kits)

Summarising the data it can be said that the knowledge transfer from scientific world into industry is insufficient.

3. What designers wish

On the other hand the programmers are strongly interested in improving their knowledge. They expect that tools with "built-in" ergonomic knowledge for user interface design will improve the usability of their products.
In a second study we asked for the expectations of designers regarding tools and other types of support. Questionnaires were sent to all German software firms registered in the ISIS Software-Report (1990) with a total return of 44 completed copies.
They were asked about external sources of support available in present and what they wish to have in future. At first we asked for the general type of support (e.g. by documents, other persons, software etc.).

Table 4
External support in present and expected in future by different sources of information.

support by	present	future
colleagues	80%	91%
training / courses	14%	86%
guidelines	57%	86%
computer-based support	21%	81%
examples (positive/negative)	27%	77%
information system	7%	73%
local expert	11%	39%

The difference between present and expected in future is impressive. This can be underlined with the next table where we asked for the kind of presentation of information for different topics. Table 5 presents some detailed results for design problems within the layout of visual displays.

Table 5
Kind of presentation of support-information needed for different design problems.

visual aspects of the interface	paper-based	computer-based
coding	26%	44%
icons / symbols	15%	44%
graphic illustration	14%	57%
textual information	17%	50%
colours	13%	53%
highlighting	30%	40%
data structuring	19%	48%
windows	14%	53%

4. Possibilities of support

There are different possibilities of support. One idea is to develop a knowledge based system to design the interface more or less automatically (Weisbecker & Kern 1991), another possibility is to guide the designer in the whole process of software development (Gorny & Viereck, 1991). In our opinion the demand expressed in the third column of table 4 and in table 5 will be met adequately by a combination of a computer system and a textbook. Both are in the first stage of development. While the interactive system is intended to consist of a collection of positive and negative examples with annotations showing the possibilities and the limits of software ergonomics the textbook will present some background knowledge in cognitive ergonomics and applied psychology. Both the system and the textbook will be developed in co-operation with practitioners of system design. The rapid prototyping approach will be used.

A first draft of the textbook has already been tested with regard to text comprehension and effectiveness. To analyse the effect of the textbook we tested it by using an evaluation task developed by Molich & Nielsen (1990). Two groups (labelled B and D in the table 6) of subjects had to look for design errors and deficiencies in a simple user interface. Table 6 presents the results in comparison with a control group and data gained in other investigations. The data of the experimental group are similar to the results we found after a training course in software ergonomics of three days (group C).

Table 6
Knowledge in software ergonomics of different groups of (A = nation wide contest - no limitation in time and external support (Molich & Nielsen), B = after reading the textbook, C = after attending a three days course in software ergonomics, D = control group)

sample	A	B	C	D
percentage of errors and deficiencies found:	37,3%	22,5%	28,6%	15,4%

But only reading a textbook is obviously not sufficient. Therefore further work is directed to develop a computer-based information and consulting system, including a collection of positive and negative examples. At the same time the textbook will be permanently improved.

• This research is supported as part of the project WEDA by the *Work and Technology* program of the Federal Ministry of Research an Technology. Project No. 01 HK 790/8

5. References

Aschersleben, G. & Zang-Scheucher, B. (1989) Der Prozeß der Softwaregestaltung - eine Bestandsaufnahme in Wissenschaft und Industrie. In S. Maaß & H. Oberquelle (Eds.) Software-Ergonomie '89 (S. 244-253). Stuttgart: Teubner.

Gorny, P. & Viereck, A. (1991) Ein Software-Ergonomie-Expertensystem. In D. Ackermann & E. Ulich (Eds.) Software-Ergonomie '91 (S. 152-161). Stuttgart: Teubner.

Maaß, S., Rosson, M. B. & Kellogg, W. A. (1987) Benutzerfreudlichkeit, Systemkonsistenz und andere schwer definierbare Prinzipien: Interviews mit Systementwicklern. In W. Schönpflug & M. Wittstock (Eds.) Software-Ergonomie '87. Nützen Informationssysteme dem Benutzer? (S. 417-427). Stuttgart: Teubner.

Molich, R. & Nielsen, J. (1990) Improving a human-computer dialogue. Communications of the ACM 33, No. 3: S. 338-348.

Weissbecker, A. & Kern, P. (1991) Unterstützungswerkzeuge zur benutzergerechten Gestaltung der Mensch-Maschine-Schnittstelle. In M. Frese, Ch. Kasten & B. Zang-Scheucher (Eds.). Software für die Arbeit von morgen. Ergänzungsband (S. 361-372). Berlin: Springer

WORK WITH DISPLAY UNITS 92
H. Luczak, A. Çakir and G. Çakir (Editors)

Mental workload in "small-scale" user interfaces

Robert Baggen, Ronald Schwarz and Rainer Wieland-Eckelmann

Projektgruppe MenBIT, Bergische Universität-Gesamthochschule Wuppertal, Gaußstr. 20, W-5600 Wuppertal 1, Germany

Abstract

The paper introduces PROTOLAB, a collection of empirical procedures for the evaluation of "small-scale" user interface prototypes. The procedures are used to assess working memory load associated with the work on two prototypes. As a result of different design principles, the prototypes elicit different amounts of load. The PROTOLAB tools reliably measured these differences.

1. THE PROBLEM

"Small-scale" user interfaces represent the physical base of interaction between users and computerised machinery such as laser printers, video recorders etc. In contrast to their "large-scale" counterparts (i.e. computers with Cathode ray tubes and typewriter keyboards) small-scale interfaces do not offer large scopes for interface design; they are usually sized to fit in small cases or to have valuable prices. As an important part of our daily work routine, small-scale interfaces should not be neglected in software ergonomic research. Concepts like "task-orientation" or "user-centered design" should not only be applied to bulky computer programs but also to our erverydays struggle with photo copy devices or laser printers.

To ease the application of this concepts, we need (a) theory-based guidelines for the construction of appropriate small-scale interfaces, (b) empirical methods to test existing or yet to be constructed new small-scale interfaces, and (c) evaluation standards. The following paper will address the second, that is, we want to introduce the concept of PROTOLAB, discuss in detail some of the experimental procedures we developed, and report empirical results we obtained in the analysis of two prototypes of a small-scale interface.

2. THE CONCEPT OF PROTOLAB

PROTOLAB is the short name for an applicational laboratory we set up for the analysis of user interface prototypes. Within PROTOLAB, various methods based on current theory and research on mental workload can be used to assess the appropriateness of interfaces for the user and the task to be solved. These methods provide data from three sources: Performance, subjective ratings and physiological measurements.

Within the *performance* domain, techniques are used for the empirical assessment of mental workload. The first one is based on the dual-task paradigm and measures mental workload on several dimensions of cognitive functioning. This subject will be addressed later. The second is based on observational data. It is used to assess mental workload in situations where an objective assessment of the user activity associated with the interface is impossible. Unfortunately, this is often the case when user interfaces are studied.

Subjective data are collected with paper and pencil methods. That is, questionaires are given to subjects working on the prototypes several times during their work. The questionaires are based on the concepts the ADACL (Thayer, 1978) and the NASA-TLX-Scale (Hart & Staveland, 1988). Modifications of this scales enable us to measure directly mental, emotional and motivational components of the subjectively experienced workload (for details see Wieland-Eckelmann, 1992). In order to improve the assessment methods for subjective ratings, we developed a so-called Auditive Statement Reaction System (ASRS). This computerised system renders the possibility of an online-assessment of subjective ratings by literally asking the subjects questions about their state. The subjects answer the questions via a special keyboard. The system is currently used to assess the workload of drivers on highway tours.

In the realm of *physiological* data heart rate and their variability is used as an indicator of workload.

3. THE ASSESSMENT OF WORKING MEMORY LOAD

In the literature on mental workload the working memory is regarded as a central processing unit involved in nearly every goal-directed action carried out by man. Thus, working memory load can be regarded as a valid indicator of mental workload.

3.1 Experimental setup for the assessment of working memory load

The *decay rate of a memory image* in the presence of additional memory items is used to assess memory load. The more additional load, the faster the decay of the memory image. Imagine you want to memorize a telephone number. Soon after you have read the number, the memory image starts to decay, and this decay is the more pronounced the more additional items you keep in mind. To prevent forgetting the number, you may do some rehearsal of the digits. This means, you give priority to the task of memorization of the telephone number in order to keep it under any circumstance. This would slow down the decay process and you remember the number correctly for a longer period of time. But it will cost capacity that is taken from the task you are currently doing.

At this moment, your memory task starts to *intrude* the main task you are doing. However, an ideal measurement task that is constructed for the purpose of workload assessment should not systematically intrude the main task at all. This is important in situations, where main task performance cannot be measured or controlled. We invented several precautions to prevent the subjects from doing rehearsal as a cause of intrusion (see Figure 1).

First, we only use short tones of medium pitch as stimuli to be kept in mind. After a decay period the subjects hear a second tone that is either equal or slighty different in pitch to the first one. The subjects have to judge whether the first or the second tone is higher in pitch and to press a foot lever accordingly. About seven of these trials appear during one minute of work on the main task. Since the pitch of the tones is varied in very fine steps, the subjects are unable to label a tone with a certain identity. When numbers or letters were used as stimuli, this labeling would take place as the first action in a rehearsal strategy. *Second*, the duration of the decay period is varied in a random order, so that the subjects are unable to anticipate its end.

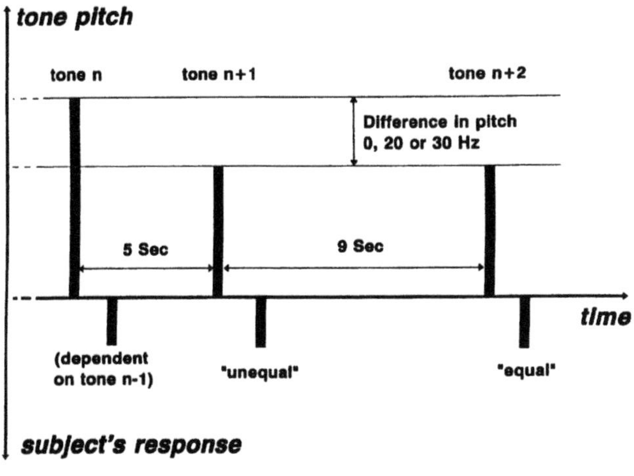

Figure 1. Experimental setup for the memory task.

With the construction of this measurement task we hope to have a tool that indicates load on working memory by means of performance data with a minimal and controllable amount of intrusion. A task with these features would not require performance assessments of the main task when used in a dual-task setup. This is very important since small-scale interfaces normally do not allow an automatic assessment of the ongoing action in the main task.

3.2 Empirical test of the procedures: Mental load in two small-scale user interfaces

Two prototypes of a small-scale user interface constructed for a programable device that is used for the industrial production of bread were tested with our memory task. Operating the first, *machine-controlled dialogue interface,* subjects had to enter the parameters for the baking process by means of a numeric keypad. Besides baking times and temperatures the user could decide whether to use several additional functions to control the baking process. The second, *function key-controlled interface* provided different keys for the activation of the baking process. The numeric values of the parameters had to be entered via a numeric keypad, too. However, it was up to the user to choose an order of programing the various functions.

During the experiment, 30 subjects had to work on eleven *baking programs*. It was assumed that memory load for the function key-controlled interface, requiring a considerable amount of action-scheduling and memorization of functions and parameters, would be higher compared to the dialogue interface.

3.3 Results of the empirical test

Reaction latency and the correctness of the subjects' judgements are the data to be presented for the memory task (MT). Since the subjects had to judge whether two successive tones were equal or different in pitch near detection threshold, the data were analysed in the framework of *signal detection theory* (SDT).

The ordinate of Figure 2a shows the d′-parameter of SDT. The abscissa shows the decay time, that is, the time elapsing between the first and the second tone. As a parameter of detection performance, the d′-parameter should decrease with increasing decay time since the quality of the memory image decreases with decay time. The data in figure 2a were analyzed by fitting a log-linear model (Bishop, Fienberg & Holland, 1975) to the cell frequencies of correct and false responses. The statistical data presented refer to the significance of the parameters of this model.

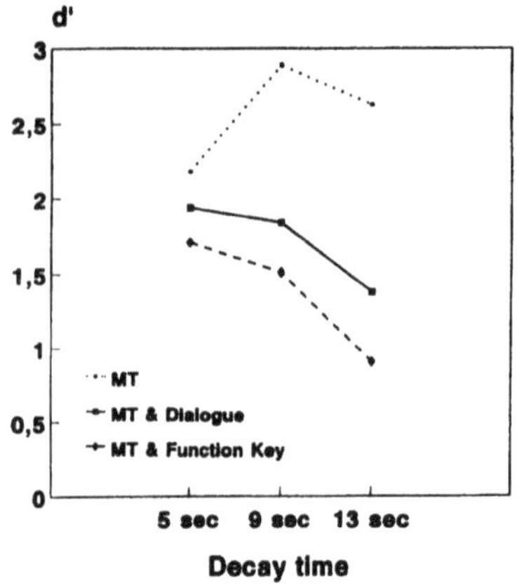

Figure 2a. d′-Parameter for the nine experimental conditions.

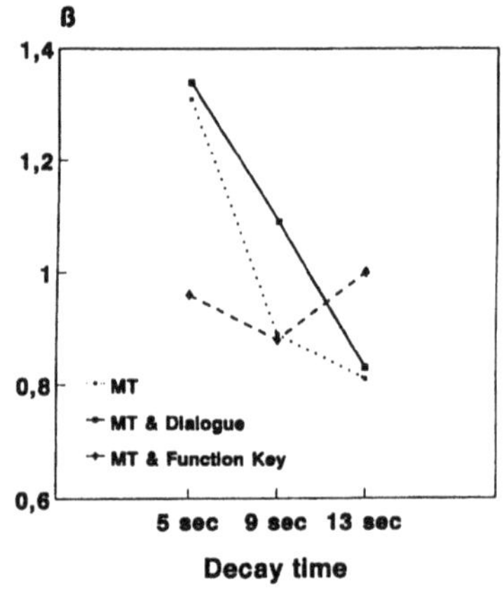

Figure 2b. ß-Parameter for the nine experimental conditions.

The top line of the diagram shows the *d′-parameters* for single-task performance. Although d′ rises with increasing decay time, this change was not statistically significant. That is, decay time does not affect the performance in this task when it is performed alone. The two lines below show the d′-parameter when the memory task is performed simultaneously with the programing of the prototypes. The average d′ in these dual-task conditions is significantly different from the d′ with the memory task alone (Log-Lin-Parameter: $P=0.29$, $z=5.61$, $p<.01$). Furthermore, increasing decay time leads to a decrease of the d′, as hypothesized earlier ($P=-0.19$, $z=-3.99$, $p<.01$). The subjects working on the second prototype with higher memory load achieved a lower d′ ($P=0.20$, $z=2.61$, $p<.05$). However, in order to serve as a measurement tool that can assess different loads on working memory, the amount of decrease in d′ must be different for different loads. This means, that "kind of prototype" and decay time should interact in their influence on d′. And this was actually the case ($P=-0.27$, $z=-2.08$, $p<.05$).

The *β-Parameter* of SDT reflects the decision strategy adopted by the subjects. The ßs for the nine conditions are shown in figure 2b. Apparently, there is some tendency for the subjects in the MT and the MT+dialogue condition to lower their ß with increasing decay time. On the other hand, the subjects in the MT+functional key interface condition mantained their strategy throughout the experiment. This result might be caused by the different amount of workload the subjects had to cope with. In the first conditions, the total workload was low enough to allow an adjustment of the decision strategy to changes in the probability of occurrence of the different stimuli, but the subjects in the MT+functional key condition were unable to adapt their strategy accordingly due to the high amount of total load.

Besides the d′- and the ß-parameter as indicators of detection performance, the *reaction latency* might be covarying in a regular fashion with the nine conditions. In detail, if reaction latency is high, when the d′-parameter is high and vice versa, one might argue, that the d′-parameters earlier presented might be the result of some speed-accuracy-trade-off and not of different memory loads. To address this question, we did some statistical analyses of reaction latency. As expected, we found no systematical variation of reaction latency with the experimental conditions.

4. SUMMARY

As a part of PROTOLAB, the dual-task-technique and in particular the working memory task used in this experiment has proven to be a useful tool for the evalution of workload in small-scale interfaces. An analysis of the *intrusion effects* revealed that further improvements of the memory task would allow an intrusion-free measurement of mental load, provided longer measurement periods and decay times can be used. For further results and a more detailed discussion see Baggen, Schwarz & Wieland-Eckelmann (1992). Further applications of this technique will address this issue as well as the measurement of other components of mental load, for instance load on perception or motor functions.

5. REFERENCES

Baggen, R., Schwarz, R., Wieland-Eckelmann, R. (1992) Prototypische Arbeitssysteme auf dem Prüfstand mentaler Beanspruchung: Das Anwendungslabor PROTOLAB. In GfA (Hrsg.) Bericht zum 38. Arbeitswissenschaftlichen Kongreß an der Technischen Universität Braunschweig, Braunschweig, 25.-27.3.92.

Bishop, Y.M., Fienberg, S.E., Holland, P.W. (1975) Discrete multivariate analysis: Theory and practice. Cambridge: MIT Press.

Hart, S.G., Staveland, L. (1988) Development of NASA-TLX (Task Load Index): Result of empirical and theoretical research. In P.A. Hancock & N. Meshkati (Eds.) Human mental workload. Amsterdam: North Holland.

Thayer, R.E. (1978) Toward a psychological theory of multidimensional activation (arousal). Motivation and Emotion, 2, 1-34.

Wieland-Eckelmann, R. (1992) Kognition, Emotion und psychische Beanspruchung. Göttingen: Hogrefe.

The research presented in this paper was supported by a grant from the Federal Ministry of Research and Technology (BMFT). Grant No. 01 HK 469 was given to PD Dr. R. Wieland-Eckelmann.

WORK WITH DISPLAY UNITS 92
H. Luczak, A. Çakir and G. Çakir (Editors)
1993 Elsevier Science Publishers B.V.

Information presentation and diversified dialogue in advanced process control user interfaces.

Jon Øyen Hol

Man–Machine Systems Research, Institutt for energiteknikk, OECD Halden Reactor Project, P. Box 173, N–1751 Halden, Norway

Abstract.

This paper presents some of the challenges that emerge when current computer based information presentation and handling is introduced in process control rooms. A few guidelines are given, and some current and prospective research issues are mentioned.

INTRODUCTION.

Today, there is in practice no technical design restriction in design of information presentation and user interaction. In today's process control and supervision (PC&S) there is therefore a dramatic change in that computerized operator support systems with sophisticated information presentation is being introduced. One of the challenges is to limit the diversity of the user dialogue, i.e. the modes and means for information presentation and response to it, that may be caused by the combination of new and old information presentation design, and user information handling.

INFORMATION PRESENTATION.

In PC&S of modern plants, information presentation must be simple and unambiguous. It must not only be ergonomically and qualitatively correct for user friendliness, it shall also serve to inform about all the multitudes of process states and conditions, and to advice, emphasize and prioritize. In our laboratories the challenge is to find a «design formula» that combines relevant ergonomic factors with the need to present diverse and integrated information so that essentials are correctly interpreted and understood immediately. So far the formula describes adherence to overall consistency in layout of all displays, and careful and considered use of icons and symbols.

Let us have a look at two very different presentations and see what diversity that may be involved. The first one, in figure 1, are varieties of the simple icons most universally used for fans and pumps. They represent movement and pressure change. The second one, figure 2, is a Rankine Cycle diagram, a modification of the Carnot cycle. It describes the thermodynamic characteristics of a heat transfer power engine where a phase transition from liquid to steam phase and the reversal from steam to liquid take place.

For fans and pumps only three elements altogether are used: the circle, arrow and triangle. Both represent movement, but for the control room operator they have very different functions in the process, in that fans move gases (normally air), pumps move fluids. And pumps are not simply pumps: a centrifugal pump is designed to move great fluid quantities against low head pressures, a piston pump is designed to move rather small quantities against extremely high head pressures. Thus fans, centrifugal pumps and piston pumps must be supervised and controlled differently. To differ in presenting the two pump types, a tail is added to the arrow.

When changing the relative position of the arrow or the triangle, different operational states can be shown. As shown in table 1a and 1b, *running* and *stopped* are but a few of the needed diversity in presenting pump information:

Table 1a
Static pump information

– pump type	– other pump characteristics
– pump capacity	– process identification code
– pumping direction	

Table 1b
Dynamic pump information

– pump stopping, switched off	– pump operational, i.e ready for start–up
– pump stopping, not switched off	– pump not operational
– pump stopped, switched off	– pump tripped
– pump stopped, not switched off	– pump tripped, and in alarm
– pump stopped and in alarm	– current pump capacity (if relevant)
– pump starting	– current control mode (if relevant)
– pump running	– standby spare (if relevant)
– pump running and in alarm	

A contrast to a simple icon is the Rankine Cycle diagram in figure 2. For any power plant using heat (e.g. fossil or nuclear fuelled) with liquid/steam/liquid phase transition the diagram is designed for an overall supervision of the plant thermodynamic characteristics. It describes the process in an entropy–temperature diagram, a so called S–T–diagram. Figure 2 is from our full scale simulation of a Pressurized Water Reactor (PWR) power plant, the NORS simulator. The diagram tells that operation is undisturbed at full power. It can hold the following information:

- The saturation curve for water and steam in the S–T space.
- The modified Rankine diagram for the secondary circuit in the S–T–space.
- The diagram for the primary circuit cycle shown in terms of temperature and degree of subcooling.
- The pressurizer temperature.
- The temperature difference between the primary and the secondary circuits.
- The level of the pressurizer, the steam generators, the feed water tanks and the condensers.

In using the diversity to present information, as illustrated by the relative simpleness of the pump icon and the sophisticated, information–packed Rankine Cycle diagram, one puts a vast span in the requirement to the control room operator to perceive, interpret, understand and diagnose.

It should also be said that use of colour, either separately or in combination with form, give a still added dimension in diversity. Further, one can add the dynamic use of colour change, still either separately or in combination with form. This will increase even more the span put upon the requirements to the control room operators' faculties to do a correct and safe task performance. Since this is an issue of working with display units, the dimension of sound is only mentioned. So also the dimension of information merging through using the emerging «multimedia» techniques. In this way the span in requirements to the control room operators' faculties may seem endless. However, sound and «multimedia» can be used to simplify and improve the possibilities for perceiving and understanding.

To find the limit of this span in various work situations is also what we search for in our laboratories, as a dimension in our «design formula».

INFORMATION REQUEST AND HANDLING.

In PC&S information request must be simple and direct, not exceeding 3 to 4 actions to obtain the desired information, and with a prompt response (< 2 sec). The same is also valid for access to information handling, e.g. to alter presentation parameters; to merge, store, zoom, pan, etc. An action is defined here as to press a button once, or one pointing (i.e. positioning the cursor and press the «read»–button). These requirements are based on the fact that in PC&S one deals with a «live» process that may very suddenly demand full attention, quick and correct decisions, and a follow–up to ensure restoration of desired conditions. This makes the work of control room operators comparable to that of aircraft pilots, flight controllers, and money–dealers in a hectic financial market.

The possibilities, or the traps, to diversify lie in the combination of buttons and pointing devices. The challenge for designers is to find a «once–and–for–all»–procedure for all information requests and access to information handling. Regardless of the procedure(s) selected, the questions: «Where am I?», «How do I get what I want?» and «How do I proceed from here?» must always be promptly answered.

Until recently, with a relatively directly referred PC&S dialogue, these questions were relatively easy to answer with techniques like use of format naming and indication of allowed selections in a menue. But now, because of the complexity of the modern plants and the requirements to optimal production availability, cost and environment protection, the need to add COSSs (Computerized Operator Support Systems) has emerged. COSSs may be systems like ASA (Automatics System Analyzer), CFMS (Critical Functions Monitoring System), COPMA (Computerized OPerations MAnual), DD (Detailed Diagnosis), DISKET (DIagnosis System using Knowledge Engineering Technique), DP (Detailed Prognosis), EFD (Early Fault Detection) and SPMS (Success Path Monitoring System). Even in the names themselves is displayed a diversity which calls for a common process related dialogue basis, and a rethinking in the modes and means for information merging in the formats to limit the necessary dialogue volume. These COSSs are currently implemented in our laboratory at a prototype level, we are therefore on the verge to start work on a common dialogue reference.

But regardless of the mode of selecting particular information, there is one major rule: Require only one action for returning to a common «point of return».

Some safety related issues require direct requests, regardless of information complexity, and at least two independent means for requests and handling. One of the direct means for access to such information can be through dedicated function buttons. The other can be the usual procedure; in that way one can use the familiar ways and means. A third can be through pointing only, for keyboard independence.

Some important system induced information presentation may overrule the user's information requests and handling. This may be the case for alarm presentation and overview information. But otherwise the design philosophy is that the user, and not the system, is the master.

A major part of our work is to find job situation adapted procedures for information requesting and access to information handling, for inclusion in our «design formula».

PROCESS CONTROL AND SUPERVISION (PC&S)

In PC&S there is not much room for human error due to availability and cost requirements. The process is usually in round–the–clock operation through which there is a diversity of task performances and work situations. A "global" dialogue pattern prevails: i.e. address, actuate and observe the response; this pattern must also be followed in all dialogue design. A detailed task analysis must decide the design of the format layout and information content. Main design criteria are consistency and task performance adaptation.

There must never be any doubt about the information and dialogue reference to process, one must know precisely what one deals with. For experienced operators this is normally given by the information itself, novices need some «help–functions». Process response must also be unambiguous. It shall preferably be done in the displayed information, not through additional displays, except for safety reasons. For PC&S we have already a rather detailed «design formula».

CONCLUSION.

We do not fully know yet how to adapt new technological possibilities into user interface design. However, we know rather well where to look for the answers. From our more than 20 years experience in «Working With Display Units», and the successive development of our «design formula» we know that almost all the diversity to be introduced in PC&S interfaces shall be in the modes, means and content of information presentation, not in the user actions. The user actions shall be as simple as:

address, actuate and observe.

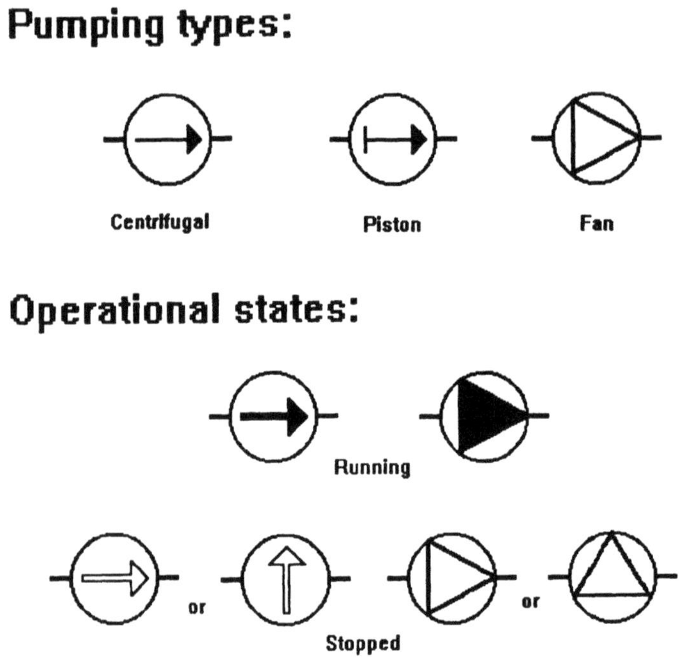

Figure 1. Diversity in pump information presentation.

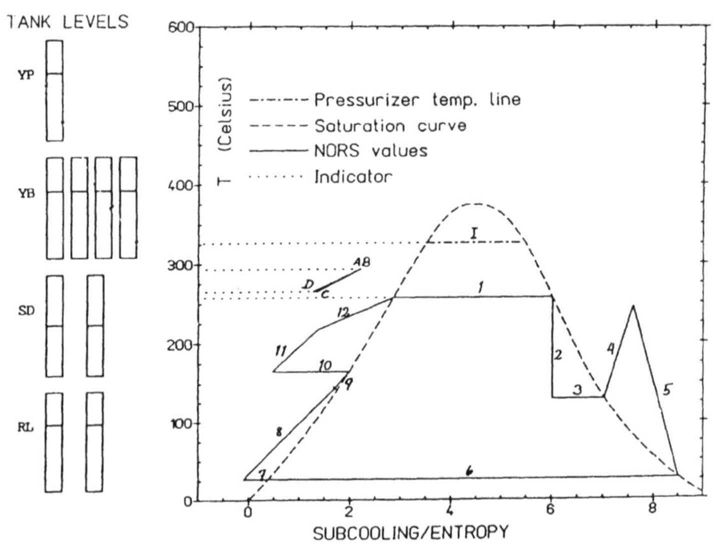

Figure 2. The Rankine Cycle diagram, showing a normal process condition.

WORK WITH DISPLAY UNITS 92
H. Luczak, A. Çakir and G. Çakir (Editors)

Beyond the Desktop - Software Ergonomics in Real Time Systems

A. M. Heinecke

Universität Hamburg, FB Informatik / ANT, Troplowitzstr. 7, D-2000 Hamburg 54, Germany

Abstract

Software Ergonomics mostly deal with office applications. In order to determine whether results obtained by studies of office systems can be transfered to real-time systems the differences between these classes of applications have to be analysed. The crucial factor is timeliness: in process control it puts demands not only to the response time of the system, but also to that of the user. Combining an action-oriented model of the operator in process control with a model of user interfaces we obtain a framework for the design of ergonomical user interfaces in real-time man-machine systems.

1. INTRODUCTION

1.1 Software Ergonomics

Early conferences on man-machine systems were held in the 1960s, and in 1969 the International Journal of Man-Machine Studies appeared for the first time [1]. However, only when new computers with powerful graphics opened new ways of human-computer interaction in the 1980s, interest in software ergonomics grew, and important series of international conferences have been established.

Since then, software ergonomics have become an interdisciplinary area of research aiming at an ergonomic design of data processing systems. As this includes questions like task adequacy and functionality of an application we should prefer the term "software ergonomics" to "human-computer interaction", although the latter is mostly used in the same meaning.

A lot of theoretical and empirical work has been done which led to several national and international standards or draft standards, company style guides, and other recommendations. There are several models dealing with different aspects of human-computer interaction.

1.2 Real Time Systems

According to [2] a real-time system is "any system in which the time at which output is produced is significant. This is usually because the input corresponds to some movement in the physical world, and the output has to relate to that same movement. The lag from input time to output time must be sufficiently small for acceptable timeliness. ... Real-time systems are usually considered to be those in which the response time is of order milliseconds; interactive systems are those with response times of order seconds ... . Examples of real-time systems include process control, embedded computer systems, point-of-sale-systems, and computer-aided testing."

Obviously this definition is based on the response time of the computer system only. Thus a lot of very different systems become subsumed under real-time systems. By far the most important application of real-time systems is process control. Many conferences on real-time systems deal more or less with process control only. Most series of these conferences on real-time systems started earlier than those on software-ergonomics.

1.3. Importance of Software Ergonomics in Real-Time Systems

As errors in operating real-time applications like process control may cause huge damage in terms of money and even human lives, one should expect that user interfaces and operating procedures of real-time systems would have been a focus of conferences on software ergonomics, but in fact software ergonomics and real-time systems seem to be two areas which have rather few interest in each other. Only a small part of the contributions to conferences on software ergonomics deals with real-time applications (typically less than 10%). On the other hand, there are very few papers in classical conferences on real-time systems covering aspects of man-machine interaction (typically less than 20%).

This seems to suggest that there are no problems in human-computer interaction with respect to real-time systems or, at least, that there are no problems that are different from those in any other application. In order to find out whether this is true it is necessary to examine how software ergonomics deal with time, as time makes the difference between interactive and real-time systems, if we follow the definition given above.

2. TIME IN HUMAN-COMPUTER INTERACTION

2.1. Time as a Criterion for Usability

Interactive systems must respond to the user's input within a certain time. The length of the tolerable *response time* depends on the type of input. A complex database query may need several minutes of execution, whereas a movement of the mouse must be echoed on the screen immediately. Response time is an important factor for the acceptance of a system by the users.

The time a user needs to perform a certain task with an interactive system indicates the quality of the system with respect to this task. In many studies *task performance time* has been used in order to determine the best of several input devices, menu layouts, means of information presentation, or ways of interaction. In most cases results of such studies cannot be generalized as they refer to a single task or at best to a certain class of similar task.

2.2. Time as a Part of Information

Frequently *data* are *related to* periods or moments of *time*. For example, in office systems we may have data like sales in certain months or years, in process control we may have measurements at certain moments. Such data can be presented by different diagrams like bar graphs or curves. Usually there is no difference between diagrams where data is a function of time and diagrams where data is a function of other values.

In information systems which relate to the physical world data are often valid only for a certain period of time. Often it is necessary to hold such *time dependant data* for a period of time which is longer than that in which data remain unchanged. In some databases this problem is delt with by time stamps. In other applications we may have different versions. From the view of software ergonomics it is important that the user always knows whether data shown on the screen are valid for the given period or moment of time. For example, in many real-time systems it is possible to call a status report showing the current states of all processes in memory (running, dormant, waiting for a semaphore and so on). If such a listing remaines unchanged on the screen until another output becomes produced, states of some processes may have changed meanwhile. Thus the user may get an incorrect view of the system.

Whereas the latter two topics apply to real-time applications and other applications as well, *information about temporal behaviour* of processes appears only in real-time systems in the wider sense. In [3] the problems of operators in perceiving such temporal data and in developing temporal strategies have been described. Unfortunately, so far there has been rather no research in ergonomical presentation of data related to temporal structures of processes, although similar problems occur in the visualization of project planning.

2.3. Timeliness

As stated in the definition a real-time system has response times of order milliseconds.

However, this does not refer to the user interface but to the process interface. From the user's point of view a real-time system appears as an interactive system. The *response time of the system* to user inputs must be of order milliseconds only if these inputs are to influence processes. In other cases it may be longer.

In real-time applications like process control timeliness requires not only small response times of the system but also small *response times of the user* or operator. Depending on the physical processes monitored by the system the operator has to react correctly within a certain time in order to avoid damage. From the view of software ergonomics this makes the difference between real-time systems and interactive systems.

3. REAL-TIME MAN-MACHINE SYSTEMS

3.1 An Action-oriented Model of Process Control

If there are demands of timeliness on the computer system and on the user as well, we shall speak of real-time man-machine systems. Unlike as in office applications, where the user acts and the computer system reacts, in real-time man-machine systems the rolls of acting and reacting part may change. Especially in process control the operator has to *react* to unpredictable events reported by the system. Besides phases like start-up or close-down process control is often a monitoring task (Figure 1). The operator has to perceive data displayed by the control system, to decide what has to be done, and to carry out the necessary actions (perception - decision - manipulation).

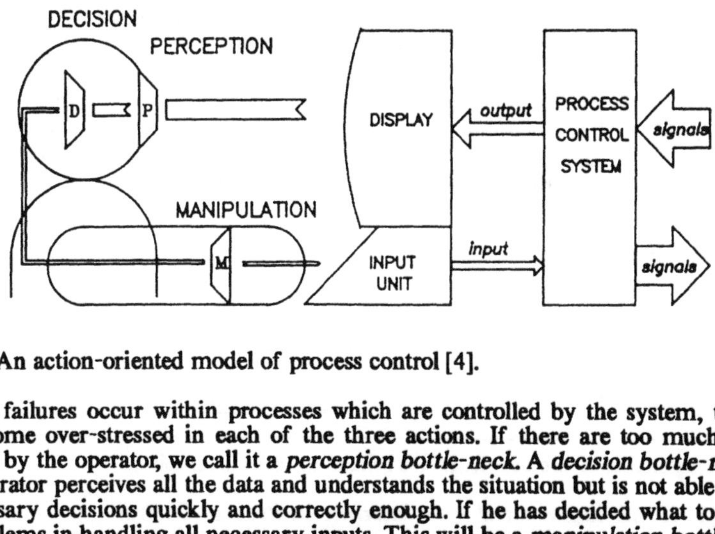

Figure 1. An action-oriented model of process control [4].

When failures occur within processes which are controlled by the system, the operator may become over-stressed in each of the three actions. If there are too much data to be perceived by the operator, we call it a *perception bottle-neck*. A *decision bottle-neck* occurs, if the operator perceives all the data and understands the situation but is not able to make up the necessary decisions quickly and correctly enough. If he has decided what to do, he may have problems in handling all necessary inputs. This will be a *manipulation bottle-neck*.

3.2. A Framework for User Interfaces in Process Control

As a structuring frame for the design of user interfaces for process control we use a model of the user interface based on the IFIP model of user interfaces [5]. According to this model there are four main parts (i/o interface, dialogue interface, tool interface, and organizational interface) for which the objects of design can be studied in detail (Figure 2).

In order to describe all of these design objects the four main parts can be organized in a hierarchy of components and sub-components like it has been done for CAD user interfaces [6]. All structural and dynamical aspects of the user interface can be classified according to these components. Their actual design determines the properties of the user interface.

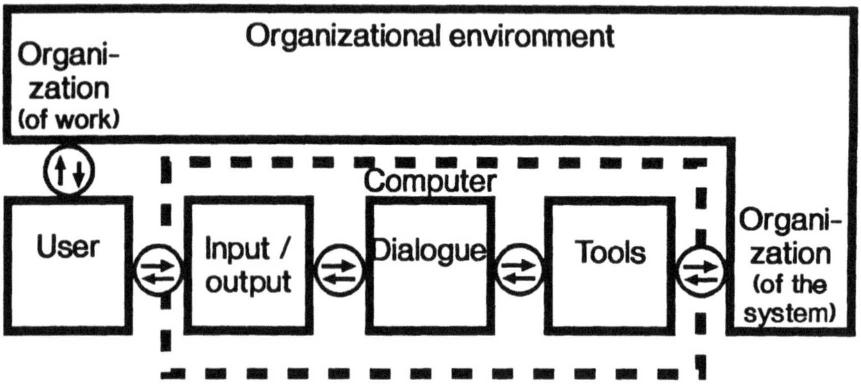

Figure 2. A model of process control user interfaces.

A major goal of the design of user interfaces for process control must be the avoidance of over-stress of the operator. That means, the user interface must be designed so that it eases perception, decision and manipulation in order to allow the operator to react timely and correctly.

Combining the user interface model with the action-oriented model of process control we can determine how each component of the user interface can contribute to the achievement of the goal of correct and timely process control (Figure 3).

Tasks / Components of the UI	Perception	Decision	Manipulation
Input/Output			
- I/O Devices	Speech output for alarms		Trackball instead of mouse
- Codings	Text for messages	Graphical status displays	
- Screen Layout	Message window	History window	Buttons instead of menus
...			
Dialogue			
- Style	Acknowledgement procedure		Control by direct manipul.
...			
Tools			
- Individualization	User's native language	Annotations	User- defined function keys
- Functionality for the task	Messages	Decision aids	Emergency buttons
...			
Organization			
- Organization of work		Training by simulation	
...			

Figure 3. Components of the user interface related to tasks (examples).

3.3. Concepts for an Ergonomical User Interface in Process Control

Research on user interfaces for process control has concentrated mainly on the input/output part and less on the dialogue part. Studies dealing with the tools or the organization are rather rare. There are very few attempts for integrated approaches covering all the components with respect to the basic tasks of perception, decision, and manipulation.

The ALCOSY Alarm and Control System has been developed as a prototype of a small process control system. It aims at reducing the operator's workload by facilitating decisions in critical situations, by providing a consistent way of man-machine interaction, and by providing means for individualization with respect to the user's needs.

ALCOSY combines four basic concepts for a control system, namely messages with decision aids, emergency displays, multi-level process control, and adaptability, within a uniform interaction environment based on a window system with direct manipulation by means of a trackball (for a detailed discussion and for figures see [7]). By these concepts we try to fulfil the demands put to the components of the user interface by the three basic tasks.

For example, a failure in the technical process activates a textual message indicating the technical sub-system the message comes from, the priority of the message (alarm or warning), the nature of the failure, the possible effects of the failure, and the recommended actions. The message appears at a defined location of the screen within a message window. Priority and technical sub-system are also given by speech output. The message window contains push-buttons for acknowledgement and for further information. Thus the concept of messages with decision aids uses the design of different components of the user interface in order to avoid bottle-necks in decision, perception and manipulation as well.

4. CONCLUSIONS

On the one hand, we have shown that there are substantial differences between real-time man-machine systems and other applications: in process control the operator has to respond to the system, and he has to do that within a certain time. On the other hand, models and methods of software ergonomics that have been developed mainly for office systems can be used in real-time systems, too. By combining the IFIP User Interface Model with the action-oriented model of process control we have tried to establish a framework for an ergonomic design of user interfaces in process control.

In the past, the design of process control systems has often been done by control engineers and computer scientists. Software ergonomics have concentrated on office applications. Although there has been some interdisciplinary research, a lot is still to be done. There are many open questions of visualization and graphical interaction in real-time systems [8] which need the efforts of scientists from different fields like informatics, psychology, control engineering, and ergonomics. This demand results from another difference between real time man-machine systems and other applications: Errors due to deficiencies in the design of user interfaces for process control may cause a lot more damage than those in office applications.

5. REFERENCES

1 Gaines, B.R.; 1985: "From Ergonomics to the Fifth Generation: 30 Years of Human-ComputerInteraction Studies". In: B. Shackel (Ed.), "Human-Computer Interaction - Interact 84. Proceedings of the IFIP Conference". North-Holland, Amsterdam.

2 Illingworth, V. (Ed.); 1990: "Dictionary of Computing, 3rd Edition". Oxford University Press, Oxford.

3 Decortis, F. and V. de Keyser; 1988: "Time: the Cinderella of Man-Machine- Interaction". In: J. Ranta (Ed.); 1989: "Analysis, Design and Evaluation of Man- Machine-Systems 1988, Selected Papers from the Third IFAC/IFIP/IEA/IFORS Conference". Pergamon Press, Oxford.

4 Heinecke, A.M.; 1985: "Konzeption eines ergonomischen Prozeßleitsystems mit veränderlicher Mensch-Maschine-Schnittstelle". In: H.-J. Bullinger (Ed.); 1985: "Software-Ergonomie'85, Mensch-Computer-Interaktion". Teubner, Stuttgart.

5 Dzida, W.; 1987: "On tools and interfaces". In: M. Freese, E. Ulich and W. Dzida (Eds.); 1987: "Psychological Issues of Human- Computer Interaction in the Work Place". North-Holland, Amsterdam.

6 Heinecke, A.M.; 1992: "Recommendations for ergonomical CAD user interfaces". In: P. Brödner and W. Karnowski (Eds.); 1992: "Ergonomics of Hybrid Automated Systems III, Proceedings of the 3rd Conference on Human Aspects of Advanced Manufacturing and Hybrid Automation". Elsevier, Amsterdam.

7 Heinecke, A.M.; 1988: "A Desktop Style User Interface in Process Control". In: I.M. MacLeod and A.D. Heher (Eds.); 1989: "Software for Computer Control 1988, Selected Papers from the Fifth IFAC/IFIP Symposium". Pergamon Press, Oxford.

8 Heinecke, A.M.; 1990: "Visualisation and Graphical Interaction in Process Control Systems". In: A. Finkelstein, M. Tauber and R. Traunmüller (Eds.); 1990: "Human Factors in Analysis and Design of Information Systems". North-Holland, Amsterdam.

WORK WITH DISPLAY UNITS 92
H. Luczak, A. Çakir and G. Çakir (Editors)

A product oriented approach to quantify usability attributes and the interactive quality of user interfaces.

Matthias Rauterberg
Work and Organizational Psychology Unit, Swiss Federal Institute of Technology (ETH)
Nelkenstr. 11, CH-8092 Zurich, Switzerland

Abstract
Four different measures based on a product oriented view of user interfaces are introduced. Different types of user interfaces can be described and differentiated by the powerful concept of "interaction points". Regarding to the interactive semantic of "interaction points" (FIPs), 4 different types of FIPs must be discriminated. Based on the concept of interaction points, the dimensions "feedback", "interactive directness" and "flexibility" can be quantified. The results of a theoretical and an empirical validation of 4 quantitative measures are presented and discussed.

1. INTRODUCTION

One of the main problems of standards (e.g. ISO) in the context of software ergonomics is, that they can not be measured in a quantitative way. The scope of our paper encloses the product "interactive software". Today there are 4 different views on human computer interaction to measure interactive qualities (see also [10]; [1]:651).

(1) The user performance view: usability can be measured by examining how the user interacts with the product; all kinds of usability testings with "real" users are subsumed here [5].
(2) The *user oriented view*: usability can be measured in terms of the mental effort and attitude of the user (-> questionnaires and interviews).
(3) The *product oriented view*: usability can be measured in terms of the ergonomic attributes of the product (-> quantitative measures); all heuristic evaluations carried out by ergonomic experts investigating a concrete software product fall in this category, too.
(4) The *formal view*: usability can be formalized and simulated in terms of mental models; Karat (1988) describes formal methods in the context of "theory based" evaluation.

These 4 different views can be classified by the two dimensions "user" (u) and "computer" (c), which are really (r) or virtually (v) involved in the measurement: (1) = u.r & c.r, (2) = u.r & c.v, (3) = u.v & c.r, and (4) = u.v & c.v. Till today nobody knows, how these 4 different views can be successfully combined (see [4]). Nevertheless, "there are invariable errors or misconceptions which will be discovered in any process of having users test a system that even the most insightful of designers would miss. It is a necessary experience to become aware of the fact that none of us knows everything about how the human mind functions" ([5]:895).

2. A DESCRIPTIVE CONCEPT OF INTERACTION POINTS

To come up with a set of metrics of usability based on the product oriented view, a concept of descriptive terms, which can be counted, is necessary. The granularity of the descriptive terms must be on a medium level: not to specific (e.g. "push button", "menu option", etc.), and not to general (e.g. "transparent", "flexible", etc.). We need a granularity level, on which we can describe the different types of user interfaces ("batch", "command", "menu", "desktop") in a uniform and precise way, which is powerful enough and easy to go.

The interaction space (IS) consists of two different interlaced spaces: the object space (OS), and the function space (FS). OS encloses all perceptible objects (RO) and all hidden objects (HO), which users can grasp and bring into the actual dialog context; the same situation is valid for FS: we have to distinguish between perceptible functions (RF) and hidden functions (HF). A dialogue context (DC) contains a subset of the union of OS and FS.

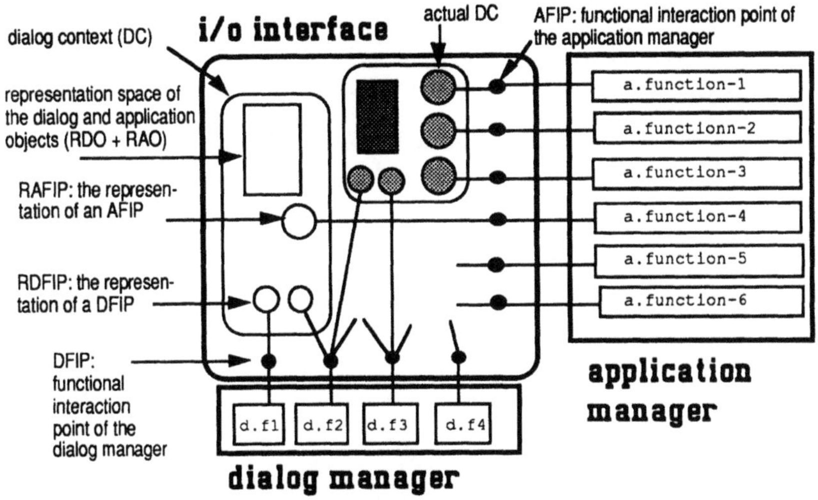

Figure 1. A schematic presentation of the i/o interface, the dialog and the application manager of an interactive system with a two level menu tree.

Belonging to the distinction of an interactive system in a dialog and an application manager [3], we distinguish between two types of objetcs and two types of functions: dialog object (DO) and application object (AO), and dialog function (DF) and application function (AF). Each function has a functional interaction point (FIP): AF –> AFIP, DF –> DFIP. RF is the set of all implemented representations of FIPs. A perceptible AFIP is called a RAFIP, a perceptible DFIP is called a RDFIP (see Figure 1 and 2). These perceptible structures can have a visible, audible and/or tactile representation. RO is the set of all implemented representations of DOs (e.g. button, icon, window, etc.) and AOs (e.g. text document, grafic, data base, etc.). A perceptible AO is called a RAO, a perceptible DO is called a RDO. An AFIP changes the state of an AO, and a DFIP changes the state of a DO. All DFIPs are more or less "interactive overhead". DFIPs are only suitable to handle the constrained interactive ressources (e.g. screen space).

The complete set of all description terms is defined as follows:

$IS := OS \cup FS$; $DC \in IS$; $OS := RO \cup HO$; $FS := RF \cup HF$;

$RO := RDO \cup RAO$; $HO := DO \cup AO$; $RF := RDFIP \cup RAFIP$; $HF := DFIP \cup AFIP$;

$RDFIP := \{(df,rf) \in DFIP \times RF: rf = \delta(df)\}$; $RAFIP := \{(af,rf) \in AFIP \times RF: rf = \alpha(af)\}$

δ := mapping function of a df $\in$ DFIP to an appropriate rf $\in$ RF.

α := mapping function of an af $\in$ AFIP to an appropriate rf $\in$ RF.

$RDO := \{(do,ro) \in DO \times RO: ro = \mu(do)\}$; $RAO := \{(ao,ro) \in AO \times RO: ro = \nu(ao)\}$

μ := mapping function of a dialog object do $\in$ DO to an appropriate ro $\in$ RO.

ν := mapping function of an application object ao $\in$ AO to an appropriate ro $\in$ RO.

The intersection of RF and RO is sometimes not empty: $RF \cap RO \neq \emptyset$; in the context of graphical interfaces are icons elements of this intersection: e.g. RDFIP "copy" $\equiv$ RDO "clipboard", RAFIP "delete" $\equiv$ RAO "trash".

The "interaction point (IAP)" introduced by Denert (1977) is not differentiated enough to appropriately describe graphical user interfaces; an IAP is more or less the same as the "dialog context (DC)" discussed in this paper (see Figure 1 and 2).

If both mapping functions δ and α are of the type 1:m(any), then the user interface is a command interface; the command interface has only one rf$\in$RF: the "command prompt" (e.g. the topmost RAFIP in Figure 2). If both mapping functions δ and α are of the type 1:1, then the user interface is a menu or direct manipulative interface; each f∈FS FIP is related to a perceptible structure RF on the i/o interface. One important difference between a menu and a direct manipulative interface is the "interactive directness": a user interface is 100% interactively direct, if the user has fully access in the actual dialog context to all AFIPs [7]. Good interface design is characterized by optimizing the multitude of DFIPs (e.g. "flatten" the menu tree [8]) and by allocating an appropriate RDFIP to the remaining DFIPs.

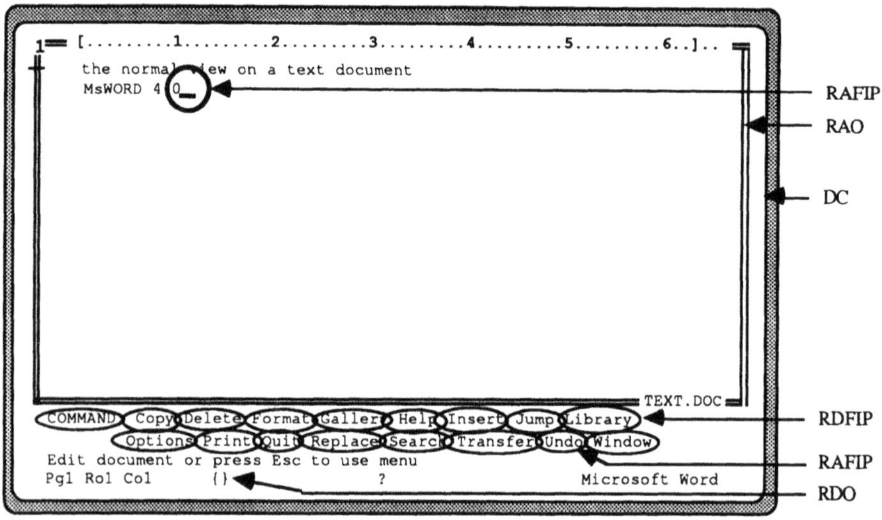

Figure 2. An actual dialog context (DC) of the textprocessing program MsWord with the representation space of the interactive object (RAO: text document; RDO: clipboard), and the representation space (RF: marked by circles) of the interactive functions (RAFIP: text entry point, undo; RDFIP: menu options).

2.1. A quantitative measure of "feedback" of the function space (FFB)

In the context of an actual dialog state the user must know, what he can do next. To support the user in this sense, different kinds of representational structures for functions (RF: e.g. menues, icons) have been developed. If each functional interaction point (FIP) has his own representational interaction point (RF), then the user has 100% feedback (FFB) of all available functions. To estimate the amount of "feedback" of an interface, we calculate a ratio: "number of RFs" (#RFIP = #RAFIP + #RDFIP) divided by the "number of FIPs" (#FIP = #AFIP + #DFIP) per dialog context (see Formula 1). This ratio quantifies the average "amount of feedback" of the function space (FFB). [D = number of all different dialog contexts]:

$$FFB = 1/D \sum_{d=1}^{D} (\#RFIP_d \;/\; \#FIP_d) \quad * \; 100\% \qquad (1)$$

2.2. A quantitative measure of "interactive directness" (ID)

The physical limitations of the i/o-interface (-> screen size) is one reason, not to present all available functional interaction point (FIPs) with a specific representation on the screen (RF). So, the user has to navigate through menu structures (= activating DFIPs) to come down to a DC with the desired AFIP. The average length of all possible sequences of dialog operations (PATH) from the top level dialog context down to DCs with the desired AFIP is the basic idea for a good quantitative measure of "interactive directness" (ID): the reciprocal value of the average path length (= number of dialog steps). An interface with the maximum ID of 100% has only one DC with path lengths of 1 dialog step. [P = number of all different dialog PATHs]:

$$ID = \left\{ 1/P \sum_{p=1}^{P} lng(PATHp) \right\}^{-1} * 100\% \qquad (2)$$

2.3. A quantitative measure of "flexibility" of the dialog interface (DFD)

The number of ways to leave a dialog context (DC) is a precise measure of "dialog flexibility" ("fan" degree). To quantify the flexibility of the dialog manager we calculate the average number of DFIPs per dialog context (DFD). [D = number of all different dialog contexts]:

$$DFD = 1/D \sum_{d=1}^{D} (\#DFIP_d) \qquad (3)$$

2.4. A quantitative measure of "flexibility" of the application interface (DFA)

To quantify the flexibility of the application interface we calculate the average number of AFIPs per dialog context (DFA). A modeless dialog state has maximal dialog flexibility (eg. "command" interfaces). [D = number of all different dialog contexts]:

$$DFA = 1/D \sum_{d=1}^{D} (\#AFIP_d) \qquad (4)$$

3. VALIDATION OF THE QUANTITATIVE MEASURES

First, a fictive example: we have an application manager with 625 AFIPs. Three different interface types are implemented: (1) a command interface with 1 RF (the "command prompt") and 1 DFIP (e.g. a transparency operator like "ls" of UNIX); (2) a menu interface with a strict hierarchical menu tree (3 levels: 1 DC on level-1 with 5 DFIPs [down], 5 DCs on level-2 with 6 DFIPs [5 down, 1 up] per DC, and 25 DCs on level-3 with 1 DFIP [up] and 5 AFIPs per DC); (3) a desktop interface with a complete net structure (5 DCs with 125 AFIPs and 4 DFIPs per DC). FFB of the menu and the desktop interface is 100%; each $f \in HF$ has a $r \in RF$.

Table 1
Comparison of command, menu and desktop interfaces of the fictive example relating to the quantitative measures FFB, ID, DFA, and DFD.

	#DC	#AFIP	#RAFIP	#DFIP	#RDFIP	FFB%	ID%	DFA	DFD
command	1	625	1	1	0	0.2	100.0	625.0	1.0
menu	31	625	625	60	60	100.0	33.3	20.2	1.9
desktop	5	625	625	20	20	100.0	55.6	125.0	4.0

The command interface is the most direct interface (ID=100%) with the highest amount of flexibility (DFA=625), but with more or less no "feedback" (FFB=0.2%). The ID of the desktop interface with the net dialog structure is higher than the ID of menu interface with the hierarchical menu tree.

Second, to validate the quantitative measures (FFB, ID, DFA, DFD) in a more general sense, we need a real product with different interfaces and an empirical investigation. We compared a menu interface (CUI) with a desktop interface (GUI) of the same application manager: a relational data base management system [9]. The results of the product oriented description of these 2 interfaces with the introduced terms are shown in Table 2. The main result of this empirical investigation is, that the mean task solving time with the GUI is significantly shorter than with the CUI interface (see for more details [9]). One reason for this empirical outcome is the high "interactive directness" (ID=50.5%) and the great "dialog flexibility" (DFD= 21.6) of the GUI. The great influence of the dimension "flexibility" is in accordance with the other results presented in [9]. Interesting is the fact, that the GUI supports the user with less "visual feedback" (FFB= 67%) on average than the CUI (FFB=73%). This high amount of FFB of the CUI is caused by 22 small DCs with FFB= 100%; the GUI has only 14 DCs with FFB=100%.

Table 2
Comparison of a menu and a desktop interface of a relational data base management system relating to the quantitative measures FFB, ID, DFA, and DFD.

	#DC	#AFIP	#RAFIP	#DFIP	#RDFIP	FFB%	ID%	DFA	DFD
menu	36	434	36	362	161	73.0	27.7	12.1	10.1
desktop	27	438	38	583	396	67.0	50.5	16.2	21.6

CONCLUSION

Using the 4 quantitative measures for "feedback", "interactive directness" and "flexibility" to measure the interactive quality of user interfaces we are able to classify the most common types: batch, command, menu, desktop. The command interface is characterized by high interactive directness, but this interface type has a very low amount of visual feedback. Only graphical interfaces (GUIs) can support the user with sufficient interactive directness and high flexibility. The presented approach to quantify usability attributes and the interactive quality of user interfaces is a first step in the right direction. The next step is a more detailed analysis of the relevant characteristics and validation of these characteristics in further empirical investigations. In the context of standardization we need criteria to test user interfaces for conformity with standards.

REFERENCES

[1] Bevan, N / Kirakowski, J / Maissel, J (1991) What is Usability? in: Human Aspects in Computing: Design and Use of Interactive Systems with Terminals; (Bullinger, H-J.; ed.); Amsterdam: Elsevier; 651-655.

[2] Denert, E. (1977) Specification and design of dialogue systems with state diagrams. in: International Computing Symposium 1977; (Morlet, E. & Ribbens, D.; eds.); Amsterdam: North-Holland; 417-424.

[3] IFIP (1981): Report of the 1st Meeting of the European User Environment Subgroup of IFIP WF 6.5. German National Center for Computer Science (GMD), P.O. 1316, D-5202 Sankt Augustin (Germany).

[4] Jeffries, R. & Desurvire, H. (1992) Usability testing vs. heuristic evaluation: was there a contest? *SIGCHI Bulletin* 24(4), 39-41.

[5] Karat, J. (1988) Software Evaluation Methodologies. in: Handbook of Human-Computer Interaction; (Helander, M.; ed.); Amsterdam: Elsevier; 891-903.

[6] Kirakowski, J. & Corbett, M. (1990) Effective Methodology for the Study of HCI. in: Human Factors in Information Technology, vol. 5; (Bullinger, H. & Polson, P.; eds.); Amsterdam: North-Holland.

[7] Laverson, A., Norman, K. & Shneiderman, B. (1987) An evaluation of jump-ahead technique in menu selection. *Behaviour and Information Technology* 6(2), 97-108.

[8] Paap, K. & Roske-Hofstrand, R. (1988) Design of menus. in: Handbook of Human-Computer Interaction; (Helander, M.; ed.); Amsterdam: North-Holland; 205-235.

[9] Rauterberg, M. (1992) An empirical comparison of menu-selection (CUI) and desktop (GUI) computer programs carried out by beginners and experts. *Behaviour and Information Technology* 11(4), 227-236.

[10] Rengger, R. (1991) Indicators of usability based on performance. in: Human Aspects in Computing: Design and Use of Interactive Systems with Terminals; (Bullinger, H-J.; ed.); Amsterdam: Elsevier; 656-660.

WORK WITH DISPLAY UNITS 92
H. Luczak, A. Çakir and G. Çakir (Editors)

Multi-modal interaction - An introduction

Pierre Falzon

Laboratoire d'Ergonomie, C.N.A.M., 41 rue Gay-Lussac, 75005 Paris, France
falzon@cnam.cnam.fr

Abstract
The objective of this text is to provide an introduction to the theme of multi-modal and multi-media interactions and interfaces. There is quite often some confusion in the use of the terms "modes", "modalities" and "media". The first section presents some tentative definitions. The second section focuses on synergic multi-modal interaction, and deals with interaction between modes. The following section is concerned with within-mode variation.

1. Mode, medium, modality : some definitions

1.1. Mode and modality
A modality is an operator that can be applied to a core proposition. The application of various modalities yield various sentences.

Proposition : [eat (Mary, ice cream)]

Sentence	Modality
Mary eats an ice cream	assertive, present
Mary ate an ice cream	assertive, past
Mary does not eat an ice cream	negative, present
Will Mary eat an ice cream ?	interrogative, future
An ice cream was eaten by Mary	assertive, past, passive

1.2. Mode and medium
Here are tentative definitions :
- a medium is a technical or physical means; it is defined
  - either by the type of human sensor or human organ it calls for
  - or by the type of device by which it is captured or produced
- a mode is defined by the code it uses : its vocabulary, syntax, semantics

For instance :
- "natural language" is a mode, that can be used with different media :
  - on the device side : keyboard input, screen output, speech recognition, speech synthesis ;
  - on the human side : (hand- or type-) writing, speech, hearing.
- "gesture" is a medium, that can be used in the production of different modes : sign language (as for the deafs), graphic codes, technical drawing.

The confusion stems from bijection cases, in which a single medium seems to correspond to a single mode. I will here concentrate on modes rather than on media.

2. Interaction between modes

2.1. Exclusive vs synergic multimodal interaction

These concepts are borrowed to Coutaz and Caelen (1991).

Exclusive multi-modality designates situations in which modes do not interact. For instance, in an HCI context, different software may run in different windows (e.g. a text editor, a spreadsheet, a graphic editor, etc.). The interface may be said to be multi-modal, but there is no interaction between modes. The user, if a sufficiently long time is considered, will be using several modes, but that should be considered as time-sharing rather than as true, simultaneous multi-modal interaction.

Even if a single software allows the user to use several modes (imagine for instance a software with text-editing, computational and graphic capabilities), these modes may be independent : specific commands will be used to do computation, others for producing a drawing, still others to write text.

Thus, many systems are multi-modal, but only in the sense that they allow different modes to be used at different moments, independently. Of course, this is indeed one way in which we use modes : we switch from one mode to another according to the needs of the situation. We may use the same mode for long periods (natural language for instance, when reading a novel).

Synergic multi-modality refers to situations in which modes interact :
- a single production uses several modes, or
- what is emitted cannot be understood without integrating the productions done in several modes.

Modes are there used in a more interactive fashion. This does not forbid the use of each mode in isolation. For instance a click on an icon will activate the corresponding object. But the user can also click on an icon, then type "delete it", with the effect that the object will be deleted. Both modes are then used to build meaning.

Synergic multi-modality can take on different forms. Here is a non-exhasutive list :

- stress (or phatic aspects : intonation, gesture). Consider for instance how intonation modifies the following utterance :
  "You should not do that"
  "You should not do that !"
- modalization (e.g. by intonation or gesture)
  "I should do that." (assertion)
  "I should do that ?" (question)
- valuation : spatial information, anaphoric reference
  "Last sunday, I caught a trout that long !" + gesture
  "Put this there" + click
- argumentation through performative assignment : examplification, demonstration (see Robert & Falzon in this book), formatting characteristics of texts (see Tazi and Virbel, 1985).
- commented demonstration : this type of synergic multi-modality appears quite often in advisory dialogues. The advisor demonstrates how to perform an action, providing comments while the action is being executed.

2.2. Synergic multi-modal natural interactions

The following observations result from a study of computer-mediated human-human dialogues using both typed and graphical interactions, in a problem solving situation of network design (Falzon, 1991a).

A first observation is that classic phenomena studied in multi-modal research do appear in these dialogues. First, graphical resolution of deixis ("put this there") is indeed present. Second, subjects switch easily from one mode to the other (A types something, B answers with some graphical action, A types something else). Third, context is constituted by the whole dialogue, irrespective of the mode used : there is not a verbal context and a graphical context, but a dialogue context. In fact, verbal references are even made to information inferred from the drawings. Here is a typical example, which exhibits this phenomenon.

A. Go ahead, draw
B. [*B draws*]
A. Let me tell you that you are far beyond the distances from the right-hand segment.

Other observations point at some phenomena that are less studied. First, part of the dialogue aims at clarifying the links between what is drawn and what is discussed : defining some graphical objects, agreeing on what is left implicit, etc. The following extract provides an example of that behaviour.

A. Can you give me a first idea of solution ?
B. Yes. [*B draws*] My cable is not visible, I draw it aside.
A. Get rid of the network of floor shafts, we will assume we know it now.

Second, explanations may make use of both language and graphics, as the second intervention of A in the example below shows.

A. Generally, that kind of shaft is located in the floors ; it allows for instance the telephone connections to arrive in the center of the rooms. Do you see what I mean ?
B. Not really, could you draw me one ?
A. [...] I draw what this could be in a small part of the building over there. [*A draws*] Do you understand ? According to your description, there are access floor outlets every 1.5 m in every room. I draw some of these. [*A draws*] Here you are.

There are then many ways in which language and graphics may interact. A better knowledge of their natural uses would be beneficial to the design of multi-modal interfaces.

3. Variation in mode usage

3.1. The use of graphics

A frequent belief is that each mode is used in an homogeneous way. This is not what observations show, as the two following examples will demonstrate.

The first example concern the use of graphics (the figures appearing in this section have been kindly provided by Françoise Darses). Consider the succession of graphical productions of an architect, while he is designing a house. After an initial phase of discussion with the client, which aims at eliciting the main constraints (cost, location, needs and tastes, etc.), the architect begins to draw. The nature of these drawings varies a lot over time. The architect begins with very rough sketches of the different rooms, drawn as intersecting shapes, with fuzzy boundaries (Fig. 1). Fuzziness is here an advantage : the architect does not wish to be constrained by too precise a drawing ; this is of course in strong contradiction with the vast majority of graphical editors.

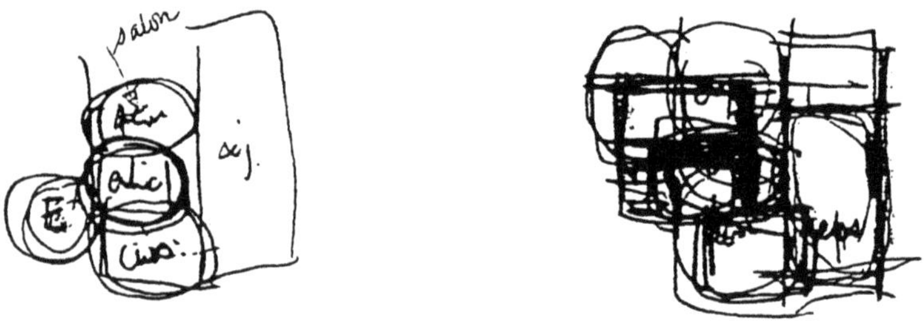

Figure 1

After a while, another type of drawing appears : rooms are now better defined (although the architect is not yet using a ruler), communications between rooms are mentioned, relative surfaces get more precise (Figure 2).

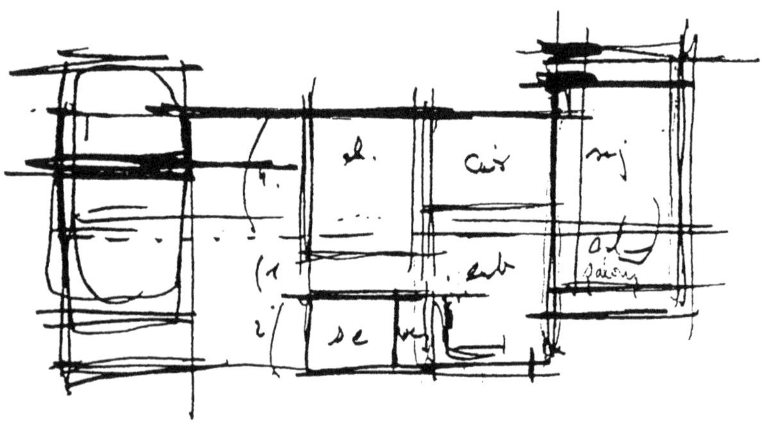

Figure 2

Up to now, the drawings are planar and global : this means that the architect uses an *horizontal* representation of the *whole* building. From then on, and according to problem solving needs, drawings may be partial (some of them may represent only a part of the building) and make use of other angles of representation (Figure 3) : vertical views of the front of the building for instance, or three-dimensional simulations of a part).

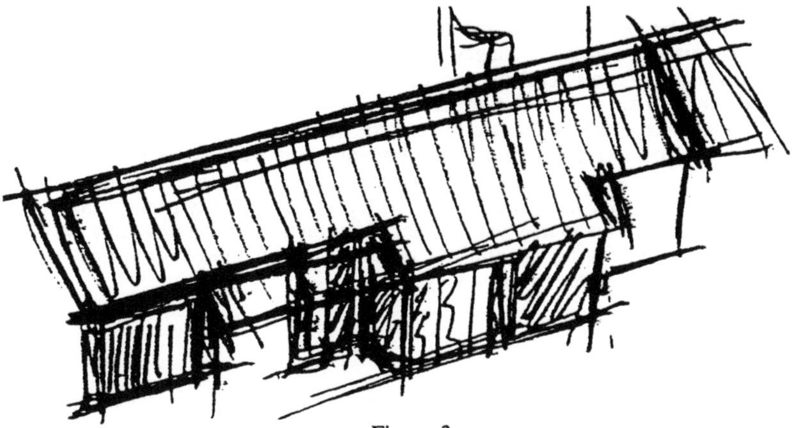

Figure 3

At the same time, the horizontal representation gets more and more precise, up to the point when the architect judges that a solution has been reached (Figure 4).

This example has been developed at some length to indicate that, although productions are mostly graphical (very few verbal indications appear), they use different graphical modes. At the moment, no existing system would accomodate and coordinate these different modes.

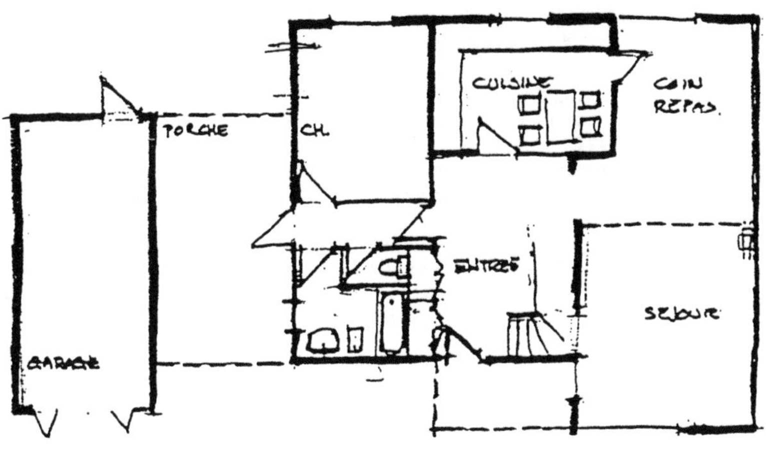

Figure 4

3.2. The use of language

A second example can be found in verbal interactions. We tend to believe that there exists only two kinds of languages : formal languages, which take several forms (programming languages, command languages, various codes), and natural language, which is considered to be an homogeneous body. This is not what observation shows (Falzon, 1989 & 1991b). First, the natural language of experts in a domain differ a lot from the natural language of the layman. Technical dialects ("operative languages") are gradually built by the experts. After a while, the teaching of these operative languages to the trainees becomes a necessity for the acquisition of expertise in the domain. Second, according to the level of complexity of the situation met, the language changes : experts who may use a technical jargon most of the time may switch back to natural language when facing an unusual problem. Again these variations in language production are not accomodated by present systems.

4. Conclusion

Most present days systems propose exclusive and stable modes : in each sub-world, only a specific mode can be used (no synergy between modes) and each mode is to be used in a stable way (no within-mode variation).

This is not what natural interaction exhibits : human beings mix modes, and use each mode in a varied way. The definition of systems which take these characteristics into account is a challenge for the next years.

References

Coutaz, J. & Caelen, J. (1991) A taxonomy for multimedia and multimodal user interfaces. *Proceedings of the ERCIM workshops*. INESC, Lisbon, Portugal, Nov. 14-15, 1991.

Falzon, P. (1989) *Ergonomie cognitive du dialogue*. Grenoble, France : Presses Universitaires de Grenoble.

Falzon, P. (1991a) Multi-modal interactions and interactions between modes in MMI2 design dialogues. Proceedings of the Venaco Workshop on Multi-Modal Dialogues, Maratea, Italy, September 1991.

Falzon, P. (1991b) Cooperative dialogues. In J. Rasmussen, B. Brehmer and J. Leplat (Eds.) *Distributed decision making. Cognitive models for cooperative work*. Chichester, U.K. : Wiley.

Robert, J.M. & Falzon, P. (1993) How do human tutors help learners ? *In this book*.

Tazi, S. & Virbel, J. (1985) Formal representation of textual structures for an intelligent text-editing system. In V. Dahl & P. Saint-Dizier (Eds.) *Natural language understanding and logic programming*. Amsterdam: North Holland.

WORK WITH DISPLAY UNITS 92
H. Luczak, A. Çakir and G. Çakir (Editors)

MULTIMODAL INTEGRATION IN MMI2: ANAPHORA RESOLUTION & MODE SELECTION

JL Binot, L. Debille, D. Sedlock, B. Vandecapelle[a] and H. Chappel, M.D. Wilson[b]

[a]BIM, kwikstraat 4, 3078 Everberg, Belgium

[b]SERC RAL, Informatics Department, Chilton, Didcot, Oxon OX11 OQX, United Kingdom

Abstract

The paper describes the approach taken in the MMI2 ("Multi Modal Interaction with Man Machine Interfaces for knowledge based systems") demonstrator to integrate multiple interaction modes between the user and the system for a computer network design task. This integration is achieved through five design principles which together assure a high degree of flexibility in the (combined) use of multiple modes in knowledge base interaction.

1. Introduction

The MMI2 system (Binot et al, 1990) demonstrates an approach to multimodal cooperative dialogue between user and computer system. The user can input to the system through English, French or Spanish natural languages, command language, by direct manipulation on a graphical display or through design gestures with a mouse. The system can output through the natural languages, graphical display, or non-verbal audio. The interaction of these modes with the underlying KBS for designing computer networks is governed by five principles:

1) there is a meaning representation formalism, common to all modes, which is used as a vehicle for internal communication of the semantic content of interactions inside the interface and also used as a support for semantic and pragmatic reasoning.
2) mode integration is mainly achieved by an integrated management of a single generalised discourse context.
3) there are different model theories for the evaluation of symbols in the meaning representation formalism for the application domain and for the interface domain.
4) The effect of formally evaluating communication actions against a domain can cause side effects in the other domain.
5) Informal processing of dialogue may be performed for user utterances (by the informal domain expert) and system output (by the communication planning expert).

One of the objectives of the demonstrator is to investigate multimodal integration. Given the design principles behind MMI2 this paper will describe the two major classes of multimodal integration: the integration of user input through anaphora resolution, and the integration of modes for system output.

2. Anaphora and deixis resolution

Dealing with anaphora in multimodal contexts is a powerful means of integrating modes. It allows users to select for each part of their commands or requests the appropriate mode without losing the possibility to reference across modes. An example situation is where a user wants to add a disk to each of a number of machines on the network. Without intermodal anaphora, the following options would be open to him:

1) a series of NL commands repeating 'Add a disk to <machine-name>'
2) a series of graphical actions adding a disk icon to each machine

With the availability of intermodal anaphora, the user can perform such actions much more efficiently by selecting the machines in the graphical display and then issuing a command in NL:

User: Add a disk to these machines.

Anaphora resolution across modes adds an additional level of difficulty over and above the usual complexity of identifying valid antecedents from the context and establishing anaphoric relations. The additional difficulty stems from the fact that the system is forced to deal with non-textual modes; modes in which notions such as 'establishing a context' and 'mentioning an object' take on quite different meanings. In NL, for a user to mention an object and thus make it part of the context and available for later reference, is to either name the object (MachineX567) or to describe it (the machine to the left of the server). Graphical object selections however are less predictable than their NL counterparts as to their intended interpretation. When a user clicks on the graphical display, his intention can be any of the below:

1) reference to a particular location on the screen (xy coordinates of pixel clicked on)
2) reference to the graphical icon displayed where the click occurred
3) reference to the domain object represented by the icon

Another significant difference between textual and graphical modes is the role focus plays in the process of reference resolution. Textual focus (i.e. the topic or theme) is strictly tied to the actual time of interaction. Once the user changes the topic, the previous one goes out of focus until explicitly mentioned again. On the other hand, the graphical display remains present throughout the interaction. It would seem impossible to force the user to ignore this display as a possible visual context for NL reference at any time.

Both considerations have contributed to a design decision with respect to the way MMI2 manages the dialogue context. Most systems that deal with anaphora resolution, implement a specialised structure to represent dialogue history, discourse structure, focus shifting, antecedent stack etc. In MMI2, we have adopted a different approach: every interaction is simply stored as it comes from or is sent to the different modes. The complexity is shifted from the extraction procedures that manipulate the internal representation and construct the discourse structure to a body of rules that retrieve context related information on demand by the anaphora resolver. This approach has the following advantages:

- It economises on time and space. Since the retrieval rules are only activated when an anaphor is detected and needs resolving, all the time spent analysing input and output that never gets invoked in contextual interpretation is saved. As for space, storing a discourse representation that makes explicit a lot of information that is implicit in user and system interactions will necessarily take up a lot more space than simply storing the user and system interactions themselves.

- It is more practical and more flexible from the point of view of software design. Extracting a particular discourse representation for the purpose of contextual interpretation is almost necessarily biased by the kind of dialogue phenomena one intends to handle. Transferring the complexity to a dedicated antecedent retrieval rule component and storing the dialogue history as a simple transcription of the dialogue interactions themselves avoids the risk of being forced to change the basic context representation to accommodate further development in one or the other context based interpretation module.

In the context of multimodal systems, resolution often has to deal with a type of anaphoric relation that increases the importance of the previous advantages even more. It is a fairly frequent phenomenon that anaphoric elements are used in NL, yet no suitable antecedent is explicitly present in the context. The resolver then has to try and construct an antecedent itself, given what is explicitly present in the context, and given a number of rules on how to build valid antecedent-anaphor relations. This process of creative antecedent retrieval is called 'accommodation'. One example of accomodation occurs in the following pair of interactions

User: <clicks on a machine icon in the graphical display>
User: What does the disk cost?

where the conceptual relation 'part of' is implicitly validated as an anaphoric relation. The multiple interpretation possibilities of the graphical click also give rise to accommodation. In this example, it is the type of the anaphor and reasoning over the type of antecedent it requires that allows the system to make a decision as to the meaning of the user click. Finally, the persistence of visual focus leads to a more or less permanent supply/stock of antecedents which can be invoked at any time if called for.

With such a multitude of possibilities for antecedent construction and creative anaphoric relation definitions, extracting all relevant contextual information from every interaction would lead to a large body of information which would be costly on processing time and storage space and potentially very difficult to manage.

The decision to store interactions directly rather than constructing a special discourse representation is partly made possible by the design principle of MMI2 that the same representation language (CMR) is used by all modes, i.e. all 3 natural languages, as well as command language and the graphical modes. This uniformity has the considerable advantage of not only allowing the resolver to deal with anaphora in all 3 natural languages in the same way but also permitting the antecedent rules to search without distinction through context coming from textual and graphical modes.

3. Integration of modes in system output.

Whereas the integration of user input from different modes was mainly brought about through the application of the first two design principles behind MMI2, the integration of modes for system output is mainly due to the third and fourth principles. For example, the question (a) is a communication action which would result in a CMR representation which would be evaluated against the application domain and produce a reply (b) which would also be a communication action. In contrast, the question (c) would be evaluated against the interface domain which represents the visualisation of graphs and other interface aspects of the system to produce a reply (d).

(a) User: What is the cost of the network?
(b) System: 13000 Sterling.
(c) User: How many graphs?
(d) System: 3

Example (e), which would appear to be evaluated against the application domain, is in MMI2 evaluated against the interface domain also. In the design KBS used for MMI2 the exact spatial locations of objects were not represented. Therefore it is necessary to interrogate the graphical display to provide the semantics for the spatial relation 'on the left of' and to determine which machines are on the left of a server.

(e) What machines are on the left of the server?

A command such as (f) requires data to be acquired from the application domain about the computers that exist and their costs, but the evaluation of the 'displaying' of this data takes place in the interface domain, with the result that a bar graph is displayed. The communication action in reply to this command is an acknowledgement that it has succeeded in natural language (g). The display of the bar graph is the consequence of successfully updating the 'displaying' in the interface domain.

(f) Display a bar-graph of the cost of the computers.
(g) System: ok

Further complexity arises for a command such as (h) which would be evaluated against the application domain to make it true that a Sparc SLC existed in Room23, but a side effect of updating the application domain would be to update the interface domain so that the icon of a Sparc SLC appeared in Room23 in the display on the screen. In this example, the reply to the user resulting from the command arises from the success of the update to the application domain and would be (g) which would be a communication action by the system. There would be no communication action by the system corresponding to the graphical update of the icon on the screen since this was a side effect of the update to the application domain, and was not explicitly asked for by the user. If instead of (h) the user had typed (i), the update would have failed since the design KBS does not know about Cray computers. The answer to the user resulting from the failed update would then be (j), which is an appropriate communication action as a reply to the failure in the application domain, and no side effects occur in the interface domain. Through the use of side effects in one domain from operations in another, system replies remain consistent with the force of the user's input whilst also causing changes in other modes than that used to express the communication action of the reply.

(h) User: Add a Sparc SLC to Room23.
(i) User: Add a Cray XMP to Room23.
(j) System: No way.

Despite the power of multimodal integration offered by the use of side effects and the use of evaluation over separate domains, some examples require a further informal communication planning provided by the fifth principle. For example, the question (k) would result, after formal evaluation in the application domain, in the answer (l) which makes no use of the multimodal facilities available. In some task circumstances what the user would like to see would be the room where the machine is located highlighted on the graphical display. In order to achieve this the communication planning expert must add to the formally produced answer which is already a communication action for the natural language mode, an additional communication action for the graphics mode which will highlight the room.

(k) User: Where is Machine4?
(l) System: Room3.

Even when the form of the answer is presented in a single mode, the choice of this mode can be made by the communication planner. For example, the answer to the query:

(m) User: Which computers are in which rooms?

will produce a list of pairs of computers and rooms after formal evaluation in the application domain. Both natural language and graphics are capable of presenting this type of information, and the communication planning expert chooses the mode which will more effectively present it to the user. In this case the mode would be graphics and the graphics mode itself would then decide on the most effective form of graphical presentation and would select a table, which would then be presented to the user.

One last example appears at first consideration to introduce the informal domain expert into the choice of which mode to use for presentation. The informal domain expert stores plans for completing tasks and has identified that for executing (n), the network must be designed and the building described. These preconditions are stated as system desires which the communication planner attempts to fulfil. It decides that the way to express this request to the user is to use both a natural language request and to provide a graphical tool in which the user should answer that request. Therefore although it may appear that the informal domain expert is choosing modes as a result of planning information, it is in fact the communication planning expert again which is choosing the mode as a result of the system need which has been identified from the plans.

(n) User: Put the network in a building.
(o) System: Describe the building specifications <Displays tool to draw the building>

4. Conclusion

The first four principles appear to be sufficient to govern multimodal interaction in most cases without having to resort to the freedom offered by the informal approach of the fifth principle. However, both for some principled occasions such as the selection of the most effective presentation mode, and some conventionalised ones (as in example (o) above) informal communication planning beyond that provided by the first four principles is required. Future work should include basic cognitive science and ergonomics research to redescribe those aspects of the informal communication planning in a formal way.

5. References

- Binot, J-L., Falzon, P., Perez, R., Peroche, B., Sheehy, N., Rouault, J. and Wilson, M.D. (1990). Architecture of a multimodal dialogue interface for knowledge-based systems. In Proceedings of Esprit '90 Conference, 412-433. Kluwer Academic Publishers: Dordrecht.
- Bolt, R.A. (1984) The Human Interface: where people and computers meet. Lifetime Learning Publications: Belmont, Calif..

The work reported in this paper was partly funded by the CEC (Esprit project 2474, MMI2).

WORK WITH DISPLAY UNITS 92
H. Luczak, A. Çakir and G. Çakir (Editors)
1993 Elsevier Science Publishers B.V.

Cognitive Attitudes and Speech Acts in Situations of Man-Machine Communication

Anne-Lise Fréchet and Jean Caelen

Institut de la Communication Parlée
46 avenue Félix Viallet
38031 Grenoble cedex
France

Abstract

This article describes a dialogue in the context of multimodal human-computer communication. We think that it is possible to infer the user's intentional states from the chronological analysis of the actions he has planned.

1. INTRODUCTION

Based on Conversation Analysis or Dialogue Analysis, many authors focus on the problem of goals, intentions etc., for the design of human-computer interfaces and take into consideration the user's cognitive functions for a better interaction with the computer. An intelligent human-computer interface provides between human people and computer a system which is able to adapt dynamically to the user and enables him to communicate effectively. This double adaptation has to reckon with the user's abilities and performances in the context of the demanded task. Multimodal human-computer communication is based on the principle of an exchange of composite messages, through different channels (voice, gestures, vision, etc.).

In this article, our interest is in the prediction of the user's intentions and goals, concerning the problem to be solved and in the deduction of the dialogue and communication rules (on principles of negotiation, cooperation, mutual reaction, etc). Nobody knows whether multimodal dialogue can benefit from human to human conversation analysis or not. So, in a first step, considering only voice and gestures, we attempt : 1) to describe structures and patterns in the organisation of the interaction, from linguistic data contained in the corpus that has been registered in situations of problem solving, 2) to describe task planning and activity control with regard to intentions and more generally cognitive attitudes, 3) to establish links between discourse pragmatic markers relevant to communication acts and these cognitive attitudes in a multidimensional perspective, 4) to find relations between utterances and actions that reflect the user's tacit reasoning through the discourse structure.

2. THE ACT OF COMMUNICATION

Ethnomethodologists claim that conversational structures are normative, socially organised procedures. On the other hand, cognitive psychologists claim that behaviour can be explained by reference to cognitive or mental states, but they ignore social rules. With Austin and Searle, communication is intention causing action (via speech acts) [1].
The different modalities of communication convey linguistic and extra-linguistic information and complement one another. The search for users' intentions goes far beyond the problem of comprehension. In this case, the computer has to infer the goals the speaker wants to reach, in spite of approximations, linguistic ambiguities and the redundancy of multimodal information. We call this problem "illocutionary interpretation".

2.1. Our empirical model

More precisely, in the case we consider the addressee is the computer, the act of communication in the sense speaker-addressee is essentially illocutionary. The prior intention (first intention oriented by the task to be executed) generally evokes a plan of action that can be broken down into tasks, sub-tasks and/or scripts. For Searle intentions in action are sufficient to explain utterances and gestures. We think that more sophisticated representation would be useful in order to embed social rules, psychological attitudes, linguistic performance and competence of the speaker, etc. So, we distinguish intentions among cognitive attitudes. To simplify, we assume that a speaker's verbal and gestual acts P_i (physical component) are linked to his intentional states E_i of which they are the direct reflection. These speech acts are linked by temporal relations according to the discourse structure. Intentions can be considered as nodes of a graph whose arcs are the actions a_j. Actions are task-driven. This intermediary level contains the mental component i.e. cognitive attitudes organized in bijection to the physical component. The deepest level, the third one contains the plan of activity which is task driven. We have complete replications about actions on arcs from the first plan to the third one. It is obvious that this model – in which an utterance contains only one intention – is easier to implement in the context of human-computer interaction, but this model is also more simplified. For our application, this is not a restriction insofar as the dialogue is of a reactive type.

2.2. Experiment

In our experiment, the computer is only reactive and the problem is to analyse the act of communication in order to infer the goals pursued by the user through his cognitive attitudes and intentions. Subject and observer both face the screen of the computer. The software is a voice signal editor. The subject handles the mouse and the keyboard while speaking. He comments his intentions and actions. The observer is someone who's familiar with the software, he triggers the subject's comments without helping him. All exchanges are tape-recorded and then orthographically transcribed.

3. METHODOLOGY OF ANALYSIS

3.1. Training from the empirical model and data

Our model is empirical so it cannot be formalized nor described with prior explicit knowledge. The only means we have to define it is the training from real situations and ad hoc corpora. We adopt the following stages :
(1) Survey and collect corpora (speech + gestures),
(2) Study the corpus in order to obtain analysable data,
(3) Segment into speech acts,
(4) Label the data with appropriate dialogue markers,
(5) Code the intentional states according to the realized task, from the illocutionary interpretation of speech acts,
(6) Find the plan,
(7) Search for relationship between intentional states and dialogue markers.

Most of these stages are still done manually.

3.2. Cognitive attitudes

Cohen and Perrault [2] [3] used a number of modal functions in order to describe the speaker's cognitive attitudes, such as : believe, want, know. We introduced others, in our concern for descriptive precision. These are :

a (x)	: act on x	(action on x)
b (x)	: believe x	(personal belief)
d (x)	: desire x	(expression of a wish)
j (x)	: judge x	(evaluation)
th (x)	: think x	(estimation)
P (x)	: perceive x	(sensorial aspect of knowledge)
k (x)	: know x	(shared knowledge)
w (x)	: want x	(expression of a goal)

These eight functions enable us to summarize the user's cognitive attitudes. They give us information on his mental state, his behaviour, his attitudes and his anticipation faculties in order to conduct the dialogue in a satisfactory way. Three functions act on predicates (act, perceive, want) and five functions act on propositions (believe, desire, judge, think, know). Note that "desire" can be considered as a weakened form of "want". In our concern for precision, we keep these two terms anyway.

3.3. Speech acts

The taxonomy of speech acts initially suggested by Austin [4] and Searle [5] has often been revised since according to the needs of analyses or of domains of application. We will follow this tradition by introducing our own definitions for greater convenience and adapting to the type of discourse we have analysed. The different speech acts are : assertive, directive, commissive, expressive, declarative, expectative and metadiscourse.

3.4. Structure of discourse

About human to human dialogue, the Geneva School [6], [7] defines the hierarchy intervention, exchange and negotiation (initiative, reaction, evaluation). Our context is simpler because we have to deal with a reactive type dialogue. We call it reactive because the computer never takes any initiatives : it only reacts to the user's commands if they are well formed. The phases of the dialogue which we keep are the following : opening, continuation, closing (all three split up into initiative, evaluative and reactive), incidence (temporary giving up of an activity during its execution, before taking it up again later), and rupture (definitive giving up). A plan starts with an opening and finishes with a closing.

4. ANALYSIS AND RESULTS

4.1. Analysis presentation

We present the analysis results and their formalization in different columns of a chart. A session using a signal editor utility divides into several sections, whose biggest section is the plan (long term control to reach objectives). Each plan splits up into different structures, explained with arborescences (middle term strategy). Script, the elementary unit of action, contains verbal productions divided into speech acts. This atomic entity, often equivalent to a clause, designates short term actions. The presence of a gesture using the keyboard or the mouse is indicated by a cross. Discourse occupies an other section of the chart. We show linguistic markers extracted from the script, then we determine the nature of the speech acts and the different discourse phases. Then, we have the mental states section. Concerning intentions we determine, for each script, whether the intention is a "prior" or "in action" intention. Cognitive attitudes and strategies are specified. The last column describes the software interventions.

4.2. Results and discussion

The realization of a complex task requires from the user an effort of complex reasoning in order to reach the final goal. If the user is familiar with the task (as in the case of an expert), the planning will be logical and linear since the software cannot answer two commands at the same time. Verbal linearization and multimodal interaction don't seem to be any trouble in this case. It will become so if the system controls several tasks in parallel.

If the user hesitates in the organization of his actions, we observe during the course of actions, incidences, verbal hesitations, or ruptures. Disorganized searching, due to the absence of planning, may result in lengthening the frames in an anarchic way.

The location of linguistic markers is important because they link units of activity and they convey the anchoring of the language in the enunciative context or in the process of communication [8]. Their role is either argumentative (*tout d'abord, mais*, etc.) or logical (*donc, et*, etc.).

The most frequent speech act is the assertive act (57 %). The less frequent acts are declarative (2 %) and expectative (3 %). The frequency of the other acts is the following : directive (16 %), commissive (10 %), expressive (8 %) and metadiscourse (4 %).

A plan generally starts with an initiative opening and less frequently with an

evaluative opening and for only one speaker the plan starts with a reactive one. A plan generally finishes with an evaluative closing and less frequently with an initiative one. Continuation is of recursive type and can be either initiative, reactive or evaluative.
Concerning cognitive attitudes, we remark that every "a" generally appears after "d" or "w". Moreover "j" or "k" can intervene at any moment. On the other hand, a sequence of two "d" functions denotes a changing of intention with rupture. The sequence of operators that would allow us to measure the efficiency of action is [(w+d).a] (+ means "or", . means "and") since to desire or to want leads directly to an action. This type of behaviour characterizes the user who controls the domain of activity and the interface. Looking more closely, we have to make sure that the sequence [(v.a)*] (* means "recursive") does not hide loops.

5. CONCLUSION

We have defined a model for analysis based on the observation of users in situations of communication and problem solving. This empirical model links the task to the plan of activity and to several cognitive components – intentional states, cognitive attitudes – through speech acts that are the outer marks of the act of communication. Firstly we divided the multimodal aspect into two : the oral non-operative dialogue and a set of operative gestures, in order to enable us to study a particular type of dialogue allowing the user to verbalize his actions in an explicit way. Secondly, we hope to use a Wizard of Oz technique to study real multimodal dialogues. Results already show the effectiveness of this model since it is possible to explain without ambiguity each phase of the discourse, to extract a strategy from it and to draw lessons for the design of human-computer interaction. But an important problem remains : can our model accept automatic detection and labelling of speech acts and cognitive attitudes for automatic learning ?

6. REFERENCES

[1] J. R. Searle, *Intentionality*. Cambridge U. P., 1983.

[2] P. R. Cohen, *On knowing what to say : Planning speech acts*. Ph.D. Thesis, Technical Report n°118, Department of Computer Science, University of Toronto, January 1978.

[3] Ph. R. Cohen, C.R. Perrault, Elements of a Plan-Based Theory of Speech Acts. *Cognitive Science* 3, pp. 177-212, 1979.

[4] J. L. Austin, *How to do things with words*. Oxford U. P., 1962.

[5] J. R. Searle, *Speech Acts*. Cambridge U. P., 1969.

[6] E. Roulet, *L'articulation du discours en français contemporain*. P. Lang-Berne, 1985.

[7] J. Moeschler, *Modélisation du dialogue, représentation de l'inférence argumentative*. Hermès ed., 1989.

[8] D. Bassano, Opérateurs et connecteurs argumentatifs : une approche psycholinguistique. *Intellectica*, pp. 149-191.

WORK WITH DISPLAY UNITS 92
H. Luczak, A. Çakir and G. Çakir (Editors)
1993 Elsevier Science Publishers B.V.

How do human tutors help learners ?

J.-M. Robert†, P. Falzon††

† Ecole Polytechnique de Montréal, Département de génie industriel, Case postale 6079, Succ. A, Montréal, Québec, Canada H3C 3A7

†† Conservatoire National des Arts et Métiers, Laboratoire d'ergonomie et de neurosciences du travail, 41 rue Gay-Lussac, 75005 Paris, France

Abstract
This study examines how human tutors help subjects learn a computer application in the context of learning by exploration. Its goal is to analyze the tutors' styles and strategies in order to help designing the didactical module of intelligent tutoring or coaching systems. Six subjects paired to six tutors participated in the study. They had to use a new word processor for making a series of modifications to a letter shown on the screen of the computer, in an hour, and without reading any documentation. They were asked to explore the new application as much as possible, but could also request help from a tutor. Results show that at least three different tutoring styles could be observed during the session: exploration-oriented, teaching-oriented, and exploration/teaching-oriented. The adoption of a style results from a mutual and constant adaptation between the tutor and the subject, and from the task difficulty. These styles correspond to three learning modes adopted by the subjects. Tutors also used various strategies for helping subjects: cues/short answers, confirm/infirm, reformulation, recall, recapitulation, demonstration, generalization, example, analogy, repetition, and questions. Finally, tutors often help subjects pursue sub-optimal procedures for completing a task. As a conclusion, we indicate some promising research directions for the future.

1. INTRODUCTION

This study examines how human tutors help subjects learn a computer application in the context of learning by exploration. Its goal is to identify and analyze the means used by the tutors for helping the subjects, in order to define design principles and guidelines for the didactical module of intelligent tutoring or coaching systems (ITS, ICS). This module has the crucial role of deciding when, and how to help subjects to acquire knowledge. Unfortunately it has been neglected so far, as compared to the expert and the user modules in ITS and ICS (e.g., see the systems SOPHIE by Brown et al. 1982, EdCoach by Desmarais 1990, and LMS by Sleeman, 1982). The didactical principles guiding the responses of these systems are defined intuitively rather than on experimental results. This situation is similar to the one encountered in knowledge-based systems (KBS) where the explanations offered to the users are often considered inadequate (e.g., Johnson & Johnson, 1991).

In this study, the natural dialog between tutors and learners is used as a reference for defining the dialog between a learner and an ITS or ICS. Although these two types of dialogs differ in several respects (the natural dialog is both verbal and non verbal, visual and auditive, whereas the human-computer dialog is non verbal and visual), research has shown that human-human

dialog can be a valuable source of reference for human-computer dialog (Falzon, 1989). Accordingly, we conducted a study that allowed us to collect verbal and non-verbal dialogs between human tutors and learners, and thus to investigate how tutors help learners with a new computer application.
We chose a learning-by-exploration situation because, generally, this learning mode is the source of important difficulties for the learners of new computer applications (Carroll & Rosson, 1988; Robert, 1989). As such, it creates numerous opportunities of exchanges between the learner and the tutor, and contains multiple examples of natural help.

2. METHOD

Subjects. Six subjects participated in the experiment. They had no experience with Microsoft (Ms) Word 4.01 (English version) which runs on the Macintosh, but knew at least another word processor. Only 2 subjects were familiar with a mouse, and 4 with menus. All were students at Ecole Polytechnique de Montréal; five were between 20 and 23 years old, and one was 44 years old. Six tutors, who were paired to the subjects so as to have six teams of two persons, also participated in the experiment. They had a minimum of 2 years of experience with Ms Word; actually 3 tutors had 2 years of experience, 1 had 3 years, and 2 had 5 years. They had no particular training or experience in tutoring. Their age varied between 21 and 30 years.

System. The Macintosh system was used in this experiment because its direct manipulation user interface with menus, icons, windows, and a mouse, lends itself very well to exploration.

Task. For the subjects, the experimental task consisted in making 48 modifications to a 24-line letter shown on the screen of the computer, in one hour, by exploring as much as possible without reading any documentation about Ms Word. These modifications were concerned with content changes (i.e., insert, move, delete, replace, modify characters (fonts, style, size), break lines, merge lines, make a table, create a footnote, use the scrapbook), and text formatting (i.e., justify text, indent, modify margins, modify interline, use the tabs). To a large extent, the categories of modifications are the same as the ones used by Roberts (1980) for evaluating different text editors. For the tutors, the task consisted in helping the subjects to make the modifications, but only after a subject's request.

Procedure. First, the subject and the tutor read a brief text about the goal and the procedure of the experiment. Then, they were also given a copy of the initial letter, a copy of the final letter including all the modifications, and the list of all the tasks to be made. Once they had read this material, they completed a brief questionnaire on their age, training, occupation, and computer knowledge. The subject, who was asked to think aloud during the session, was encouraged to explore Ms Word as much as possible but was also allowed to ask questions to the tutor whenever it was felt necessary. The tutor, who was somewhat isolated from the subject to prevent intimidation, was instructed to play a reactive role only, i.e. provide help only when it was requested and only on the topic mentioned in the subject's question or comment; so he/she was not allowed to initiate dialogs, nor to provide non-requested information. In some situations, the experimenter intervened either to insure that the subject and the tutor did not engage in too long exchanges, or to encourage subjects to request help when they seemed too hesitant to do so. The learning sessions were videotaped, and the subject-tutor dialogs were recorded and transcribed for an in-depth analysis.

3. RESULTS

Results are based on verbal and non-verbal protocol analysis of the subject x tutor interactions. Protocols contain information on the time, the task to be done, the system state, the subject's question, the tutor's response, the subject's actions following the response, the subject's degree of success with the task, and general comments from the experimenter. Here, the results bear upon the tutors' styles and strategies for helping the subjects; other results (e.g., on the learners' performance, the rate of agreement between tutors) appear in Bouchard (1991) and Robert & Bouchard (1991).

3.1 Tutoring styles

At least 3 different tutoring styles could be observed among the tutors: exploration-oriented, teaching-oriented, and exploration/teaching oriented (a mixed style). In the first style, the tutors, encouraged or not by the subjects and to some extent influenced by the instructions, played a very minor role: they remained passive, they gave very little information, and did not exert control over the session, in order to let the learner think, explore further and discover by him/herself. In the second style, the tutors behaved in an opposite way on each of these points. They played a major role: they were active, they provided much information that was not strictly requested by the subjects, and exerted control over the session. In the third style, which is the most common, the tutors stood between these two extremes on each of these points. They adapted to the context, at one time by being passive or giving little information when they considered the learners did not need help or needed a minimal one, at another time by being active and giving more information when they considered the learners needed more help. Exploration-oriented tutors tend to provide short, incomplete, and indirect information as opposed to teaching-oriented tutors. These three tutoring styles directly correspond to the three learning modes used by the learners. An ideal situation is the matching between a tutoring style and a learning mode (e.g., both exploration-oriented). Otherwise, adjustments are required either from the tutor, from the learner, or from both.

The important individual differences that exist between tutors seem to depend on both the tutor's personal preference for a tutoring style, the subject's personal preference for a learning mode, and the task difficulty. It is impossible to weigh the contribution of each factor because it varies greatly from one situation to another. In some cases, one finds a rather dominant tutor who tends to impose his/her own tutoring style to the subject. In other cases, one finds a dominant subject who also tends to impose his/her own learning mode to the tutor. Yet, in other cases, a subject encounters difficulties such that he/she is forced to request more help than he/she would be inclined to, and the tutor is led to give more help that he/she would be inclined to. The most striking result, which represents a tricky challenge for ITS or ICS, is the mutual and constant adaptation of the subject and the tutor to each other, to the task difficulty, and to the evolving context. Indeed, the tutor and the subject take into account the style of their partner, the task difficulty, and the information that has been requested or provided so far during the session, and constantly adjust to this context for the sake of a smooth interaction and of a better performance at the task. This behaviour corresponds to an intelligent adaptation that is also expected from ITS or ICS. It stresses all the importance of a flexible and intelligent approach for helping subjects.

3.2 Optimal vs sub-optimal procedures

Tutors did not always propose optimal procedures when helping subjects to perform a task. Indeed, where there was a choice of procedures in the application for doing a task, and when the subject was already engaged in a valuable (but not optimal) procedure, they often proposed to pursue that procedure and make it operational instead of starting with a new one and not take into account the work accomplished up to this point. This strategy corresponds to what can be called a "local optimization" instead of a global one.

Such an approach has also been proposed in the context of computer programming (Maïs,1989). It seems quite desirable in several situations, where one is more interested in the result than in the procedure, where we want to show the alternative procedures available in a system for doing a task, or where it is important to acknowledge the work done so far by the person for encouraging exploration and improving satisfaction towards the system. However, it represents an extra challenge for ITS and ICS since the work done by the subject has to be evaluated and problems have to be diagnosed, if any.

3.3. Helping strategies

The tutors used a variety of strategies for helping the subjects. These strategies are not mutually exclusive and can thus be combined in the same answer. They are classified according to the first two tutoring styles described above. They bear upon concepts as well as procedures.

Exploration-oriented tutoring strategies

- *Clues/Brief answers.* The tutor does not answer the question directly, nor completely; instead he/she provides clues or gives a short answer that will hopefully lead the subject to think carefully, explore further, and discover the answer on his/her own. For instance, a subject wanted to type text into the scrapbook, but did not know its role, nor the procedure for using it. He asked: [S stands for subject, and T for tutor]

S: What is the scrapbook ?
T: Click on the apple (icon menu).

- *Confirm/Infirm.* The tutor just confirms or infirms the subject's hypothesis or proposition about the relevant actions to do for performing a task. This strategy was frequently used during the session; it is considered more rapid than asking the tutor to produce the answer, and allows the subject to control the dialog and be active. For instance, a subject wanted to move something; he selected a piece of text and the "Cut" command from the "Edit" menu; then he asked the tutor:

S: Now, I guess that I have to return into the "Edit" menu ?
T: Yes
S: And then, paste, maybe ?
T: Yes.

Teaching-oriented tutoring style:

- *Reformulation.* The tutor expresses in different words what has just been said. The answer (content, syntax, terminology, length, ...) is adapted to the subject's level of knowledge. For instance, the tutor explained how to select text for having it bold, and said: "When you want to select a piece of text for being able to do an operation on it, you must drag; there are several technics, one of them consists in taking the mouse and dragging it from the beginning until the end. To drag means that you holds the mouse down at the beginning and you move it until the end".
- *Recall.* The tutor reminds the subject of notions that have already been presented and that are considered as pertinent to the current task. The goal is to help the subject learn. For instance, in several situations where the task required the selection of a command from the menu, the tutor said: "You select the text first, then a command from the menu".
- *Recapitulation.* On his own initiative, the tutor states explanations that have been given earlier during the session. The number of recapitulations and the amount of detail vary greatly from one tutor to another, and from time to time. Obviously, the goal is to reinforce the subject's learning. For instance, after having explained that one must select text before the command that applies to it, and following a question on how to center a word, the tutor said: "OK, to center, you understood the operation principle, that is you must select the text to which you want to apply a command".
- *Demonstration.* As a complement to or a partial replacement of a verbal answer, the tutor shows how to do something by giving a demonstration with the system. There are several cases where the tutors did something themselves with the system instead of asking the subject to do it. For instance, a subject was not using the mouse correctly; so the tutor grabbed the mouse and made a short demonstration to show how to hold and use it. Another tutor explained how to use the tabs in the ruler; he grabbed the mouse and used a few tabs.
- *Generalization.* The tutor adds information that goes beyond what is asked in the question, and identifies other situations the answer also applies to. For instance, after having explained how to select an object on the screen, the tutor said: "This selection procedure applies to a character, a word, a line, a paragraph".
- *Example.* The tutor uses examples to illustrate the answer in order to make it more explicit and be better understood by the subject. For instance, at the end of a long explanation on positioning the cursor with the mouse, the tutor said: "For example, if you want to move the cursor at the end of a line, you simply click the mouse at the end of the line. It is like that that you move the cursor in the text".

In all tutoring styles:

- *Analogy*. The tutor makes analogies with something encountered previously in the session or that is considered known to the subject. The analogy is often used as complement to an answer. To a subject who was trying to reverse two addresses within a letter and who was already familiar with the WordPerfect editor, the tutor said: " It is the same philosophy with this editor (...) Actually, the equivalent to "move" are the commands "cut", "copy", and "paste" in the Edit menu". To a subject who had succeeded in moving a piece of text with the "cut" and "paste" commands, and who still had text to move, the tutor said: "It is the same procedure (...)"
- *Repetition*. During a learning session, it happens that the tutor must repeat an explanation once or several times because the learner did not understand correctly. For instance, a subject had problem to reverse two addresses in a letter by using the "cut" and "paste" commands. The tutor had to repeat three times how to perform the task with these two commands. A repetition can be quite similar to or slightly different from the initial answer. It can also be presented in one shot or step by step while the subject executes the procedure.
- *Questions*. The tutors often asked questions to the subjects, not only for knowing their goal, but also for having them confirm something for being able to pursue the dialog with the conviction that the subjects had understood correctly. This strategy is effective for better controlling the communication with a partner. For instance, while there were several windows opened on the screen in front of the subject, the tutor said: "You click into the text window behind. You see this text window ?" In another situation, after a long explanation on positioning the cursor with the mouse, the tutor said: "Do you understand ?"

3.4 Multi-modal interaction

The tutors and the subects did not only communicate verbally, even though the verbal exchanges remain the most important way to communicate with each other. They also used gesture for pointing at the screen and designating objects of reference they were talking about (e.g., icons, menus, piece of text). Moreover, as mentioned above, some tutors even made a demonstration to show how to operate a system component (e.g., the mouse, the tabs in the ruler) in order to convey information more effectively to the subjects. These various communication modes for the tutors (voice and gesture) could run in parallel or in rapid alternance to each other so that the tutor could verbally explain what to do while pointing at objects on the screen or manipulating them with the mouse. The subjects then received auditive and visual information at the same time; moreover, the visual information was not only static (e.g., T: "See the tabs in the ruler"), sometimes it was made dynamic through animation made by the tutor (e.g., T manipulates the tabs with the mouse). This natural behaviour of human tutors suggests the use of multi-media interfaces in ITS or ICS.

4. CONCLUSION

This study has shown that human tutors adopt different tutoring styles and use various strategies for helping subjects. The adoption of a particular tutoring style results from a mutual and constant adaptation during the session between the tutor and the learner, and from the task difficulty. Here flexibility is crucial among tutors for being able to offer adequate help. Besides, the tutors often helped subjects pursue a sub-optimal procedure for completing a task, instead of proposing a new (and optimal) one. Moreover they also used gesture for communicating with the subjects, either for designating objects on the screen or for giving a demonstration about the operation of some system components. It is clear that all these characteristics of the tutors' behaviours require a level of intelligence that is much behond the reach of many ITS or ICS. Yet, they represent interesting challenges for R & D on intelligent operator assistance.

The next step of this study (see Falzon & Robert, 1993) will consist in making an in-depth analysis of the verbal communications between the tutors and the subjects (e.g., content, form, timing), and of the close articulation between requests and help. This will allow us to show the different types of utterances and their succession within the subject's and the tutor's discourse, and the step-by-step coupling of these utterances from the subject and the tutor. These results will help to design better didactical modules for ITS and ICS.

5. REFERENCES

Bouchard, S. (1991). Analyse du comportement des tuteurs humains dans un contexte d'apprentissage par exploration. Master's dissertation in applied sciences, Université de Montréal. Unpublished document.

Brown, J.S., Burton, R.R., De Kleer, J. (1982). Pedagogical natural language and knowledge engineering techniques in Sophie I, II and III, in Sleeman, D., Brown, J.S. (Eds.). Intelligent Tutoring Systems, London: Academic Press, pp. 227-282.

Carroll, J.M., Rosson, M.B. (1988). Paradox of the active user, in Carroll, J.M. (Ed.). Interfacing Thought. Cognitive aspects of human-computer interaction. Bradford, Cambridge, pp. 80-111.

Desmarais, M. (1990). Architecture et fondements empiriques d'un système d'aide assisté par ordinateur pour l'édition de texte. Doctoral dissertation in psychology, Université de Montréal. Unpublished document.

Falzon, P. (1989). Ergonomie cognitive du dialogue. Presses de l'Université de Grenoble, France.

Falzon, P., Robert, J.-M. (1993). Natural advisory interaction in a HCI context (running title). In preparation.

Johnson, H., Johnson, P. (1991). Empirical investigation of different dialogue styles, in Bullinger, H.-J. (Ed.). Human aspects in computing: Design and use of interactive systems and information management. Elsevier, pp. 915-919.

Maïs, C. (1989). L'adaptation de l'aide à l'utilisateur: aider les programmeurs occasionnels à opérationnaliser leurs plans sous-optimaux. Thèse de doctorat en psychologie cognitive, Département de psychologie, Université de Provence Aix-Marseille I.

Robert, J.-M. (1989). Learning a computer system by unassisted exploration. An example: the Macintosh, in Klix, F., Streitz, N., Waern, Y., Wandke, H. (Eds.). MACINTER II - Man-Computer Interaction Research. Elsevier, Amsterdam, pp. 461-477.

Robert, J.-M., Bouchard, S. (1991). Investigating how computer users and human tutors interact with one another, in Quéinnec, Y., Daniellou, F. (Eds.). Designing for Everyone. Taylor & Francis, London, pp. 555-557.

Roberts, T.L. (1980). Evaluation of text editors. Palo Alto Research Center, Report SSL-79-9, Palo Alto, California, November.

Sleeman, D. (1982). Assessing aspects of comptetence in basic algebra, in Sleeman, D., Brown, J.S. (Eds.). Intelligent Tutoring Systems, London: Academic Press, pp. 185-199.

WORK WITH DISPLAY UNITS 92
H. Luczak, A. Çakir and G. Çakir (Editors)

AUXA: A Development Tool for Help Systems

Erdmuthe Meyer zu Bexten[a] and Claudio Moraga[b]

[a]Fraunhofer Institute of Microelectronic Circuits and Systems,
Finkenstr. 61, W-4100 Duisburg 1, Germany

[b]University of Dortmund, Department of Computer Science,
Otto-Hahn-Str. 16, W-4600 Dortmund 50, Germany

1. INTRODUCTION

The computer aided design of very large scale integrated circuits uses a collection of sophisticated tools. Their complexity grows both with the steadily increasing requirements of the users and the high efficiency of the supporting workstations. For such a complex work the users need effective support in form of a textual and graphical information service. *Help system* is the name given to a service of this kind. Since the design tools have a high complexity it becomes apparent that the necessary help system offered to the designer, also exhibits a high complexity. The implementation of complex help systems cannot be done without a development tool.

At the Fraunhofer Institute of Microelectronic Circuits and Systems and the University of Dortmund (Department of Computer Science) such a *help development tool*, called AUXA (**AUX**ili**A**r-System) [1, 2], has been implemented and used e.g. for the help system of the Computer Aided Simulation System CASSY [2]. AUXA supports the development of help systems based on the hypertext concept.

2. MAIN COMPONENTS OF AUXA

A help development tool is a system to produce applications specific help systems. It consists of the following three components

- *input language*
- *display tool*
- *consistency checker*

which are discussed below.

2.1. Input Language

The input language provides commands to introduce a hypertext oriented syntactical structure into the help text under development. Two views of a help text are distinguished: a programmer's and a user's view. The main concern of the programmer is to prepare the appropriate display of help texts. To support this, ten commands are available to the programmer. A help information together with the required commands for its display will be called *processable help text*. The users only see the displayed help text (i.e. without commands) where the references are emphasized in bold face or button shape. The syntax of this language is easy to learn because there are only four control and six special commands. The control commands define the layout of the window, labels, references and the membership of references to an *index*. The index contains all references defined by the help system programmer. The special commands and their performance are listed below:

- **OPEN** allows reading available help files.
- **PIC** links graphic files to text files to generate a combined help display.
- **SYS** establishes a communication with the operating system without leaving the help system.
- **LAST** and **GOTO** are branching commands. With LAST the program goes (back) to the former label, with GOTO, to a given label.
- **QUIT** closes every possible help text. With this command the help system will be left.

A special converter adapts information texts available as LaTeX file (e.g. paragraphs of a manual) to be used as help texts.

Excerpt from the Input Language Syntax

The following BNF-grammar shows an excerpt from the syntax of the processable help texts. The symbols `spc` and `newline` define the line oriented structure of the language.

```
<help text>              ::=  <window configuration> { <entry> }+
<window configuration>   ::=  <number> <space> <number> <space> <name>
                              <space> <name>
<entry>                  ::=  newline { <label> }+ { <command label> }
                              <text entry>
<label>                  ::=  newline . <name> . |
                              newline . <name> . I { spc <name> }
<command label>          ::=  newline .# <command> #.
```

```
<command>            ::=  <open> | <sys> | <quit> | <pic> | <last> |
                          <goto>
<text entry>         ::=  newline { <word> }
<word>               ::=  <name> | <reference> | <pic in text> |
                          spc | newline
<reference>          ::=  <bold delimiter> <name> <bold delimiter> |
                          <button delimiter> <name>
                          <button delimiter>
<bold delimiter>     ::=  @
<button delimiter>   ::=  |
<pic in text>        ::=  <pic delimiter> <name> <pic delimiter>
<pic delimiter>      ::=  #!
<space>              ::=  { spc }+
<name>               ::=  { <character> }+
<number>             ::=  { <digit> }+
<digit>              ::=  0|1|...|9
<character>          ::=  A|...|Z|a|...|z| <digit> |:|,|+|-| ...
```

2.2. Display Tool

The display tool uses the commands of the language to show the help text according to the hypertext concept. The help text is presented in a special window following the OSF/Motif guide lines. The window is divided in the three areas:

- *menu bar*
- *working field*
- *button row*

Special points of the menu bar at the top of the help window allow among other things the navigation through the help system. An example of these points is the browser, which characterizes the last selected references on the path to the current help information. In the working field both textual and graphical help informations can be shown. References are highlighted by using buttons or a bold font. The most selected options of the menu functions are additionally represented as buttons with pictures in the button row. These are: 'Index', 'Browser', 'Last Item', 'Search', 'Printer' and 'Exit'. The index can be shown in two different representations: lexicographically sorted or in form of a hierarchical structure. With the browser the user obtains a trace of his navigation. The trace (corresponding list of references) is shown in a special window and covers the last ten visited help texts. By activating the button 'Last Item' the user can return to the former help text. The search button allows the user to look for a special reference. By selecting the button 'Printer' the text actually present in the help window will be printed. To leave the help system the user must press the 'Exit' button.

2.3. Consistency Checker

The consistency checker guarantees that the author of a help system writes the selected help text and the proper commands in the right way to ensure correct behaviour of the whole system. The following aspects are tested particularly:

- Syntax of basic and special commands
- Semantic check of processible help texts
  (e.g. multiple appearance of a label, empty help texts, or unreferenced labels)
- Semantic check of the special commands OPEN, PIC and GOTO
  (missing target objects: text file, picture file and target label)

3. EXAMPLE

The following section shows a small example of a processible help text including a picture. Figure 1 illustrates the displayed help text.

```
80 20 ENGLISH white

.interface types.
The dimensions of distance from user goals and @degree engagement@ form
a space of @interfaces@ within which we can locate some familiar
types of interfaces.  Direct manipulation @interfaces@ are those
that minimize the distances and maximize engagement.
As always, the distance between @user intentions@ and the interface
language depends on the nature of the task the user is per-
forming.

#!engagement.xbm#!

|Quit| or |Index| ?
```

The development tool AUXA can be used in all user interfaces based on the X-Window system and OSF/Motif or Open Look.

Acknowledgments

The authors wish to thank Markus Stark, Inka Kloster, Ulrike Jarnuczak, Andrea Faust, Sabine Eberling, Jorge Aragon and Andreas Pothmann (students at the University of Dortmund, Department of Computer Science) for the prototype implementations of these concepts.

4. REFERENCES

1 E. Meyer zu Bexten, J. Büddefeld and C. Moraga: *Die Signalbeschreibungssprache SIBA eingebunden in eine ergonomische Benutzeroberfläche*, Workshop, 2. Dresdner Informatiktage, 04.-08.02.91 in Dresden, S. 14-21, Hrsg: Technische Universität Dresden, Fakultät Informatik, 1991.

2 E. Meyer zu Bexten: *Eine Simulationsumgebung für signalverarbeitende Systeme*, Dissertation, Universität Dortmund, Fachbereich Informatik, Shaker Verlag, Aachen, 1992.

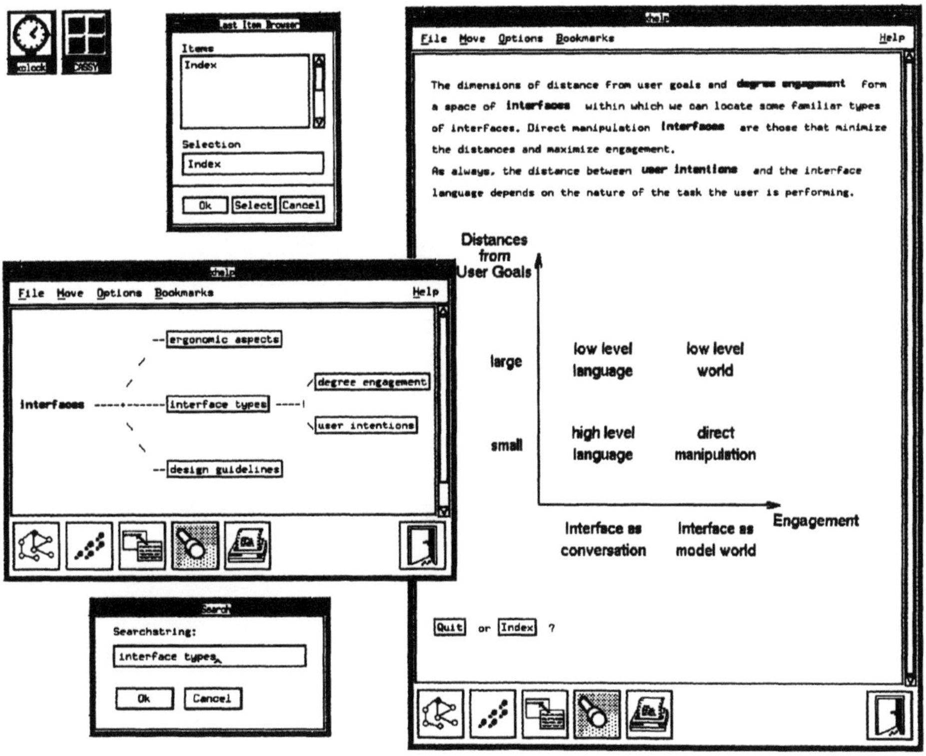

Figure 1. Help window with different contents.

WORKLOAD, STRESS AND STRAIN

WORK WITH DISPLAY UNITS 92
H. Luczak, A. Çakir and G. Çakir (Editors)

WORK ORGANIZATION AND HEALTH ASPECTS OF WORK WITH VDU:s

Carl Åborg(1), Gunnar Aronsson and Margareta Dallner(2)

(1)The Swedish Foundation for Occupational Health and Safety for State Employees, S-371 87 Karlskrona, Sweden

(2)National Institute of Occupational Health, S-171 84 Solna, Sweden

Abstract

The aim of the study was to analyze the relationship between work organization, type of VDU-work and mental and somatic symptoms.

The study group consists of two different samples of State employed VDU-users, whose work environment and health were examined through questionnaires. In total, 5.771 people filled in the questionnaires.

The results showed that work conditions, and the consequences of computerization, vary considerably, between groups with different VDU tasks and between women and men. The amount of symptoms increased with the number of hours per day spent at VDU work. Women reported a larger number of symptoms than men.

1. INTRODUCTION

Computer technology is now transforming working life and affects everyone within a company. The consequences vary between occupational groups and between men and women.(1-2)

The aim of the study was to analyze the relationship between health complaints on the one hand and type of VDU activities and time spent daily at VDU work on the other. Other questions were: Are there differences between the work situations of men and women, and how is gender related to health complaints?

Type of VDU-work was classified into five different categories: Data entry(DE), Data acquisition(DA),Interactive communication (involves both data entry and data acquisition)(DE+DA), Word processing(WP) and Programming/CAD(Computer-Aided Design)(Prog).

2.METHOD

The population of the study consists of all those people who, over two different two-year periods, responded to questionnaires on VDU work, issued by the Swedish Foundation for Occupational Health and Safety for State Employees. The Foundation is the organizer of occupational health service for state employees in Sweden, and have local occupational health care centres spread over the country.

During the first period, August 1985 to August 1987, 3.247 state employed VDU-users at 83 different working places filled in the questionnaires. During the second period, August 1988 to August 1990, a new sample of 2.524 VDU-users from 55 different working places were examined by the same questionnaires.

A number of standardized, well-tested questionnaires were used.(3) The questionnaires contains questions on job content, physical and psycho-social work environment and mental and somatic health symptoms.

Data collection was conducted through the local occupational health care centres.

3.RESULTS

The data analysis from the first sample of 3.247 people showed that work conditions vary considerably, both between groups of users and between women and men. The data entry group reported a greater number of somatic and mental symptoms. The amount of symptoms increased with the number of hours per day spent at VDU work. Women reported more somatic and mental symptoms than men.

Data from the new sample of 2.524 people have been classified and analyzed in the same way.

Some results from this second part of the study are reported here. The results confirm the earlier findings, that the consequences of computerization vary between groups and between men and women.

3.1 Figures

Figure 1 and Figure 2 show that the distribution of types of VDU work, and of time spent at a VDU, is strongly gender related. In figure 3 psychological complaints is based on an index of questions concerning concentration, restlessnes, tension, irritation, anxiety, depression or sadness. It shows the differences between men and women and between groups with different VDU tasks.

Figure 4 is based on questions concerning all kinds of eye-symptoms, such as red, teary or dry eyes. It shows the clear increase of eye-symptoms with time spent at a VDU.

Figure 5 shows how the incidence of neck problems differ between men and women, and how the problems increase with increasing number of hours per day at VDU work.

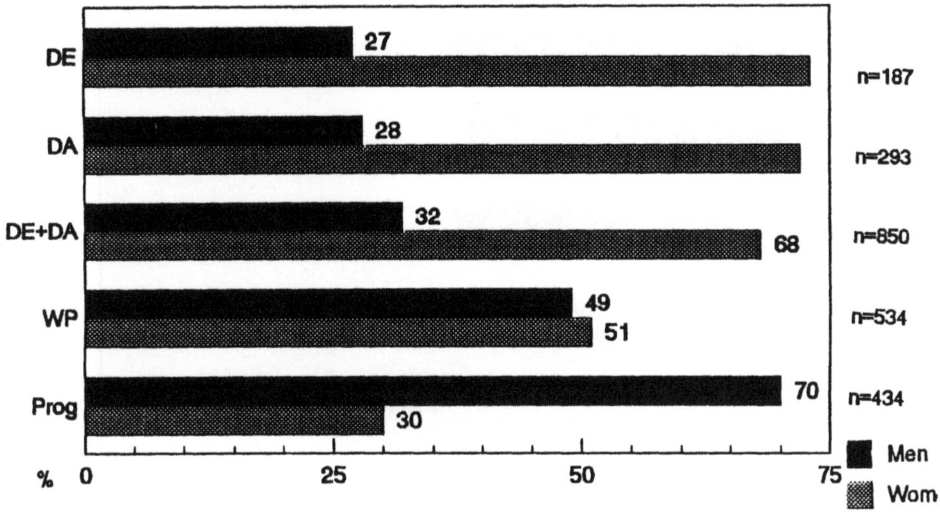

Figure 1. Type of VDU work, gender distribution (n=2.524, women=1.381, men=1.039)

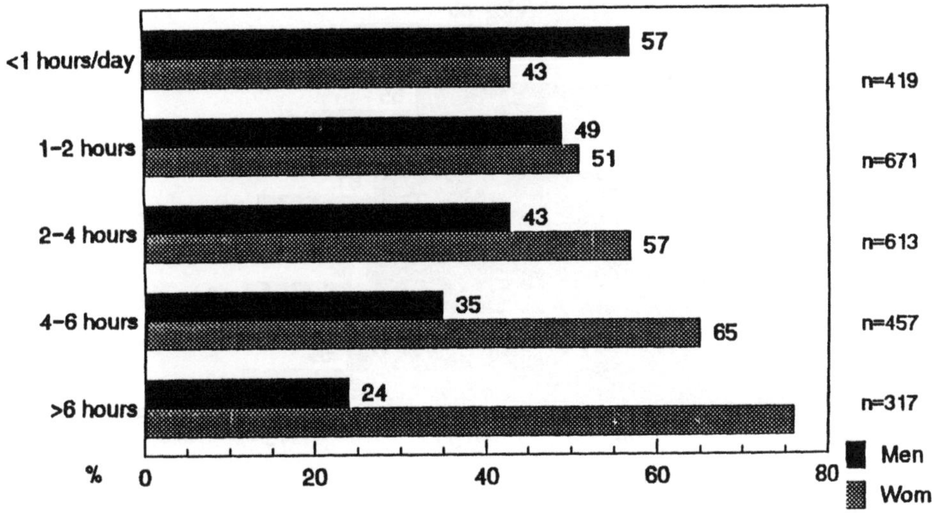

Figure 2. Hours per day at a VDU, gender distribution (n=2.524, women=1.381, men=1.039)

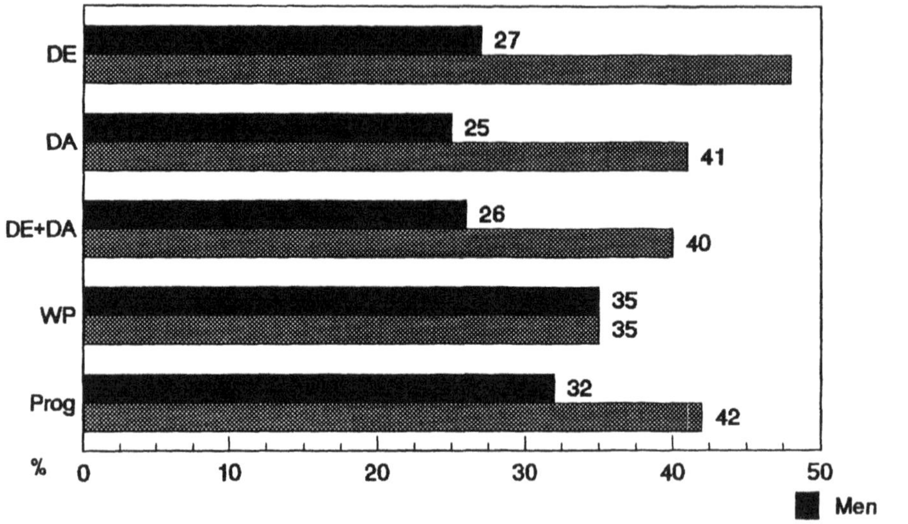

Figure 3. Psychological complaints (n=2.524)

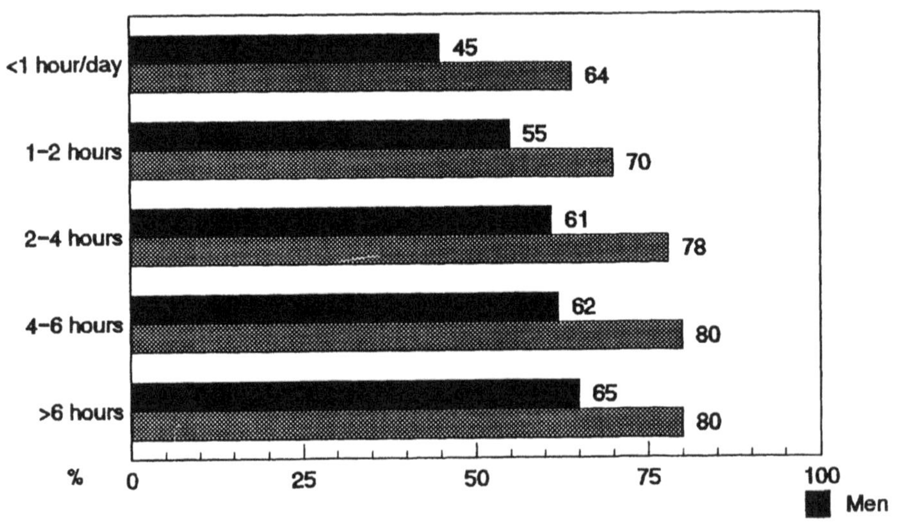

Figure 4. Eye-symptoms (n=2.524)

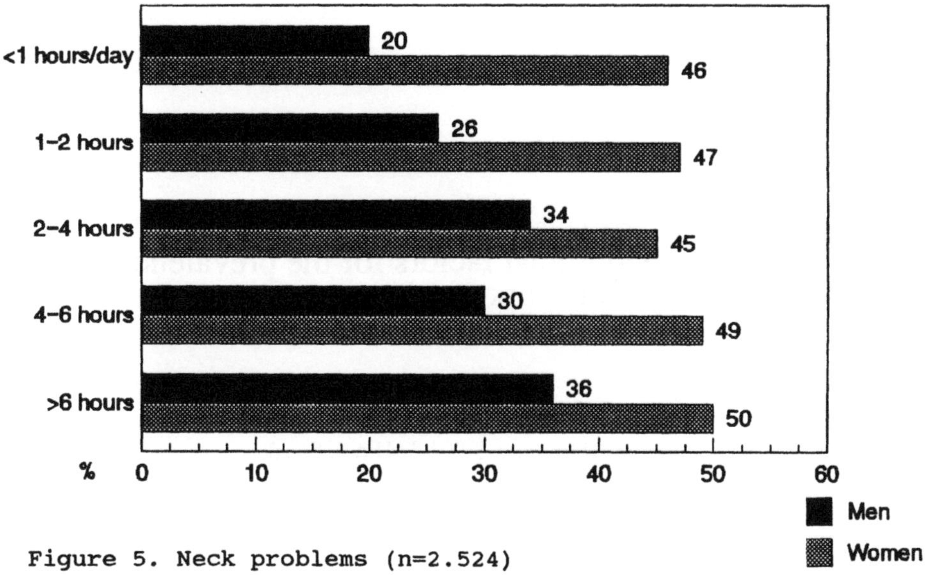

Figure 5. Neck problems (n=2.524)

4. CONCLUSIONS

There clearly are winners and losers from computerization. Most of the losers are to be found among women with repetitive data entry or data acquisition work 6 hours or more per day at a VDU.

To support the losers to become winners the work organization has to be changed.

The increased level of symptoms of ill-health with increasing number of hours per day at a VDU strongly supports the work towards a redistribution of job tasks.

5. REFERENCES

1 Aronsson,G.,Åborg,C.,Örelius,M.(1988)Datoriseringens vinnare och förlorare.Arbete och Hälsa,27. (Winners and losers of computerization)

2 Bauer,H.,Aronsson,G.,Åborg,C.,Örelius,M. Health aspects of work with VDU:s.,in Berlinguet,L. and Berthelette,D.(eds) (1990)Work with Display Units 89, Elsevier Science Pub., North-Holland.

3 Kvist,L.(1991)Referensdata, allmän del,Statshälsan. (Reference data. The Swedish Foundation for Occupational Health and Safety for State Employees.)

WORK WITH DISPLAY UNITS 92
H. Luczak, A. Çakir and G. Çakir (Editors)

The Office Illness Project in Northern Sweden. The significance of psychosocial factors for the prevalence of skin symptoms among VDT workers. A case referent study.

J. Höög and N. Eriksson

Department of Sociology, Umeå University, S-901 87 Umeå, Sweden

Abstract

This case/referent study is a part of the multidisciplinary project *The Office Illness Project in Northern Sweden*. From a initial questionnaire study among 6000 office workers, 75 VDT workers with skin symptoms and 75 without such symptoms were selected for a case referent study. The reported symptoms are erythema, itching, pricking and burning sensations in facial skin. The data contains a questionnaire filled out by all 150 individuals and interviews with representatives of the workplaces. The purpose of this part of the project is to investigate the importance of psychosocial and organizational factors in explaining prevalence of skin symptoms among VDT workers.

The results show that psychosocial factors, especially workload, social relations and social support are of importance for prevalence of skin symptoms among VDT-workers.

1. INTRODUCTION

During the past 10-15 years environmental issues in office work have been given increased attention. One topic that has gained interest is skin problems among VDT workers, which have been reported from Sweden (1), UK (2), USA (3) and Japan (4) . In different studies it has been found that selfreported skin symptoms are more prevalent among VDT workers than among other office workers (5). In the basic questionnaire in The Office Illness Project it was found that office workers with more than 4 hours daily VDT-work reported a significant higher frequency of skin symptoms (OR 2.5) than employees with no VDT-work.

Even though an exposure-response relationship between VDT work and skin symptoms can be stated, no definite explanation of the causes has been found. Electrostatic fields, electric and magnetic fields, psychosocial and psychogenic factors have all been pointed out as risk-factors.

Today it seems as if a multifactorial explanation is most likely. One relevant factor in this complex is the psychosocial work environment, which deals with the interaction between the individual and the work environment. It includes questions concerning work content, work organization and social relations at the workplace and how the individual experience these factors. Our main hypothesis is that a poor psychosocial work environment can be a riskfactor as such, as well as it can make the individual more liable to other riskfactors which in turn may be a part in the etiology of facial skin symptoms.

The part of the work environment that deals with psychological and social questions has been given more attention since the mid-seventies. The reason to this is that, firstly, the physical work environment overall has become "better". Secondly, we are getting more aware of the importance of a "good" psychosocial work environment when discussing health and well-being among employees as well as efficiency in organizations. This awareness has also lead to higher demands from employees and their unions concerning the psychosocial work environment.

2. MATERIAL AND METHODS

Data collection

This case referent study is a part of *The Office Illness Project in Northern Sweden* (6). Officeworkers from three different cities in the county of Västerbotten in northern Sweden were selected. A proportional stratified sample of offices were drawn from each city. Only workplaces with at least 10 employees were included. Employees that had spent more than half their working time in the office during the preceding three month were included. A questionnaire was mailed to these 5 986 office workers. The data collection were accomplished during the period october to december 1988. The return rate was 97.5 %. Aproximately 13 % were excluded mainly because they were absent during the current period. Of the remaining 4 943 questionnaires, 3 200 were VDT-workers.

The study population in this case referent study consists of 150 individuals (75 cases, 75 referents). The data contains a second self-administered questionnaire distributed to cases and referents, with a return rate of 92 %, and interviews with representatives of the organizations concerned. The purpose with the interviews were to get some information about the organizations where the respondents work.

All respondents spent most of their time at work in one single room and they worked with VDT's at least one hour per day.

Cases were defined as office workers with VDT-work more than one hour daily who reported apperance of sensory and visual facial skin symptoms at least weekly during the preceding three month. The symptoms were itching, stinging, tight or burning sensations in facial skin and dry or flushed facial skin. Referents were VDT-workers without such symptoms. Cases and referents were matched by age (+/- 5 years), sex and residential area.

Data analysis

Using factor analysis, several indices were constructed to facilitate the analysis. The independent variables were classified into a limited number of categories, normally three, of equal size if possible.

The influence of different factors on the risk to have facial skin symptoms was calculated using the EGRET package. Crude odds ratios (OR) were calculated from fourfold tables in a bivariat analysis. A five percent level of significance were used. In the multivariat analysis odds ratios (OR) with 95% confidence intervals were calculated from a logistic regression model (matched analysis).

The dimensions of the psychosocial work environment we have focused are psychological demands at work, work control, social support (from co-workers as well as from supervisors), information, organizational factors (culture, changes, economy), work satisfaction.

Because of the limited space in this article we will concentrate on factors that seems to be of greater importance for the prevalence of facial skin symptoms among VDT workers than others. Risk-levels will be presented both as crude odds ratios and after confounders are held under control. In the matched analysis only discordant pairs are computed which restricts us to assess only one confounder at a time.

The confounders used have been selected from other parts of the project and they all have shown significant effects on the prevalence of skin symptoms (7). The first is atopy, a dichotomous variable with the category has/have had asthma/rhinitis used as an risk-indicator. The second is type of screen on fluorescent tubes at the workplace, a dichotomous variable with tubes with glas or plastic screens used as risk-indicator and metallic screen as reference category. The third is electric field in room measured in five points in the room, given as field strength (E) with the SI unit volts per meter (V/m). The mean value of these measurements was taken as the general level for a room. The variable was divided into three categories. Levels over 30 V/m constitute the risk category and levels below 13 V/m reference category. The fourth is the VDT related magnetic field from the vertical deflection (Extremely Low Frequency, ELF). The variable was divided into three categories. Levels over 0.29 uT constitute the risk category and levels below 0.18 uT the reference category. The fifth is VDT exposure measured as time in front of a VDT. A dichotomy was used with more than four hours daily VDT work constituting the risk category. The sixth confounder is heating system with electric heating as the risk category.

3. RESULTS

The first presented measure in table 1 below is a construction based on two indices. The first refers to perceived amount of work, the second to support from supervisors. The new measure was divided into three categories. Those who reported that they had a high workload *and* a lack of support from supervisors, constitute the risk category (25% of the sample). Those who reported low or moderate work load and high support from supervisors constitute the reference category (50% of the sample). (Table 1).

Table 1. Relative Risk (OR) and Confidence Intervals (CI) for facial skin symptoms due to psychosocial riskfactors. Different confounders held under control.

Variable		Confounder					
OR CI	Crude	Atopy	Fluores-cent tubes	Electric field in room	Magnetic field near VDT	Vdt-exposure	Heating
Workload and support from supervisor	**4,3** 1,2-16,1	**4,7** 1,3-17,2	**2,7** 0,6-10,3	**6,2** 1,5-25,8	**4,8** 1,2-18,8	**5,8** 1,4-24,1	**3,2** 0,7-14,6
Relations to co-workers	**4,4** 1,1-17,3	**5,4** 1,3-22,7	**7,5** 1,3-42,2	**4,8** 1,2-19,4	**4,3** 1,0-17,7	**4,4** 1,1-17,1	**4,8** 0,9-26,7
Appreciation from supervisor and co-workers	**2,5** 0,9-6,6	**3,5** 1,1-10,7	**1,8** 0,5-5,8	**2,9** 1,0-8,7	**2,9** 1,0-8,8	**3,6** 1,1-11,4	**2,8** 0,8-9,2

We found a significant higher risk among those who reported high work load and low support from supervisors (crude OR 4.3, CI 1.2-16.1). The excessed risk remained after controlling for different confounders. The level was significant higher except when controlling for type of screens on flourescent tubes and type of heating system.

The second presented measure is an index based on two items; the first refers to co-worker relations, how you get along with your co-workers, and the second to which extent you and your work-mates discuss things concerning work. The index (relations to co-workers) was divided into three categories. The fourth quartile constitute risk category and the first quartile was used as reference category. We found a significant higher risk (OR 4.4, CI 1.1-17.3) for skin symptoms in the high-risk group with relatively bad relations to co-workers compared with the low-risk group, the category with relatively good relations to co-workers. This effect remains at a significant level after controlling for possible confounders, except for type of heating system (Table 1).

The third measure is an index based on five items and it refers to the respondents perception concerning appreciation, valuation and feedback from supervisors and co-workers. The index was divided into three groups of the same size. We used the upper third as risk category and the lower third as reference category. Those who felt that their work had a low "status" in this sense showed an increased risk (OR) of 2.5 (CI 0.9-6.6). The high level found in the risk category remained when confounders was taken into account. Again the risk-level was lower when controlling for types of screens on flouresent tubes (Table 1).

4 DISCUSSION

The results show that different combinations of work demands and support from supervisors have a strong impact on the prevalence of skin symptoms. Office workers with a reasonable work load and a good support more seldom experience these symptoms. Apparently, the *combination* of high workload and lack of support seems to be unhealthy, direct or indirect.

Social relations at the workplace and communication with co-workers also seem to be strong factors. Those with bad relations more often show symptoms. Obviously the "climate" in the office has some effect on human health.

The third factor tested here - valuation and appreciation of ones worktask - is also of importance. Employees who feel that their job is not respected and their performance is not appreciated by supervisors and co-workers, more often report facial skin problems. Thus percieved social status at work might be reflected in health status.

These results are quite stable even when confounders are controlled for. However there are two confounders that seem to make the results more uncertain - "Fluorecent Tubes" and "Heating System". These confounders are a little problematic though. Firstly, we can't exactly be shure of which other factors in the buildings they represent. Secondly, the distribution among the categories is very skew and the number of missing cases is high and this in combination with the matched analysis leads to unreliable results.

Thus we can conclude that the psychosocial work environment, especially the parts concerning demands, support, appreciation and social relations bear a relation to the risk of having facial skin symptoms among VDT-workers. The interpretation of these connections could be that those factors themselves cause the symptoms as a stress reaction and also makes the individual more sensible to other risk factors. It is too early at this point though to make certain statements of the relations between the different risk factors and the symptoms. Still a lot of research has to be done before statements of that kind will be adequate. What the results from this study allows us to state though, is that psychosocial factors seem to be too important for an understanding of the problem to be excluded from the research agenda.

5. REFERENCES

1. Stenberg, B.(1987). A Rosacea-like skin rash in VDU-operators. In: Knave, B., Widebäck, P.G. (Eds). Selected papers from the international scientific conference: Work With Display Units, Stockholm 12-15 May 1986. Amsterdam, Elsevier Science Publishers BV p 160-164.

Knave, B. et al (1985). Work with Video Display Terminals among office employees. I. Subjective symptoms and discomfort. Scandinavian Journal of Environmental health, vol 11 p 457-466.

2. Rycroft R.J.G. & Calnan, C.D. (1984). Facial rashes among Visual Display Units operators. In: Pearce, B.G.(Ed). Health hazards of VDT's ? Chichester, John Wiley & Sons p 13-15.

3. Fisher, A.A.(1986). "Terminal" dermatitis due to computers (Visual Display Units). Cutis vol 37 p 153-154.

4. Matsunaga, K., Hayakava, R. & Hisanaga, O.(1988). Facial rash in Visual Display Terminal operator. (In Japanese, Abstract in English). Ann Rep Nagoya Br Hosp vol 22 p 57-61.

5. Knave, B. et al (1985). Work with Video Display Terminals among office employees. I. Subjective symptoms and discomfort. Scandinavian Journal of Environmental health, vol 11 p 457-466.

Berg, M. (1989). Facial skin complaints and work at Video Display Units. Epidemiological, clinical and histopathological studies. Acta Derm Venerol suppl 150.

6. Stenberg, B. et al (1991). Inomhusmiljö och hälsa bland kontorsarbetare i Västerbotten. En enkätstudie av upplevd hälsa samt exponeringsförhållanden i arbete och bostad. Stockholm. National Institute of Occupational Health, Undersökningsrapport nr 11.

7. Sandström, M. et al (1991). Inomhusmiljö och hälsa bland kontorsarbetare i Västerbotten. Elektriska och magnetiska fält: en fall-referentstudie bland bildskärmsarbetare.Stockholm. Institute of Occupational Health, Undersökningsrapport nr 12.

Stenberg, B. et al (1992). Inomhusmiljö och hälsa bland kontorsarbetare i Västerbotten. Studiens bakgrund, syfte och uppläggning. Stockholm. National Institute of Occupational Health, Undersökningsrapport nr 17.

WORK WITH DISPLAY UNITS 92
H. Luczak, A. Çakir and G. Çakir (Editors)
1993 Elsevier Science Publishers B.V.

The Psychophysiological Rationale and Empirical Basis for End-tidal PCO_2 as an Index of Stress-Health Effects in Computer Work

Lawrence M. Schleifer[a] and Ronald Ley[b]

[a]Office of Human Resources Modernization, Internal Revenue Service, HR:H:TWD, 1111 Constitution Avenue, Washington, D.C. USA.

[b]Department of Psychology and Statistics, State University of New York at Albany, 1400 Washington Avenue, Albany, New York USA.

Abstract

Schleifer and Ley (1) recently reported that end-tidal PCO_2 (peak concentration of carbon dioxide in a single breath of exhaled air) can discriminate among psychophysiological states of VDT data-entry work and relaxation, and that end-tidal PCO_2 may be useful in indexing the stress-health effects of human-computer interactions. Despite its promise as a index of psychophysiological activity in computer work, respiratory parameters such as end-tidal PCO_2 have been neglected by work-stress researchers in favor of more familiar variables such as heart rate, blood pressure, and catecholamine levels. The tendency to overlook breathing parameters has been fostered by the treatment of respiration as a source of artifact or a confounding variable in psychophysiological studies of cardiovascular functioning. In addition, work-stress researchers are often unfamiliar with or misunderstand the psychophysiological principles of breathing or are unacquainted with the methods involved in PCO_2 monitoring and measurement. This presentation provides an elaboration and clarification of the psychophysiological rationale and empirical basis for end-tidal PCO_2 as an index of stress-health effects in computer work (1-2).

1. INTRODUCTION

Psychophysiological techniques have been used in an attempt to define the biological and physiological mechanisms through which the stress effects of human-computer interactions may impair health. Johansson and Aronsson (3), for example, found that computer response delays and unscheduled system down-time result in elevated blood pressure and increased catecholamine production. Floru et al. (4) reported decreased heart rate and increased heart-rate variability associated with mental fatigue while performing a repetitive, data-entry task. Tanaka et al. (5) observed higher levels of noradrenaline excretion after VDT work using small letters on the CRT screen. Schleifer and Okogbaa (6) reported increased blood pressure and decreased heart-rate variability under VDT data-entry work with monetary incentives.

One psychophysiological parameter that has received little attention by work-stress researchers is respiration. The neglect of respiratory parameters (e.g., breathing frequency) is not surprising, however, given the general tendency in psychophysiology to "treat respiration as a nuisance variable" (7, p. 284). Respiratory parameters have been monitored in psychophysiological research primarily to determine artifact or to partial-out its effects on the cardiovascular system, prompting Hassett (8) to observe that "respiration may be the most underrated variable in current psychophysiological research" (p. 73).

Recently, however, signs of a renewed interest in respiration among psychophysiologists have appeared. Suess et al. (9), for example, investigated hyperventilatory stress responses to threat of electric shock. Grossman (7) noted a strong theoretical and empirical rationale for the reciprocal effects of stress, respiration, and cardiovascular function. Ley (10,11) has proposed a stress-hyperventilatory theory of panic attacks. Schleifer and Okogbaa (6) have raised the possibility that reductions in heart-rate variability under monetary incentives for VDT data-entry work may be the result of stress-induced increases in breathing frequency that, in turn, lead to a suppression of the respiratory sinus arrhythmia (RSA). Further signs of the growing interest in the relationship between respiration and emotional activity are Ley's (12) assertions that "breathing may well be the bridge between psychology and physiology" (p. 37) and that "respiratory psychophysiology has achieved the status of an independent field of research" (p. 2).

2. RATIONALE AND EMPIRICAL BASIS

Based on a hyperventilatory model of stress, Ley (2) has proposed using respiratory parameters, such as end-tidal PCO_2, to index the stress effects of VDT-computer work. End-tidal PCO_2 refers to the percent of peak concentration of carbon dioxide in a single breath of exhaled air at the end of the expiratory phase, and is considered to be a near-perfect estimate of partial pressure of CO_2 (PCO_2) in arterial blood (13,14).

Under stressful conditions, breathing exceeds metabolic requirements for oxygen (i.e., overbreathing or hyperventilation); this excessive ventilation leads to an excessive loss of CO_2, which results in a disproportional reduction in end-tidal PCO_2 concentrations. Moreover, hyperventilation can occur regardless of whether the rate of respiration is rapid or slow (2,12,15). [Hyperventilation or breathing that exceeds metabolic demands for oxygen should not be confused with hyperpnea (voluminous breathing or tachypnea (rapid breathing) which occur in response to increased metabolic demand (e.g., physical exercise)].

Cardiovascular effects that accompany hyperventilation include decreases in blood concentrations of CO_2 which, in turn, leads to vasoconstriction and ischemic impedance of regional blood flow to the brain and heart (7). Severe hyperventilation can lead to a reduction in the amount of oxygen that hemoglobin can release to the body tissue (i.e., hypoxia). Somatic symptoms associated with hyperventilation include heart palpitations, dyspnea, dizziness, and trembling (16,17).

Grossman (7) cites over 20 studies that demonstrate a relationship between situational stresses (e.g., heat stress, threatening imagery, threat of shock, mental workload, and pain) and respiratory function. While a few studies have not found a relationship between stress and respiratory function (i.e., respiration frequency) (18,19,20), most studies have. More importantly, Suess et al. (9), for example, reported that end-tidal PCO_2 decreased from baseline among 27 of 29 subjects who performed a perceptual-judgment task under threat of electric shock for making too many errors. Reductions in end-tidal PCO_2 were accompanied by increases in heart rate and self-reported anxiety scores. And Ley and Yellich (21) found significant differences in end-tidal PCO_2 concentrations between high and low test-anxious subjects.

Several other studies have reported an inverse relationship between the magnitude of stress and arterial PCO_2 and end-tidal PCO_2 (22-26). Conversely, end-tidal PCO_2 levels have increased under conditions of quiet adaptation, also suggesting a linear relationship between stress and arterial PCO_2 tension (9,27).

With respect to computer work, Schleifer and Ley (1) reported that end-tidal PCO_2 decreased significantly under VDT data-entry relative to a baseline relaxation period and a progressive muscle relaxation period. In addition, end-tidal PCO_2 was a more sensitive indicator of psychophysiological states of relaxation and computer work than respiration frequency, heart rate, or heart rate variability. Schleifer and Ley also reported that the low intrinsic variability of end-tidal PCO_2 observed in this study suggests that this respiratory indicator is sensitive to small variations in psychophysiological activity. Overall, the findings of this study support the premise that end-tidal PCO_2 is an index of psychophysiological activity during human-computer interactions.

A significant advantage of end-tidal PCO_2 over other psychophysiological indicators is its unique ability to discriminate stress effects in VDT-computer work from the physical effects of repetitive keying. Stress effects in VDT-computer work are indicated by reductions in end-tidal PCO_2 (i.e., breathing that exceeds metabolic demands for oxygen). By comparison, heart rate, respiration rate, or other measures of ventilation such as minute volume increase as a result of either stress or physical activity, thus inextricably confounding one effect with the other. While the physical demands of VDT-computer work are relatively light, Lee and Park (28) cite several studies (29-32) including their own research (28), which indicate that even the physical load effects of a binary choice reaction task (i.e., finger tapping) can significantly alter heart rate and heart rate variability. In this connection, end-tidal $PC0_2$ holds promise of being a single, reliable and valid measure of stress that is independent of physical effects of work.

3. CONCLUSIONS

End-tidal PCO_2 is a promising index of psychophysiological activity in human-computer tasks. Further research is needed to determine the utility of this index in discriminating the cognitive and emotional demands of the same task performed at different levels of difficulty, as well as in differentiating between the cognitive and emotional demands of various types of tasks (e.g., programming vs. data entry). In addition, the well-established effects of respiratory parameters on cardiovascular function (see 7) suggest that monitoring variations in end-tidal PCO_2 may contribute to an improved understanding of the cardiovascular stress-health effects of human-computer tasks.

REFERENCES

1 SCHLEIFER, L. M., and LEY, R. In press, End-tidal PCO_2 as an index of psychophysiological activity during VDT data-entry work and relaxation, Ergonomics.

2 LEY, R. 1987, Respiratory activity as an index of stress in video display terminal work, Contract No. 87-11615 (National Institute for Occupational Safety and Health, Cincinnati, OH).

3 JOHANSSON, G. and ARONSSON, G. 1984, Stress reactions in computerized administrative work, Journal of Occupational Behavior, 5, 159-181.

4 FLORU, R., CAIL, F., and ELIAS, R. 1985, Psychophysiological changes during a VDU repetitive task, Ergonomics, 28, 1455-1468.

5 TANAKA, T., FUKUMOTO, T., YAMAMOTO, S., and NORO, K. 1988, The effects of VDT work on urinary excretion of catecholamine, Ergonomics, 31, 1753-1761.

6 SCHLEIFER, L., and OKOGBAA O. 1990, System response time and method of pay: Cardiovascular stress effects in computer-based tasks, Ergonomics, 33, 1495-1509.

7 GROSSMAN, P. 1983, Respiration, stress, and cardiovascular function, Psychophysiology, 20, 284-300.

8 HASSETT, J. 1978, A primer of psychophysiology, (W. H. Freeman, San Francisco).

9 SUESS, W., ALEXANDER, B., SMITH, D., SWEENEY, H., and MARION, R. 1980, The effects of psychological stress on respiration: A preliminary study of anxiety and hyperventilation, Psychophysiology, 17, 535-540.

10 LEY, R. 1985a, Agoraphobia, the panic attack, and the hyperventilation syndrome, Behavior Research and Therapy, 23, 79-81.

11 LEY, R. 1985b, Blood, breath, and fears: A hyperventilation theory of panic attacks and agoraphobia, Clinical Psychology Review, 5, 271-285.

12 LEY, R. In press, Breathing and the psychology of emotion, cognition, and behavior, in B. Timmons & R. Ley (eds) Functional Disorders of Breathing (Plenum Press, London).

13 HARDONK, H. and BUEMER, H. 1979, Hyperventilation syndrome, in P. Vinken and G. Bruyn (eds) Handbook of Clinical Neurology. Volume 38. Neurological Manifestations of Systemic diseases (North Holland, Amsterdam), 309-360.

14 JONES, N. L., ROBERTSON, D. G., and KANE, J. W. 1979, Difference between end-tidal arterial PCO_2 in exercise, Journal of Applied Physiology, 47, 954-960.

15 LEY, R. 1991, The efficacy of breathing retraining and the centrality of hyperventilation in panic disorder: A reinterpretation of experimental findings, Behavior Research and Therapy, 29, 301-304.

16 SINGER, E. P. 1958, The hyperventilation syndrome in clinical medicine, New York State Journal of Medicine, 58, 1494-1500.
17 LEWIS, B. I. 1959, Hyperventilation syndrome, California Medicine, 91, 121-126.
18 COHEN, H. D., GOODENOUGH, D.R., WITKIN, H. A., OLTMAN, P. GOULD, H., and SHULMAN, G. 1975, Effects of stress on components of the respiratory cycle, Psychophysiology, 12, 372-380.
19 DUFFY, E. 1962, Activation and Behavior, (Wiley, New York).
20 STERNBACH, R. A. 1966, Principles of Psychophysiology (Academic Press, New York).
21 LEY, R. and Yelich, G. 1991 End-tidal PCO_2 as an index of test anxiety, Supplement to Psychophysiology, 28, 38.
22 BECKMANN, K. 1915, Uber Anderungen in der Atmungsregulation durch psychische und phramkologische Einflusse, Deutsches Archiv fur Klinische Medizin, 117, 419-437.
23 DUDLEY, D. L., HOLMES, T. H., MARTIN, C. J., and RIPLEY, H. W. 1964, Changes in respiration associated with hypnotically induced emotion, pain, and exercise, Psychosomatic Medicine, 26, 46-53.
24 DUDLEY, D. L. MARTIN, C. J. and HOLMES, T. H. 1964, Psychophysiological studies of pulmonary ventilation, Psychosomatic Medicine, 26, 645-660.
25 GARSSEN, B. 1980, Role of stress in the development of the hyperventilation syndrome, Psychotherapy and Psychosomatics, 33, 214-225.
26 MOTTA, P. E., FAGIANI, M. B., DOLCETTI, A., BELLONE, E., and BORELLO, G. 1971, Modificazioni dei gas nel sangue nello stato ansioso di media gravita, Archivio per le Scienze Mediche, 128, 111-119.
27 NAIFEH, K. H., and KAMIYA, J. 1981, The nature of respiratory changes associated with sleep onset, Sleep, 4, 49-59.
28 LEE, D. H. and Park, K. S. 1990, Multivariate analysis of mental and physical load components in sinus arrhythmia scores, Ergonomics, 3, 35-47.
29 RUYSSENAARS, N. J. M. G. 1970, Sinus arrhythmia as mental load, sinus arrhythmia and neuroticism, Report, Laboratory of Ergonomic Psychology (TNO).
30 MULDER, G. and MULDER-HAJONIDES VAN DER MEULEN, W. R. E. H., 1973a, Mental load in a binary choice reaction task: an evaluation of some scoring methods, Acta Psychologica, 36, 239-251.
31 MULDER, G. and MULDER-HAJONIDES VAN DER MEULEN, W. R. E. H., 1973b, Mental load and the measurement of heart rate variability, Ergonomics, 16, 69-84.
32 LUCZAK, H. 1979, Fractioned heart rate variability. Part II: experiments on superimposition of components of stress, Ergonomics, 22, 1315-1323.

WORK WITH DISPLAY UNITS 92
H. Luczak, A. Çakir and G. Çakir (Editors)
1993 Elsevier Science Publishers B.V.

Speed and accuracy variability as an indicator of fatigue and boredom in a VDT data-entry work

C. S. Pan[a], R. L. Shell[b], and L. M. Schleifer[c]

[a]This paper is based on the first author's doctoral dissertation written at the University of Cincinnati. The data for this study was collected while the author was a guest researcher in the Division of Biomedical and Behavioral Science, National Institute for Occupational Safety and Health, Cincinnati, Ohio, USA. Present address: Department of Mechanical, Industrial, and Nuclear Engineering, University of Cincinnati, Cincinnati, Ohio 45221-0072, USA

[b]Department of Mechanical, Industrial, and Nuclear Engineering, University of Cincinnati, Cincinnati, Ohio 45221-0072, USA

[c]Formerly Research Psychologist, Division of Biomedical and Behavioral Science, National Institute for Occupational Safety and Health, Cincinnati, Ohio, USA. Present address: Human Resources Modernization Branch HR:H:TWD, Internal Revenue Service, 1111 Constitution Avenue NW, Washington, D.C. 20224, USA

ABSTRACT

Twenty-four data transcribers entered numeric data from tax forms at a video-display terminal (VDT) for three consecutive workdays under one of the following work management conditions: Electronic Performance Monitoring (EPM) or No Electronic Performance Monitoring (No EPM). Self-ratings of fatigue and boredom were assessed at periodic intervals. The speed (keystrokes) and accuracy (errors) of task performance were recorded on a continuous basis. Irrespective of the EPM and No EPM conditions, there was an increase in fatigue and boredom from the morning to afternoon work sessions. Correspondingly, there was a significant increase from the morning to afternoon work sessions in the variability of speed performance under the No EPM condition. Trend analyses revealed a correspondence of the linear trend for fatigue and boredom with the linear trend for accuracy variability across the morning work periods under the EPM condition. Also, trend analyses indicated a correspondence in the linear effects of fatigue and boredom with the linear effect of speed variability across the afternoon work periods under the No EPM condition. These findings suggest that performance variability may be a useful indicator of fatigue and boredom effects in a data-entry task.

1. INTRODUCTION

Concern regarding the stress effects of fatigue and boredom in repetitive office work has increased with the use of computers to monitor work performance and enforce compliance with performance standards in data entry, tele-marketing, and customer service operations [1, 2, 3]. In addition to the possible negative effects on worker health, fatigue and boredom also can reduce the consistency or stability of task performance [4, 5].

The first objective of this study was to determine whether performance variability (speed or accuracy) in a computer-based data-entry task is a useful index of fatigue and boredom under the following work-management conditions: Electronic Performance Monitoring (EPM) or No Electronic Performance Monitoring (No EPM). Secondly, the objective of this study was to determine the effects of EPM work management vs. No EPM work measurement on the relationship of fatigue and boredom with performance variability.

2. METHOD

Twenty-four female data transcribers in good physical condition (ages 18-40) were recruited from a clerical-secretarial agency. The subjects entered numeric data into a computerized data base from simulated tax forms (11 lines per form) via an video-display terminal (IBM 3163) under one of the following randomly assigned task conditions: (1) EPM Work Management (14 subjects): Subjects were instructed to perform a numeric data-entry task and to meet the following speed and accuracy performance standards: 200 keystrokes per minute and 6 errors per minute. Compliance with the performance standards was enforced using electronic performance monitoring and performance feedback of keystroke production and error rates. (2) No Work Management (10 subjects): Subjects were informed to perform the data-entry task at their normal rate of speed and level of accuracy. There were no performance standards and no performance feedback was provided under this task condition. Subjects participated in the study for three consecutive days. Each day consisted of a morning and afternoon session. Each session was further divided into three, 40-minute work periods.

Keystrokes and errors per minute were captured and stored in a continuous data base file. Time to complete each form and errors per form were calculated and used as indicators of speed and accuracy, respectively. The fatigue scale was a modified version of a similar scale selected from the Profile of Mood States [6]. The boredom scale was developed at the University of Michigan, Institute for Social Research [7]. Subjects were instructed to rate the extent of their fatigue and boredom using a response format ranging from 1 (hardly at all) to 5 (a great deal).

Performance variability was measured using the statistical variances of the average time to complete one form and average errors perform over a given work period (log speed variance and log accuracy variance). The data analyses focused on only the session and period time intervals of three working days to provide for the most meaningful and minimal number of comparisons in evaluating the correspondence between performance variability and mood state.

3. RESULTS

3.1. Fatigue and Boredom: Session Effects

Analyses of variance on repeated measures revealed significant session effects for fatigue [$F(1, 22) = 25.73$, $p < .001$, one-tailed test] and boredom [$F(1, 22) = 24.38$, $p < .001$, one-tailed test], indicating that the mean self-ratings of mood state increased from the morning work session to the afternoon work session. Since there was no session*condition interaction for fatigue and boredom, the session effects were comparable for both the EPM and No EPM work management conditions.

3.2. Speed Variability: Session*Condition Effects

There was a significant session*condition interaction for speed variability [$F(1, 22) = 3.44$, $p < .05$, one-tailed test]. The increase in speed variability from the morning to afternoon work sessions was greater for the No EPM condition than for the EPM condition. Moreover, the increase in speed variability under No EPM from the morning to afternoon sessions corresponded with the increases in fatigue and boredom over the same time interval.

3.3. Accuracy Variability: Session or Session*Condition Effects

There was no significant session or session*condition effects for accuracy variability.

3.4. Period Effects

3.4.1. Fatigue. Trend analyses showed a significant linear trend for both EPM [$F(1, 13) = 3.96$, $p < 0.04$, one-tailed test] and No EPM work management conditions [$F(1, 9) = 14.63$, $p < .002$, one-tailed test] across the afternoon work periods, indicating an increase in fatigue for both the EPM and No EPM work management conditions as a function of time spent performing the data-entry task. Also, trend analyses revealed a significant linear trend for both EPM [$F(1, 13) = 3.42$, $p < 0.05$, one-tailed test] and No EPM work management conditions [$F(1, 9) = 7.09$, $p < .02$, one-tailed test] in which fatigue increased across the morning work periods.

3.4.2.Boredom. Trend analyses showed a significant linear trend for both EPM [$F(1, 13) = 7.91$, $p < .01$, one-tailed test] and No EPM work management conditions [$F(1, 9) = 17.69$, $p < 0.002$, one-tailed test] across the morning work periods, indicating an increase in boredom for both the EPM and No EPM work management conditions as a function of time spent performing the data-entry task. Also, trend analyses revealed a significant linear trend for the No EPM work management condition [$F(1, 9) = 31.65$, $p < 0.0002$, one-tailed test] across the afternoon work periods, indicating an increase in boredom for this group as a function of time spent performing the data-entry task. No significant effect of work period on boredom was found, however, for the EPM work management condition.

3.4.3. Speed Variability. Under the EPM work management condition, there was no significant trend for speed variability across the work periods. However, trend analyses revealed a linear effect for speed variability under the No EPM [$F(1, 9) = 8.26$, $p < .01$, one-tailed test] work management condition across the afternoon work periods, which slightly paralleled the moderate linear increases in fatigue and boredom observed during these periods.

3.4.4. Accuracy Variability. Under the No EPM work management condition, there was a quadratic trend [$F(1, 9) = 5.43$, $p < 0.03$, one-tailed test] for accuracy variability across the morning work periods. In addition, trend analyses revealed a linear trend for accuracy variability under the EPM work management condition [$F(1, 13) = 3.51$, $p < .05$, one-tailed test] across the morning work periods, which corresponded with linear increases in fatigue and boredom observed during these periods.

4. DISCUSSION

The results of this study indicated that fatigue and boredom increased significantly from the morning to afternoon work sessions for both the EPM and No EPM conditions. Correspondingly, there was an increase in speed variance from the morning to afternoon work sessions for only the No EPM condition. Apparently, speed performance variability is a better indicator of fatigue and boredom under No EPM work management than under EPM work management.

Compared to the No EPM work management condition, the EPM work management condition resulted in significantly lower variability in speed performance from the morning to afternoon work sessions. This finding may be related to the timely performance feedback of EPM work management. EPM can track performance on an individual basis and enforce compliance with a performance goal [8]. Performance feedback enhances motivation for maintaining consistency of the speed performance. Therefore, if a worker receives regular performance feedback, it may be possible to maintain low performance variability in a repetitive and short-cycle task.

The results of the trend analyses for period time intervals suggest moderate linear correspondences between performance variability and self-reports of fatigue and boredom. Therefore, time-dependent linear trends across the work periods provided useful comparisons for displaying the degree of fatigue and boredom as a function of speed or accuracy variability under the EPM and No EPM work management conditions, respectively.

Overall, the results of this study suggest that performance variability may be a useful indicator of fatigue and boredom effects in a data-entry task. Research is needed to replicate the findings of this study and to characterize the fatigue and boredom effects and indicators for other short-cycle and repetitive work tasks.

5. REFERENCES

[1] Office of Technology Assessment, Congress of the United States. (1987). *The electronic supervisor: New technology, new tensions* (OTA-CIT-333). Washington, DC: U. S. Government Printing Office.

[2] Smith, M. J., Carayon, P., & Miezio, K. (1987). Electronic monitoring and job stress. In G. Salvendy, S. L. Sauter, & J. J. Hurrell (Eds.), *Social Ergonomic and Stress Aspects Work with Computers* (pp. 33-42). Amsterdam: Elsevier Science Publishers.
[3] Schleifer, L. M., & Shell, R. L. (1992). A review and reappraisal of electronic performance monitoring, performance standards and stress allowances. *Applied Ergonomics*, *23*(1), 49-53.
[4] Murrell, K. F. H. (1962). Operator variability and its industrial consequences. *Int. J. Prod. Res.*, *1*(2), 39-55.
[5] Henning, R. A., Sauter, S. L., Salvendy, G., & Krieg, E. F. (1989). Microbreak length, performance, and stress in a data entry task. *Ergonomics*, *32*(7), 855-864.
[6] McNair, D. M., Lorr, M., & Droppleman, L. F. (1971). *The Profile of Mood States*. San Diego, CA: Educational and Industrial Testing Service.
[7] Caplan, R. D., Cobb, S., French, J. P. R. Jr., Harrison R. V., & Pinneau, S. R. Jr. (1975). *Job Demands and Worker Health*. Washington, DC: U. S. Department of Health, Education and Welfare.
[8] Schleifer, L. M. (1991). *Electronic performance monitoring: Stress prevention strategies*. Unpublished project protocol, Cincinnati: National Institute for Occupational Safety and Health.

WORK WITH DISPLAY UNITS 92
H. Luczak, A. Çakir and G. Çakir (Editors)

Practice-oriented recording of stress factors in office workplaces and occupational health monitoring

W.Hilla

Central Health Service, AUDI AG,
8070 Ingolstadt, FRG

The recording and analysis of complex stress factors in office workplaces is a constant challenge for industrial scientists, ergonomists and occupational health specialists. In this context particular attention must be given to activities involving visual display units, which are being used increasingly as work aids.
The "classical" methods used for recording stress factors, developed in the main according to strict scientific principles, often fail in practice due to their complexity, particularly with regard to the up-dating procedures required. For this reason a practice-oriented assessment questionnaire has been developed at the Audi company to describe the requirements imposed by office workplaces.
In many cases, however, the acceptable limits for certain criteria cannot be exactly defined. In such cases, comparison with strain data obtained from occupational health check-ups can be used in order to evaluate the correlation between conspicuous strain patterns and particular stress factors. Records of health complaints in the form of epidemiological analyses can be regarded as the main information giving an early indication of particular strain parameters. But the method of proceeding from a consideration of stress factors to a consideration of strain factors is not the only approach.
Reference to the stress situation in the case of conspicuous patterns of health complaints can enable occupational health monitoring to render more differentiated and significant information. The methods described should preferably be integrated within an organizational procedure that provides not only the required flow of information, but also ensures that the necessary action can be taken, including initiatives affecting work-place design which may be required in particular cases.

The recording and analysis of complex stress factors in office workplaces is a constant challenge for industrial scientists, ergonomists and occupational health specialists. In this context particular attention must be given to activities involving visual display units which are beeing increasingly used as a means of performing office tasks. The visual display unit is becoming an ubiquitous piece of office equipment, whereas in the past he typical kind of work performed with display units was mainly limited to workplaces specially set up for the purpose. This type of work often involved (and still does involve) a very much reduced spectrum of activities, with the emphasis on the recording of data, such as keying in texts or information copied from invoices and the like. With very little communication required and a virtually constant workload, these activities are performed in the seated position with the resulting need to maintain a fixed posture. For this reason efforts in this field up to present have been concentrated on the optimum ergonomic design of the equipment used for typical display unit work. However, due to the increasing automation of data recording and the increasingly widespread introduction of VDUs as office equipment, the stress factors encountered have now changed significantly. The VDU as a work aid is penetrating into more and more activities in all areas of the office work process, ranging from traditional filing tasks to communication and scheduling, or the production of documentation for presentations. At the same time, with job content becoming more flexible (through job enlargement and job enrichment), there are more communication tasks to be performed and the work in general is subject to changing requirements.

In this context the "classical" methods used for recording stress factors, developed in main according to strict scientific principles, and designed for specific and uniform tasks, are not well suited for practical purposes. Additionally, they often involve a large amount of work to record the required data, particularly as regard the necessary updating procedures. For this reason a practice-oriented assessment questionnaire has been developed at de AUDI company to describe the requirements imposed by office workplaces. The factors considered include both objective parameters (measurable values, etc.) and a subjective assessment of criteria for which no measurement techniques exist or can be effectively used.

The checklist in this questionnaire consists of separate "modules":
For the work surroundings there are modules to cover work space, including lighting and furniture. Parameters related to the display unit itself are covered by modules for the display screen, keyboard and software. Additional criteria include noise as a disturbing environmental factor, and the amount of time spent working with the display unit. Other specific factors, such as how the work is organized and how asks are assigned, are not covered by the routine analysis, especially since the factors can hardly be evaluated in terms of stress. The relevance of this information to subsequent strain effects can be estimated primarily from the health data obtained from prophylactic examinations. The assessment process is performed by a suitably qualified "expert" in cooperation with the employee concerned, in order to ensure that the information-gathering process is standardized as far as possible, and at the same time to obtain as much valid information as possible regarding the work requirements. For example, the module entitled "Display Units" has been constructed with simple questions requiring Yes/No answers, as you can see. These assessments are carried out when new office workplaces are established, and in cases where particular concentrated stress factors are identified as a result of occupation-related health problems. The results of the assessments indicate the need for possible workplace design measures, although no direct automatic procedure is involved. Instead, a differentiated investigation is made to determine whether in fact there is a substantiated need to take action. The results of a pilot survey of 94 office workplaces in our Ingolstadt factory can be considered as an example. On the basis of variations from the ideal norm it is possible to identify conspicuous stress factors. Doubtlessly, the problems emerging in this context are in many cases already known, but nevertheless the quantification of these problems helps to substantiate the need for measures to improve workplace design.

One problem encountered is that the acceptable limits for several criteria cannot be exactly designed. In such cases, comparison with health data can be used in order to evaluate the relevance of conspicuous stress patterns to subsequent strain effects. For this purpose an occupational health service working on a prophylactic basis will need parameters that provide an early indication, giving pointers towards unsuitable, strain-producing conditions at the workplace before the actual occurance of any manifest disorders. Data on health complaints are very sensitive an can therefore be used predominantly for this purpose. However, it is extremely important to ensure standardization of the recording situation and the recording methods; this possibility is available specifically as part of the anamnesis in the (routine) preventive occupational health examinations. The main data assessed in this way, with the emphasis placed on conditions or complaints that are relevant to stress factors, are derived from complaints related to the locomotive system and psychomental forms, and are thus equally suitable for health monitoring of both production and office personnel. On the basis of epidemiological criteria it is possible to derive pointers for further analyses and intervening measures from the evaluation of complaints and disorders. The health data compiled from prophylactic occupational health examinations for employees working with visual display units have been analysed as a practical example. In global terms the predominant complaints are related to headaches, complaints in the vicinity of the cervical spine and complaints related to the vegetative system; these are likely to be the limiting criteria, whereas the distribution of complaint is otherwise largely inconspicuous. Visual complaints related to work with display units are within a range of about 3 - 4 %, although no standardized data are available here for comparison, unlike the case with the other type of complaint. On this basis, as a continuation of this general assessment, evaluations related to particular target groups will be carried out in order to identify concrete cases where particular types of stress are predominant.

As a practical example, this is the profile of complaints compiled for a group of computer console operators. Their task consists of controlling and trouble-shooting the operation of programmes on main-frame computers, and they work mostly in a dedicated computer centre. These specific stress factors applicable in this case are the widely varying work requirements, in many cases with tasks to be performed inside very limited time schedules. In addition, they have a changing work rhythm in a

three-shift system, with occasional periods of stand-by duty. In consequence, in this particular case, it is not the locomotive system that constitutes the limiting criterion, but the condition of the psycho-vegetative system. A corresponding result is shown by the profile of complaints from prophylactic occupational health examinations, with a clear emphasis on psychological an vegetative complaints reported by the subjects. The control group used was selected according to the "matched-pairs technique", taking account of the relevant standardization criteria. As a result of the conspicuous findings in this case, measures are now being implemented to improve the work situation. The problem would not have been apparent (or certainly not to this extent) had the analysis been based exclusively on stress factors with the emphasis on ergonomic aspects. For the purpose of health monitoring applied to office work places, it is therefore basically desirable to adopt an integrated approach to the observation of both stress and strain factors. For investigation of stress factors, information systems serve to identify and roughly classify the subject data. More detailed information can be provided from additional data compiled with the aid of the checklist presented here. The results should be evaluated on the basis of existing experience in the field of occupational health. By relating such data to the strain situation it is possible to investigate the relevance of conspicuous stress patterns.
But the method of proceeding from a consideration of stress factors to a consideration of strain factors is not the only approach. By recording and analysing the stress situation in the case of conspicuous patterns of health complaints it is possible for occupational health monitoring to render more differentiated and significant information. The methods described should preferably be integrated within an organizational procedure that provides not only the required flow of information but also ensures that the necessary action can be taken including initiatives affecting workplace design which may be required in particular cases.

As regards the investigation and evaluation of physiological parameters, the measurement of vision functions has been institutionalized as an examination method used in all cases: not just as part of a specific prophylactic examination for persons working with display units, but increasingly as part of the general prophylactic occupational health examinations. The aim is to obtain and compile information on the condition of subjects for individual occupational health consultation (individual medicine), an in addition for purpose of epidemiological analyses (group medicine). Additionally, this makes it possible to ensure optimum vision capability, if necessary by obtaining any vision aid that may be necessary in individual cases. From the socio-medical point of view, the selection of persons as being suitable for working with display units on the basis of vision capability must be regarded critically: in any case this is not necessary for practical purposes. Primary importance must be given to the measures needed to design the layout of the workplace so that optimum vision capability of the person using it is not an essential requirement. Another consideration is that, due to the changing stress conditions in office workplaces, the main stress factor is not the processing of the information the operator views on the display unit, and not the act of viewing itself. Admittedly, this does not apply entirely to all workplaces with display units, as for example CAD systems with their own very specific tasks. In general, however, future requirements for the design of workplaces will not be concerned with "typical" display unit workplaces, but office workplaces where the staff make a wide use of modern information systems with the associated visual display units.

WORK WITH DISPLAY UNITS 92
H. Luczak, A. Çakir and G. Çakir (Editors)

Longitudinal studies on job stress among software engineers

Yuko Fujigaki

Dept.of Information Science,
Univ. of Tokyo
3-8-1 Komaba, Meguro-ku, Tokyo 153, JAPAN
TEL:81-3-3467-1171 EX.675, FAX:81-3-3465-2896

To investigate the relationship between job pressure and engineers' stress, a longitudinal study, an observation of the job content and stress in each individuals for six months, is conducted. As stress measures, subjective rating method and the physiological measure were used. The work-content of each day and each weeks were also surveyed using a diary-style. The results showed that stressors, such as time pressure, quantitative workload, fluctuate over time and that they affect on the engineers' stress. It is suggested that the fluctuation of the work-pressure, quantitative workload, and work characteristics should be considered in the longitudinal studies on job stress.

1. Introduction

The aim of this study is to investigate the relationship between job pressure and workers' stress of software engineers in longitudinal studies. Software development work is one of the most stressful works in Japan. Although the software engineers are one of the workers who use the VDU in their working time, the contents of their work with VDU is vastly different from those of general users of VDU. To investigate the effect of VDU on workers' health, the research question , "How do they work with VDU?", is more important than the question, "Whether do they use VDU or not?".

The previous study showed that the workload of software engineers varies due to the software development stage.(Fujigaki, 1990a) It is indicated that effective aiding system for requirement-definition stage, system-design stage and debugging stage is need to reduce their workload. It is also showed that the contents of projects and working environment affect the stress of engineers.(Fujigaki, 1990b) To reduce the workers' stress, we also tried interactive approach in working group for two years. (Fujigaki, 1991) However, these studies are conducted based on group-level. The time series of work-content, job pressure, and their relationships with stress in each individual engineers are not surveyed. Considering these points, this research mainly aims to investigate job stress and work-content in each individuals in longitudinal studies.

2. Method

The work-contents and stress reaction of 10 subjects who belong to three different projects were surveyed every two weeks during a half year. The work-content of each day and each weeks were surveyed using a diary-style. The subjects reported the work-contents of every 15 minutes using codes.

As the stress measure, subjective rating method and the physiological measure were used. Subjective rating method is categorized into 6 categories; depression, anxiety, pain, arousal, drowsiness, and busyness. As the scale of depression, the SDS(Self-reported Depression Scale) developed by Zung(1965) was used. As for physiological measure, we got urine sample of 10 subjects during their working time. The heat rate measure was used for 3 subjects, one for each 3 projects.

3. Results

Fig-1 shows the change over time in the score of depression, level of adrenalin, and subjective rating on busyness in one subject. Whereas the horizontal axis shows the time: the month/date, the vertical axis shows the standardized score of depression, and the level of adrenalin. The solid line shows the standardized value of adrenalin divided by the value of nor-adrenalin and the dotted line shows the standardized score of depression. The horizontal band shows the subjective-rating of busyness. The black band means"very busy" and diagonal-band means "a little busy".

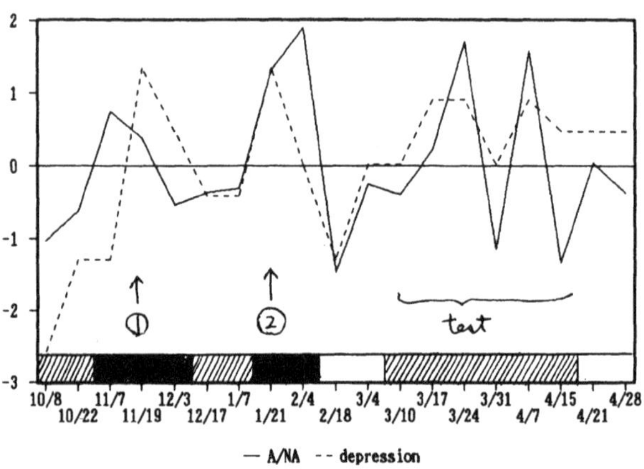

Fig-1. Change over time in standardized score of depression, in level of adrenalin, and in subjective-rating of busyness(band) of subject-A. "very busy" "a little busy"

In this figure, at point 1), the subject engaged in the detail-design stage having deadline of specification at the end of November. He was also busy at the point 2), with the deadline of program-specification near at hand. During March and April, he worked hard to test more than 100 modules.

Thus the work content and work pressure change over time according to the development stage. The score of depression, the level of adrenalin, and the rating of busyness also change according to this work content and work pressure.

Fig-2 shows the change over time in the score of depression, level of adrenalin, and subjective rating on busyness in another subject. In this figure, at point 1), the subject engaged in the system-design stage having deadline of specification at the middle of November. He was also busy at the point 2), with the deadline of a temporary system. At the middle of march, there was a final deadline of the whole system.

This figure of another subject also shows the change in the work content and work pressure over time. The score of depression, the level of adrenalin, and the rating of busyness also change according to the work content and job pressure.

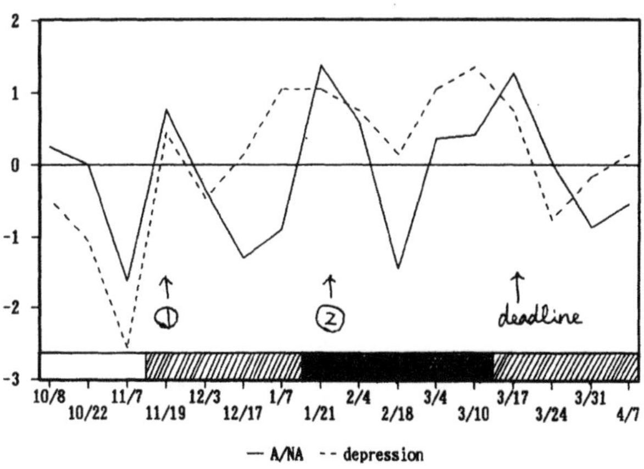

Fig-2. Change over time in standardized score of depression, in level of adrenalin, and in subjective-rating of busyness(band) of subject-B. ■"very busy" ▨"a little busy"

4.Discussion

From the results of the longitudinal stress survey among software engineers, we can point out next two points.
/ Stressors (time pressure, quantitative workload, etc.) fluctuate over time according to the work content change.
/ These stressors affect the stress of engineers.

4-1. Intervention for software engineers
The previous studies mainly focused on the group intervention to reduce the stress of engineers.(Fujigaki, 1990,1991) However, this study showed that stress reaction of each engineer changes according to the work-content, time pressure, quantitative workload. Although it is indicated that stress of engineers differ among each project and among each individuals, there is a time that every engineers show the high stress level, the time which close to the deadline. For effective intervention to reduce the stress, a surveillance of quantitative workload and of time pressure before the deadline for each project/individuals is considered to be important.

4-2. General implications for longitudinal stress studies
For the time-flame of the stress research, Frese and Zapf(1988) showed one of the excellent models. They insisted the initial impact and the effect of exposure time of the stressors. Their model is very effective for the rapid environmental change, for example, the introduction of new system, such as VDU work, in each work situations. Most of the studies on effects of VDU use consider only two kind of state: non VDU-use and VDU-use. The researchers assume that the strength of stressor due to the VDU use is constant.(Fig-3a) They consider the initial impact of VDU use where the state changes from non VDU-use to VDU-use and they consider the exposure time in the state of VDU use.

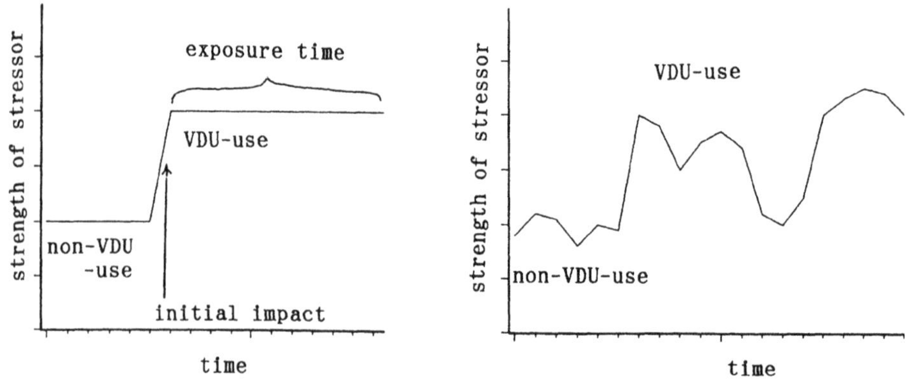

Fig-3. Time Series of Strength of Stressor
a:constant model(left), b:fluctuation model(right)

Most of the studies assumes that the strength of stressor of these two states(non-VDU-use and VDU-use)is constant. However, in real life, the strength of stressor in each state is fluctuating according to the change of the work-pressure, quantitative workload, or job content(Fig-3b). This tendency is often seen in the software development work. There is a effects of fluctuation of stressor after the state shift to the VDU-use. Fluctuation of stressor means change of work content, change of work pressure, change in quantitative overwork, etc.

The model of Frese and Zapf is very effective for the rapid environmental change, since they assumed the "start" or "end" of the stressor. The start of VDU-use can be one of the "start of stressor". We can consider the initial impact of stressor only in the case that the start of stressor is clear; like the case of start of VDU-use. However, in consideration of the fluctuation of stressor in normal working life mentioned above, there is no such clear "start " of stressor. The end of the stressor will be recognized at the time of deadline. Therefore, the concept of "initial impact" is not clear in these fluctuation in real working life.

We can suggest that the fluctuation of the work-pressure, quantitative workload, and work content should be considered in the longitudinal studies on job stress. It should also be considered the amplitude and frequency of this fluctuation.

There emerge the question whether the deviation in stressor (differential factor) or cumulative effect of stressor (integral factor) is more important. Further studies should be done on this point.

1)Fujigaki,Y.; 1990a. A Study of Mental Workload of Software Engineers, In L.Berliguet and D.Berthelete(edited), Work with Display Unit 89 Elsevier(North-Holland), 395-402.

2)Fujigaki,Y; 1990b. Stress Analysis of Software Engineers for Effective management, In K.Noro and O.Brown(edited), Human Factors in Organizational design and Management-3, Elsevier(North-holland),255-258.

3)Fujigaki, Y.:1991. Interactive Approach to Reduce the Stress of Working Group in Information Technology. In Y.Quennec and F.Daniellou(edited), Designing for Everyone, Taylor and Fransis, 1265-1267.

4)Zung, W.W.K.:1965. A Self-rating Depression Scale. Arch. Gen. Psychiatry, 12: 63-70

5)Frese, M. and Zapf, D.:1988. Methodological Issues in the Study of Work Stress: Objective vs Subjective Measurement of Work Stress and Question of Longitudinal Studies. In Cooper and Payne(edited), Causes, Coping, and Consequences of Stress at Work, John Wiley and Sons,Ltd, 375-411.

6)Fujigaki, Y:1992. Occupational Stress of Software Engineers(ed. in Japanese), Publication of the Institute for Science of Labour, 1-177.

WORK WITH DISPLAY UNITS 92
H. Luczak, A. Çakir and G. Çakir (Editors)

LONGITUDINAL STUDIES OF JOB DESIGN AND VDT USE: OVERVIEW AND SYNTHESIS

Pascale Carayon

Department of Industrial Engineering
University of Wisconsin-Madison
Madison, WI 53706 USA

Abstract

Recent longitudinal studies have examined the dynamic relationship between job design, VDT use and worker stress. The following issues have been addressed: characteristics of the change process and their effect on worker stress, effect of technological and organizational change on quality of working life, time effects of job design on worker stress, and comparison of short-term and long-term reactions to VDT use. Some of the conceptual and methodological implications of the dynamic study of job design and VDT use are explored.

1. INTRODUCTION

In the past twenty-five years, there have been many studies of VDT use and job design. The majority of these studies are cross-sectional. They either compare VDT users to non-VDT users (Smith et al., 1981), examine different groups of VDT workers (Huuhtanen and Leino, 1992), compare VDT workers who use VDT's for varying amount of time (Westlander and Aberg, 1992), or study the impact of various computer problems (Carayon-Sainfort, 1992). Some consistent effects have emerged from these studies. For instance, the effect of VDT tends to be more negative on low-level jobs than on professional and managerial jobs (Smith et al., 1981; Huuhtanen and Leino, 1992). But there have also been many inconsistencies as to the negative or positive effect of the VDT on job design and stress. For some, the VDT is a source of stress, while, for others, the VDT makes their job easier and more efficient. The following question has been raised: is the VDT the cause of the stress problems? The answer to this question is both yes and no. The VDT can have both direct and indirect effects on job design, quality of working life and stress (Smith, 1987). It then becomes important to understand and conceptualize the contingency factors that can help explain how VDT use affects or is related to job design and quality of working life. Furthermore, it is important to examine the relationship between VDT use and job design over time. This paper will examine recent longitudinal studies of VDT use and job design, and highlight conceptual and methodological challenges in the conduct of such longitudinal studies.

2. LONGITUDINAL STUDIES OF VDT USE

Many papers were presented at the WWDU'92 conference that described findings from longitudinal studies of job design and VDT use. Some studies examined the characteristics of the change process that can affect job design and the quality of working life. Fujigaki (1992) studied the link between stage of software development process, job stressors and worker stress. Other studies examined the effect of a change on job design and quality of working life. Jarvenpaa (1992), Gard and colleagues (1992) and Beuschel and Kling (1992) studied the effect of technological change on different groups of workers using a variety of methodologies and measurements. Huuhtanen and Lindstrom (1992) compared a change in information technology to an organizational change.

All of these studies demonstrate the importance of time factors. Fujigaki showed that stressors can vary in amplitude and frequency over time. Jarvenpaa showed differences between short-term and long-term effects of the implementation of office automation. Huuhtanen and Lindstrom showed that employee evaluation of the change of information technology tended to become more negative over time. Gard and colleagues demonstrated that the effects of computerization were positive for some of the stress outcomes, but not for others. Beuschel and Kling showed that key changes unfold over long periods of time. At the WWDU'92 conference, Frese (1992) has described some of the conceptual and methodological implications of longitudinal studies of job design and VDT use.

These studies and others (e.g., Korunka et al., 1992) demonstrate that the relationships between people and their working environment (including the VDT) are dynamic. Studies conducted at the University of Wisconsin-Madison provide additional conceptual and empirical evidence for this (Carayon, 1992; Carayon et al., 1992; Carayon, 1993).

The relationship between job design and worker strain may not be stable over time, that is the work factors that influence worker stress may not be the same work factors that influence worker stress at another time (Carayon, 1992; Carayon et al., 1992). If these results are replicated, they can question the validity of cross-sectional studies. In addition, we need to re-think the way we conceptualize the relationship between job design and worker stress. The effects may not be direct, nor simple, nor linear. We need to consider not just one or two job design factors, but a variety of job design factors that can interact with each other or influence each other in complex ways to affect worker stress (Smith and Sainfort, 1989).

We do not know a lot about the time effects of job design on worker stress. Unlike theories of stress and life events, models of job design and stress assume that job design factors are <u>chronic</u> stressors (e.g., Karasek, 1979). Recently, a study of computer users showed that workers exposed to low job control over a period of three years reported higher stress than workers exposed to high control or to varying levels of control over that same period of time (Carayon, 1993). Longitudinal studies are needed to examine the "daily hassles" (DeLongis et al., 1982) faced by computer users that can lead to high levels of stress over time. These daily hassles could include computer-related problems such as computer slow response time and computer breakdowns (Lindstrom, 1991) or poor work factors such as low control, high work pressure and high cognitive demands (Smith and Carayon, 1993).

3. CONCEPTUAL AND METHODOLOGICAL IMPLICATIONS

Since the technological environment changes very rapidly, technologies and tools used by workers change very often. Therefore, understanding the relationship between people and their working environment in a dynamic way is even more important. We need to develop theories and methods to examine the relationships between people and their working environment over time. The following are some of the conceptual and methodological issues of importance to longitudinal studies of job design and VDT use.

3.1 Conceptual Issues

- study of technological or organizational change:
  Do the effects last over time?
  Are there transient effects, such as resistance to change or honeymoon effect, that can affect the validity of the results?
  Can we differentiate between the acute stressor (e.g., technological change) and chronic stressors that may result from this acute stressor (e.g., increased workload)?
  Do people adapt or adjust to the change over time?
- time-models of stress effects:
  Frese and Zapf (1988) have proposed different time-models of stress effects. How can we design longitudinal studies that examine these different models? These models assume that the cause of stress is constant, and has a beginning and an end. This may not be true (Fujigaki, 1992). How can we modify or adapt these models to take into account variations in the strength of the stressor?
- temporal shapes of the stressor and the stress effects:
  Kelly and McGrath (1988) have proposed different temporal shapes for examining the variation of the stressor or the stress effects over time. How can we adapt these models to the study of VDT work?
- temporal shape of the relationship between job design and worker reactions:
  The relationship between job design and worker reactions may change or evolve over time (Carayon, 1992; Carayon, 1993). Are the effects of job design and VDT work on stress chronic, long-term or transient and variable?

3.2 Methodological Issues

- measurement of worker stress:
  How can we measure both short-term and long-term stress effects?
  What time dimensions (e.g., frequency, duration and severity) should we use to measure worker stress?
  How long, when and how often should we take measures of stress?

- **time intervals between measurement:**
  How wide should the temporal window be between the various measurements? How many measurements should we take?
- **sample:**
  How can we reduce attrition?

4. CONCLUSION

To study time takes time! Therefore, we cannot see the outcomes of longitudinal studies right away. This may deter researchers and funding agencies to conduct longitudinal studies of VDT use. However, given the importance of time factors, the number of people using VDT's and the extent of the job stress problem, these studies are necessary. However, we cannot wait for these studies to be done before changing work. Job design principles have been developed to (re)design work to fit worker needs and reduce stress (Smith and Sainfort, 1989). Actually, one class of longitudinal studies is highly recommended, studies of the effectiveness of job (re)design interventions.

5. REFERENCES

Beuschel, W. and Kling, R. (1992) "Computerization and workplace transformations" In WWDU'92 Abstract Book, edited by H. Luczak, A.E. Cakir and G. Cakir, TUB, Berlin, Germany, p.F.23-F.24.

Carayon, P. (1992) "A longitudinal study of job design and worker strain: Preliminary results" In Stress and Well-Being at Work: Assessments and Interventions for Occupational Mental Health, edited by J.C. Quick, L.R. Murphy and J.J. Hurrell Jr., American Psychological Association, Washington, D.C., pp.19-32.

Carayon, P. (1993) "Chronic effect of job control, supervisor social support and work pressure on worker stress among office workers" to be published in the proceedings of the APA/NIOSH Conference on Occupational Stress.

Carayon, P., Yang, C.-L. and Lim, S.-Y. (1992) "Examining the relationship between job design and worker strain over time: A longitudinal study of office workers" Under review.

Carayon-Sainfort, P. (1992) "The use of computers in offices: Impact on task characteristics and worker stress" International Journal of Human-Computer Interaction, 4(3): 245-261.

DeLongis, A., Coyne, J.C., Dakof, G., Folkman, S. and Lazarus, R.S. "Relationships of daily hassles, uplifts and major life events to health status" Health Psychology, 1(2): 119-136

Frese, M. (1992) "Conceptual and methodological issues in studies on stress and VDT use" In WWDU'92 Abstract Book, edited by H. Luczak, A.E. Cakir and G. Cakir, TUB, Berlin, Germany, p.F.21.

Frese, M. and Zapf (1988) "Methodological issues in the study of work stress: Objective vs. subjective measurement of work stress and the question of longitudinal studies" In Causes, Coping and Consequences of Stress at Work. edited by C.L. Cooper and R. Payne, John Wiley & Sons, pp.375-411.

Fujigaki, Y. (1992) "Longitudinal studies on job stress among software engineers" In WWDU'92 Abstract Book, edited by H. Luczak, A.E. Cakir and G. Cakir, TUB, Berlin, Germany, p.F.17-F.18.

Gard, G. and colleagues (1992) "Stress and qualification of administrative computer work" In WWDU'92 Abstract Book, edited by H. Luczak, A.E. Cakir and G. Cakir, TUB, Berlin, Germany, p.F.22.

Huuhtanen, P. and Leino, T. (1992) "The impact of new technology by occupation and age on work in financial firms: A 2-year follow-up" International Journal of Human-Computer Interaction, 4(2): 123-142.

Huuhtanen, P. and Lindstrom, K. (1992) "Satisfaction with the implementation of new information technology among banking personnel in 1988 and 1990" In WWDU'92 Abstract Book, edited by H. Luczak, A.E. Cakir and G. Cakir, TUB, Berlin, Germany, p.F.20.

Jarvenpaa, E. (1992) "A longitudinal study of the implementation of office automation" In WWDU'92 Abstract Book, edited by H. Luczak, A.E. Cakir and G. Cakir, TUB, Berlin, Germany, p.F.19.

Karasek, R. (1979) "Job demands, job decision latitude, and mental strain: Implications for job redesign" Administrative Science Quarterly, 24: 285-307.

Kelly, J.R. and McGrath, J.E. (1988) On Time and Method. Sage Publications, Beverly Hills, CA.

Korunka, C., Karetta, B. and Weiss, A. (1992) "The conversion to new technologies: Psychological and physiological stress reactions related to aspects of the conversion process - An interdisciplinary longitudinal study" In WWDU'92 Abstract Book, edited by H. Luczak, A.E. Cakir and G. Cakir, TUB, Berlin, Germany, p.F.7.

Lindstrom, K. (1991) "Well-being and computer-mediated work at various occupational groups in banking and insurance" International Journal of Human-Computer Interaction, 3(4): 339-361.

Smith, M.J. (1987) "Is the VDT technology stressful?" WWDU'86, Stockholm, Sweden.

Smith, M.J. and Carayon, P. (1993) "A 'balance' model for examining psychological job stress in VDU work" this volume.

Smith, M.J. and Sainfort, P. Carayon (1989) "A balance theory of job design for stress reduction" International Journal of Industrial Ergonomics, vol. 4, pp.67-79.

Smith, M.J., Cohen, B.G. and Stammerjohn, L.W. Jr. (1981) "An investigation of health complaints and job stress in video display operations" Human Factors, 23(4): 387-400.

Westlander, G. and Aberg, E. (1992). Variety in VDT work: An issue for assessment in environment research. International Journal of Human-Computer Interaction, 4(3):283-301.

WORK WITH DISPLAY UNITS 92
H. Luczak, A. Çakir and G. Çakir (Editors)

Computerization and Workplace Transformations

Werner **Beuschel**[a] and Rob **Kling**[b]

[a]University of Dortmund, Computer Science, 4600 Dortmund 50, Germany, beuschel@iug.informatik.uni-dortmund.de

[b]University of California, Information & Computer Science, Irvine, CA 92717, USA, kling@ics.uci.edu

Abstract

This paper summarizes two independent research efforts, focused on desktop computers and on expert systems. Both studies aimed at computerization processes at the workplace. They were guided by similar theoretical assumptions, based on the relevance of observing social processes in a longitudinal way. Thus, it seems useful to articulate insights and conclusions which are supported by findings of both studies in order to analyze the transformations taking place and to articulate open questions for further research with regard to computerization issues.

1. INTRODUCTION

Diverse computing innovations were introduced in the 80's into numerous and diverse offices in the US at an amazing pace. There were many high expectations, both technologically utopian and anti-utopian, that this new wave of computer technologies would lead to dramatic changes at all organizational levels.

Desktop computing was a major innovation, while expert systems were introduced into a comparatively small number of workplaces. The Desktop Computerization project (headed by Rob Kling) and a study of expert systems development (headed by Werner Beuschel) were both conducted at the University of California, Irvine. These research efforts sought to investigate the nature of actual changes in worklife which were attributable to computerization.

Methodologically, the desktop study emphasized a mixture of surveys and case studies of desktop computerization and work in over 40 work groups between 1986 and 1990. The expert systems study employed in-depth case studies of system design rationale and organizational integration in two large companies between 1989 and 1991.

2. OVERVIEW OF THE PROJECTS

2.1 The Desktop Computing Project

Desktop computerization is a potentially powerful catalyst for changing modern work organizations. Some people argue that computerization is leading to major transformations in the character of work. There are some compelling examples about how desktop computerization has transformed the work of some specific occupations: laptop computers and telecommunications have transformed the workstyles of many journalists and travelling salesmen; fast spreadsheets have altered the workstyles of many accountants and financial analysts; word processors have changed the way that many managers and professionals work with their secretaries or the "typing pool."

Changes like these are not universal. For the past several years a group of researchers at UC Irvine has been studying how worklife changed in workgroups that have adopted desktop computing [cf.1-8]. The term "desktop computing" was used in the context of the project for any computing equipment which is available to workers on or near their desks: terminals, microcomputers, dedicated word processors, or engineering work stations. The study focused on work groups: small numbers of people who work for the same supervisor, usually in close proximity to each other.

The research group has been studying desktop computing since the mid 1980s. Through interviews and surveys important insights into the complexity of the relationship between computers and work were developed. In 1987 work groups were selected to participate in an annual survey based on the amount of computer equipment they used. The researchers looked for work groups who used computers a great deal in their work, expecting these would be the places to find most changes in the way that people worked.

One striking change that took place over the three year period of the survey was the dramatic increase in the presence of computers in these workplaces. When the annual survey began in 1988, these work groups used computers for a major part of their work week - on average 16 hours per week. Many people shared computers with co-workers. By 1990, their usage had increased by almost a day of work, to an average of 23 hours per week! Professional as well as clerical workers alike spent half of their work week working on computers. Not only were work groups using computers more frequently, they were also using computers or terminals to do a greater variety of different tasks. By 1990, computers were used, on average, for 14 different tasks such as word processing, data entry, and searching records. By 1990, 82% of workers had computers on or near their desks which they rarely shared.

These changes in computer use illustrate the dynamic quality of computerization. Work groups constantly added on new equipment or additional software packages, or system applications. The technological changes were often minor (e.g. upgrading to a newer version of a wordprocessing package), but ongoing. In some cases, the technological changes were more dramatic -- including the implementation of whole new systems, or conversion from PCs to MACs. People are often most aware of changes in technology, because it is visible. The newer equipment is often faster and more capable than older equipment. Supervisors expectations also changed with the growing presence of computers. They expected more professional quality documents, greater accuracy, and speedier work from their staffs. However, the increased use of computers and increased supervisors' expectations did not always lead to better work.

2.2 The Expert Systems Study

The variety of expert systems investigated in two case studies of organizations in California filled in niches of system applications. The expert systems were about to become part of already existent systems and networks. Not in an imperative top-down manner as envisioned by some of the pioneers in the field, who saw whole organizations governed by artificial intelligence systems. Rather a kind of 'functional extension' to EDP systems took place. This made it important from the research perspective to take a closer look how technology and organizational aspects would interact and how the development process was organized [9].

Practices for design, transfer and use of small expert systems in different areas, oil production and office work, were analyzed [10,11,12]. The examples showed clearly the emphasis of most managers and system developers to reach an integration of technical and organizational change. Despite this approach unforeseen outcomes with regard to organizational and social issues occured during the development processes, though on a small scale.

This effect can be explained by showing that, regardless of managerial precautions, the applied development practices create ambiguities, which are likely to lead to organizational turbulences. These are provoked due to slightly shifting boundaries of competency between work groups or between users and computer.

Shifts in competency can be understood, if we interpret the development of expert systems as an intervention into a work process, whith the aim of reconstructing professional knowledge. The fact that the reconstruction as such does not become very obvious to the participants during the development phases can be linked to an idealizing view in the underlying theory of expert systems. This theory -- most often implicitely -- contributes to a static view of terms like "knowledge" or "organization", rendering inflexible knowledge bases. Thus, changes in the workplace are covered up rather than making them the subject of discussion and negotiation. Along this line of argumentation, the discrepancy obetween hidden social assumptions in the theory versus practical -- situational -- requirements, the relatively low degree of interpenetration of industrial and commercial areas with expert systems may find its explanation.

The case studies point to the limits of development practices which are based on an idealizing theory of human knowledge. Contradicting an often heard belief, the cases also speak for the continued necessity of training efforts in the context of expert system developments.

The important practical lesson to be learned from these and other examples is that the more human knowledge -- and not just number crunching -- is the subject of computerization, the more organizational efforts will be necessary in order to reach the goal of a usable system. As important as software implementation seems to be organizational implementation.

3. RESULTS SUPPORTED BY BOTH STUDIES

Some common ideas emerge of both of these studies with regard to the transformation of workplaces and the quality of work:

A. Computerization rarely transforms work in a coherent and uni-directional way. In most cases changes in work organization and control are neither as frightening nor as empowering as one might expect from envisioning the computer as a tool for purposive organizational change.

B. Computerization projects differ in key social elements, such as issues of control over technology and the support for enskilling workers. Contingencies like these make a major difference in the resulting quality of worklife. Further different approaches to computerization reflect different "social logics."

C. Although it appears that computerization has changed few organization-wide structures, it still presents a variety of challenges and options at the work group level with regard to these multiple logics.

D. Key changes in work organization unfold over periods of years, not just weeks or months. This observation has important theoretical and methodological consequences.

4. FURTHER RESEARCH QUESTIONS

Important questions about how to characterize the various logics of computerization and how to extrapolate to future applications arise. If we ask which insights we could gain from the investigations for future research we have to further explore the social dimensions of computerization projects:

- *Control:* Who gains, who loses in terms of power and control in current main computerization scenarios under which circumstances?
- *Design goals and rationales:* What supports and influences the main metaphors/visions system designers pursue in their application design and how does this add up to a design rationale within an organization?
- *User empowerment:* What fosters and what hinders participation in the development process, and are there idiosyncracies concerning projects using desktop or expert system computerization?
- *Skill changes and training:* Which skills are needed in these computerization processes, and how is the distribution of chances to acquire new skills for different roles in the office affected?

5. REFERENCES

The Desktop Project:

1 George, J., Kling, R. and S. Iacono (1990): The Role of Training and Support in Desktop Computing. In: Kaiser, K.M. and H.J. Oppeland (eds.): Desktop Information Technology: Organizational Worklife in the 1990. North Holland: Amsterdam.

2 Kling, R. (1990). More Information, Better Jobs?: Occupational Stratification and Labor Market Segmentation in the United States' Information Labor Force. The Information Society, 7(2): 77-107.

3 Kling, R. (1992): Behind the Terminal: The Critical Role of Computing Infrastructure in Effective Information Systems' Development and Use. In: Cotterman, W. and J. Senn (eds.): Systems Analysis: A Research Perspective. Wiley: N.Y.
4 Kling, R., & Iacono, S. (1989a). Desktop Computing and the Organization of Work. In Forester (ed.): Computers in the Human Context. MIT Press: Cambridge, Massachusetts.
5 Kling, R., & Iacono, S. (1989b). The Institutional Character of Computerized Information Systems. Office: Technology and People, 5(1), 7-28.
6 Kling, R., Iacono, S., & George, J. (1990). Occupational Power, Patterns of Desktop Computer Use, and Quality of Worklife. In K. Kaiser, & H. Oppeland (Ed.), Desktop Information Technology: Organizational Worklife in the 1990s. Elsevier/North Holland: Amsterdam.
7 Zmuidzinas, M., & Kling, R. (1989). Changes in Computer Use and Work Life: Simple contrasts from surveys of desktop computing users 1988-1989. Public Policy Research Organization Working Paper.
8 Zmuidzinas, M., Kling, R. and J. George (1990): Desktop Computerization as a Continuing Process. Proc. of the 11th Annual Conf. on Information Systems, Copenhagen, Denmark, Dec. 1990.

The Expert Systems Study:
9 Beuschel, W. (1991): What will impact assessment teach us about expert systems design? In: Van den Besselaar, P., Clement, A. and P. Järvinen (eds.): Information System, Work and Organization Design, Elsevier: Amsterdam: 63-72.
10 Beuschel, W. (1991): Organizational Advantages and Obstacles of Development Practices for Expert Systems - Two American Cases. In: H.-J. Bullinger (ed.): Expertensysteme in Produktion und Engineering, Springer: Berlin Heidelberg New York: 179-197.
11 Beuschel, W. (1991): AI meets the company: Case Studies on the Organizational Impact of Expert Systems. In: H.M. Hamza (ed.): *Proc. of the Ninth Int. Conf. Applied Informatics*, Acta Press: Anaheim Calgary Zurich: 473-476.
12 Beuschel, W. (1991): Expertensysteme im Betrieb - Fallstudien in den USA zu Auswirkungen auf Arbeitsorganisation und Qualifikation. Discussion paper FS I 91-5, Wissenschaftszentrum Berlin, Berlin.
13 Beuschel, W. (1992): Replacement, Reconstruction and Enhancement: The Impact of Expert Systems Re-examined. In: Luczak, H., A.E. Cakir, G. Cakir (eds.): Work With Display Units, Proc. of the Third Int. Scientific Conference, Berlin: G42-43

Acknowledgments: Research of the Desktop Project was funded by a National Science Foundation grant #IRI-87-09613; the Expert Systems Study was executed under a sholarship grant by the German Science Foundation.

APPLICATIONS IN OFFICE AND INDUSTRY

WORK WITH DISPLAY UNITS 92
H. Luczak, A. Çakir and G. Çakir (Editors)

Eye-Contact Video Communication System

Takashi Toriizuka, Tetsuri Inoue, Kageyu Noro

School of Human Sciences, Waseda University
2-579-15, Mikajima Tokorozawa Saitama, Japan

Abstract

The spread of ISDN has increased the office use of teleconferencing systems. Given the mounting popularity of the B-ISDN in recent years, teleconferencing systems will find increasing usage in a variety of applications. However, conventional teleconferencing system has one problem concerned with eye-contact. This problem has been solved by using new system which enables eye-contact communication.

1. INTRODUCTION

1-1. Communication

Communication means the state that each parson is not only a server of informations but also a reciever. Various signs exist as the means of information, for example the gesture, the expression, the word and so on. We must select some of these as a communication tool. Among those tools " Language" is the most popular. Like this, to use language as a tool of communication is called verbal communication. On the other hand, to use tools excluding language as a communication tool is called non-verbal communication. While verbal communication is mere a language information, non-verbal communication is a communication sued to human senses such as a sight etc. So non-verbal communication includes more informations compared with verbal communication. Thus it could be said that non-verbal communication is more important than verbal communication. It is said that the important working in such non-verbal communication will be done concerning faces like an eye-contact or an expression. For instance, one report says that non-verbal communications concerning faces occupy 55% and verbal communications like languages do 7%, in normal conversations between two parsons.

1-2. Remote Communication

Though it is obvious that non-verbal communication performs an important role in case of communication like conversation, non-verbal communication like an eye-contact or an expression can be transmitted in the faced conversation but cannot be done in the not-faced conversation for example remote communication. The telephone has been a main current in the remote communication. Though the telephone is an epochal remote communication tool, it cannot transmit non-verbal communications. However in recent yeas, teleconferencing system has been developed as a remote communication tool.

2. VIDEO COMMUNICATION SYSTEM

2-1. What is Video Communication System?

The system which uses image as a communication medium is called video communication system like teleconferencing system. Fig. 1 shows one teleconferencing system. This system is very epochal system because it enables to transmit non-verbal communication, which has not been able to transmitted, by using video images.

The spread of the Integrated Services Digital Network (ISDN) has increased the office use of teleconferencing systems. Given the mounting popularity of the broadband ISDN in recent years, teleconferencing systems will find increasing usage in a variety of applications. Teleconferencing systems were applied to conduct tele-trials some time ago and are faced with various demands. One problem is concerned with eye contact.

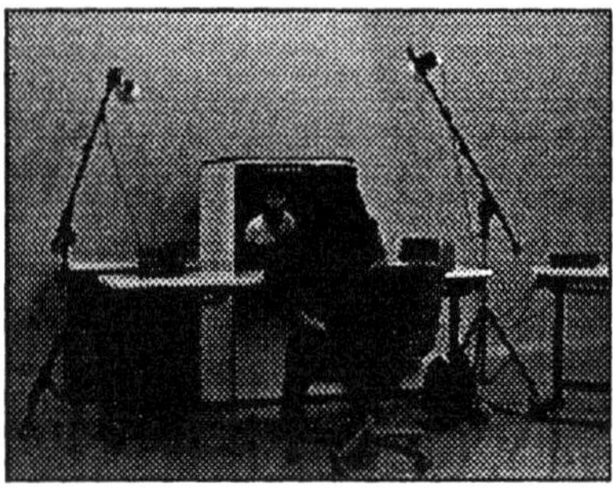

Fig.1 Teleconferencing system

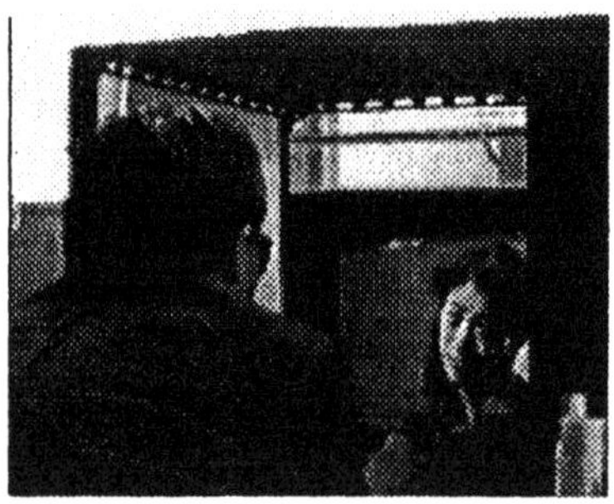

Fig.2 Eye-contact video communication system

2-2. Conventional Video Communication System

Fig. 3 shows a model of teleconferencing station in current use. If the angle ν between the camera and monitor is large, the conferees cannot converse with eye-contact. The large angle ν is a serious obstacle to facial non-verbal communication like eye-contact communication. Fig. 4 shows the image in this system. The conferee seems to watch to the under completely in the image of conventional video communication system whose ν is large enough as shown in Fig. 3. Therefore conferees cannot converse with eye-contact each other, moreover the expression transmits vaguely because of the angle ν. So a big improvement might be necessary to use this system as a virtual communication system.

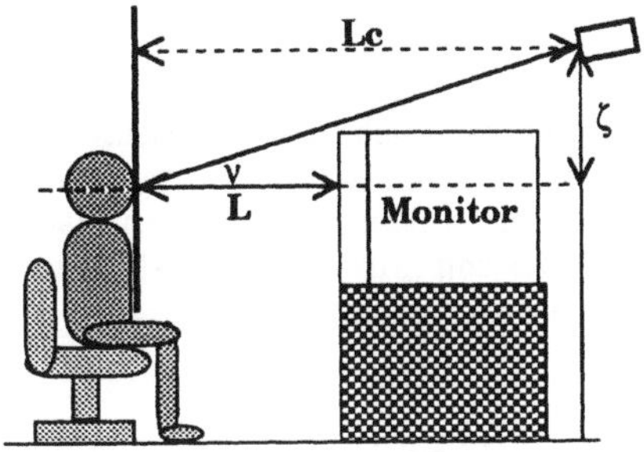

Fig.3 Model of conventional video communication system

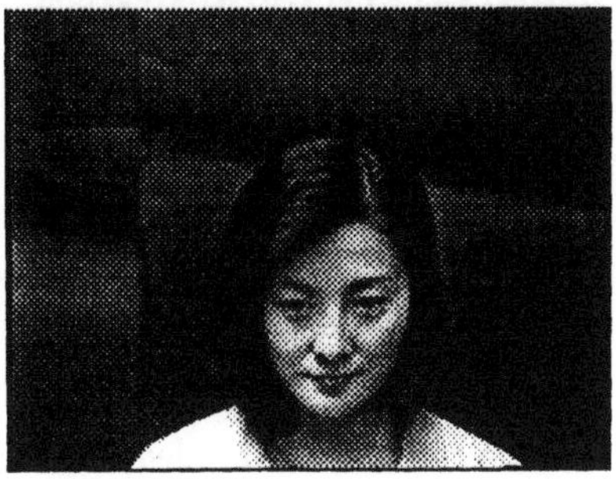

Fig.4 Image on conventional telecpnferencing system

2-3. Eye-Contact Video Communication System

The solution to this problem calls for the development of a teleconferencing system that allows the conferees to converse with eye contact. The eye-contact problems was resolved by integrating the camera and monitor with the aid of a half-mirror (Fig. 5). That is, the eye-contact video communication system was made (Fig. 2). The originality of this system is in the use of the half-mirror. Half-mirror plays a role of mirror when the background is bright and plays a role of glass when the background is dark. By using the characteristic of half mirror like the above, the camera was identified with the monitor. So the conferees have been able to watch the camera with watching the monitor. Therefore, the conferees have been able to transmit non-verbal communication such as the eye-contact or the expression by using this eye-contact video communication system (Fig.6).

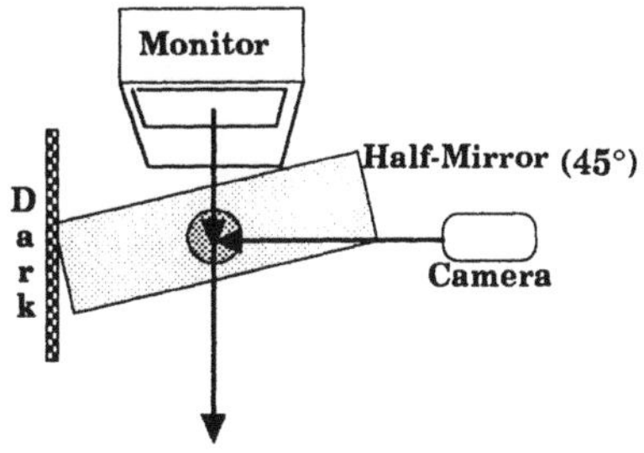

Fig.5 Model of eye-contact video communication system

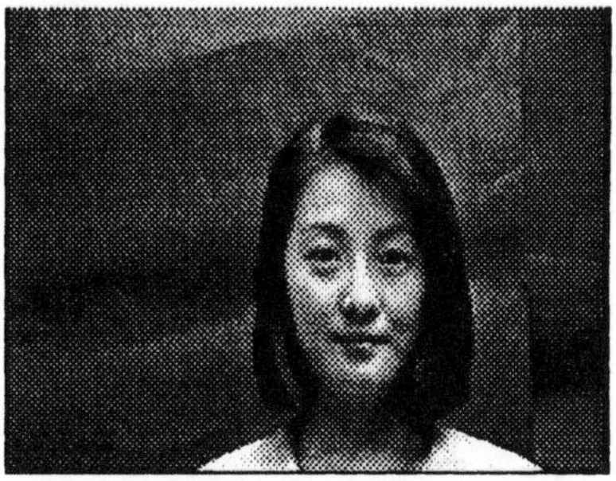

Fig.6 Image on eye-contact video communication system

3. EVALUATE EXPERIMENT

3-1. The Aim of Experiment

Though eye-contact video communication system which enables facial non-verbal communication, are there any differences between a conventional video communication system and an eye-contact video communication system in case of video communication? Here, the eye-contact video communication system was evaluated in comparison with a conventional teleconferencing system.

3-2. Experimental Method

The conventional video communication systems (**condition 1**) or eye-contact video communication system (**condition 2**) were set up in two laboratories. The height of the monitor is the same as the height of conferees' eyes. Two laboratories were tied with a coaxial cable and each camera and each monitor were connected with the cable. The subjects were made to talk freely for 10 minutes. During 10 minutes, sampling time is defined as 4 minutes after 4 minutes from the start of experiment. After this experiment finished, their eye aversion rate and blinking rate were counted and analyzed, based on the video tape. The reason for counting their eye aversion rate and blinking rate is that they are important indexes in personal psychology.

3-3. Results and Discussion

3-3-1. Eye-aversion

The number of times one conferee turned the eyes away from the other conferee during their conversation increased with the new teleconferencing system (Fig.7). People are said to intentionally turn the eyes toward and away from each other when they talk. The eye aversion rate data show that the new teleconferencing system can provide for more natural communication between the conferees.

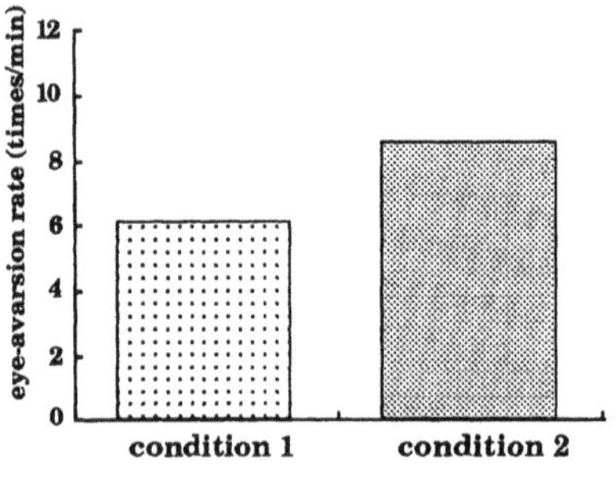

Fig. 7 Eye-avarsion rate par minutes ($p<0.05$)

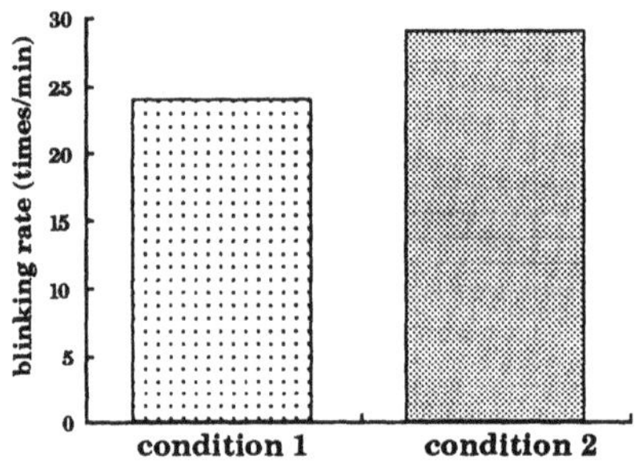

Fig. 8 Blinking rate par minutes ($p<0.05$)

3-3-2. Blinking

It is known that people blink the eyes when they think. The blink rate was 45 blinks per minute under condition 1 and 33 blinks per minute under condition 2 (Fig.8). The blink rate data suggest that the conferees thought more and more earnestly talked when they used the new teleconferencing system.

4. CONCLUSION

Non-verbal communication such as the eye-contact or the expression plays a very important role on most communications in spite of its delicacy. However, the eye-contact or the expression had not been able to been transmitted because of its delicacy by using conventional video communication system. But the eye-contact video communication system has solved that problem. Therefore, it is guessed that the video communication system will spread more and more because of developing this eye-contact video communication system. Make-up consultation and divination by the features were performed by using the eye-contact teleconferencing system, indeed. The most frequent of the opinions the subjects had of the eye-contact system was that they could watch the delicate facial expression of the other conferee and though as if they were actually meeting with each other. This opinion points to the capability of the eye-contact system to convey the facial expressions and feelings of the conferees. Depending on the virtual communication system like the eye-contact video communication system, this kind of paformances have been achieved. As described in Introduction, teleconferencing systems are finding use in a variety of applications. The research of video communication systems is expected to assume increasing importance. The eye-contact communication system discussed here will occupy an important position among the video communication systems. One of the human dreams is being achieved. So for example, the day, when we can do video party between Tokyo and Berlin, might have come.

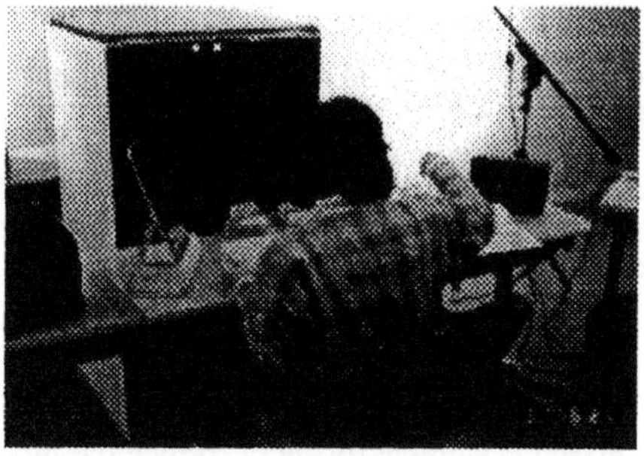

Fig. 9 Make-up consultation

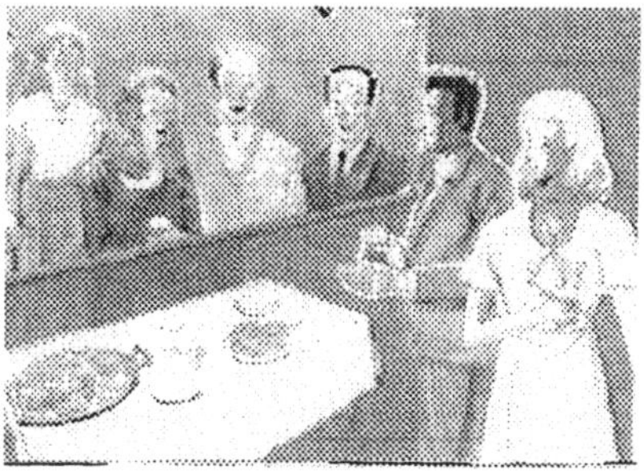

Fig. 10 Teleparty
By using eye-contact system, we can do video party between Tokyo and Berlin

WORK WITH DISPLAY UNITS 92
H. Luczak, A. Çakir and G. Çakir (Editors)

Development of a User Interface for Epilepsy Diagnosis

Inga Tschiersch[a] and Hartmut Haubrich[b] and Klaus Henning[a]

[a]Department of Cybernetics (KDI), University of Technology (RWTH) Aachen, Rolandstr. 7-9, D-W-5100 Aachen

[b]Applied Measuring Technique and Process Automation ltd. (AMEPA), Jülicher Str. 320, D-W-5100 Aachen

Abstract
This presentation deals with the development of a user interface for a computer supported entropy analysis of electro- encephalograms (EEG) to localize an epileptic focus.

1. CRITERIAS FOR A USER INTERFACE

Usually physicians have neither studied the entropy function based on information theory, nor are they trained in handling a complex computer program [1] . Therefore the development of the user interface requires great care [2] . Only a user interface suitable for physicians guarantees that using the entropy function supports the diagnosis. Otherwise this tool would make the problem more complex for the physicians than working without it.Therefore a user interface for physicians has been designed considering the following three aspects.

1.1 Software-Prototyping

Only the users are able to decide which user interface is suitable for them. Hence the physicians have been integrated into the development of the user interface at an early stage. Their needs have been directly taken into consideration. During the development process they got used to the new method of diagnosis and accepted it.

1.2 Modelling

The user interface represents elements familiar to physicians. The visual display represents a model of the problem. This model consists mainly of elements familiar to physicians from their work and only a few elements are explicitly derived from the entropy function.

1.3 Adaptability

The interface allows the physicians to work on different levels of abstraction. The physicians are able to get all information about the analysis, even the theoretical entropy curves and the parameters from information theory. The userinterface supports the physicians to learn the new method. The user can reduce the medical elements and increase the theoretical level refering to the entropy function. Thus the physicians feel responsible for the analysis because they are able to control the computer program and not vice versa.

2. EPILEPSY DIAGNOSIS

On the following paragraph a short introduction is given to epilepsy diagnosis supported by entropy function.

An epileptic focus is a region within the brain, where epileptic fits start in a special case of epilepsy. If medical treatment is not succesful and the focus can be localized, its surgical removal can be considered. This is a serious and irreversible operation, all consequences and implications should be examined well [3] . To localize the epileptic focus the medical experts analyze visually the epileptic activity detected by electrodes and traced by an electroencephalogram (EEG).

One tool to support the EEG-analysis is the entropy function as developed by Henning [4] and Mars [5] . The entropy function is based on information theory. Similar to the well known cross-correlation it measures statistical dependence and delay times. Because of the large amount of data the analysis needs to be aided by a computer program [6,7] . Figure 1 shows five entropy functions of consecutive samples of the signals recieved at the adjacent electrodes no.3 and no.10, which show the statistical dependence between the signals arriving at electrodes no.3 and no.10, similar - maybe epileptic - patterns of the electrodes. The peaks are at small positiv delay times, which indicates that the epileptic signals are received earlier by electrode no.3 than by electrode no.10.

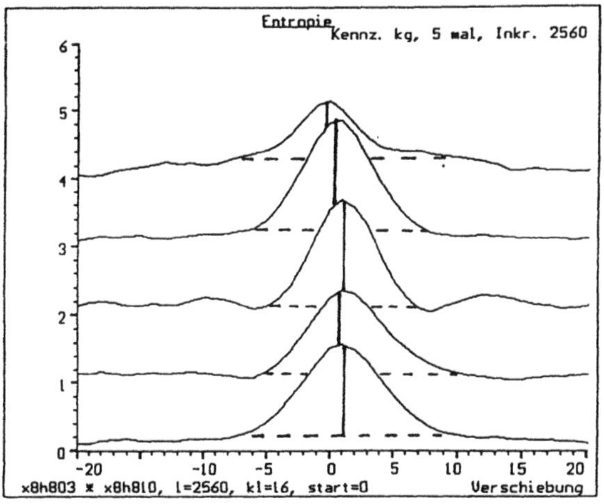

Figure 1 . Entropy-function of a sequence of sample.

3. DEVELOPMENT OF THE USER INTERFACE

The figure 2 constitutes the developed display representations of this project. The display shows a model of the brain. Therefore the diagrams map the arrangement of electrodes at the brain.

The following design elements were proposed by physicians involved in the project. To reduce complexity the information is distributed into three figures. Figure 2a shows the average dependence between the electrodes and Figure 2b shows the chronological development of the statistical dependence. Several lines connect the electrodes. The thickness of the lines is related to the statistical dependence. Therefore an "area of blackness" indicates an epileptical focus in a qualitative way.

The chronological development of the delay time is represented in Figure 2c. The line´s deviation from the centre is proportional to the delay time.

Physicians used to the entropy function can adapt further the user interface to their needs and experience. The representation of Figure 2d integrates all information about the development of statistical dependence and delay time. Thus it is possible for physiciancs to work on a fairly abstract level of the entropy function (Figure 1).

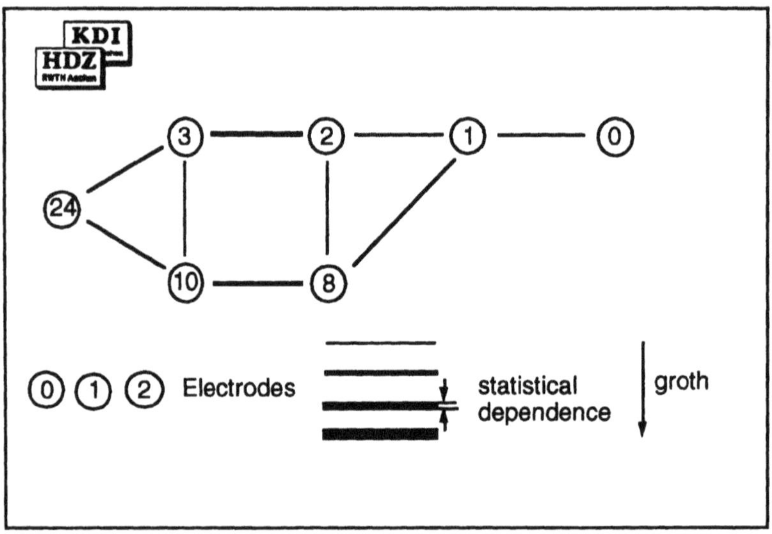

Figure 2a . Display representation of the average statistical depence.

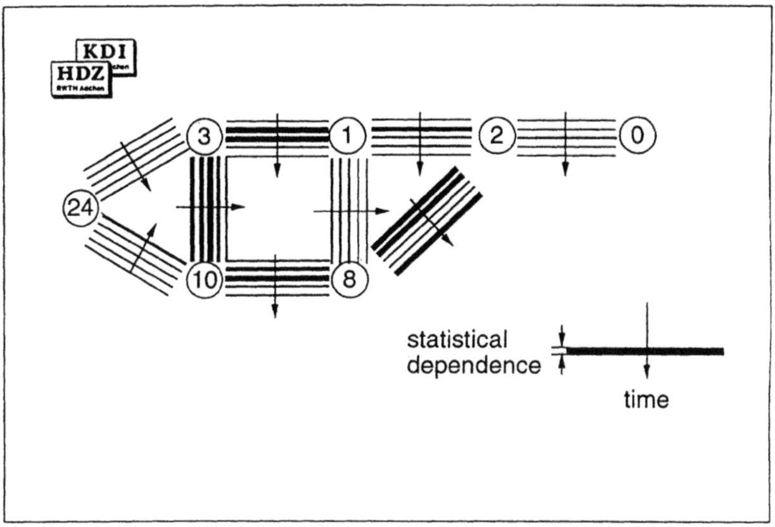

Figure 2b . Display representation of the chronological development of the statistical dependence.

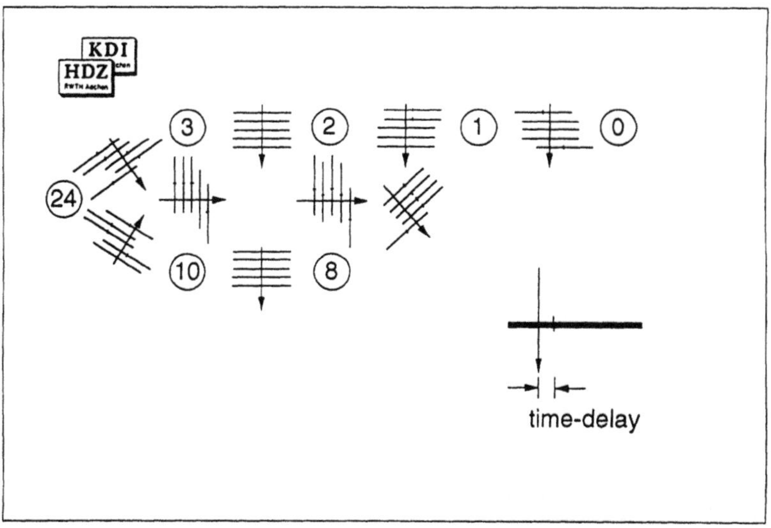

Figure 2c . Display representation of the chronological development of the time delay.

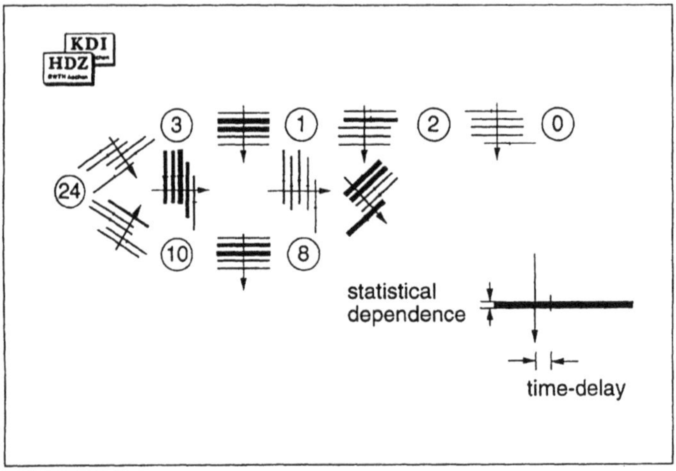

Figure 2d . Display representation of all information.

Hence the aspect of software-prototyping, modelling and adaptability support the design of an easy-to-understand interface for an extremly complex mathematical algorithm.

4. ACKNOWLEDGEMENT

The authors would like to thank Prof. C.E. Elger, Dept. of epileptology, Universitätsnervenklinik Bonn, for his cooperation, suggestions and support.

5. REFERENCES

1 B. Thull and M. Langen and G. Rau, Ansatz eines Dialogmanagers für ein intensivmedizinisches Informationsystem, in [8]
2 M. Dahm et al., DIBA- der digitale Bildarbeitsplatz für die Medizin, in [8]
3 H. G. Wieser and C .G. Elger, Presurgical Evaluation of Epileptics, Springer, New-York, 1987
4 K. Henning, Die Entropie in der Systemtheorie, Postdoctoral Thesis, Aachen, 1980
5 N.J.I. Mars, Computer-Augmented Analysis of Electroencephalograms in Epilepsy, Thesispaper, Leiden, 1982
6 S. Kutscha, Statistische Bewertungskriterien für die Entropieanalyse dynamischer Systeme, VDI Verlag, Düsseldorf, 1989
7 H. Haubrich and S. Kutscha and K. Henning, Localisation of Epileptogenic Sites by Means of Dynamic Entropy Analysis, 1st europ. conf. on biomedical engineering, Nizza, 1991
8 D. Ackermann and E. Uhlich (eds.), Software-Ergonomie ´91, Benutzerorientierte Software-Entwicklung, Stuttgart, 1991

WORK WITH DISPLAY UNITS 92
H. Luczak, A. Çakir and G. Çakir (Editors)

Ergonomic Investigation of Agricultural Videotex Information System

K. Landau, Yt. Huang, M. Zeraschi, P. Werny [1)], M. Harkin [2)]

[1)] Department of Ergonomics, University of Hohenheim, Fruwirthstrasse 48,
7000 Stuttgart 70, Germany
[2)] ORCA Computer Ltd., L-9161 Ingeldorf, Gd. Duchy de Luxemberg

Abstract

This paper reports the main investigation results of the Project "Agricultural Videotex Information Ergonomics", which was carried out in five EC countries, England, Ireland, Germany, Portugal and Spain. The principal objectives of this project were to find the reasons for agricultural users' dissatisfaction with VTX information systems, to determine the weakness of the user interface in the agricultural VTX information system and finally to provide some ergonomical recommendations for the agricultural VTX system designers.

1. Introduction

Videotex (VTX) is a mass medium that can be used for individual dialogue. It has opened up a completely new potential for the transmission of information. VTX is a medium offering a wide range of facilities such as transmission and reception of special news and information, data processing, VTX dialogue, creation of private user groups etc.

These facilities are however only being used to a limited extent. The introduction and use of these facilities are in many cases generously subsidised with public funds. VTX was thought to solve problems in the flow of information through the permanent access facility it offered. In fact, VTX has in the agricultural sector, as elsewhere, failed to establish itself alongside other media.

The reason for the low level of market penetration achieved by VTX to date appears to be that potential users were reluctant to subscribe because the amount of data offered was inadequate. Similarly, the potential suppliers of data and services were reluctant to participate because the number of VTX subscribers was too low [1].

Very little research has been devoted to software ergonomics and cognitive psychology in the design of man-machine dialogues in VTX systems [2]. In agriculture, where some work has been carried out [3], it was found that a large proportion of the end users were dissatisfied with the VTX system even after having worked with it for as long as one year, because they still found it difficult to understand and use. User-oriented dialogue design in VTX systems has been neglected in the past. Recommendations for the design of the masks failed to take account of the dynamics of interaction with the user. The selective improvements of the user interface can only be introduced after the lacking information on the conditions under which

VTX systems are used in important fields of application, e.g. agriculture, has been obtained and analysed.

An EC research project involving England, Ireland, Portugal, Spain and Germany was therefore devoted to investigating the shortcomings of the VTX system in those countries and to identify potential improvements in the farmer-VTX interface.

In order to reflect the range of user types, main enterprises and end-user technical equipment, twenty users of videotex in Ireland, Portugal and Spain were selected for a preliminary questionnaire. Case studies were carried out on ten users, a subset of the questionnaire survey sample, in each of these countries. The purpose of these case studies was to appraise how the system users were able to find both familiar and unfamiliar information on their videotex system and to try to establish the influence of software ergonomics on their ability to use the videotex systems with regards to efficiency and ease of use. Consequently this would help to determine areas where improvements could be made.

2. Analysis of weaknesses

2.1 Method

This analysis of weaknesses is based on the results of a survey carried out in four EC countries. The sample sizes in these four countries were 15 in Germany, 20 in Ireland, 20 in Portugal and 20 in Spain. The survey comprised a total of 37 questions, some of which were divided into several subsections. A preliminary test was carried out to check the validity and reliability of the survey procedure. This survey aimed to obtain information from agricultural users on the following points:

1) Data on use of the VTX system by farmers;
2) Data on the farmer's expectations from VTX;
3) Data on ease of use of the VTX system and the clarity and simplicity of the aids available to the farmers;
4) The verdict of the respondents on the quality of the available VTX services.

The survey also collected data on the hardware used, time of VTX installation, relative importance of VTX compared with other information sources, and the subjective appraisal by the user of his competence in working with VTX.

2.2 Results

In the survey 86% of the farmers used some form of dedicated VTX terminal. Philips terminals were used most frequently in Portugal and Minitel most frequently in Ireland. Only 14% of the users in the sample were using either a PC with software or a TV set with adapter.

The categories of information most frequently used varied from country to country, depending on the range of information offered by the relevant national VTX network. However, certain categories of information such as market information, weather information, plant health and agrometeorological information had a high rate of use among the farmers in all four countries.

The data for all countries and information categories showed that 63% of all respondents were highly proficient at retrieving information from the VTX system. Of all users 88% rated VTX "important" or "very important" as a source of information. And 53% of them perceived the system's 24-hour availability as the main benefit. The opportunity to conduct a dialogue came second with 31% of users, followed by time-saving in third place with 36% of users and greater convenience compared with other information sources for 27% of users. The wide range of information offered by VTX and VTX as a sole source of information came lower in the list of perceived benefits, but were mentioned by 35% and 29% of users respectively.

The negative aspects varied from country to country. The following points show some general opinion of the respondents to the weaknesses of the systems.

- **insufficient training**: Of all respondents in Ireland, Portugal, Spain and Germany 63% stated that their introduction into VTX had been only demonstration of how to use the system. Among them 17% received no training at all. Portugal was the only country in which all respondents had received some training, and it was also the only country in which professional training facilities were available.
- **poor organisation**: Dialogue between VTX users would be encouraged by the formation of organised user groups. Only 12% of the respondents in all four countries stated that a user group existed in their district. The remaining 88% stated that no user group existed or that they were unaware of the existence of such a group.
- **too little regional information**: One factor of particular importance to farmers is the availability of a local or regional service offering specific information. The farmers were dissatisfied with these services. They would like more information to be provided.
- **software ergonomics**: Overall satisfaction with VTX varies according to the ergonomics of the VTX software or, in other words, the ease of use. Of respondents in all four countries 43% reported difficulties in use, whilst 49% complained that there were too many menus and 25% complained about delays in information retrieval at busy times of day. Other 19% were dissatisfied with the speed of information retrieval and that they were sometimes cut out of the system.
- **user feedback**: Of respondents in all four countries 36% criticised the fact that it was not possible to made suggestions or comments on the VTX system. A further 39% stated that this facility existed, but they did not use it. Ireland was the only country in which 100% of the respondents knew of the suggestion facility, but 60% stated that they did not use it.
- **other weaknesses**: Other weaknesses stated by the respondents were high cost for investment and maintenance, instability of the system, only rudimentary arrangements for a European VTX link-up, response time too long, updating rates too low etc.

These strengths and weaknesses apply in varying degrees to the individual national VTX systems, but there were always complaints about difficulties in using the system.

3. Benchmark tests

3.1 Method

The aim of these benchmark tests was to assess the performance of respondents trying to carry out a series of information retrieval tasks on their normal videotex system. The respondents were rated according to their skill in retrieving both familiar and unfamiliar information. The tests ought to identify the points at which users experienced difficulties with the system, whether these difficulties arose in familiar or unfamiliar areas and whether any of the difficulties were caused by deficiencies in the ergonomic design of the system or of the information provided.

Benchmark tests were carried out in the field under the actual working conditions on the farms, and not in the laboratory. This meant that there was only limited scope to control the trial conditions.

The template for the benchmark design was created by Orca Computers Ltd. The Irish Agriline system was used as the model and this was adapted to suit the systems available in Portugal and Spain. The benchmark tests were completed by eight respondents in Ireland (two respondents were unable to complete the benchmark tests due to time pressure) and nine respondents in Portugal (one respondent could not complete the benchmark tests because of a telecommunication's problem) and ten respondents in Spain.

The following variables were determined in the benchmark tests with the help of a computerised video documentation of work flow and time measurements performed in accordance with time and motion study criteria:

1) Success rate (SR): SR is an indicator for the simplicity and clarity of the VTX system.
$$\text{SR}=\frac{\text{no. of targets successfully reached}}{\text{total no. of targets}}$$
2) Probability of correct menu choice (PCC): PCC is an indicator for both the versatility and the simplicity and clarity of the VTX system.
$$\text{PCC}=\frac{\text{no. of correct menu choices}}{\text{total no. of choices}}$$
3) Efficiency (E): The efficiency variable (E) makes is possible to identify deviations from the optimal algorithm.
$$\text{E}=\frac{\text{minimum no. of menu pages per target}}{\text{actual no. of pages accessed}}$$
4) Number of pages accessed (NP): NP is an indicator for the menu depth.
5) Search time (ST): ST illustrates the system's versatility and the qualities of the hardware and software.
$$\text{ST}=\frac{\text{total time taken to retrieve target}}{\text{no. of pages accessed}}$$
6) Time spent in search (TS): TS indicates the influence of all aforementioned factors.

These performance parameters would also be affected by the qualities, skill and ability of the user. In order to avoid any great discrepancy in accuracy, only three comparative categories were defined:

- 50% slower than the "expert user"
- slower than the "expert user"
- quicker than the "expert user"

3.2 Results

Success rate:

In Ireland 25% of the respondents had a success rate of 100%, 62.5% of them had a success rate over 90%. In Portugal and Spain the respondents had even better results (see table 1).

The fact that the success rate was high in all VTX systems shows that the retrieval of both familiar and unfamiliar information appeared to present no problems for the respondents.

Table 1: Success rate of the respondents

Ireland		Portugal		Spain	
Respondents	Success rate	Respondents	Success rate	Respondents	Success rate
25%	100%	67%	100%	100%	100%
62.5%	90%	33%	94%		
12.5%	85%				

Probability of correct menu choice:

The comparison of the parameter PCC for the various VTX systems shows clearly the effect produced by the comprehensive and complex range of information available from the Irish system. Although it is reasonable to assume that the Irish users are extremely experienced because they have been using the system longest, the mean value here for this parameter is the lowest (82.04 of 25 targets) and there is a substantial standard deviation (18.22) in the results.

The Portuguese system comes second (84.75 of 16 targets). The highest number of correct menu selections is to be found in the Spanish system (91.15 of 13 targets), despite the fact that the users there have relatively little experience. The reason for this is the simplicity of information available.

Efficiency:

The percentage of respondents who were as efficient as or more efficient than the expert was 77% for Irish system, 75% for Spanish system and 30% for Portuguese system. The Irish users were very experienced at operating their system and deviated very little from the optimal path despite the wide range of information offered and the risk of getting lost. The Spanish sample registered a similar high level of proficiency despite the fact that their training and experience was inferior, as demonstrated by other investigating methods. The only explanation for this similar level of proficiency is thus the simplicity of the Spanish VTX system. The Portuguese sample registered low efficiency levels, apparently the result of a combination of relatively short experience and a relatively complex system.

Average search time per page and no. of pages accessed:

Of the Irish respondents 37% were quicker than the expert in average search time per page, and 34% were quicker in time spent in the search process. 72% of the respondents accessed the same number of pages as the expert.

The probable reasons for this high level of proficiency are that the Irish system offers a wide range of useful information and the respondents use it frequently. They are therefore skilled at using the system and in the methods and sequences necessary for retrieving information. The Irish system offers the widest range of information of the three systems investigated.

For the Spanish system the majority of respondents were slower than the expert and had to access more pages than the expert. The Spanish system is slower and less complex than the Irish and Portuguese systems.

The Portuguese respondents were the slowest of the three. There are several reasons for this, such as the slowness of the system and the poor telecommunication links.

4. Checklist interview

4.1 Method

The purpose of this ergonomic checklist is firstly to ascertain where users of the videotex system experience difficulties or where they are not satisfied with the performance of the system taken from an ergonomic point of view. Secondly, it is aimed to establish how well the users are informed about the system and what it is able to do.

The design of the checklist, based on a checklist developed by Ravden and Johnson (1989) [4], took account of the fact that the respondents were not computer experts and that the checklist should be understood by a range of users including farmers, farm managers, agricultural services and agricultural information providers.

The checklist consists of eight sections, each section taking a different aspect of the videotex system.

1) **Section One**: ***Visual comfort and screen layout***
This section looked at the display of information and the ease of finding and entering information.
2) **Section Two**: ***Representational consistency***
This section looked at the consistency of information display and function keys.
3) **Section Three**: ***Ease of operation***
This section concerned with the ease of operating the videotex system and the ease of understanding instructions, commands and informational text.
4) **Section Four**: ***Error recognition and correction***
This section asked about the ease of preventing or correcting an error and the ability of the system to inform the user whether an error has been made.
5) **Section Five**: ***Appropriate functionality***
This section asked about the ease of moving within the system, the ease of finding desired information and the ease of comprehension of the system functions.

6) **Section Six**: ***User guidance and support***
   This section concerned with the availability of user guidance and support and the ease of using the help facility.
7) **Section Seven**: ***System usability problems***
   This section asked questions regarding specific areas of use of the system.
8) **Section Eight**: ***Open questions***
   This section asked general but more personal questions about the system and gave the respondents the opportunity to make any comments that they had not expressed or that they wanted to emphasise.

The checklist was answered by seven respondents in Ireland (three respondents were unable to complete the checklist due to time pressure) and ten respondents in both Spain and Portugal. The checklist was also answered by two videotex system experts from each of the three countries and their answers were used as a basis by means of which the answers of the respondents could be compared.

Although it is not possible to make a direct comparison between certain aspects of the three VTX systems due to the variety in complexity of the individual systems, an attempt has been made to obtain an overall impression from the respondents sampled and to try to establish possible similarities with regards to ergonomic problems within the three different systems examined.

4.2 Results

The satisfaction levels of the respondents with their individual system are shown in the figure 1. In general, the respondents were satisfied with their individual system. The segments and details with which the respondents were dissatisfied are analysed. Some ergonomical recommendations for the VTX system designer are made on this basis.

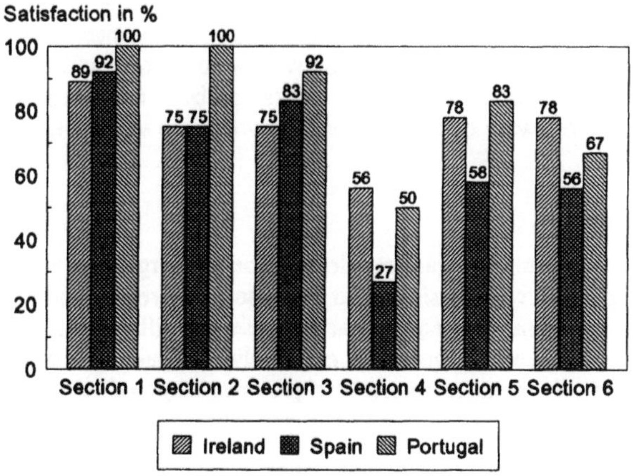

Figure 1. Level of satisfaction with the VTX system

Visual comfort and screen layout:

The majority of respondents was satisfied with the way of entering information and the clarity of displayed information. The respondents had different opinion about the background colour. Over 50% of the Spanish and Irish respondents prefered light colour over dark background, and 50% of the Portuguese respondents had the same opinion. The Spanish and Portuguese expert preferred however dark colour over light background.

Representational consistency:

The Irish respondents were considerably less satisfied with the consistency of information display and function keys of the system than the Portuguese and Spanish respondents. The reason is that the cursor was not always at the same place on the screen and its position had to be identified before being able to proceed.

Over the half of the Spanish respondents mentioned that colour was used in the VTX system inconsistently. The majority of the Spanish and Portuguese respondents thought it would be helpful if the colour used in VTX system was coded with a standardised meaning.

Ease of operation:

The satisfaction level in this section is high. In Ireland it was found that 43% of the respondents had difficulties in understanding informational text as a result of too many technical words being used.

The Spanish expert had the opinion that the experienced videotex user cannot make use of short-cuts with the help of special symbols or input commands.

Error recognition and correction:

The respondents were least satisfied with the error messages and error correction. In Ireland 56% of the respondents, in Portugal 50% and in Spain only 27% were satisfied with the error correction. The reason for the dissatisfaction is that none of the three systems allowed the system user any double-checking of an important command before the system carrying it out. Part of the respondents did not know how to correct an input error and the system gave the user no feedback on whether all errors had been corrected or not. In Spain only a few respondents were aware of the help facility, which shows how to correct an input error.

Appropriate functionality:

In all videotex systems information was considered to be well organised and all information necessary to completing a task was considered to be present. In Ireland and Portugal the use of special words and expressions does not appear to cause any difficulties. However 66% of the Spanish respondents answered this questions negatively. In Spain 67% of the respondents found if difficult to undo an action, to return to a previous stage of screen or to call up a desired page.

User guidance and support:

The Spanish respondents were the least satisfied among the three countries. This can be explained by the fact that only 11% of the Spanish respondents have a user's guide. There was also a general lack of awareness of the help facility. In Spain the help facility is not so extensive as that available in Ireland and Portugal. The Portuguese experts were also dissatisfied with the user guidance.

System usability problems:

Most of the respondents and all experts had no problems learning how to use the system. They did not think that there were too many colours used on the screen, but 80% of the Irish respondents found no improvement in ease of use when colours were used. The Irish expert found if difficult to call up the help facility and the system response time too long.

Open questions:

In this section came a variety of personal opinions given in the answers. The following are some of the more frequent observations made about the individual system, which were similar to the answers given in the first survey (analysis of weakness) but had more details about the shortcomings of the system.

The positive aspects in Ireland were the quick availability of information and the access to market information. In Spain these were the ease of use, systematic design, 24-hour service and the wide access to agricultural information. In Portugal these were the ease of getting up-to-date information, the ease of access to information and the clarity of menus.

The negative aspects in Ireland were the high cost and the inability to move in the system after pressing a wrong key. In Spain the respondents complained the difficulties obtaining a line, slowness of the system and that too many pages had to be gone through to access the desired information. In Portugal these were the slowness of system and the low updating rate of information.

The mistakes most often made by the respondents when using VTX system were hitting wrong keys, using wrong page number and misspelling.

5. Discussion

From the results it can be said that there do not appear to be any overwhelming problems or difficulties experienced by the respondents and any major lack of knowledge with regard to system capability. Difficulties are experienced in various areas and shortcomings of the systems and suggestions for improvements are varied.

Individual problems experienced are not always the results of the system but more the result of technical difficulties which affect the performance of the system. These technical difficulties are beyond the control of the system designers, for example the line problem. However, the areas needing improvement and consideration have be determined and analysed.

For agricultural users of VTX systems the designer must always take into consideration that most of them have no experience in using the system. It is consequently of permanent importance that information is clearly presented, simple to understand and that help is available either in the form of a manual or in an easily understandable computer help facility.

The questions of training users to be more efficient is another problem area. A user can be informed initially as to what is available and given an introductory training session - this information does not necessarily remain at the forefront of the users memory. Errors will always be made and therefore a successful and easy-to-use error correction facility is necessary.

Clarity of information and ease of comprehension and use are vital to the success of videotex as a source of information. The majority of videotex users use the system because it is a quick and easy method of obtaining up-to-date information and the system should be designed to encourage this and not to hinder it.

References

1 Kohler, C.U., BTX in der Landwirtschaft, DLG-Mitteilungen, Heft 20, 1986.

2 Landau, K., Man-machine interfaces in agricultural data processing applications, the green telematics challenge - proceedings of workshop held in Brussels, 9-10 June. , Luxembourg, 1989.

3 Schiefer, G., Akzeptanz und Nutzung von BTX in landwirtschaftlichen Betrieben, Deutscher Bauernverband e.V. (Hrsg.), Bildschirmtext in der Landwirtschaft, Bonn, 1985.

4 Ravden, S.J. and Johnson, G.I, Evaluating Usability of Human-Computer Interfaces, A Practical Method, New York, 1989.

WORK WITH DISPLAY UNITS 92
H. Luczak, A. Çakir and G. Çakir (Editors)

Video & Hypermedia for Communication between Groups

H. Miyamoto[a], T. Toriizuka[b], T. Inoue[b] & K. Noro[b]

[a]Department of Computer Science, Chiba Institute of Technology
2-17-1, Tsudanuma, Narashino 275 Japan

[b] School of Human Sciences, Waseda University
2-579-15, Mikajima, Tokorozawa 359 Japan

Abstract

In our days, as decentralized offices both in space and time become more and more common, the communication between humans through machine, or the communication between human and machine has become more important topics of research. Video & hypermedia communication will be one of the ultimate forms in such circumstances.

Here, we introduce a concept of "hyper communication" which is under development at the Research Committee of Human Interface, supported by JEIDA. Cognition of 3D vision, video conference and large screen display are discussed to illustrate the technological basis for hyper communication with their drawbacks and proposed solutions. Issues in ethics are also discussed in conjunction with human factors and a guideline for things to do and things not to do is proposed which will become important in the age of hyper communication.

1. INTRODUCTION

Along with the progress of microelectronics, an industrialized society where the productivity had the priority, came into a new stage: an information oriented society. There, in addition to the information, new functions, new materials and newly developed structures raise the values of the products. And due to the progress of the industrial science, those industrial products came to have more functions, higher quality and lower prices. However, with a greater number of functions, a product may become more difficult to use; for example, in the case of *high tech* products such as office automation equipment and personal computers, when the operation is very abstracted, every operation looks alike and it is very difficult to carry it out intuitively; the users tend to feel more stressed.

In this paper, we discuss why video & hypermedia are needed for a better human interface in group works with its appropriate usage. To improve the quality and quantity of information exchanges in communication, technological basis for hypermedia communication should be surveyed in conjunction with human factors. Three examples are discussed from the view point of human factors. Issues in ethics should be treated when this kind of hypermedia communication is used; a guideline for things to do and things not to do is pointed out for a healthy and sound human life to avoid harming somebody inadvertently through hyper communication.

2. WHY VIDEO & HYPERMEDIA ARE NEEDED FOR A HUMAN INTERFACE IN GROUP WORKS? ITS APPROPRIATE USAGE; HOW TO IMPROVE THE QUALITY AND QUANTITY OF INFORMATION EXCHANGES IN COMMUNICATION

2.1. Human Interface Committee of JEIDA and its activities since establishment

Human Interface Committee of the Japan Electronic Industry Development Association (JEIDA) , a non-profit organization composed of major electronic manufacturers in and out of Japan, is an official committee for improving ergonomics associated with VDT and other human-computer interfaces in Japan. The committee is working to pursue the ideal picture of human-computer interface in line with future technological renovations and to establish guidelines for the development of human-computer interface systems in the 1990s. The committee is now undertaking researches on the need for hypermedia in group work interface and proposes its correct use.

In the first half of the 1980s when visual display terminals (VDTs) were introduced, the committee gathered overseas information and cooperated with the Ministry of International Trade and Industry (MITI) in preparation of related materials. In 1989, the committee placed its basic focus on ergonomics, expanded its scope of topics, and initiated many-faced activities.

2.2. Hyper communication is a key tool of office communication in the 1990s: its purposes.

The word "hyper communication" means communication utilizing five senses and intuition of humans; there the human characteristics are even taken into account. It is used for communication between humans and computers, or between humans through computers.

With conventional electronic information processing systems for office work relationalization and productivity improvement, it's humans that must approach the system and not vice versa. The hyper communication system, however, has interfaces natural to the humans and serves as an intelligent tool to aid the humans in their creative activities.

2.3. The human Interface Committee consists of two sub-groups

The first group handling this program from physical aspects prepared a hyper communication map composed of technological factors, human factors, environmental factors, and basic research. The basic technological systems and recent topics of hyper communication are illustrated. The second group handling this program from psychological aspects compiled the results of past studies about telecommunication as a media usage pattern for hyper communication, transactional analysis as a research method for clinical psychology, and ethical standards to be observed in connection with hyper communication.

2.4. Future plans

The Human Interface Committee is searching for the ideal picture of human-computer interface and preparing guidelines for system development in the 1990s. Particularly, the committee is preparing system development guidelines concerning the effective use of a display screen, diversification of input and output methods, utilization of hypermedia, and introduction of groupware.

3. TECHNOLOGICAL BASIS FOR HYPER COMMUNICATION AND HUMAN FACTORS

Video teleconference among multi points, Computer Assisted Design (CAD) system using virtual reality, to name but a few, are all examples of hyper communication although they are yet at premature stage. Some potential technological tools for hyper communication are surveyed and analyzed from the view point of human factors (Table 1).

Table 1
Potential technological tools for hyper communication

DataGlove
Camera for HDTV
3D Digitizer using Magnetic Technology
Communication Aids using Synthesized Voice
High-Definition Display for Multimedia
Input/Output Devices for Disabled Persons
Recognition of Hand Gesture
CG and Color Representation
Image Data Compression Technology
Voice Recognition System
B-ISDN
Personal Display
DataSuit
Navigation System using Optical Fiber-based Gyroscope
Application of Fuzzy-Set Theory
Neural Network Technology
Virtual Reality
Hologram for 3D Display
Support Technology for Video Teleconference
3D Display for Bi-directional Communication

4. COGNITION OF 3D VISION, AND ITS APPLICATION TO HYPER COMMUNICATION

Stereoscopic images can convey a far greater amount of information than by conventional 2D images. As such images can provide 3D virtual space and virtual objects, 3D system may become an effective tool in hyper communication. Three dimensional spaces reproduced by stereoscopic images are, however, virtual spaces and are different from real ones which we ordinarily feel. In order to use such stereoscopic 3D images effectively, researches on the following points become important; how humans see, perceive, feel stereo images, and react to them, and the use of stereo images from the viewpoint of human factors.

4.1. Principle of 3D image and cognitive characteristics of human vision

Stereoscopic 3D images use the binocular disparity, one of the important information of 3D vision in human visual system as shown in Figure 1. The space and objects reconstructed by images can be calculated from the disparities between the images. With this technique, to provide an image of an apple, for example, which the observer wants to grasp, it is necessary to set the binocular disparities and viewing distance so that the reconstructed apple image may come within reach of the observer.

Stereoscopic 3D images are superior to conventional two-dimensional images in depth discrimination when the objects are slightly different in depth as illustrated in Figure 2. To use such 3D images more effectively, it is important to make clear the cognitive characteristics of human vision to the images and to choose parameters for image setting carefully.

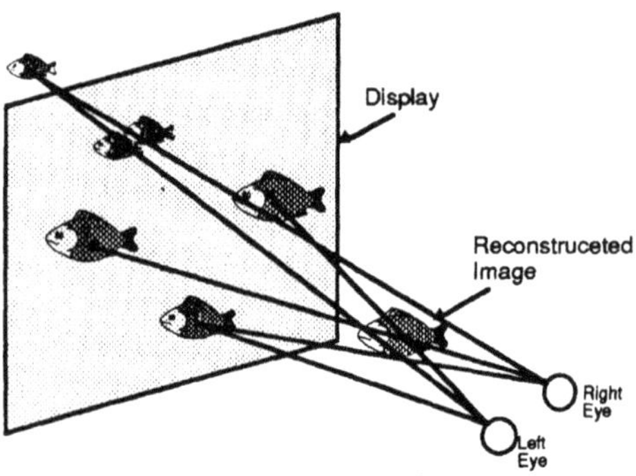

Figure 1. Stereoscopic 3D display

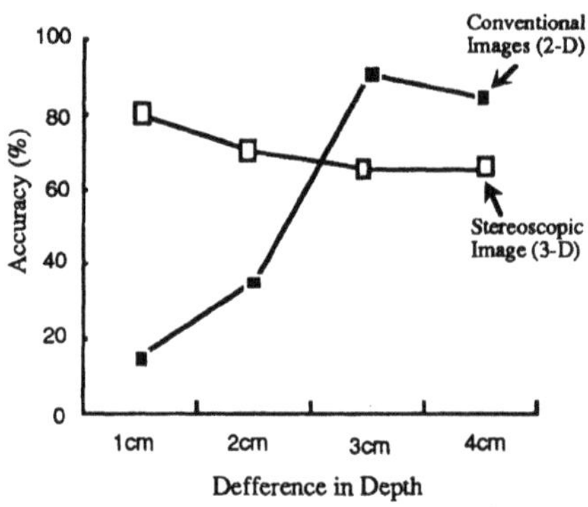

Figure 2. Experimental result of accuracy in depth discrimination

4. 2 Three-dimensional vision and virtual reality

Virtual reality system, a system giving a sense of reality although it is virtual one, is now widely studied in various fields. Virtual reality system transmits the visual or other sensory information to humans, and makes the virtual environment or virtual space in which the humans can react to such information. As stereoscopic 3D image can provide such a sense of reality, its application field will extend more and it will find its application in the fields of virtual CAD system, video art, supplementary tool for relaxation or rehabilitation.

5. USAGE OF A LARGE SCREEN DISPLAY SUCH AS 110"; SHALL MEN RESPOND IN THE SAME WAY AS WITH THE CONVENTIONAL DISPLAY?

Since several years ago, video displays of larger size have been used for a computer workstation, a control panel for plant surveillance, and in a video teleconference etc. Now, large screen displays as large as 110" are more and more used for presentation in a group work. In those cases, one might think that these displays differ only in geometrical scale, as far as viewing angles are the same, and that they can show the same amount of information, or in some cases, the larger the screen size is, the more information it can provide. But, shall men respond really in the same way to such a large screen display?

5.1. Use of large screen display in group works

We carried out experiments to see if there are any differences in eye movements of a subject seeing a video display screen of different size and with the different angle of view;

1) a conventional 14" display,
2) a 110" large screen display of rear projection type with the same angle of view as that for the 14" display,
3) the same 110" display with the doubled angle of view.

5.2. Comparative experiments

As the first task, a set of mazes of 29 by 40 squares were prepared and used at random during the experiments. Subjects (4 students) were requested to find and follow the right way from the entrance to the exit of the maze on 14" or 110" screen video display. When he/she failed to follow it or came to a dead end, he/she had to go back to the most recent point where he/she lost the right way, and started again until he/she arrived at the exit. In this experiment, the subjects were not permitted to use a pointer for a land mark in the maze.

As the second task, 14 short sentences starting with a different Japanese alphabet, were prepared and randomly placed. The same subjects as those participated in the first task were requested to sort and arrange these sentences by a simple mouse operation, so that the first character of each sentence is aligned in Japanese alphabetical order.

5.3. Reactions depend on the nature of information displayed

Numbers of fixation points per 1000 frames obtained by analyzing eye movements of a subject with Eyemark Recorder, are shown in Figure 3 as an example. In the first task, even though the viewing angle is kept unchanged, the results differs considerably between 14" conventional display and 110" large screen display, while in the second task, the difference between these two conditions is small. These preliminary experiments suggest that we react differently to images or texts on a video display depending on its size, even though the viewing angle is the same. The difference in reaction depends on the nature of the information displayed. It is thus important to consider this point when we design images or texts on a large screen display.

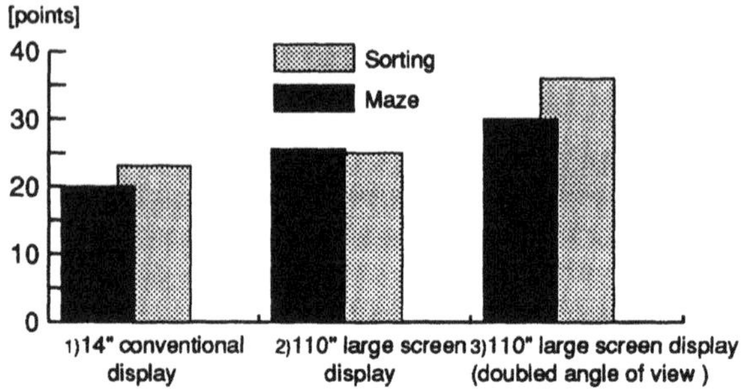

Figure 3. Numbers of fixation points per 1000 frames

6. PROBLEMS OF VIDEO CONFERENCE FROM THE VIEW OF POINT OF HUMAN FACTORS AND ITS SOLUTION

Video conference system is one of the communication systems with which we can share information with the persons in distance and can do complex work with them cooperatively and efficiently. With the conventional communication systems (for example, facsimile or e-mail), we transmit only logical and verbal information. With the video conference system (for example, teleconferencing system), in addition to them, visual information can also be exchanged between persons on the visual terminals. As the video conference system thus provides a new form of the communication systems among distant people, this system will be an effective tool of cooperative works.

6.1. What kind of functions are required for the video conference system?

The video conference system may provide an excellent communication means if we can communicate each other as if we met in person. In order to realize such video conference system, what kind of functions shall be required for the system? Examples of required functions are listed in Table 2. This is a list made by a Japanese company when it introduced the video conference system. It shows that the system is required to provide conditions similar to an ordinary conference. It should be noted that there is a strong demand for the sense of reality in the video conference.

Table 2
Requirements of Video Conference System

Conference can be set up at any time.
Conference can be held among several different places.
Voice of conferees can be clearly recognized.
Facial expression of conferees can be clearly recognized.
Conference shall have the sense of reality.

6.2. Levels of communication and problems of present system

Table 3 shows functions to be achieved according to levels of communication. Only the first level of communication is satisfied by the present video conference system. We carried out experiments changing lighting conditions to the conferees as well as the eye contact between conferees in the video conference system, but both are not yet well resolved in the present system.

Table 3
Levels of communication and the required functions of the system

1. Words and signals	Movement of a conferee's mouth can be recognized
2. Will and feelings	Facial expression of a conferee can be conveyed
3. Atmosphere in surroundings	Delicate atmosphere can be transmitted well

6.3. Various possible forms of video conference system in the future

Although present video conference systems are used only by a limited number of persons in limited situations, various applications could be expected if the system can satisfy the above conditions.

In Figure 4, various forms of the video communication system are shown according to the number of the persons and the distance of communication.

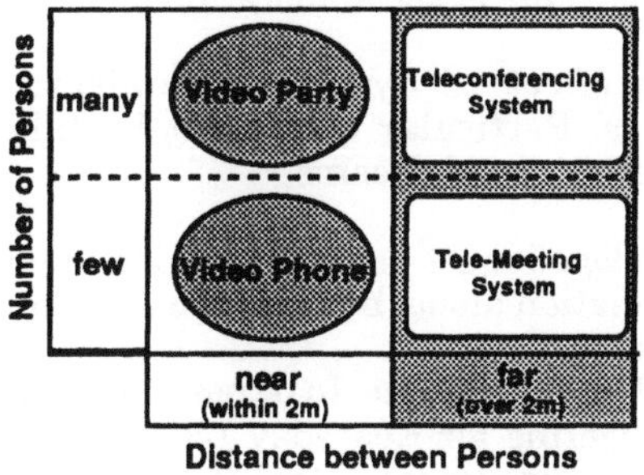

Figure 4. Various forms of video communication system

7. ETHICS IN THE USE OF HYPER COMMUNICATION

Technology has played an important role in advancing the 20th century to the present stage. Criticism has been leveled at technology a few behind the progress of technology. This delay has not allowed the criticism to be made fully used of in improving the technology. The ethical standards have been established after reflecting on this point.

Present information technology must be friendly to users or readily usable by everybody without any trouble, must improve the capability of individual persons, and must not interfere with human activities. As the information technology tends to make equipment too complex and difficult to use, it should be particularly noted that such equipment is very demanding on elderly or physically handicapped people. Another thing to be recognized is that the spread of the information technology is increasing the complaint of mental stress, which is known as techno-stress in various parts of society.

7.1. A guideline for things to do and things not to do for a healthy and sound human life

Ethical standards to be observed in the development and diffusion of hyper communication and hypermedia are described as draft version in a JEIDA report[1] as follows:

1) *Responsibility for environment and society*
   Considering new media, for example, we must not only tout the convenience and novelty of the new media, but also consider the effect of the new media on the health, comfort, mental stress, and physical stress of users.
2) *Responsibility for improvement in human capability*
   Users must be informed of to what degree they can expect their capability to improve when they utilize the new system or equipment to be developed.
3) *Responsibility for principle of justice*
   New scientific terms like fuzzy-set theory and neural network theory are used too casually. The electric appliance industry is beginning to worry about this trend. Some manufacturers think it easier to advertise their products using *big words* rather than to spend time for conducting painstaking research. They must take note of social morality.
4) *Responsibility for future*
   We must always consider the effect of hyper communication and hypermedia on the future of users. Particular care must be taken lest children lose their humanness, creativity, and dreams.
5) *Responsibility for human*
   Equipment and systems to be developed must promote the rich humanness of users, and must not pursue automation alone, but also provide users with a sense of participation and satisfaction.

Compilation of these ethical standards is significant. In Japan, the University of the Air has been broadcasting "Engineering for Everyday Life" as one of the elective subjects for social industry course students from April 1992.

8. CONCLUSIONS

A concept of hyper communication has been presented which means communication utilizing five senses and intuition of humans, by taking the human characteristics into account. Human factors related to each potential technological tool has been studied to realize an effective hyper communication system. An ethical guideline is pointed out as ethics will become important in the age of hyper communication.

1 Japan Electronic Industry Development Association: New Office System Survey Report 1991, Tokyo, pp.155-181.

WORK WITH DISPLAY UNITS 92
H. Luczak, A. Çakir and G. Çakir (Editors)

Human-Centered Development of Knowledge-Based Systems[1]

M. Kloth[a], M. Hoenen[a], M. Geenen[b] and B. Busch[b]

[a]Fraunhofer-Institute for Materialflow and Logistics, Joseph-von-Fraunhofer-Str. 2-4, W-4600 Dortmund 50, Germany

[b]University of Bonn, Informatik III, Römerstr. 164, 5300 Bonn 1, Germany

Abstract

The focus of this presentation is the description of an alternative software development method that considers human-oriented criteria to ensure the user's qualifications. Different modes of use shall satisfy the needs of qualified users. Finally, we give an example of some modes of use. The chosen domain is logistic-planning.

1. PROBLEMS IN THE USE OF SOFTWARE

Todays knowledge-based systems often are not useful to handle complex tasks. In several presentations and interviews with users we identified problems in the use of knowledge-based systems. These problems concern the user's qualification, the quality or efficiency of work or the quality of products. Some of them are caused by decisions during the development of the systems.

They can be considered as mismatches between the user's skills and needs, the user's task, the system, and the surroundings. Some of them could have been avoided or overcome by adequate decisions (e.g. concerning modes of use - see 3) during the development of the system.

For example, the user of a system for the configuration of process control computer systems had to interrupt configuration for two or three days when new components were needed that still had to be specified in the knowledge base by the maintenance - instead of inserting it himself. He also could not obtain information why the system would not accept certain components in a certain place. So, instead of checking it out by looking possible reasons in the documentation, he first tried all other components. Or the users of a system

---

1 This paper is based on the hitherto results of two research projects the authors are involved in. These projects are entitled "Design of Expert Systems Ensuring Qualification and Quality" and "Ensuring Qualifications and Quality as a Goal in the Process of Designing Expert Systems". Both are part of a research initiative comprising six cooperating projects with the theme "Changes of Knowledge Production and Knowledge Distribution by Expert Systems" sponsored by the Federal Ministry of Research and Technology (FRG).

about public aids implemented for the support of credit consultations did not know how to interprete certain questions or how to classify certain facts concerning a question. They also resigned about altering facts because the undo function was too difficult to handle.

In regard to the problems of the validation and verification of expert systems (see also [1]) we demand that the users of knowledge based systems shall be skilled enough to proof the adequacy of the systems use and the correctness of the results.

Experts using expert systems that are designed as monotonic problem solvers (see 3) as described above are strongly restricted in their praxis. The dominance of this mode of use turns out to be problematic considering human-oriented criteria based on ergonomics [2, 3, 4], e.g., freedom of action and choice, absence of strong time restrictions, opportunity for variations, possibilities to structure the work and preserve of direct social contacts. The problem-solving mode of use is the result of the employer's intentions -- standardization of procedures (one-best-way) and conservation of knowledge -- as well as the developer's ambitions and concepts -- simulation of experts and formalization of knowledge. In consequence systems are built that reduce the scope of actions, determine the procedures and obtain extensive competences of the user. For example, in many domains (consulting, planning, design) a usual practice is slightly varying a case until there is an acceptable solution. We found expert systems that did not allow users to change comfortably inputs and thus prevented them from experimenting and optimizing solutions.

2. ALTERNATIVE CONCEPTS AND METAPHORS

Other concepts and metaphors as tool [5], workshop [6, 7] and working resources [8] point to the concept of *open work environments* for skilled users. In such work environments experts are able to decide by themselves which sub tasks the systems should support. However, concepts alone are not sufficient as a framework for the development of knowledge-based systems. Alternative development processes are necessary to realize the concept of an open work environment.

This paper presents an approach to transform the new concepts into a framework for knowledge-based system design. This framework can be used as an aid for human-centered development processes. The basic idea in this approach is the development of a model in the sense of an informal description of the domain and the course of actions. This model supports a far-reaching participation of users by making available a communication platform between developers and users. This joint modeling shall support transparency and validity of the development process as well as the system's usability for the user.

The modeling process helps to find an adequate distribution of tasks and functions between the user and the system. It takes into account specific requirements of individual methods of working and cooperative work. Therefor the tasks and the different ways to structure the work have to be analyzed and documented. The next step is to find out, which sub tasks shall be supported by the system and the selection of adequate modes of use for each sub task. Finally the whole system design shall allow the user to decide for each sub task and each case if he needs support in his work or not.

3. DIFFERENT MODES OF USE FOR EXPERT-SUPPORTING SYSTEMS

During the modelling process the entire variety of possible modes of use should be considered for a selection of modes adequate to the specific task, organization of work and users' qualification. For systematic reasons this variety can be described as divided in four major groups -- use for problem solving, use as a medium, exploring and modifying the system.[2]

Problem solving certainly is the purpose knowledge based systems are designed for. The most traditional and widespread mode of use for problem solving might be one we call "*monotonic problem solving*". It can be characterized by a phase of system-driven input selection (possibly partially driven by inference) followed by a presentation of a result. The designation "monotonic" is derived from the conception that such a mode of use does not allow the retraction or alteration of inputs or intermediate results. This mode of use may result from the employer's intentions and the designer's ambitions and lead to the consequences as pointed out in the beginning. Possible alternative or complementary modes of use for non-monotonic problem solving are *varying the present case* by altering inputs on the base of intermediary results presented by the system[3] or a so-called "*critiquing mode*" that allows the input of user's hypothesis for verification or completion. Another possibility is using the system for the *retrieval of similar* (solved) *cases* for further variation or a take-over of results.

These modes of use can be supported by the ones of the other groups, that contribute only indirectly to problem solving:

Exploration includes modes of use allowing users to gain information about the scope and the limits of the system and how to use it, about the elements of the knowledge base and their dependencies, and about the state of the problem solving process, e.g., what facts have been collected, why an input is prompted, how a result has been or why an expected result has not been derived. In contrast to traditional explanation components exploration is based on the user's own activity and responsibility as far as possible, e.g., offering graphical and direct manipulation facilities for investigations or supporting experiments by undo functions and freezing points.

Modifications might concern elements of the knowledge base, interaction styles or the order of the dialogue. Modification by the user could help to adapt the system more fluently to changes in the domain or to individual working styles.

The *use as a medium* means storing, retrieving or transmitting information for oneself or to or from others. Medial modes of use are the administration of a *case base*, storing or retrieving informal *background information* about questions or elements of the knowledge base (such as texts, pictures or hypertext

---

2 For overviews on possible modes of use of expert systems see [9,10], for an overview on critiquing systems see [11], for an overview on case based reasoning [12], for the principle of exploration see [13, 14].

3 This might technically afford a truth-maintenance system or a quick re-computation based on the altered input.

structures referring to author, meaning or purpose) or support of *cooperative maintenance* and modification. They might help to preserve or restore context of formalized knowledge.

4. AN OPEN WORK ENVIRONMENT FOR LOGISTIC PLANNERS

The following describes a development that is based on the above mentioned approach where different modes of use are integrated to a comprehensive system [15, 16, 17]. The application is located in the domain of logistic-oriented facilities planning. Facilities planning or, in a narrower sense, layout planning is a task, planners have to deal with during the design or redesign of factories. During this iterative process they have to work on, refine, and combine different sub tasks to a complete result: e.g., the selection of conveyer and storage technologies, the determination of the production type and structure, and the positioning of components on the basic floorspace. Repeatedly, they have to consider new requirements, goals and restrictions. Therefore they need a lot of intuition and creativity besides their domain-specific qualification to be able to integrate the requirements and restrictions which cannot be determined in advance into the solution.

The usability in the sense of an open work environment requires an adequate distribution of tasks and functions between user and system based on the above mentioned modeling results. The task distribution is oriented towards the idea of supporting the planner's strengths and not replacing him in areas he can manage better.

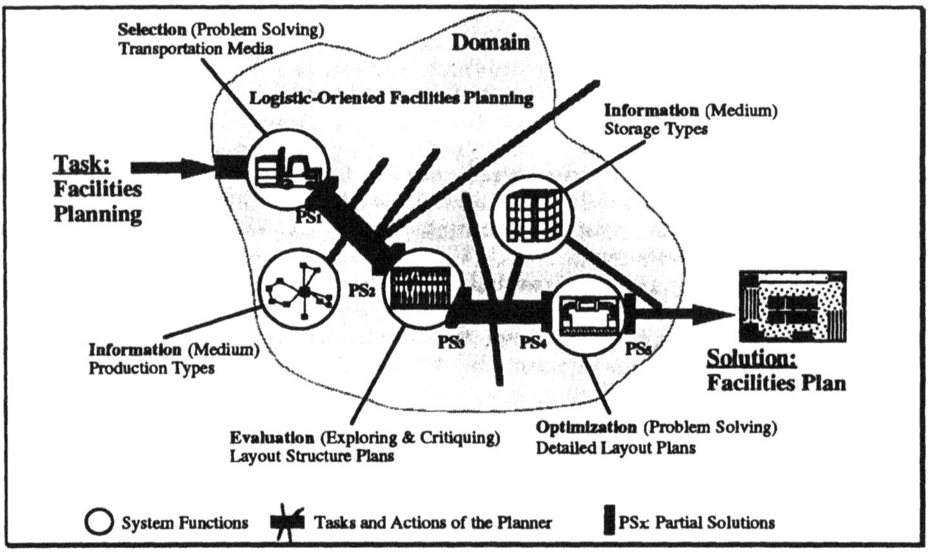

Fig.: An example for a user's choice of modes of use during facilities planning

The simultaneous offer of different modes of use for the tasks allows the user to choose how much support he needs or is able to get for each sub task. Whereas, e.g. (see figure), the user can choose the system to solve particular sub tasks that depend on detailed calculations (problem-solving of selection tasks) he himself can design intuitive and creative partial solutions which are evaluated by the system (exploring and critiquing of partial layouts). The system additionally can support the planner's decision by presenting information (system as medium concerning information about production or storage types). Other choices of modes of use lead to alternatives in the problem solving process so that the user is not restricted to "one-best-way".

This makes it possible to involve the planners qualification into the planning process and therefore to overcome the limitations of formal representation. Thereby, they can consider new and imprecise relations and goals (e.g., aesthetics and human assessments and criteria). Together with the modification mode (e.g., the adjustment of dialogue facilities and the modification of rules and functions), planners can integrate the system in their daily work to design real, practical oriented layouts. The meanings of these sub tasks are known by the user so that he is able to handle and manipulate them in a virtuoso way. The experience and the knowledge of the planner play an important role in the problem-solving process because the whole domain of facilities planning (gray hatched area in the figure) is too complex and too fuzzy to be manipulated by the system adequately.

The aim of this development is to make an open work environment available to planners in which they are able to select various modes of support depending on their different requirements and tasks. The described development process is helpful to realize the concept of an open work environment and therefore to avoid negative impacts on the user's qualification, the quality of work and the quality of products.

REFERENCES

[1] E. Steven, M. Hoenen, M. Kloth: Testability of expert systems in system development and application; to appear in: AI & Society

[2] W. Hacker: Software-Gestaltung als Arbeitsgestaltung; in: K.-P. Fähnrich (ed.): Software-Ergonomie 1987, Oldenbourg, München 1987, pp. 29-42

[3] E. Ulich: Arbeitspsychologie; Poeschel-Verlag, 1991

[4] W. Volpert: Verantwortbare Aufgabengestaltung für Informatik-geprägte Arbeitsplätze, Springer, Berlin 1990, pp. 168-177

[5] P. Ehn: Work-Oriented Design of Computer Artifacts; Almqvist & Wiksell, Stockholm 1988

[6] H. Oberquelle: Perspektiven der Mensch-Computer-Interaktion und kooperative Arbeit; in: M. Frese (ed.): Software für die Arbeit von morgen; Springer, Berlin 1991, pp. 45 - 56

[7] U. Klotz: Die zweite Ära der Informationstechnik; in: Harvard Manager, No. 2, 1991, pp. 101-112

[8] W. Volpert: Die Spielräume der Menschen erhalten und ihre Fähigkeiten fördern; in: Documentation of the conference: KI - Anspruch und Praxis im Unternehmen, 27./28. 6. 1991, Rüschlikon / Zürich

[9] Th. Herrmann, B. Busch, M. Geenen: Vielfalt von Interaktionsmöglichkeiten - Ein Gestaltungsziel bei Expertensystemen, in: D. Ackermann, E. Ulich (eds.): Software-Ergomomie '91, Teubner, Stuttgart 1991, pp. 162-171
[10] Th. Herrmann: Experts' Systems instead of Expert Systems; in: N. I. Nurminen, P. Järvinen, G. Weir (eds.): Proceedings of the Conf. on Human Jobs and Computer Interfaces, University of Tampere, Finland, 1991, pp. 305-319
[11] B. G. Silverman: Survey of Expert Critiquing Systems: Practical and Theoretical Frontiers; in: Communications of the ACM, Vol. 35, No. 4, 1992, pp. 106-127
[12] K.-D. Althoff, S. Wess, B. Bartsch-Spörl, D. Janetzko, F. Maurer, A. Voß: Fallbasiertes Schließen in Expertensystemen; in: KI 4/92, 1992, pp. 13-21
[13] H. Paul: Exploratives Agieren in interaktiven EDV-Systemen, in: B. Endres-Niggemeyer, Th. Herrmann, A. Kobsa, D. Rösner (eds.): Interaktion und Kommunikation mit dem Computer; Springer Verlag, Berlin, Heidelberg u.a., 1989, pp. 80-93
[14] Th. Herrmann: Support of Intervening Use. In: P. Brödner, W. Karwoski (eds.): Ergonomics of Hybrid Automated Systems III. Amsterdam et al.: Elsevier. pp. 289-294
[15] M. Kloth, I. Land, J. Herrmann: Ein wissensbasiertes Assistenzsystem für die Layoutplanung; in: W. Görke, H. Rininsland, M. Syrbe (eds.): Information als Produktionsfaktor; Springer, Berlin 1992, pp. 657-668
[16] B. Hellingrath, M. Hoenen, I. Guschok: Wissensbasierte Systeme unterstützen die Transportmittelauswahl; in: Fördertechnik, Spring 1992
[17] M. Kloth, M. Hoenen: Working With Instead Of At The Computer; in: P. Brödner, W. Karwowski: Ergonomics in Hybrid Automated Systems III, Elsevier, Amsterdam, London, New York, Tokyo, 1992, S. 337 - 342

WORK WITH DISPLAY UNITS 92
H. Luczak, A. Çakir and G. Çakir (Editors)

Psycho-Physiological Strain in Design-Work.

A Comprehensive Investigation on Design-Work with Drawing-Board and a CAD-System.

Thomas Müller

Institut für Arbeitswissenschaft, Technische Universität Berlin,
Ernst-Reuter Platz 7, D-W-1000 Berlin 10, Germany

1. Introduction

In mechanical engineering drawing boards are replaced more and more by Computer Aided Design (CAD) systems. Such CAD systems do not only change the physical work place, they also require several new or modified working techniques. The impacts of the use of CAD on designers workload are not cleared up yet, but there are at least two contradictory tendencies:

- The (semi-) automation of several routine drawing tasks (dimensioning, hatching, copying of details) should reduce workload.
- The 'interaction-problem', e.g. the necessity of mental representation of commands, menus, and syntax of a CAD-system, in addition to the 'design-problem' itself, should increase overall workload.

Furthermore an impact of the type of the task and the skill of the designer might be suspected (Müller et al., 1989).

To find out which of these tendencies is predominant, i.e. to find out, if the use of CAD will reduce workload and stress for the designer or if it constitutes a new source of stress, laboratory experiments were carried out.

2. Methods

Design Tasks for Experiments: The design tasks for the experiments were limited to *mechanical design* (i.e. not architectural or electrical design), *geometric modelling* (no calculations or selecting of materials), and tasks being estimated to be worked out within a *time limit* of two hours. A selection of design-tasks meeting these conditions was rated by experts in several dimensions of difficulty. Three final dimensions of task-difficulty (functional aspects, production related aspects, and aspects of graphical representation) were extracted by factor analysis. Finally a set of 8 (= 2^3) tasks was selected, having extreme (high vs.

low) factor-scores in each of the three dimensions.

Test subjects: Test subjects were 20 students of mechanical engineering (male, mean age 23.3 years (s = 2.9 years) with no or minor further experience with CAD. The participants were trained before the experiments in a compact-course of 40 hours duration on the CAD-system (Beitz et al., 1990).

Analysis of the course of action: Three types of drawing activities were distinguished: (1) Activities increasing the quantitative extent of the drawing, (2) activities decreasing the quantitative extent (erasing or deleting of elements), and (3) activities of manipulation (on CAD-Systems these operations are often performed with features summarised under a menu-item called "EDIT"). The latter do not affect quantity, but usually improve the quality of the representation (for more details see Müller, 1992).

Analysis of design results: The final design results are available as drawings (hand-drawing or computer-plot resp.). The drawings are analysed according to the quantitative extend (number of drawing elements), completeness and quality (degree of fulfilment of requirements named in task).

Analysis of perceived and physiological strain: Some physiological measures (e.g. heart-rate and variability, breath-rate, and skin-conductance) were registered (for more details see Müller, 1992). Particularly the variability of heart-rate (sinus-arrhythmia) yields information about load on human information processing capacities, especially load on short term memory (Aasmann et al. 1987).

Experimental schedule: The three dimensions of task-difficulty with two levels each (see above) and the tool (drawing-board vs. CAD-system) constitute an experimental design of the 2^4-type, i.e. 16 cells. Since each subject executes half of the 8 tasks with CAD (AutoCAD, Version 2.6, English) or drawing-board respectively, 160 work sessions were carried out. The total duration is about 250 hours.

3. Results

As expected, an increase in task difficulty results in weaker quality of design and increases working-time. Surprisingly, the use of CAD has similar effects as higher task-difficulty (figure 1).

The effects of the drawing tool are understandable looking at the activities performed during work-session (table 1). Subjects are generating approximately the same quantity of elements at the two work-places. But at the CAD workplace they delete four times the number of elements and make changes on almost five times the number of elements. Defining work-efficiency as the ratio of output (progress of drawing) to input (number of operations)+), we find, efficiency is twice as high at the drawing board as with the CAD-system (table 1).

+) Efficieny = $(\Sigma_{Generate} - \Sigma_{Delete}) / (\Sigma_{Generate} + \Sigma_{Delete} + \Sigma_{Edit})$

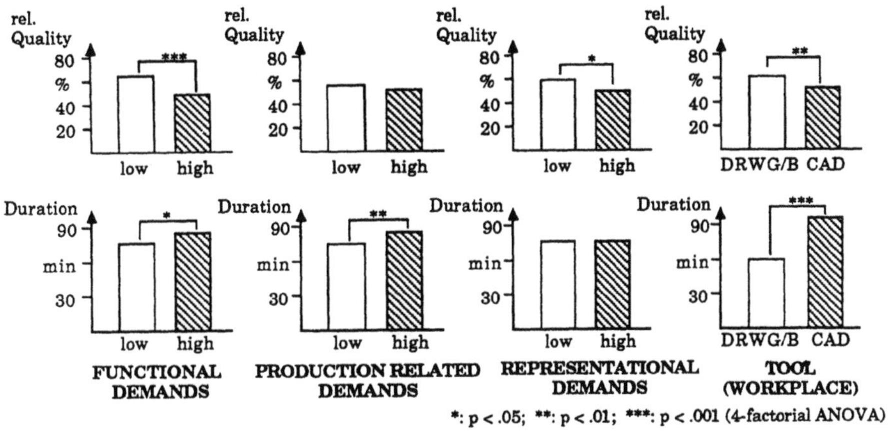

Figure 1: Quality of design results and time required by task-difficulty (3 dimensions) and tool (CAD vs. drawing-board).

According to design theory (e.g. Pahl and Beitz, 1984) different phases of the design-process can be distinguished. Such phases are embodiment design, detail design, and drawing (of a given geometry). Early phases, as embodiment design, are characterised by planning activities, search for information and creativity, later phases (detail design and drawing) by algorithmic and routine work.

Table 1: Drawing activities per work-session.

	TOOL	
TYPE OF ACTIVITY	DRAWING-BOARD	CAD-SYSTEM
Generating Element	111	134
Deleting Elements	10	45
Manipulating Elements	27	128
Efficiency	.68	.30

Figure 2 shows the number of manipulation (edit-) operations per minute by design-phase. During embodiment design three times the number of edit-operations is performed with CAD than at the drawing board. The ratio is only 1.7 during detail design and 1.2 during drawing.

Obviously there is not a general necessity for more edit-operations when working with CAD then there are at the drawing board. Furthermore, the number of edit-operations per minute at the CAD-workplace is minimum, when demands on creativity are minimum.

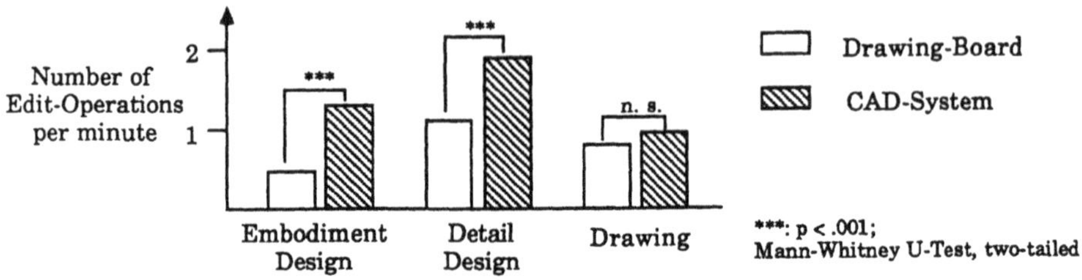

Figure 2: Manipulation ("EDIT") operations per minute by design phase.

Generally, in phases with higher (cognitive) demands the subjects made more mistakes and therefore had to make more changes.

A bottleneck in the mental capacities might be suspected, since creative problem-solving and interaction with the CAD-system use the same mental capacity. An indication for this hypothesis was found by further analysis:

Figure 3 shows the (standardised) 0.10 Hz component of power spectra of heart rate by relative drawing activity. Planning activities and other creative and cognitive activities are suspected to take place in time-sequences where subjects do not draw or draw less than average, and, vice versa, time sequences with increased drawing activities are estimated to be routine work. Effects at the drawing board are as expected: the less the subjects draw, the higher is memory load (low scores of the 0.10 Hz component indicate high load on human memory!). Quite unexpected were the effects found at the CAD-workplace. Obviously drawing itself causes load on human working memory working with CAD.

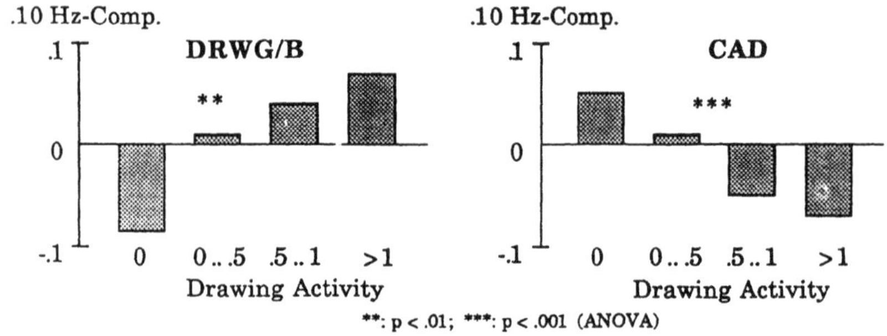

Figure 3: Z-scores of the 0.10 Hz component of power-spectra of heart rate

This is why it is suspected here that work with CAD produces a bottleneck in human working memory when design tasks are more difficult. The result is an increase of the number of errors, which require deleting and edit-operations.

4. Discussion

As pointed out, work-efficiency on drawing oriented tasks is lower with CAD than at the drawing board. Since this fact has meanwhile been proofed in several field studies with different CAD-Systems and also for experienced designers (Derisavi-Fard et al., 1989, Springer, 1992) we can be sure, that this is not a laboratory artefact. But efficiency measured here is not identical with efficiency in industrial use, since there are a lot of tasks not investigated here, where CAD will achieve higher productivity (e.g. engineering change requests, NC-programming, technical calculations).

But if it is true that this efficiency-deficits are a result of a bottleneck in human working memory greater problems may arise: If a greater partition of mental capacity is used for interaction with the CAD-system - and as we know human working memory has a limited capacity - deficits may occur in the process of problem solving in design. That would mean that we get weaker design with CAD. The laboratory experiments reported here give some indication that it is true.

So ergonomic activities are necessary to avoid that Computer Aided Design Systems become a handicap for the designer.

5. References

Aasmann, J., Mulder, G., and Mulder, L. J. M. (1987): Operator Effort and the Measurement of Heart-Rate Variability. *Human Factors*, vol. 29, no. 2, p. 161-170.

Beitz, W., Langner, Th., Luczak, H., Müller, Th., and Springer, J. (1990): Evaluation of a CAD-Course in Laboratory Experiments. *International Journal of Human Computer Interaction*, vol. 2, no. 2, p. 111-135.

Derisavi-Fard, F., Frieling, E., Hilbig, I. (1989): *Ermittlung der Belastung und Beanspruchung beim computersunterstützten Konstruieren* (VDI Fortschritt-Bericht 20/15). Düsseldorf: VDI-Verlag.

Müller, Th. (1992): *Handlungsvollzug und psycho-physische Beanspruchung bei Konstruktionstätigkeiten* (VDI Fortschritt-Bericht 1/215). Düsseldorf: VDI-Verlag.

Müller, Th., Springer, J., and Langner, Th. (1989): Job Analysis in Design Work. In: Landau, K. and Rohmert, W. (Eds.): *Recent Developments in Job-Analysis*. London, New York, Philadelphia: Taylor and Francis.

Pahl, G. and Beitz, W. (1984): *Engineering Design*. London: The Design Council.

Springer, J. (1992): *Systematik zur ergonomischen Gestaltung von CAD-Software* (VDI Fortschritt-Bericht 20/60). Düsseldorf: VDI-Verlag.

WORK WITH DISPLAY UNITS 92
H. Luczak, A. Çakir and G. Çakir (Editors)

Systematic Evaluation and Optimization of CAD Systems

J. Springer

Institute of Industrial Engineering and Ergonomics,
Aachen University of Technology, Germany

Abstract

For the development of ergonomically based design recommondations for CAD Systems field studies were carried out. The examination of different standard tasks and actual design projects was documented by video and psychophysiological data. Different strain situations were identified by cross correlation products between activities an strain reactioins. Such an analysis formed the basis for the identification of system difficiencies and recommondations for an optimization of the CAD System investigated. The recommondations were ordered into a systematics of human-computer interaction activities.

1. INTRODUCTION

Todays design departments are usually equipped with highly sophisticated CAD systems. Their application should increase the design efficiency to rationalize the product-development-process. But more and more experiences of CAD users show a gap between the goals and reality of CAD introduction (e.g. ABELN et al. 1990). Also, experiments in different design departments verify deficiencies in the use of advantages of the functional capacities of CAD systems (LUCZAK et al. 1991). This is one reason for the poor performance in performing technical drawings.

In a design department there is neither a question of the rationalization goal nor the implementation of CAD systems. Today the characteristics of a CAD system is important to improve adequacy and the adaptation to different user qualifications. But if ergonomic design rules are not taken into consideration the consequence will be a low design efficiency and a higher strain level.

Requirements on CAD systems must be based on the working condition, especially on the tasks of the designers. The task of a designer can be divided into subtasks which implies activities and operations. A task oriented systematically based analysis of a realistic design process opens the possibility to identify bottle necks and system deficiencies and to build a basis for concrete system improvements. System deficiencies are interpreted by operational characteristics and identified strain situations. One problem of such methods are the design tasks itself: they are complex and mostly the operations are not determinable. That´s the reason why ergonomic requirements were scarcely formulated to CAD system design rules. Furthermore, in existing requirements only some are based on experimental data and the most include mainly performance aspects to the work with CAD systems (HEINECKE 1991). Neither stress and strain aspects nor the characteristics of necessary design activities and operations were taken into consideration.

For the development of a requirements catalogue related to stress/strain-aspects and design activities field studies in different design departments were carried out. The methods used were firstly validated in laboratory experiments. The main focus of the experiments was a continuous analysis of the working process.

2. THEORETICAL BACKGROUND

The interaction process between a user and a computer is an interchange of signs with defined meanings. Based upon a semiotic model (MORRIS 1946) which is funded by communications theory a system of signs include syntactical, semantical and pragmatical aspects. The syntax defines the „in-between-relation" of signs, the semantics the relation to an object and the pragmatical aspect the task related goal of the information interchange.

This forms a systematically build hierarchy of an interaction process, where

- firstly the interaction goal had to be defined and the objects for the goals characterization had to be selected,
- secondly the objects had to be assigned to a defined syntax, and
- thirdly, under a technical information aspect, the signs must be interchanged by a physical way, e.g. visual, auditive, or kinesthetic information (RASMUSSEN 1983).

Such a structured user activity model is related to a correspondent functionality of a CAD system.

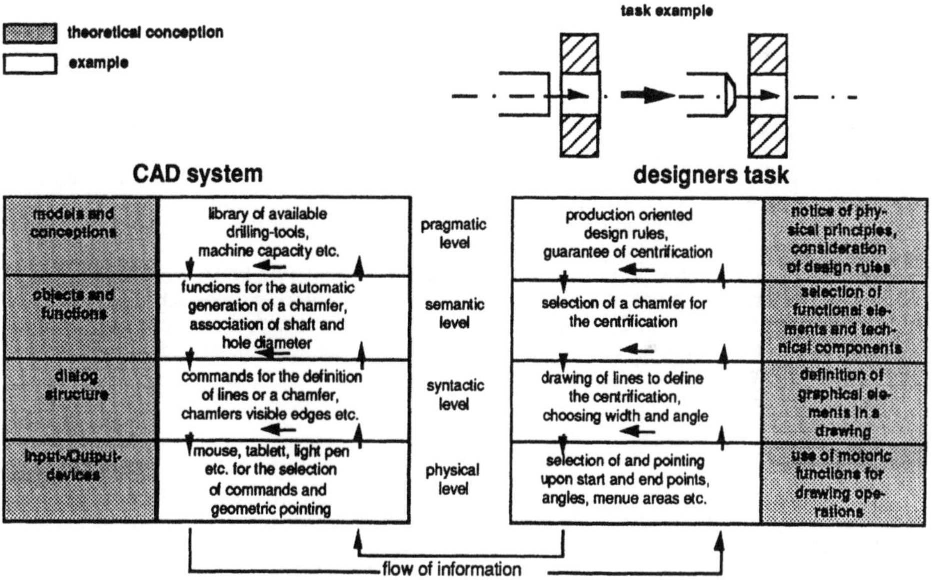

Figure 1. Example of the human-computer interaction process while performing a designers sub-task

Figure 1 shows the elaboration of a designers sub-task e.g. the ensurance of a centrification. First of all on the pragmatic level the user has to define the design goal, the production oriented design of a product part. After the formulation to ensure the centrification, on the semantic, that is the funtional level, a chamfer might be choosen as one possibility for eht entrification ensurance. Also the position and the dimensions of the chamfer are defined on that level.

In a design department normally the technical drawing represents the defined syntax for the technical communication. Therefore the syntax of the interaction process consists of the generation of lines, the selection of geometrical elements as borders, and the definition of start and end points and angles of the chamfer lines. On the physical level movements must be carried out for a selection of commands or the identification of elements. These movements are initiating commands for a generation or manipulation of the chamfer lines to represent the border lines of the centrification, that´s the syntactical level of the CAD system. The functionality of the CAD software generates the lines by electronic data and, if possible, connects for example the diameter of the shaft and the drill-hole semantically. For exapmple on the pragmatic level of the CAD system the system could proove the existance of tools for the production of such a chamfer, or the productions costs.

Shown by this example it is possible to describe all activities and operations on the users side and of the CAD sytem with the help of such a hierarchically structured systematology (SPRINGER 1991).

3. METHODS

Methods of videotechnique were used for a systematic investigation of the interaction process. The acivities were interpreted correspondent to the levels of the interaction model, e.g. the designer´s movements of a mouse to select a special point in a menu are interpreted as operations on the physical level; the execution of a function represents an action on the semantic (functional) level. The video-documented experiments were coded into a scheme representing more than 40 different activities and operations.

The strain situation of the designers was measured by psychophysiological measurements, for example heart-rate, heart-rate variability, and breath-rate. The measurements were documented on-line to the experiment and reveal to a time-based sequence of the strain situation in correspondence to the activities and operations documented by video.

As working tasks three given standard tasks of approximately 2 hours working time each, and tasks of actual design projects of approximately 4 hours working time each were processed by designers and draftsmen. The experiments were carried out with 5 subjects, each of them carried out one standard task and one design project. All tasks were elaborated with the help of the same CAD system NESCAD on SUN workstations.

4. RESULTS

Based upon an evaluation of the interactions and also upon cross correlations between the time-based psychophysiological data and measurements of the interaction process, situations of a higher strain level were investigated.

A large number of experiments with a positive cross-correlation product between Heart-Rate and different actions indicates emotional stress situations. These situations were found in correspondence to the activities of the generation of basic and complex geometrical elements (Figure 2).

A large number of experiments with a negative cross-correlation product between Heart-Rate-Variability and different activities indicates mental stress. These situations are activities of the generation of nearly all drawing elements and also the deletion of elements. In some cases, operations of manipulation indicate a higher strain level, too (Figure 3).

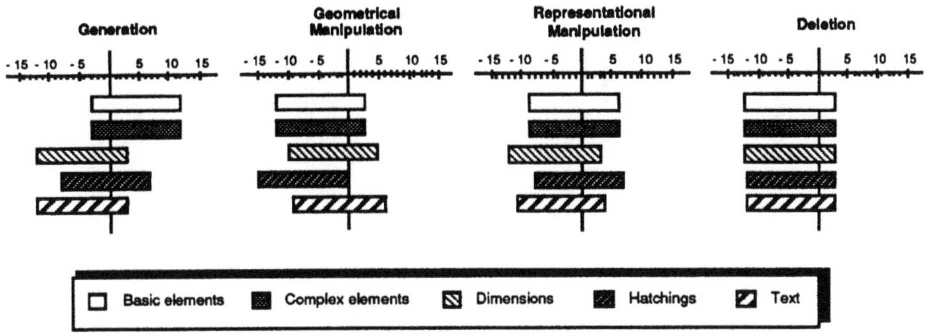

Figure 2. Number of experiments with a significant ($p < 0.10$) positive or negative cross-correlation product between different stressors and Heart-Rate

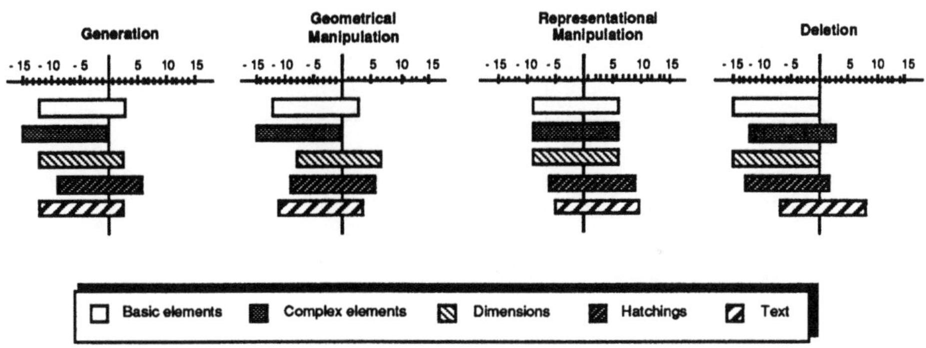

Figure 3. Number of experiments with a significant ($p < 0.10$) positive or negative cross-correlation product between different stressors and Heart-Rate Variability (ARQ)

A detailed investigation of the process of different activities were done for example by an analysis of Markov-Chains or transition-probabilities. Figure 4 shows the number of transitions between different activities. Obviously there is a high transition-probability between the use of generation, manipulation and deletion functions for basic elements as well as for dimensions and text. This indicates a stepwise elaboration of the drawing: Periods of the generation of the parts topology are different from periods where the part is dimensioned. Such a strategy implies the structure of the menu and therefore indicates design rules on the syntactical level.

	basic element generation (bg)	basic element geometric manipulation (bgm)	basic element represent. manipulation (bvm)	basic element deletion (bd)	complex element generation (ceg)	complex element geometric manipulation (cegm)	complex element represent. manipulation (cevm)	complex element deletion (ced)	dimensions generation (dg)	dimensions geometric manipulation (dgm)	dimensions represent. manipulation (dvm)	dimensions deletion (dde)	hatchings generation (hg)	hatchings geometric manipulation (hgm)	hatchings represent. manipulation (hvm)	hatchings deletion (hd)	text generation (tg)	text geometric manipulation (tgm)	text represent manipulation (tvm)	text deletion (td)
bg	500	439	21	120	9	1		3	11				5	1		1	1			
bgm	349	599	10	62	6	2		1	8	15		3	6	5			1			
bvm	9	13	17	6	2		3		1				1			1				
bd	89	68	3	86	7			6	4			8		1		3				1
ceg	5	1	4	31	7	9	18	1				1								
cegm	6				9	1	3	1			1		1		1					
cevm			1	4		13	1	1			1									
ced	2		2	8	2		4								1					
dg	4	6		2	1	1	1		322	40	19	35					5			
dgm	2	5							23	51	1	2		4						
dvm		1							10		26	3					1			
dde	3	1	1	4	1	1			37	1		5				1				4
hg	2	2		1		1			1				18	5	3					
hgm	1	1		1					1	3			1	5						
hvm					1								1							
hd				1	2							3	5			2				1
tg	2								1			1					143	2	4	13
tgm																	4	1		
tvm																			5	
td				2													12	1		12

Figure 4. Transition probabilities between the use of different CAD functions

5. DISCUSSION AND IMPROVEMENTS OF THE CAD SYSTEM

In the discussion about software ergonomic design rules there are existing some major rules, quite independent of each other, which are transparency, consistency, tolerance and possibilities of system-modification or controllability. But these design rules are not only guilty on the dialog structure. It is possible to apply the design rules to all levels of the interaction model (Figure 5, SPRINGER 1992).

design examples	transparency	consistency	tolerance	modification possibilities
pragmatic level (models and conceptions)	information about the characteristics of the models	consistency of the computer internal and the mental model	possibility of later changes of model characteristics	possibility of user defined models
semantic level (functions and objects)	clarity of the effects of a function	CAD functions consistent to design operations	reversibility of a false execution of a function	choice between different functions for the same goal
syntactic level (dialog structure)	command name clarifies the function of the command	same expression of the same parameters	possibility of an interchange of the order of parameters	choice between a menu driven or command driven interface
physical level (data input and output)	clear key-labels on a keyboard	consistent arrangement of keys on a keyboard	easy modification of key stroke faults	choice between mouse, tablett or keyboard driven data input

Figure 5. Examples for design rules at different levels of the interaction model

What type of critical phases we found, what are the weak points of the system, and what are the improvements we made to optimize the CAD system?

We found the result that the generation of elements requires a high mental effort indicated by a low Heart-Rate Variability in such phases. One possible reason on the physical level is the input of parameters, for example for the generation of lines.

In the system the designer has the possibility to define the start and/or the endpoint of the line by mouse- or keyboard-input. But if the user choose the keyboard-input he has no information about the alternatives of the parameters input. One improvement on the physical level was the implementation of soft-keys into the command-request line. On the syntactic level the user has now, in contrast to the situation before the improvements, the possibility of a free combination of the parameters, for example the input of an absolute X-coordinate, indicated by a large X, and the angle of the line. Another example for an improvement of the system consists of the permanent actual information of the user about necessary and already defined parameters.

Furthermore improvements of icons for the generational are functions used in the menu were made. For the generation of elements necessary requirements and parameters should be included into the icon much as possible and the type of the element itself should be highlighted. After the improvement the required elements are drawn consistently dashed, the element to be generated is highlighted by a continuous line. One weakness on the syntactic level was also the graphical disappearence of already defined parameters in some cases. After the optimization all numerical values, points, and/or already defined or selected elements are shown graphically, so always the designer can estimate the consequence of his input.

These are only some examples, but they might show that such an evaluation and optimization process results in a broad field of improvement ideas and therefore leads to systematically and under an ergonomic point of view „b e t t e r" designed systems.

ACKNOWLEDGEMENTS

The study was carried out by the project „Stress-/strain-analysis of design work" which is part of a multidisciplinary research group at the Berlin University of Technology financed by a grant of the German Research Association (Deutsche Forschungsgemeinschaft).

The experiments caused a high effort to the design department as well as to the subjects. The author thanks participating designers and draftsmen, and the software developers of the enterprise NESTLER for their enthusiasm and support of this study.

REFERENCES

O. Abeln, CAD-Systeme der 90er Jahre - Vision und Realität. In: Datenverarbeitung in der Konstruktion '90. VDI-Bericht 861.1. Düsseldorf: VDI-Verlag 1990.

H. Luczak; W. Beitz; J. Springer; T. Langner, Frictions and frustrations in creative-informatory work with computer aided design - CAD-systems -. In: Bullinger, H.-J. (Ed.): Human Aspects in Computing: Design and Use of Interactive Systems and Work with Terminals. Amsterdam: Elsevier 1991.

A.M. Heinecke, Developing recommendations for CAD user interfaces. In: Bullinger, H.-J. (Ed.), Human Aspects in Computing: Design and Use of Interactive Systems and Work with Terminals (Advances in Human Factors/Ergonomics 18A), Elsevier, Amsterdam - London - New York - Tokyo 1991.

C.W. Morris, Signs, language and behavior. New York: Prentice-Hall 1946.

J. Rasmussen, Skills, rules, and knowledge: Signals, signs, and symbols, and other distinctions in human performance models. IEEE Transactions on Systems, Man and Cybernetics SMC-13 (1983), 257-266.

J. Springer; Th. Langner; H. Luczak; W. Beitz, Experimental Comparison of CAD Systems by Stressor Variables. International Journal of Human-Computer Interaction 3 (1991) 4, 375-405.

J. Springer, Systematik zur ergonomischen Gestaltung von CAD-Software. Dissertation Technische Universität Berlin. VDI Fortschritt-Berichte, Reihe 20 Nr. 60. Düsseldorf: VDI-Verlag 1992.

WORK ANALYSIS, DESIGN AND STRUCTURING

WORK WITH DISPLAY UNITS 92
H. Luczak, A. Çakir and G. Çakir (Editors)

User participation in workplace design

Ritva Kukkonen and Paavo Koskinen

Institute of Occupational Health
Topeliuksenkatu 41 a A, SF-00250, Helsinki, Finland

Abstract

The participation of the workers is considered an effective method to improve the application of ergonomics during the redesign of a workplace. According to our experience, a checklist with basic instructions in ergonomics is sufficient to encourage workers to participate in the rearrangement of their workplace.

1. INTRODUCTION

In Finland muscoloskeletal disorders are a great problem among office workers. The problem has grown, in spite of ergonomic actions and instructions to workers. Ergonomic actions are usually carried out by occupational health personnel and safety personnel. The workers are usually treated as passive objects rather than active participants. This might be one reason why work communities still do not see ergonomics as an integral and continuous aspect of work.

In office work, suitable furniture and equipment give versatility to working positions and increase efficiency. In many workplaces the workers participate in the acquisition of their furniture and equipment, and in some workplaces even in the planning of their own work sites. The participation is useful, if the workers can give specifications which improve their working conditions.

Last year the Finnish Institute of Occupational Health and the Union of Commercial Employees started two joint projects during which employees were given the main role in the redesigning of their workplaces. This article deals with one of these projects, which was carried out in an office.

2. OBJECTIVE

The aim of our project was to find out whether office workers could, after a brief instruction concerning the basic ergonomic principles, analyze and assess the ergonomic arrangements of their workplace, and consequently suggest and carry out improvements. We also wanted to test, whether this kind of action is feasible at workplaces.

3. MATERIAL AND METHODS

The project comprised 44 office workers, all of whom attended a lecture on loading factors in office work. They were also given a checklist booklet for office workers, and instructed on how to use it. The booklet contained the following main items:
1) Arrange your workplace 2) Adjust your furniture 3) Place your working equipment 4) Use available facilities 5) Ensure proper working positions 6) Change working position 7) Choose your desk 8) Choose your chair 9) Check the need for improvements at your workplace.

After the instructions every worker assessed his/her workplace with the aid of the booklet. A list of the ergonomic deficiencies and possible development targets at the workplace was prepared as teamwork. The teams presented their observations and suggestions for improvements to the group including the foreman, occupational physiotherapist, technician, and the health and safety persons of the enterprise.

4. RESULTS

The biggest ergonomic problems were the lack of space in many working areas, and the lack of space on the desks. Noise was a big problem too. On the basis of their own evalution, the workers suggested rearrangements in two open plan offices in order to get larger, quiter and more suitable individual workplaces, and a proper place where to spend their pauses. They also proposed changes in the placement of noisy office machines.

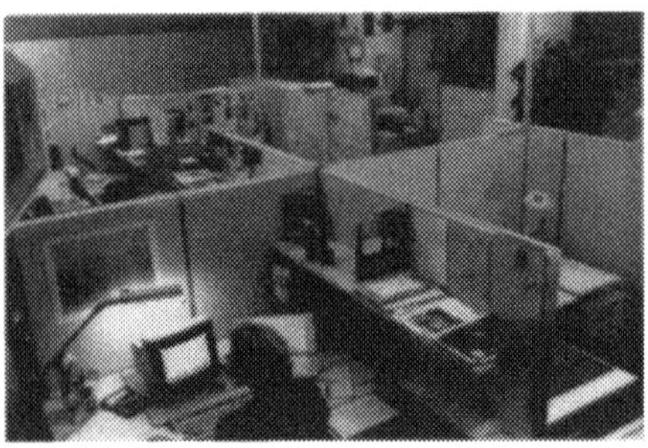

Figure 1. A cloverleaf layout througout an open plan office did not satisfy the workers.

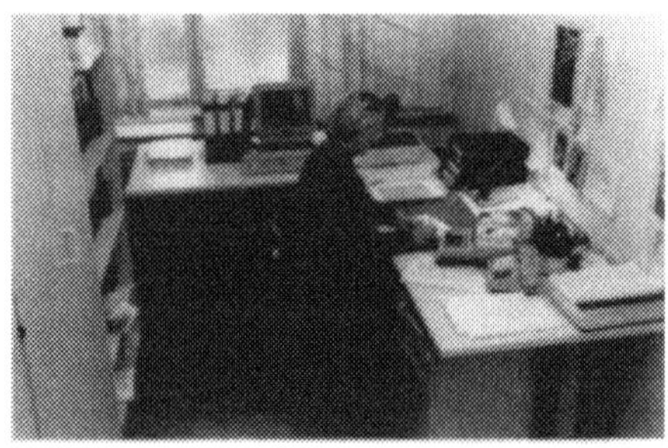

Figure 2. Rearrangements gave more space to those workers who needed it.

Half a year later I contacted the workplace in order to follow up the implementations of the ergonomic suggestions. The staff had carried out all the improvements they had originally suggested. Before the rearrangements in the office layout, the foreman drew up a rough plan on which the workers could make their own suggestions. The whole staff participated in the rearrangement. The workers were pleased that they could participate in the planning of their new computer program. The foreman as well as the workers felt that the project brought the staff members closer to each other and increased the feeling of solidarity.

5. CONCLUSIONS

Participation of the entire work community, including superiors, was crucial to the success of the project. Outside experts alone cannot improve work conditions. The employees themselves, supported by experts, must examine work conditions and futher develop them. It was essential to this training process that the workers got instructions on how to use the checklist. The workers reported the results of their workplace analyses. The staff carried out the rearrangements by themselves. According to our experience this kind of participative action is feasible at workplaces and easy to carry out. The role of the occupational physiotherapist was to give basic instruction in ergonomics and point out the loading factors in office work. The occupational physiotherapist also followed up the implementation of the suggested measures. It is very important that all the participants, especially workers and supervisors, are motivated and interested in a healthy and productive workplace.

6. REFERENCE

J. Lehtelä, R. Kukkonen, Participation in purchase of a telephone exchange - a case study. Proceedings of the 11th Congress of the International Ergonomics Association, Paris, 1991.

WORK WITH DISPLAY UNITS 92
H. Luczak, A. Çakir and G. Çakir (Editors)

Well-being and job demands after data system changes with work reorganization in the service sector

K. Lindström[a]

[a]Institute of Occupational Health, Department of Psychology, Topeliuksenkatu 41 a A, SF-00250 Helsinki, Finland

Abstract

The relationships of the characteristics of VDT use, job demands and strain symptoms to satisfaction with new VDT application and its effects on work organization were studied before and after the transition to new VDT application. The study group consisted of 319 customer service and 219 office employees from the banking and insurance sector. Satisfaction with the implemention was related to better social relations, less problems in VDT use and less strain symptoms. Bigger changes in work organization due to new VDT applications were related to more problems in VDT use, more strain symptoms and greater job pressure.

1. INTRODUCTION

The aim of the study was to describe how the satisfaction with the implemention of new VDT applications and the extent of their effects on work organization among customer service employees and office employees were related to characteristics of VDT use, job stressors and strain symptoms measured before and after the transition to new VDT applications.

During the two-year follow-up, more advanced computer technology was implemented both in the banks and the insurance companies under study.

In the first phase of the study, psychic symptoms and perceived lack of competence were related to qualitative and quantitative overload at work as well as to poor social relations. Unspecific somatic symptoms, however, were more closely related to the amount of work with visual display terminals (VDT) and various problems involved with it [1]. These results were similar to the ones in some earlier studies [2-3].

2. SUBJECTS AND METHODS

Units in which major changes in computer technology were expected during the next two years were selected from four banks and two insurance companies. The results are based on the employees who participated in both study phases, 319 customer service employees and 219 office employees.

The first survey before the transition to the new VDT applications was done in 1985 and the second survey after the transition in 1987.

The two questions indicating the criteria applied were formulated as follows in the second survey in 1987

- How *satisfied* are you *with the implementation* of new VDT applications?
- To what extent has the new VDT application *changed your work* content and organization?

3. RESULTS

During the two-year follow-up period from 1985 to 1987; the use of personal computers increased among the customer service employees. Among the office employees, both the use of personal computers as well as the use of text-processing applications increased. The total daily amount of VDT work out of the total working hours was 30 % in first study phase and 50 % in the second study phase.

The main job stressor in both 1985 and 1987 was job pressure, and the biggest change from 1985 to 1987 in job stressors was seen in job pressure and qualitative work load in both study groups. This was due to a piling up of work during the transition phase as well as changes in the job content of banking and insurance activities. As regards strain symptoms, only a minor increase was seen in psychic symptoms during the follow-up period.

3.1. Satisfaction with the implementation

Satisfaction with the implementation of new VDT applications was rather high and equal in both groups (65 %).

Among the customer service employees, the satisfaction with the implementation was related to good mastery of VDT applications before and especially after the implementation. Those reporting a slow response time of the data system after the implementation were more dissatisfied both among customer service and office employees (table 1).

Among job stressors' poor social relations were related to dissatisfaction with implementation before and after the transition among customer service and office employees (table 2). The strain symptoms correlated slightly with the satisfaction with implementation. After the transition, fatigue, anxiety and nervousness were related to dissatisfaction with implementation among office employees, but only anxiety among the customer service employees.

Table 1
Correlations between satisfaction with implementation of new VDT applications and characteristics of VDT work

	Customer service employees		Office employees	
	Before	After	Before	After
Daily amount of VDT work	-0.08	-0.03	0.10	0.04
Breakdowns, slow response time	-0.09	-0.13*	-0.09	-0.15*
Scheduling of work dependent on access to VDT	-0.02	-0.09	-0.10	-0.01
Mastery of VDT applications	0.18**	0.32***	0.01	0.12

* Statistically significant correlations

Table 2
Correlations between satisfaction with implementation of new VDT applications and job stressors

	Customer service employees		Office employees	
	Before	After	Before	After
Haste at work	0.06	0.10	-0.01	0.08
Poor coworker relations	0.21***	0.27***	0.25***	0.35***
Poor supervisory practices	0.14*	0.26***	0.23***	0.20**
Low content variety of work	0.04	-0.07	0.10	0.08

* Statistically significant correlations

3.2. Effects on work organization

The customer service employees (66 %) had experienced greater changes during the two-year follow-up in their work due to the new computer technology than the office employees (54 %).

The effects of new VDT applications on work organization were related to a great amount of daily VDT work, reported slow response times of data application, and scheduling of work dependent on access to VDT, after the implementation among customer service employees. The same pattern was found among office employees (table 3).

The effects of new VDT applications on work organization were related to haste at work and high content variety of work, only among customer service employees in 1987.

Table 3
Correlations between effects of new VDT applications on work organization and characteristics of VDT work

	Customer service employees		Office employees	
	Before	After	Before	After
Daily amount of VDT work	-0.02	0.17**	0.10	-0.30***
Breakdowns, slow response time	0.09	-0.13*	-0.09	0.15*
Scheduling of work dependent on access to VDT	0.12*	0.12*	0.18*	0.16*
Mastery of VDT applications	0.06	0.05	-0.00	-0.02

*Statistically significant correlations

Table 4
Correlations between effects of new VDT applications on work organization and strain symptoms

	Customer service employees		Office employees	
	Before	After	Before	After
Excessive fatigue	-0.01	-0.04	-0.03	0.06
Feelings of incompetence	-0.03	-0.04	0.05	0.03
Headache	0.12*	0.05	-0.09	-0.21**
Sleeping difficulties	0.05	0.04	-0.13*	-0.08
Anxiety	-0.02	-0.16**	0.08	0.00
Nervousness	0.02	-0.15**	-0.06	-0.04

* Statistically significant correlations

Among the customer service employees, the amount of change in work organization correlated to more anxiety and nervousness after the transition, and less headache before the transition. Among the office employees, the amount of change correlated to headache before transition and sleeping difficulties after the transition.

CONCLUSION

To conclude, the banking and insurance employees were rather satisfied with the implementation of the new VDT application. The perceived changes in work organization and job demands were more frequent for customer service employees than for office employees.

Those who were satisfied with the implementation generally had better social relations at work. Poor social relations before implementation predicted also dissatisfaction with the implementation and more problems experienced with VDT use and more strain symptoms after implementation. Problems in the mastery of new VDT application were more crucial for dissatisfaction in customer service work.

Those who perceived more changes in work organization generally had more daily hours of VDT work and more problems with their VDT applications, as well as more strain symptoms. They also experienced more job pressure and higher content variety at work after implementation; this was true especially for the customer service employees. This might in turn depend on the special nature of customer service work, in which social contacts are more critical and highly valued by employees.

REFERENCES

1 K. Lindström, Well-being and computer-mediated work of various occupational groups in banking and insurance. Int. J. of Human-Computer Int. No. 4 (1991) 339-361.

2 G. Johansson and G. Aronsson, Stress reactions in computerised administration work. J. of Occup. Beh. No. 5 (1984) 159-181.

3 K. Lindström and T. Leino, Assessment of mental load and stress related to information technology change in banking and insurance, In F. Klix, N.A. Streitz, Y. Waern and H. Wandke (eds.), Man-Computer interaction research, Elsevier Science Publ., North-Holland (1989) 523-533.

WORK WITH DISPLAY UNITS 92
H. Luczak, A. Çakir and G. Çakir (Editors)

Evaluation of the implementation process of information technology in offices

P. Huuhtanen

Department of Psychology, Institute of Occupational Health,
Topeliuksenkatu 41 a A, SF-00250 Helsinki, Finland

Abstract

The implementation processes of data systems were analyzed in banks, insurance companies, and industrial offices. Problems were experienced especially as regards the time and personnel resources during the change. The mastering of computer applications was lower in the occupational groups of sales personnel and supervisors. In order to improve the human side of implementation processes, new measures should be developed for adequate work-site training and social support, especially for elderly workers.

1. INTRODUCTION

The design process of information technology is of crucial importance in the planning and controlling of the effects of technology on work and well-being. Studies have shown that the new computer applications are experienced as mainly positive by different occupational groups. A follow-up study in Finnish banks and insurance companies revealed that the effects of new flexible computer applications on job complexity, autonomy, social interaction, and job appreciation were mainly positive [1]. However, the evaluation of the implementation process has not been equally positive. The most important benefits of computer systems accrue as a result of human learning [2].

Since the middle of the 80s, survey data based on standardized scales have been collected by The Finnish Institute of Occupational Health on different work places. This paper summarizes the evaluation of the implementation process of computer systems in different kinds of office work. Also the development of the training of elderly employees in the use of computer applications is discussed.

2. MATERIALS AND METHODS

Questionnaire data on the implementation were collected during 1990-91 in one bank (n=49), in three industrial companies (n=85) and in one insurance company (n=85). The evaluation of the implementation process was classified in four areas: sufficiency of information, sufficiency of training, supervisors' support, and the amount of human resources. Each area was evaluated by two to four items in the questionnaire with four answer alternatives concerning the satisfaction on the issue: (1) entirely, (2) fairly enough, (3) not quite enough and (4) not at all.

Satisfaction with training in information technology and the mastery of computer systems was earlier analyzed in different occupational groups in insurance companies.

3. RESULTS

3.1. Evaluation of the implementation process

Advance information was evaluated most positively in each branch of the office work (71-73% satisfied, Table 1). Also information about the impact of change on tasks and on the division of tasks was evaluated quite positively.

Table 1
Satisfaction with past implementation of new information technology in office tasks by branch (fully or fairly satisfied, %)

	Office work in bank (n=49)	insurance (n=85)	industry (n=85)
Information			
- advance information	71	72	73
- about impacts on tasks	71	60	73
- on division of tasks	69	59	65
Training			
- on new data system	57	63	66
- guidance in problem situations	65	66	67
Supervisors' support			
- support in problems	70	64	54
- knowledge of data systems	60	65	48
Resources			
- amount of personnel	64	64	-
- amount of time	59	50	52

Problems were experienced expecially in the amount of time to get acquainted with the new system (only 50-59% satisfied). Office employees in bank and insurance companies were more satisfied with the support given by their supervisors than their colleagues in industrial firms. Half of the workers in industrial offices felt that their supervisors should have better knowledge on the data systems used in the office.

3.2. Problems in learning

Data on different occupational groups in an insurance company have shown that sales personnel were most dissatisfied, especially with the training, but also with other aspects of the implementation process [3]. This could be seen in their evaluations of the unsatisfactory mastery of applications. In two measurements, with a two-year interval, sales personnel and supervisors, more often than the other groups, had problems in mastering the use of computers.

Previous studies have also shown that the problems of mastering the applications increase with age [1,4]. The updating of skills to fulfill the new work requirements under time pressure demands additional mental energy especially from older employees.

Based on these research findings and experiences at the workplace level, a specific intervention program was planned and carried out for elderly (over 50 years of age) sales managers in an insurance company.

The program has three aims: first, to strengthen the self-confidence and self-respect of the elderly sales managers; second, to specify and carry out individual development programs, in order to increase competence in a competitive work situation, and; thirdly, to develop the mastery of computer applications, in accordance with the specific needs of the elderly employees. This last measure was the most important improvement when the opinions of the sales managers were asked.

The program is based on intensive group work, about 15 persons per group, in one to two days' training periods. Also support at the work site will be developed. Both baseline and follow-up measurements of self-confidence, organizational commitment, and mastery of applications will be carried out.

4. CONCLUSIONS

The data presented in this paper indicate that more effort is needed as regards the human side of the implementation of data systems at work. Emphasis should be laid on both planning and learning processes.

The conclusions about coping with technological changes emphasize the fact, that it is of special importance for elderly employees that the computer applications can be integrated to each one's own work processes. The training should be based on peoples' long work experience and high work motivation. It is of crucial importance to guarantee adequate on-site social and instrumental support from supervisors, computer specialists, and coworkers. In order to master continuous changes in job contents and computer applications, sufficient mental models of the whole work process are needed.

5. REFERENCES

1 P. Huuhtanen and T. Leino, The impact of new technology by occupation and age on work in financial firms: a 2-year follow-up. Int J of Human-Computer Int., 4 (1992):2, 123-142.

2 K. Eason, Information technology and organisational change. Taylor & Francis, London, 1988.

3 P. Huuhtanen, Human side of design processes: challenge of learning. Education & Computing, 6 (1990):1-2, 23-27.

4 S.J. Czaja, Microcomputers and the elderly. In M. Helander (ed.), Handbook of Human-Computer Interaction. Elsevier, Amsterdam, 1988.

WORK WITH DISPLAY UNITS 92
H. Luczak, A. Çakir and G. Çakir (Editors)

JOB ANALYSIS OF INFORMATION SYSTEM WORKERS AT BELGACOM (BELGIAN TELECOMMUNICATION COMPANY)

CLAISSE, J.L.[a]; CORBEY, R.[a] ; DE JONGHE, C.[a], HALLOT, R.[a]

SANTE ET TRAVAIL, Occupational Health Service
Av. H. Jaspar, 128 - B-1060 BRUSSELS, BELGIUM.

Abstract

This article gives the results of an analysis of working conditions with information technology by interviewing a stratified random sample consisting 1,810 employees of BELGACOM telecommunications company. Conclusions show the impact of information technology on physical and mental complaints, work organisation and environment. Ergonomic intervention appears to be primordial yet underestimated.

1. METHODOLOGY

We have handled this project by means of interrogation of workers on the workspot. A first approach revealed 9,039 (33 % of the 28,000 employees of BELGACOM) employees working with information technology (IT) in one way or another. After stratification of this population on job-task, sex, age, seniority, language and worktools, a random sample of 1,810 employees was examined. Examination consisted of interviewing the employees on their own workspot by means of a standardized questionnaire. Following parameters were taken into account : participation in job-design and in development of job-related IT, physical environment, software, work organisation, (re)-training, physical and mental complaints or well-being.

2. RESULTS

1,678 questionnaires were completed properly, which counts for a participation of 93 %.

2.1. General data of the population

We found 76.5 % male workers in our sample, having a mean age of 39.7 years (SD : 8.6), an average seniority of 5.3 years (SD : 4.2). These data differ from most literature where the population has a female majority.

2.2. Work organisation

97.3 % starts working between 6:30 and 9:00 AM and 96.2 % stops between 3:00 and 5:30 PM. Only 1.3 % is doing shiftwork (technical maintenance and information-service). The large majority take their first break after 2 hours, in the morning (95 % between 5' and 15' of duration); a second break for lunch (82 % between 15' and 30') and third break after 2 hours in the afternoon (96 % between 5' and 15'). 96 % totalize between 15' and 120' (mean : 68' ; SD : 28') official and non-official breaks per day. Only 2 % takes no pauses (mainly in technical maintenance service).
There is a self-regulating balance between the official and non-official pauses : employees having the biggest number of official pauses don't hardly take any non-official pauses and vice versa. To a certain extent workers are autonomous in dividing several tasks among themselves.

2.3. Subjective opinion

Introduction of IT appeared to be a major change of the job of 52.5 % of the population. Only 36.0 % volunteered working with IT.

Only 51.6 % of the employees have been trained to work with IT. The others were thaught by colleagues. 34.8 % of the trained workers consider this training as adapted to their needs and 26.3 % judge it as complete. 20.8 % have a feeling that their work performance is supervised via IT. This feeling is stronger for two tasks : the information service (46.6 %) and the stock administration (40 %).
The burden of the memory (caused by memorizing codes and operating instructions) is relatively important and increases gradually with age. This increase of memory-strain (pointed out by the workers on a subjective scale) is shown in next figure.

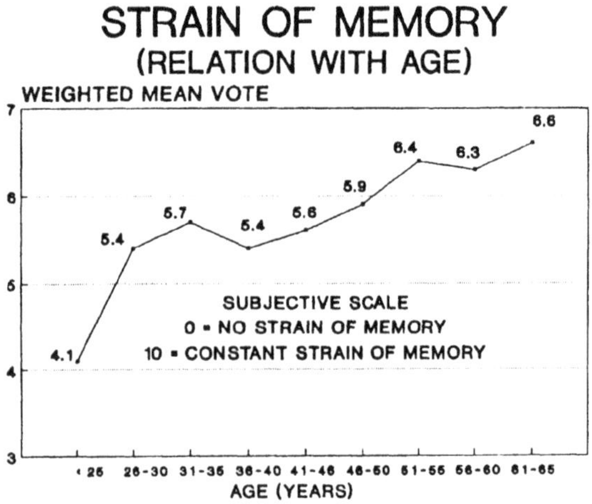

2.4. Adaptation of software

Software is little criticized. The most important remarks are : the non-adaption of the language (many programs are in english and the users are french - or dutch - speaking) ; the instructions needed to run a program cannot be transfered to another one (only 33 % thinks so).

2.5. Psychological and physical complaints

Only 48.5 % has no complaints. The most frequent complaints connected with the use of IT are : dryness and pricking of the eyes (30 %); headache (13 %); backpain 10.4 %); neckpain (8.5 %) and eyestrain (7.5 %).
The following origins of the complaints were given : inadequate lighting (reflections and dazzle) (23.3 %); non-adapted furniture (11 %); noise (printers) (6.3 %); too long continuation of work with IT (4.2 %); work organisation (4.1 %); bad quality of screens (3.8 %); inadaption of software (3.4 %).
Total complaints, headache, eyedryness and backpain are correlated with duration of work with IT (chi^2, $p < 0.001$) in next figure.

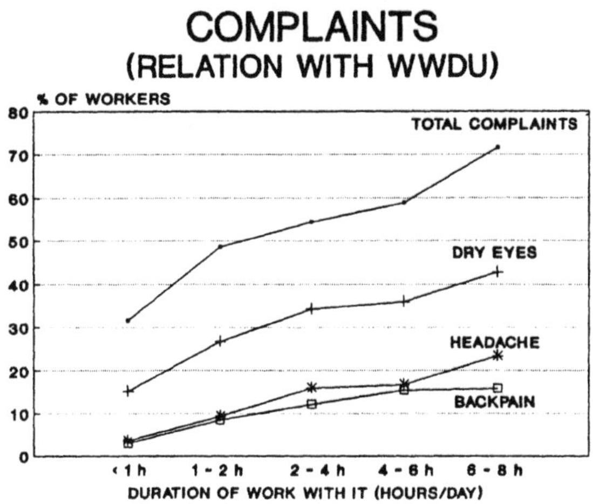

The stress, though little important overall, is also linked with the amount of time an employee is occupied with IT during the day. This progressively increasing relationship is shown in next figure.

EVOLUTION OF STRESS
(RELATION WITH WWDU)

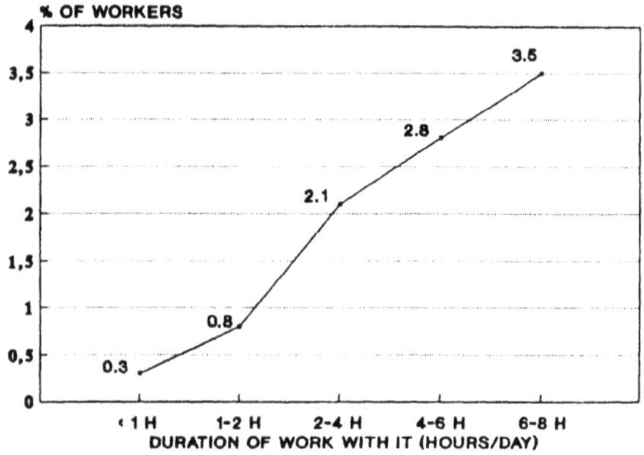

The complaints also differ largely from job to job, but a direct relationship exists between the nature of the complaints and the contents of a job (see next figure).

TYPIST-SECRETARY
(COMPLAINTS)

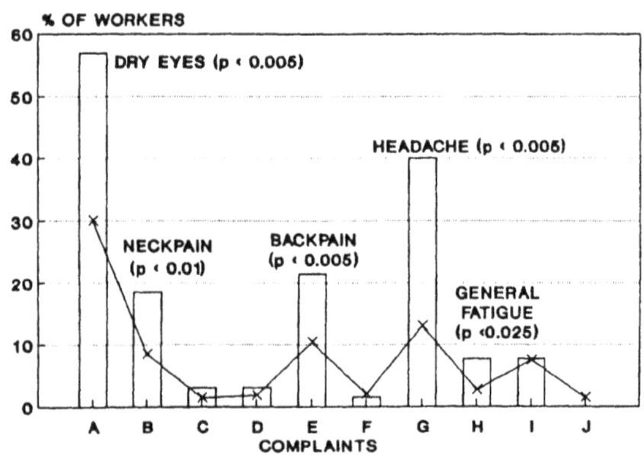

This indicates the necessity of further analysis of the secretary's job, and of the data-typist's, the information-operator's and the computer-scientist's jobs.

2.6. Visual problems

Visual problems vary with age, as is illustrated in figure below. This shows very clearly the importance of a periodical visual examination by occupational health department of those employees who work with display units regularly. Special attention should be given to workers over 45 years old, f.i. by screening them more frequently.

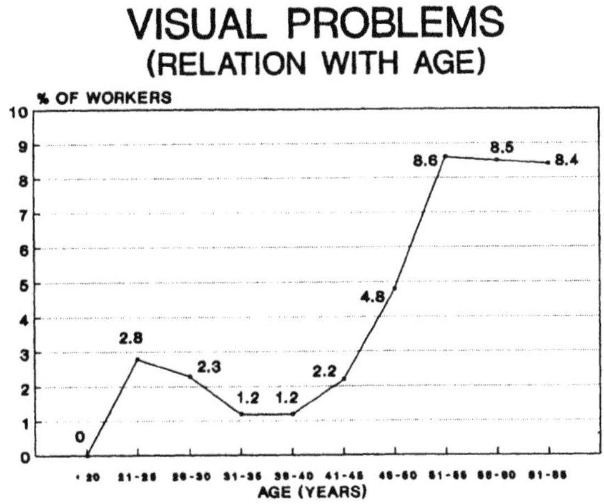

3. CONCLUSIONS

Because of a self-regulating balance between official and non-official pauses, most employees do not work for more than 4 hours a day on their display units. Nevertheless, working with IT during too long periods a day, increases the number of complaints. Therefore job organisation is primordial. Training to work properly with IT should be improved. Software instructions should be kept as simple as possible in order to avoid memory-strain which is a major complaint of the elder employee. Most common complaints are of physical nature and have a strong direct relationship with environmental and design factors of the workspot. Ergonomic intervention is the most important healing factor in reducing the discontent that can be provoked by working with IT.

STRATEGIES FOR FUTURE WWDU

WORK WITH DISPLAY UNITS 92
H. Luczak, A. Çakir and G. Çakir (Editors)

Computer keyboard evaluation using subjective questionnaires and electromyography

Kay C. Tan[a], Choon N. Ong[b], and Mui I. Koh[a]

[a]Ergonomics Laboratory, Department of Industrial and Systems Engineering, National University of Singapore

[b]Ergonomics Laboratory, Department of Community, Occupational, and Family Medicine, National University of Singapore

Abstract

Much research and development has gone into designing the QWERTY keyboard. The objectives of this research are two-folds. Experiment One employed questionnaires to the determine keyboard dimensions that are important to a user. Experiment Two assessed keyboard usability by employing the electromyography technique.

1. EXPERIMENT ONE

1.1. Subjects and Apparatus

Thirty male and twenty-eight female university staff participated in this study. They were mainly departmental secretaries and research assistants who use computers routinely as part of their daily work activities.

The objects to be evaluated were five keyboards with different keyswitch mechanisms (e.g., mechanical, spring, and rubber dome types). For experimental purpose, the keyboards were named A, B, C, D, and E. They were attached to an IBM personal computer.

The criteria for evaluation were contained in two sets of questionnaires. One is the *absolute questionnaire* which consisted of twelve items relating to: 1) typing comfort, speed, and confidence; 2) keycap size, force, stability, noise, responsiveness, and travel depth; and 3) keyboard preference and quality.

The other is the *comparative questionnaire* which was constructed to counter-check subjects' consistency in their responses to the absolute questionnaire. The items of both questionnaire were, therefore, very similar. The comparative questionnaire items concerned keyboard comfort, speed, responsiveness, confidence, and overall preference. Details of both questionnaires are given in Appendix I.

1.2. Procedure and Methodology

Subjects were instructed to use each of the five keyboards to type two passages that appeared on a computer screen. After typing on one keyboard, subjects filled-in one absolute questionnaire. For each of the twelve items, subjects had to register their opinion on a 1-7 rating scale. For example, on the item "Can type fast vs. Can type slow," subjects would put a cross in one of seven boxes. Upon completion of this questionnaire, subjects would proceed to the second keyboard and subsequently the second absolute questionnaire.

Each keyboard was introduced to the subjects in a randomized sequence. This procedure was repeated for all five keyboards. At the end of the five keyboards and their corresponding five absolute questionnaires, subjects indicated their comparative ranking of the five keyboards using the comparative questionnaire. For example, on the item "Comfort of typing," subjects would rank the most comfortable keyboard as five and the least comfortable keyboard as one. Each experiment session took approximately 50 mins to complete.

Among the attributes listed in the questionnaires, subjects were asked also to rank order them in terms of importance.

1.3. Results

Based on the average scores, the five keyboard attributes identified to be the most important were keying force, followed by keying feedback, keyboard stability, keyboard noisiness, shape of keycap, and size of keycap. The least important attributes were keyboard inclination, size, and appearance.

Of the 12 items used in the absolute questionnaire, only eight were statistically analyzed. They include: speed, comfort, appearance, restfulness, preference, responsiveness, stability, and confidence. The four questions on keycap size, noise, weight, and key travel were not statistically analyzed due to ambiguity of the questions caused by using the word "too."

Figure 1 shows the rank order of preferred keyboards indicated by all subjects. Keyboards D and E were the most preferred while keyboard B was the least preferred. A Friedman Two-Way ANOVA by Ranks test was applied on the absolute questionnaire results to find out if keyboard preference differed significantly. The results indicated significance: x_r^2 (4,56) = 20.3, $p < 0.01$.

Again looking at the absolute questionnaire data only, the Wilcoxon Matched-Pairs test showed that paired keyboards AB, AC, BD, BE, CD, and CE were significantly different in terms of keyboard preference.

Table 1 shows gender differences in keyboard preference. Based on the absolute questionnaire, the Friedman test results for both male and female subjects were significant. For the male subjects, x_r^2 (4,29) = 16.1, $p < 0.01$. For the female subjects, x_r^2 (4,27) = 12.7, $p < 0.01$. The rank order of preferred keyboards for the male subjects was keyboards D, A, E, B, and C; whereas the rank order for the female subjects was keyboards E, C, A, D, and B.

1.4 Discussion

Making comparisons among the keyboards using the absolute and comparative questionnaires, there appeared to be good representation of the crucial areas of inquiry, except for keyboard size, appearance, and inclination which were the less important attributes.

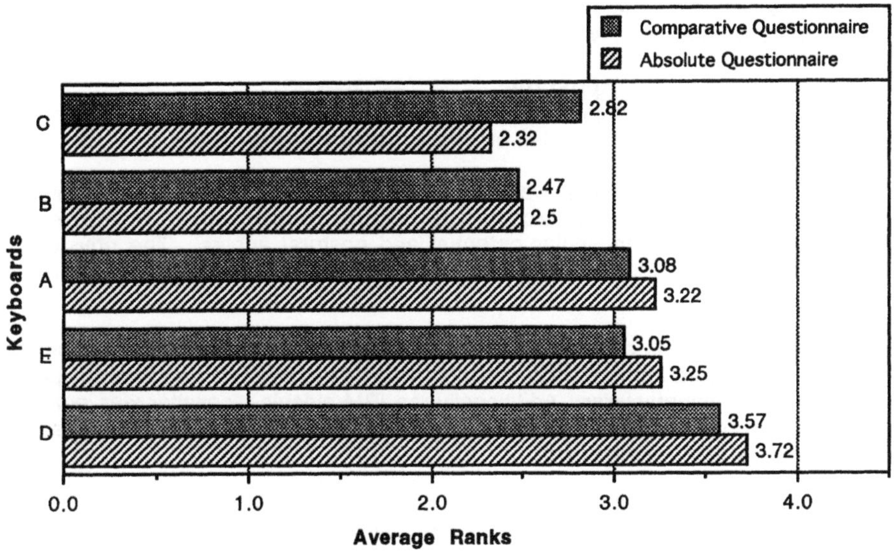

Figure 1. Rank order of preferred keyboards indicated by all subjects.

Table 1
Gender differences in keyboard preference based on the absolute questionnaire

Gender	Kbd A	Kbd B	Kbd C	Kbd D	Kbd E
Male	3.32	2.50	2.32	3.72	3.25
Female	3.15	2.08	3.19	3.02	3.56

Looking at Figure 1, the results between the comparative and absolute questionnaires showed a high degree of consistency, except for keyboard C. There seem to be gender differences in keyboard preference. Keyboard C seemed to be highly preferred by the female subjects but not by the male subjects.

2. EXPERIMENT TWO

The second experiment is an attempt to assess usability from a more objective perspective -- namely, by using the electromyography (EMG) technique. The EMG approach is a physiological one. Its usage is more focused in that keyswitch-force issues only can be evaluated. It is, furthermore, not merely a matter of "which keyboard requires the least amount of force to operate." Keyboards requiring excessive keying forces lead quickly to muscular fatigue while those requiring very little forces are prone to inadvertent actuation and increased muscular tension. Ideally, there exist a range where the keying force required is optimal.

2.1. Subjects and Apparatus

Twenty-four female subjects were recruited from the local university community. Half of the subjects had participated previously in the first experiment.

The PHY-400A physiometer was used as the main apparatus for this experiment. This is a battery operated microcomputer with a 10-channel A/D converter with sensors for measuring muscular potential and postural angles. The physiometer samples inputs (RMS value) at a rate of 400 Hz. The unit was connected to an IBM-AT standard computer.

Four keyboards with different keyswitch mechanisms were used in this experiment. Of these, three were commercially available while the other one was a prototype of a large computer manufacturer. Additionally, an IBM electric typewriter was employed as a control condition. The keyboards were named A, B, C, D, and E (the typewriter) for the purpose of this experiment.

2.2 Procedure and Methodology

Surface electrodes were attached to the left and right trapezius muscles of the subjects. Following a calibration procedure, subjects had to type on the lower half of the computer screen, a passage that appeared on the upper half. Two passages were typed using each of the five keyboards. The order of keyboard presentation was randomized and subjects had short pauses between using each keyboard.

Throughout the experimental session which lasted approximately one hr, EMG inputs and postural angles were recorded on-line for later analysis.

2.3. Results

Table 2 shows the mean percent maximum voluntary contraction (% MVC) taken of the four keyboards and typewriter at cumulative distributions of $P = 0.1$, 0.5, and 0.9. These data were analyzed using the CSS/PC Statistical Software Package (Release 2.1) by Statsoft, Inc. The Square t-test Matrix procedure was applied at each of the cumulative distribution levels.

In general, several significant differences were found. At all P-levels, % MVC required of the typewriter was statistically higher than that required of the other four keyboards. Keyboards A and C exhibited consistently lower % MVC readings than keyboards B and D (see Table 2).

2.4. Discussion

The trapezius muscles are significantly involved when a person uses a computer keyboard or typewriter. Reducing the amount of force required of these muscle sets should be one of the main goals of computer keyboard designers. As a colleague once pointed out, assuming a typical MVC of 50 kg for the average person, 10% MVC would be five kg. This translate roughly to a typist having the burden of carrying a bag of rice or jug of water and doing this eight hrs a day.

The EMG technique shows promise as a candidate for assessing keyboard usability particularly with the increasing incidence of repetitive strain injuries resulting

Table 2
Mean percent maximum voluntary contraction (% MVC) at cumulative distributions of P = 0.1, 0.5, and 0.9 for the left and right trapezius muscles

Cumulative Distribution	Kbd A	Kbd B	Kbd C	Kbd D	Typewriter
Left Trapezius Muscle					
P = 0.1	3.60	4.53	3.45	4.58	12.59
P = 0.5	6.52	7.06	6.33	7.43	16.92
P = 0.9	12.93	13.65	12.79	13.90	25.01
Right Trapezius Muscle					
P = 0.1	2.88	3.76	3.65	3.76	12.47
P = 0.5	5.88	6.90	6.47	6.98	16.68
P = 0.9	9.98	11.09	10.93	11.50	23.73

from sedentary secretarial work. Coupled with the use of questionnaires, a more complete understanding of keyboard usability issues can be realized.

3. APPENDIX I

Absolute Questionnaire: Subjects were required to place an "X" in one of the boxes of a 1-7 rating scale: 1) Can type fast/Can type slow, 2) Feels comfortable to type/Feels uncomfortable to type, 3) Feels expensive/Feels cheap, 4) Typing is restful/Typing is tiring, 5) Keys too small/Keys too large, 6) You dislike typing on this keyboard/You like typing on this keyboard, 7) Keys are responsive/Keys are not responsive, 8) Keys are quiet/Keys are noisy, 9) Keys wobble/Keys do not wobble, 10) You feel confident typing on this keyboard/You do not feel confident typing on this keyboard, 11) Keys too light/Keys too heavy, and 12) Key travel too shallow/Key travel too deep.

Comparative Questionnaire: Subjects were required to rank order the keyboards. A rank of one was given to the least favorable while a rank of five was given to the most favorable: 1) Comfort in typing, 2) Typing speed, 3) Responsiveness, 4) Noisiness, 5) Typing confidence, 6) Amount of force required, and 7) Overall preference.

WORK WITH DISPLAY UNITS 92
H. Luczak, A. Çakir and G. Çakir (Editors)

GUIDELINE ON THE VIEWING ANGLE FOR TOUCH-TYPING VDU WORKERS

M.B. Berndsen[a] and N.J. Delleman[b]

[a]Department of Work Research, TNO Institute of Preventive Health Care, P.O. Box 124, 2300 AC Leiden, The Netherlands

[b]Department of Posture and Movement Research, TNO Institute of Preventive Health Care, P.O. Box 124, 2300 AC Leiden, The Netherlands

1. INTRODUCTION

Several studies show that work with VDUs frequently causes serious neck complaints among office workers. Neck complaints are often due to factors related to biomechanics (e.g. non-optimum neck posture) and work organization (e.g. high work intensity) (Arndt 1983, Bammer, 1990, Bergqvist, 1990). One of the determinants of a good working posture is the position of the visual target, i.e. a screen or document. The location of the visual target induces the head position. The trunk position is induced by the inclination of the chair backrest. The neck posture depends on the positions of the head and the trunk and therefore, theoretically, on both the position of the visual target and of the chair backrest. Various existing ergonomic guidelines on the viewing angle show a great variety (ranging from 15° above to 45° below the horizontal).

In 1991 a study on an ergonomic guideline on the viewing angle for touch-typing VDU workers started with a laboratory experiment (Delleman & Berndsen 1992). The study was confined to the type of VDU work that induces the worker to look at one target position almost continuously, e.g. when touch-typing or using a mouse. Eight secretaries worked for almost half an hour at each of eight experimental conditions (four vertical positions for the screen at each of two chair backrest inclinations). The visual target heights tested (covering the whole range of existing guidelines on viewing angle) were related to the individual eye height: 5 cm above eye height and 10, 25, and 40 cm below eye height. The chair backrest inclinations tested were upright and 15° inclined backward (related to the vertical). Posture, subjective experiences and work performance were recorded. It turned out that at both backrest inclinations the visual target height of 10 cm below eye height showed significantly better subjective experiences than the other visual target heights. This result, corresponding with results derived among others by Grandjean et al. (1983), led to the ergonomic guideline that the viewing angle to a visual target should be 6 to 9 degrees below the horizontal when touch-typing.

The present paper focuses on the field study carried out to evaluate this laboratory-based ergonomic guideline.

2. METHODS

2.1 Subjects

In a financial organisation three experimental conditions were tested fulltime for a week each. Eleven touch-typing secretaries participated in the field study. On average they were 31.9 years old (range 25-47) and 169.9 cm long (range 165-184). One subject was male.

2.2 Independent variables

The three experimental conditions consisted of three different vertical screen positions: 5 cm above eye height and 10 and 25 cm below eye height (see figure 1). The subjects were free to use their preferred chair backrest inclination. The visual target height of 40 cm below eye height was not tested because the standard office tables offered no possibility to lower the screen.

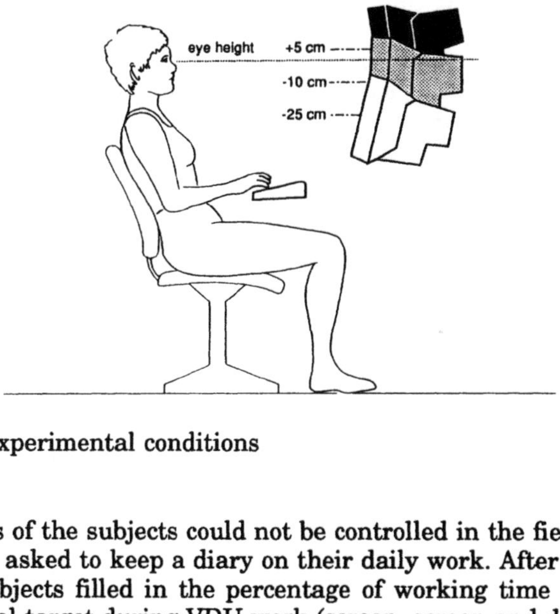

Figure 1. Three experimental conditions

Because the tasks of the subjects could not be controlled in the field experiment, the subjects were asked to keep a diary on their daily work. After each period of two hours the subjects filled in the percentage of working time worked at the screen, their visual target during VDU work (screen, screen and document alternately or document) and the position of the document.

2.3 Dependent variables and measurement techniques

In this study a limited set of dependent variables was recorded. Due to privacy considerations it was not possible to record work performance. The registration of working posture using an opto-electronic system, as performed in the laboratory study, was not possible since all subjects participated in the test simultaneously at different sites. Therefore, the dependent variables were limited to subjective experiences, i.e. local postural discomfort, perceived posture of head and neck and assessment of visual target height. All were measured in the same way as in the

laboratory study using a questionnaire. After each working period of two hours the subject was asked to rate the local posture discomfort in 19 regions shown in a diagram of the rear view of the human body (Van der Grinten & Smitt 1992). A category-ratio scale was used, ranging from 0 (no discomfort) to 10 (extremely much discomfort).
At the end of eight hours work the perceived posture of head and neck was recorded using a 7-point scale (1= very favourable, 3= favourable, 5= unfavourable, 7= very unfavourable). Also the subjective assessment of the visual target height was recorded using a 5-point scale (1= much too low, 3= good, 5= much too high).

3. RESULTS

3.1 Work intensity

The diary scores were transformed into four categories of work intensity, measured in percentage of working time worked at the screen. Some subjects scored in all intensity categories at a specific condition whereas most subjects only scored in two or three intensity categories. However, the total number of scores at each of the four categories for the whole subject group was fairly equal for all three conditions. The categories of intensity of VDU work were used to analyze the group scores on the local postural discomfort.

3.2 Local postural discomfort neck/back

Scores at midmorning (after two hours work) and end of the morning (after four hours work) for the regions neck and back were averaged. The same was done for the resulting scores at midafternoon (after six hours work) and end of the afternoon (after eight hours work). The average scores at the cluster neck-back were plotted against the categories of intensity of VDU work. This was done for morning scores, afternoon scores and working day scores (see figure 2).

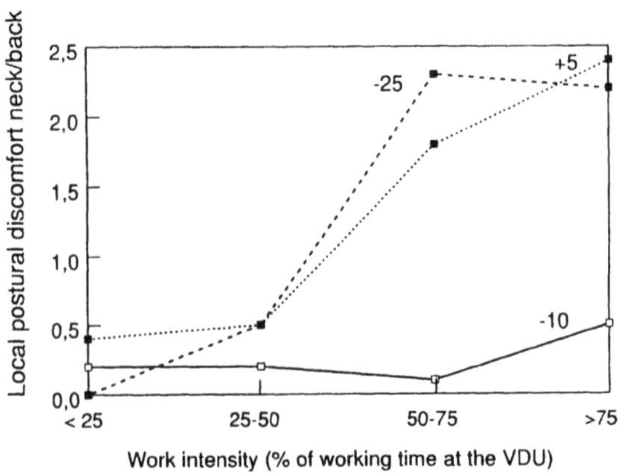

Figure 2. Local postural discomfort neck/back (working day)

The differences between the three experimental conditions were small for less intensive VDU work (defined as spending less than 25% of the working time at the screen during a period of two hours). For periods in which subjects worked intensively at the VDU (defined as spending 50% or more of the working time at the screen) the differences in local postural discomfort were considerable between the recommended screen position of 10 cm below eye height and the two other screen positions.

3.3 Perceived posture of head and neck

Independent of work intensity most subjects scored constant during the work week at a specific screen position. Eight of eleven subjects concluded the screen position of 10 cm below eye height to be most favourable. For further analysis the median score for each subject was determined. The screen position of -10 cm was assessed to induce a favourable posture of head and neck (see figure 3). The position of -25 cm below eye height induces an unfavourable posture and 5 cm above eye height a very unfavourable posture.

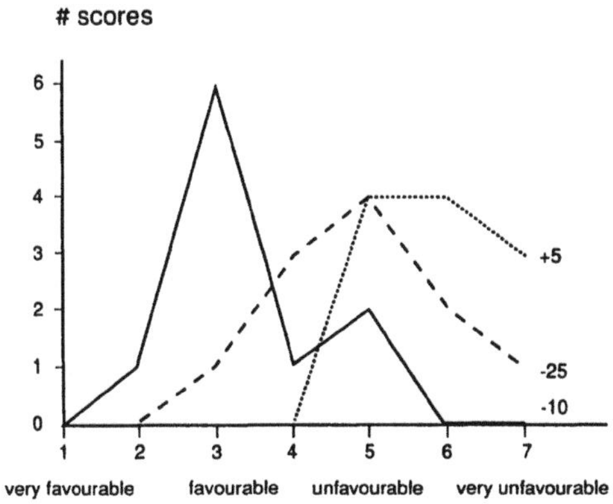

Figure 3. Perceived posture of the neck

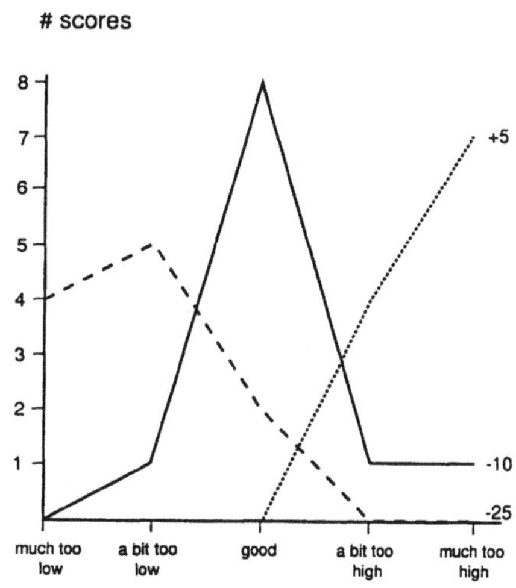

Figure 4. Assessment of visual target height

3.4 Assessment of visual target height

Similar to the scoring on experienced posture most subjects scored constant during the work week. Eight of eleven subjects judged the position of 10 cm below eye height as best. The median scores of each subject were used in figure 4. As figure 4 shows the position of 25 cm below eye height is assessed as 'a bit too low', the position of -10 as 'good' and the position of +5 as 'much too high'.

4. DISCUSSION

Carrying out an experiment in a field situation implies that the controllability of the experiment is less than in a laboratory situation. Using a diary to gather information about the intensity of the VDU work being executed by the subjects proved to be essential. The intensity of the VDU work has a considerable influence on the local postural discomfort of neck and back at the different screen positions. The -10 cm position gives less discomfort at the high intensity categories.
Furthermore, the interpretation of the results indicate that the importance of a good sitting position seems to increase with the intensity of VDU work. This supports the idea that a decrease of VDU work should be the first measure taken to prevent VDU related health complaints. If organizational measures are not feasible and workers work for a high percentage of their working time at the screen the proper position of the screen is important. The guideline stipulates that for touch-typing VDU workers the screen should be placed at approximately 10 cm below eye height.
Since the local postural discomfort is measured in relative values it can not be concluded that the perceived discomfort at the screen position of 10 cm below eye height is acceptable regardless the intensity of work. Therefore, in our opinion, it can not be stated that a visual target height of 10 cm below eye height prevents organizational measures.

REFERENCES

Arndt, R. (1983) Working posture and musculoskeletal problems of video display terminal operators - review and reappraisal, Am. Ind. Hyg. Assoc. J. 44(6):437-446

Bammer, G. (1990) Review of current knowledge - musculoskeletal problems. In: Work with display units 89, L. Berlinguet and D. Berthelette (Eds), Elsevier Science Publishers, Amsterdam

Bergqvist, U., Nilsson, B., Voss, M., Wibom, R. and Wolgast, E. (1990) Discomforts and disorders among office workers using visual display terminals - a longitudinal study, In: Work with display units 89, L. Berlinguet and D. Berthelette (Eds), Elsevier Science Publishers, Amsterdam

Delleman, N.J. and Berndsen, M.B. (1992) Computer-aided postural analysis on optimum workstation adjustment for VDU operations, In: Computer Applications in Ergonomics, Occupational Safety and Health, M. Mattila and W. Karwowski (Eds), Elsevier Science Publishers B.V., Amsterdam

Grandjean, E., Hünting, W. and Pidermann, M. (1983) VDT workstation design: preferred settings and their effects, Human Factors, 25, 161-175

Van der Grinten, M.P., Smitt, P. (1992) Development of a practical method for measuring body part discomfort, In: Advances in Industrial Ergonomics and Safety IV, S. Kumar (Ed), Taylor & Francis

WORK WITH DISPLAY UNITS 92
H. Luczak, A. Çakir and G. Çakir (Editors)

Eye movements and mental workload during process control

A. G. Fleischer, G. Becker

Universität Hamburg, Arbeitsbereich Arbeitswissenschaft,
Am Vorwerksbusch 1, D-2057 Reinbek, FRG

Abstract

The presented results provide evidence, that the task demands determine the uptake of specific visual informations. The amount of mental workload affecting the subject during the control of four simulated processes is determined by their kinetics. This effect is due to the limited capacity of the subject to deal with more than one process state within a certain time interval. With respect to the amount of information processed by the subject characteristics of the scanpath are described on the basis of the state space in order to obtain criteria which show, that the analysis of eye movements provides an appropriate tool for the evaluation of mental workload during multiple-task performance.

1. Introduction

VDU's are increasingly applied in industrial process control since they allow a large flexibility on concentrating grafical information at a single workstation. The information presented on a screen has to be visually analysed in order to achieve a decision on the action to be performed. Normally peripheral vision and the knowledge of the displayed optical structure is used to select the next position of fixation. The resulting scanpath is determined by the context and the dynamics of the process to be controlled. Therefore, the question arises to what extent mental workload can quantitatively be described by characteristics of the eye movements.

2. Methods

In order to test this approach an experimental set-up (Figure 1) was designed which allowed to record the gaze positions of a subject on a screen during the performance of a complex control task. During the experimental session the subject sat at a workstation for computer-aided design and moves a hand cursor on a horizontal graphic tablet. The current position of the hand cursor was displayed on the screen. Eye movements were recorded by means of two infrared reflecting glasses (mir1 and mir2) mounted in front of the eyes and by two cameras (C1 and C2) mounted on the left and right side of the head, respectively. The head movements were recorded by measuring the transmission time of ultrasonic pulses emitted from three sources E1, E2 and E3, mounted on top of the head, to four microphones M1, M2, M3 and M4 above the test table. From these data the X,Y,Z-coordinates of the sources could be computed.

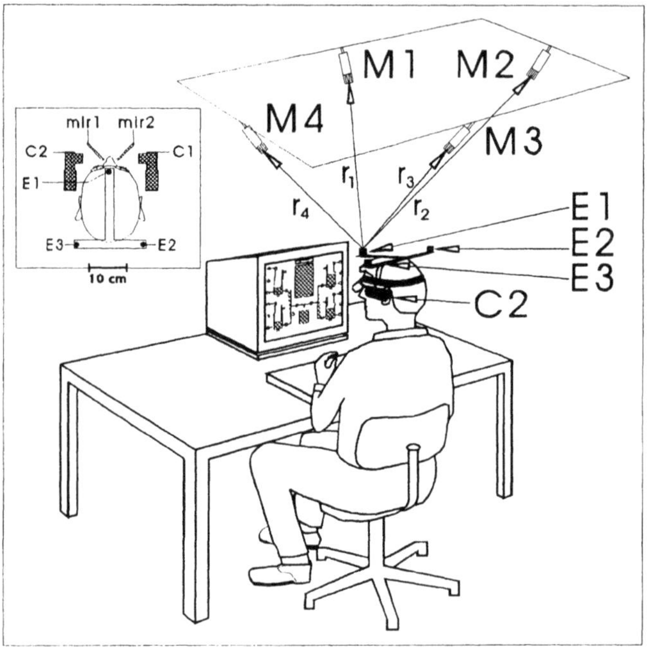

Figure 1. Experimental set-up.

During the experimental sessions trained subjects were asked to control a complex process simulation by means of cursor movements. This simulation displayed on a high resolution colour screen consisted of four process units (Figure 2). It was designed similar to the waterbath paradigm developed by [1,2]. Temperature and fluid level represent the control variables for each process unit. According to the recipe given in the upper middle part of the screen the subject was asked to mix four different fluids with a specific temperature in the large blending tank shown in the lower middle part of this diagram. These fluids were of different viscosities. This means that the rising velocity of the fluid level ranged in terms of relative units from 1 - that is slow - to 16 - that is fast. Choosing the maximal input setting a tank could be filled within 80 s by applying the slow kinetics and within 5 s by applying the fast kinetics. One recipe contained only fluids of the same kinetics.

At the beginning of the experiment the subject had to choose a certain fluid type and to try to reach the given set points of fluid level and temperature. By positioning the cursor within the corresponding setting symbol and pressing the up-key on the hand cursor the subject had to open the input valve and let a selected fluid rise up to a certain level. Underneath each tank a heater is installed which allows to reach a certain temperature of the fluid. Fluid level and temperature readout of each subsystem were represented by an analogue and a digital readout, respectively. The experimental sessions lasted two hours. The visual scanpath and all actions on the graphic tablet were recorded continuously during the experimental sessions.

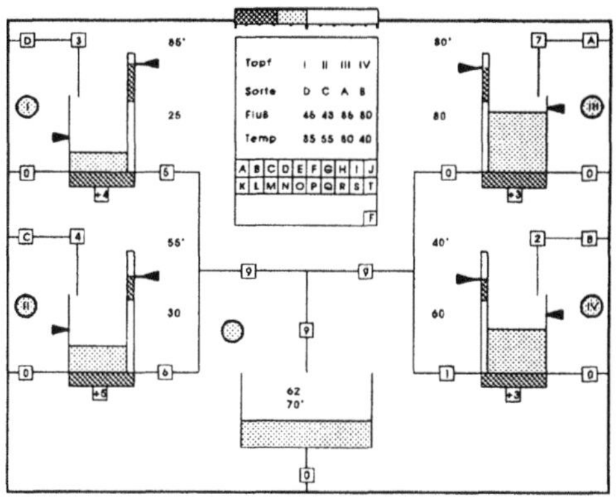

Figure 2. Display of the simulated processes. The width of the upper middle area which shows the recipe amounts to 7.8 cm.

3. Results and Discussion

From the recorded eye- and head-data the gaze position on the screen could be computed. A typical spatial distribution of the gaze positions on the screen during managing a whole recipe is presented on Figure 3a. The gaze positions are marked by black dots. The plotted time interval amounts to 4.5 min. Target areas are marked by squares, 3 cm large.

With respect to Figure 3a the allocation of attention is shown on Figure 3b. If the distribution of the gaze position on the screen is considered a three-dimensional probability distribution, contour lines can be computed. For instance, 95% of the gaze positions lie within the shaded areas, 50% lie within the darker shaded areas and 5 % within the darker dotted areas. From this picture it becomes clear that most of the attention is focussed on input and temperature settings and on fluid level and temperature readout.

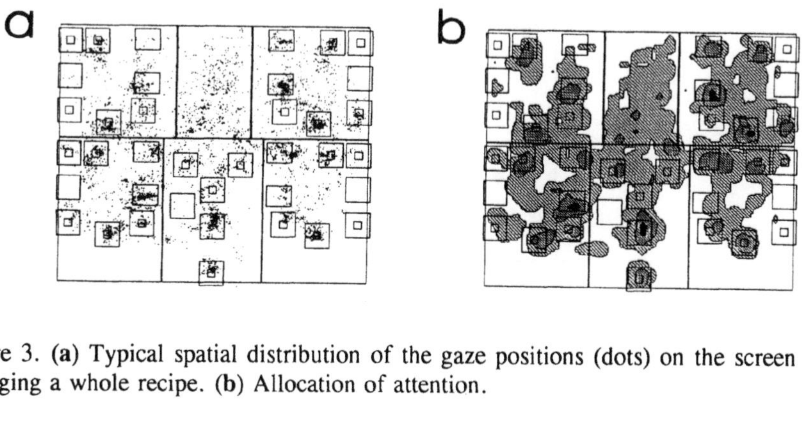

Figure 3. **(a)** Typical spatial distribution of the gaze positions (dots) on the screen during managing a whole recipe. **(b)** Allocation of attention.

However, if we want to learn more about the structure of visual information flow, we have to investigate sequences of visual information uptake with respect to the contextual structure of the working process. So first the strategies of the subjects applied during the performance of the task will be discussed.

The operator had to control four subsystems at the same time. However, he or she is only provided with a limited information processing capacity and develops certain strategies during multiple task performance. If the operator is allowed to behave freely, it is assumed that he or she chooses with respect to mental workload an optimal strategy to control the multiple task. He or she tries to avoid underload and overload, respectively.

Slow kinetics should allow the operator to control several processes in parallel, that means the minimal time interval between two required consecutive actions to control a single process is large enough to allow a shift of attention to control other processes in the meantime. In contrast, fast kinetics only allow the operator to focus his or her attention on the desired process until the set point is reached. The operator is forced to work in a serial manner. Due to limited resources for dealing with a task the shift from parallel to serial control of several processes is determined by the amount of mental workload. The operator tries to reach a balance between mental workload and the available amount of resources. Figure 4 (curve consisting of squares) shows that with increasing kinetics the subject shifts clearly his or her strategy from parallel to serial performance. 100% serial work means that the subject only concentrates on a single subsystem until it is adjusted without performing any additional control actions concerning the other subsystems.

Additionally, Figure 4 (dotted curve) shows that the required time for the final adjustment of a tank decreases with increasing kinetics. The time interval for the final control phase becomes shorter and the chance to shift attention or gaze position to an other subsystem without overshoot of the current process becomes small. Therefore, further discussion is focussed on the final control phase.

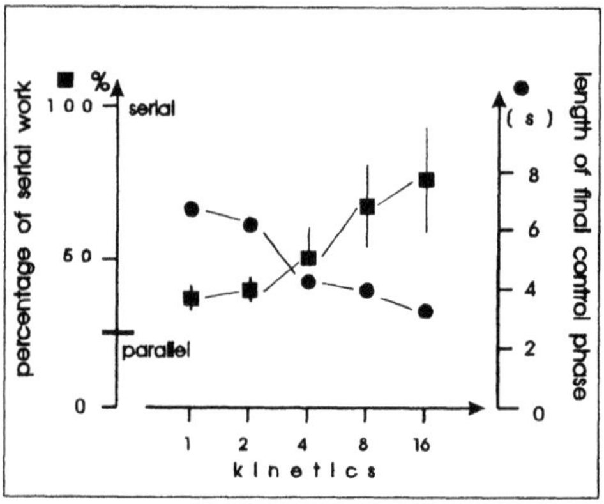

Figure 4. Shift of control strategies caused by different kinetics.

Figure 5 gives an example of the action pattern during the final adjustment of the fluid levels of all four tanks. For instance, in order to reach the required set point of subsystem I, the subject has opened the input valve to setting 7 and then increases its setting to level 8. The fluid level slowly reaches the set point. The input setting is reduced to setting 4 and then to setting 0. The set point is reached. During the final control phase one can observe an overshoot of subsystem II and III. The second part of this figure shows the horizontal and the vertical scanpath on the screen; l: left, r: right, u: up, d:down. The third part presents the cursor positions. The last part presents the actions on the keys of the hand-held cursor.

According to the state of the process saccades precede or run in parallel with cursor moves, as can be seen at arrow 2. The target is fixated until the cursor move comes to an end and the required setting is adjusted. Repetitive eye movements between input setting and fluid level readout can be seen at arrow 1. During the final control phase a complex behavioural pattern emerges from the individual control strategies and the requirements of information flow. But the question arises how to quantify the link between task demands and eye movements. This problem will be discussed on the basis of the distributions of fixation duration. From our point of view, the typical shape of the overall distribution of fixation duration (Figure 6d) is composed of specific time intervals required for the uptake of certain but not yet fully identified units of visual information.

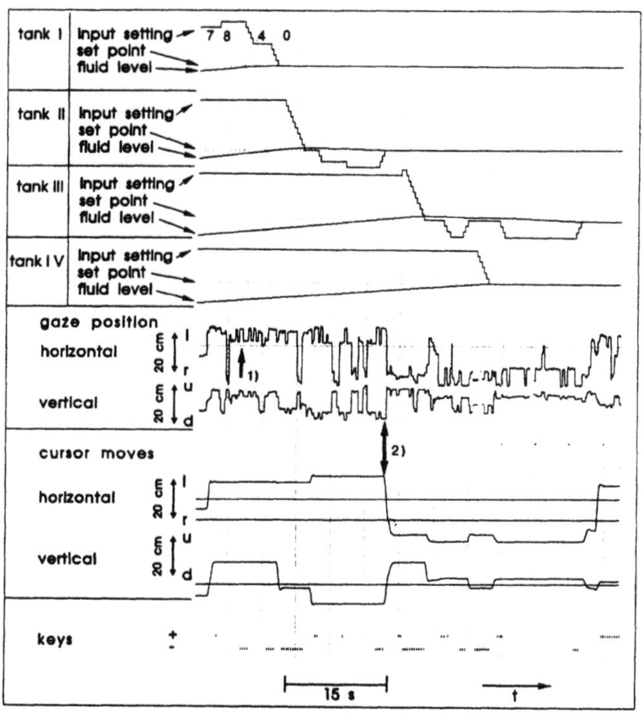

Figure 5. Action pattern during the final control phase.

Figure 5 (arrow 1) shows, that during the final adjustment of the fluid level repetitive eye movements between valve setting and fluid level readout are performed. We analysed this behavioural pattern in detail. Figure 6a shows the distribution of fixation duration during checking the valve setting. The average amounts to 320 ms and the variance is small. Figure 6b shows the distribution of fixation duration during reading the fluid level readout. The average amounts to 1000 ms and the variance is large. Figure 6c shows the distribution one obtains only considering the final control phase as a total. The obtained distribution is similar to the overall distribution shown in Figure 6d.

With respect to valve setting and fluid level readout the obtained distributions in Figure 6a and 6b differ enormously. This result lead us to the conclusion, that two different structures of visual information uptake underlie these distributions. In order to test this hypothesis, we investigated whether the average fixation duration of fluid level readout during the final control phase is affected by the kinetics of the selected fluids.

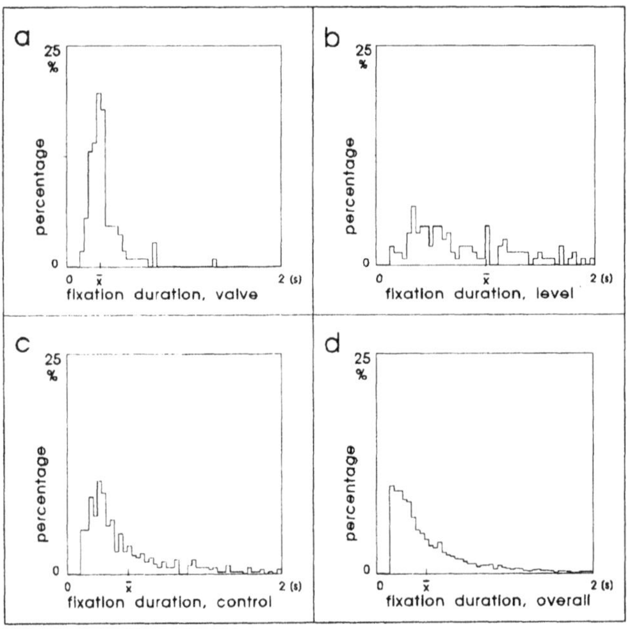

Figure 6. Distributions of fixation duration during the uptake of different visual informations.

The average fixation duration of the valve setting display remains nearly constant with respect to changing kinetics (Figure 7, dotted curve). However, as can be seen on this picture, the average fixation duration of the fluid level readout increases steadily (Figure 7, squares). We assume that this effect is caused by the limited capability of the subject to process more visual information. A minimal time interval is required to change the gaze position, to read an other part of the display and to return to the previous gaze position. If the subject has to deal with fast kinetics and if the control state is close to the set point it is likely that during this time interval the corresponding system overshoots the set point. That is why the subject avoids to change the gaze position. This observation fits to our everyday experience. For instance, during car driving we dare not change the gaze position within a critical moment.

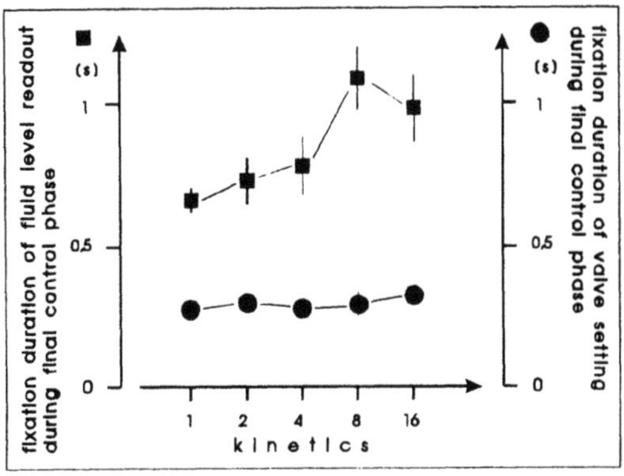

Figure 7. Average fixation time of the valve setting area and the fluid level readout, in relation to increasing kinetics of the fluids.

The presented result support the hypothesis, that a link between fixation duration and mental workload can only be expected by considering the fixation duration of specified target informations within the contextual structure of the action pattern. An effect on the overall fixation duration can hardly been expected. This is consistent with the findings during text processing [3]. Visual information is processed by sequentially fixating different targets. A minimal time interval is required to glance at an other display area. During the control of a fast process this time lack may lead to instabilities of the system state. In order to avoid these instabilities the fixation duration of the state readout is increased by the subject.

4. References

1 E.R.R.W. Crossman and S.E. Cooke, in E. Edwards and F. Leeds (eds.), The Human Operator in Process Control, Taylor & Francis, London, 1974.

2 N. Moray and I. Rotenberg, Ergonomics, 32 (1989) 1319.

3 A.G. Fleischer, Biol. Cybern., 55 (1986) 227.

Acknowledgements

Supported by the Federal Institution of Occupational Safety and Health, Dortmund, FRG.

WORK WITH DISPLAY UNITS 92
H. Luczak, A. Çakir and G. Çakir (Editors)

Kansei Engineering as Design Support Technology

Kageyu Noro

School of Human Sciences, Waseda University
2-579-15 Mikajima Tokorozawa Saitama 359 Japan

Abstract
Kansei Engineering is defined as "Design support to build into products elements that appeal to the feeling of people". Kansei Engineering is one of today's major topics . Japan has spent more than twenty years in the research and application of Kansei Engineering. Various methods have been developed, many cases have been studied, and extensive technology transfer has been made from one industry to another. Kansei Engineering is utilized to make products in many industries, including foods, breweries, apparel, automobiles, cameras, and audio-visual equipment. The concept and methodology of Kansei Engineering have become a mature technology system of Japanese origin through this technology transfer. Kansei Engineering is one of the best know-how Japan can offer to the United States and Europe.

In the United States, kansei engineering is an issue of strong interest, mainly in the automotive industry[1],[2] . It is a technology of Japanese origin. Kansei engineering is considered as design support technology that builds into products factors appealing to the feelings of users.

The concept "kansei" is reported to have been used in the lecture "Cars and People" Mr. Yamamoto, former president of Mazda Motor Corporation, presented in a seminar at Michigan University in 1986. Like "kanno kensa[3]" (sensory inspection), kansei has no apt English word to describe it. Feeling, sensibility, and comfort come to our mind as English candidates for kansei, but none of them is said to appropriately denote kansei. For this reason, kansei is used in its Japanese form. (The German words "gemut" and "gemutlichekeit" are most justes for kansei.) It is commonly thought in the United States and Europe that Japanese cars, particularly luxury models, are made excellent by kansei engineering.

Kansei engineering is a Japanese technology and is a typical example of Japanese technology transfer. It is very interesting to note technology transfer from the method of evaluating the taste of sake (sensory inspection) to the development of luxury cars. From now on, we should try to convey Japanese kansei to foreigners.

Value analysis[4]

Consider the value people have of products. Three cases can be supposed.

The Japanese people started to pay less attention to owning things in the last half of the 1970s. This phenomenon will intensify further with the progress of information society. Let C be the objective condition (quality) of a product and V be the value people recognize in the objective condition (measurable quality) of the product. Take wristwatches as examples. (The concepts described below are similar to those of value engineering (VE). The above-mentioned condition is equivalent to the function of value engineering.)

The following items are selected from among the postwar history of wristwatch technology in Japan and are taken as objective conditions (measurable qualities):

Table 1. Objective conditions (measurable qualities) of wristwatches.

C1: Waterproofness
C2: Luminousness
C3: Shock absorption
C4: Self-winding mechanism
C5: Quartz movement

Additivity holds for conditions C1 to C4. The term additivity means that waterproofness and luminousness, for example, can be added together to the product. When the values are added in this way, a linear relation is conceptually obtained between the values recognized as qualities as shown in Figure 1.

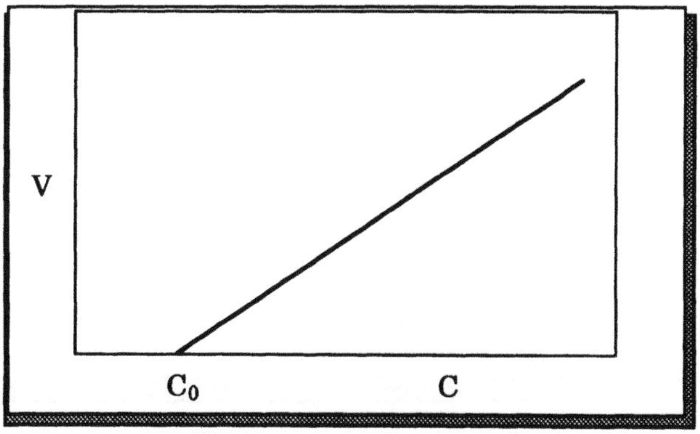

Figure 1. Additivity holds between values recognized as qualities.

If C is added one after another, V may linearly increase, but does not so in reality. There appears the stage in which V does not linearly increase with increasing C, but approaches an asymptote. This marks the beginning of the phenomenon of people showing less interest in owning goods (goods detachment phenomenon). A case in point is C5: quartz movement. When quartz watches were first launched, they were very expensive. As they were mass produced, they rapidly declined in price. Today, even cheap watches are quartz watches.

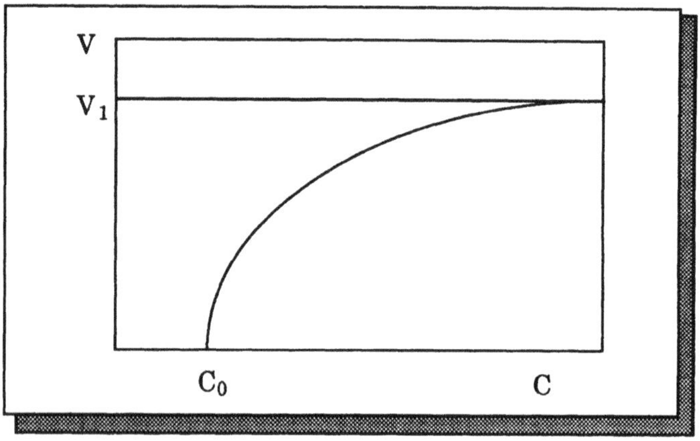

Figure 2. V does not increase with increasing C (negative acceleration) and approaches asymptote V_1.

Another functional type can be considered as shown in Figure 3.

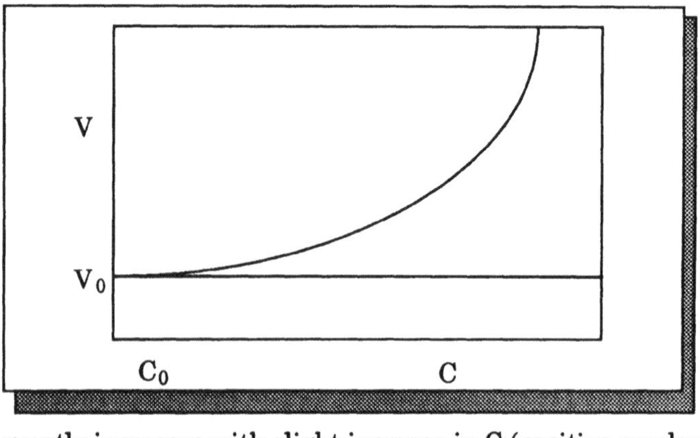

Figure 3. V greatly increases with slight increase in C (positive acceleration).

Figure 3 shows the case in which V greatly increases with slight increase in C (positive acceleration). An excellent example is a brand watch bearing a small logo. Brand neckties are another example.

Kansei quality corresponds to Figure 3. The energy for this positive acceleration is delivered as governed by the feeling of humans. This is the relationship between kansei and value. The goods detachment phenomenon frequently appears in this stage. For C often holds not for material value but for information value.

The case in which additivity holds for the values recognized as those of quality can often be regarded as being governed by rationality. This is only an incidental result and does not mean that additivity holds for all rational qualities.

The appearance of accurate quartz watches and swatches accelerated the change from the negative acceleration shown in Figure 2 to the positive acceleration shown in Figure 3. Then has come the age when attention is focused on kansei qualities. Since the 1969 invention of the quartz movement, a variety of watches have arrived on the market in a manner isolated from the process of the essential time ticking function of watches, as represented by high-grade brand watches, diver's watches, antique watches, and quartz watches of traditional design.

Figure 4 combines Figures 1 to 3.

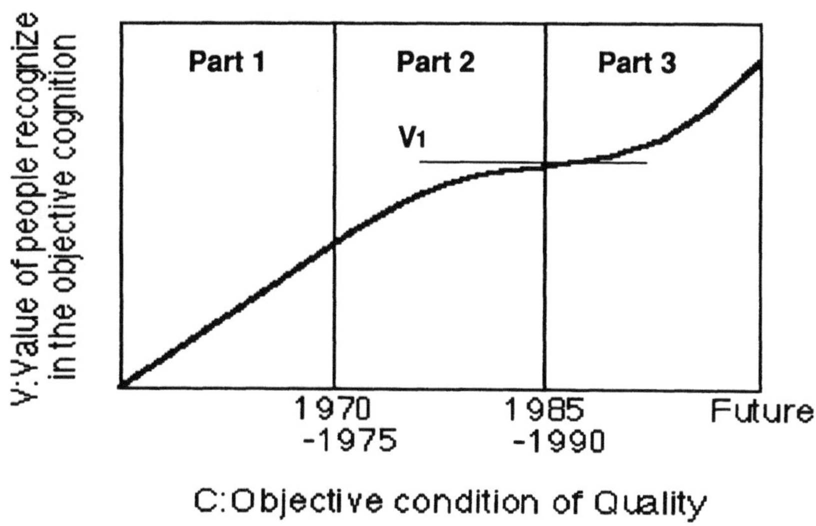

Figure 4. Changes in time and curve (connection of three curves).

The value plotted along the vertical axis is very likely to change in content in each stage. The monetary value was given priority up to the 1970s, but has been surpassed by mental affluence in recent years. The diffusion rate of main items of electric appliance exceeded 90% from 1970 to 1975 according to the Nihon Kogyo Nenkan ("Japanese Industrial Almanac"). A public opinion survey by the Prime Minister's Office shows that more people placed greater emphasis on mental affluence than material affluence in 1976 than before. This difference has continued to increase since then. These social phenomena are considered to correspond to the three curve sections shown in Figure 5. The dimension of the vertical axis indicates that people's sense of value changes with the times.

Identification and Individualization

Two measures important in consideration of modern products are taken up here. They are identification and individualization. Identification is the phenomenon of everyone wanting to own a particular product. This phenomenon can be described by the word "boom" and has been observed less and less frequently in recent years. Many individualistic products have been recently marketed as tools for diversification and individualization of people's lifestyles. Figure 5 shows the space in which many products are configured by the above-mentioned kansei-rationality axis and identification-individualization axis.

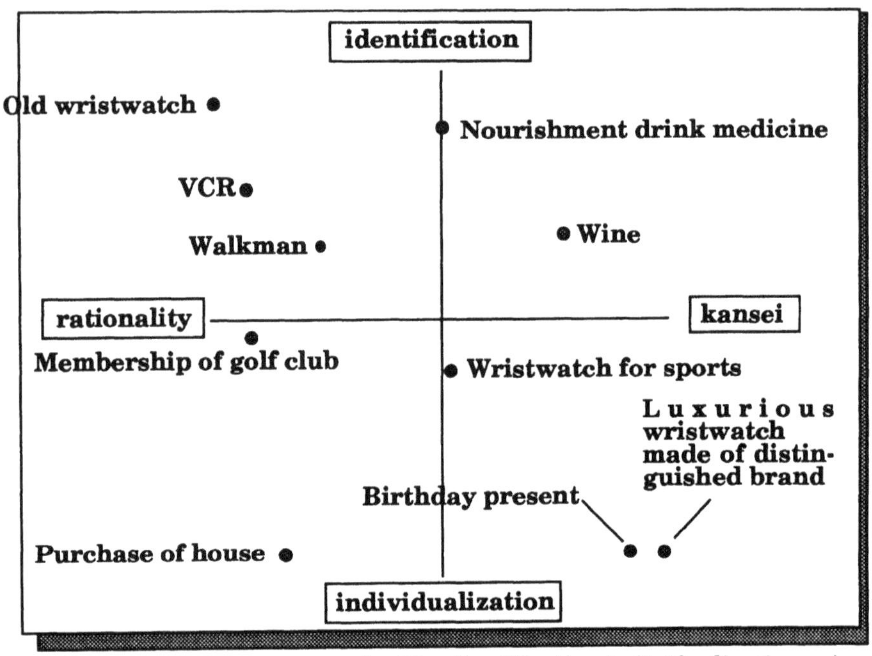

Figure 5. Product space comprised by identification-individualization axis and kansei-rationality axis[5].

People frequently cross with the identification-individualization axis and kansei-rationality axis. Depending on their living environment, people properly use "rationality" when they pursue a rational function and "kansei" when they emphasize sensory taste or personal preference. Figures 1 to 3 basically apply to identification products. In other words, many people share one type of function. Extremely speaking, each person has his or her own function as to individualization products.

Relationship with Design

Particularly great attention must be paid to the design of kansei products. It is important that designers should build their emotional experience into product design. Formerly, the functional constraints of products directly became their design constraints, and the effort expended at improving product performance left no room for product design. Today, design is made much of, and designers must build kansei into products. As design support technology, computer-aided design (CAD) has facilitated the approach to kansei. As an example, take the styling of audiovisual equipment, telephones, and cars. The design of kansei products in these fields is impossible without CAD.

Kansei Clinic

The difference in the individuality or personality of people works as important factor for the rationality and kansei discussed above. The kansei and rationality of individuals can be evaluated by the method called the kansei clinic.

REFERENCES

[1] J.Gephart,Jim Wise,the last reneissance man,Profile Pacific Northwest Laboratory,U.S.Department of Energy,September/October 1992 p4,5

[2] K.Larson,Kan-sei engineering:science with a sigh,Profile Pacific Northwest Laboratory,U.S.Department of Energy,September/October 1992 p7,8

[3] K.Noro,Kanno kensa Guidebook,Japanese Standard Association,Tokyo 1991

[4] K.Noro,Ergonomics for Everyday Life, Text for University of the Air,Tokyo,1992

[5] Dentsu Marketing Strategy Research Committee,Spending based on kansei or rationality,Nihon Keizai Shinbun Inc.,1985 p68,69

WORK WITH DISPLAY UNITS 92
H. Luczak, A. Çakir and G. Çakir (Editors)

Chaos: Introduction and Applications

Glenda Eoyang[a] and Susan Dray, Ph.D.[b]

[a]President, Excel Instruction, Inc., 1313 5th Street SE, Suite 332, Minneapolis, MN 55414, United States

[b]Director of Human Factors, IDS Financial Services Inc., IDS Tower 10, Minneapolis, MN 55440, United States

Abstract

Today's change is different in kind from changes of the past. Organizations experiencing today's rapid and continuous change require a new paradigm to cope with and manage complex, nonlinear dynamics. We present a description of the qualitative change in organizations, introduce chaos science as a mechanism for understanding change, and present some fundamental steps that can guide organizations toward effective, productive work within chaotic systems.

1. INTRODUCTION

Change is a way of life in corporations today. Even our understanding of change is changing. We are not experiencing change as a temporary state between two stable, but different, organizational structures. Rather, current changes are leading corporations into unstable, constantly evolving structures. In this paper, we will define some of the characteristics of this new state of affairs. We will introduce a new model for thinking about and working within such structures. This new model comes from the field of chaos science, the study of complex, nonlinear systems. Finally, we will demonstrate how this new model can be applied to help individuals cope with the unpredictability of constant change.

2. TOMORROW IS DIFFERENT FROM YESTERDAY

Changes in organizational and technical aspects of corporations that are currently espoused lead to increases in interdependency and complexity in organizations. For example:

- Business is undergoing fundamental restructuring. Organizations that were structured by stable criteria, such as product line or geographic area, are restructuring on the basis of cross-functional teams, which introduce new interdependencies and complicate existing interdependencies among corporate groups.
- Decentralized work groups have increasing decision making authority, so that control of organizational behavior is not as predictable as it was when all decisions came from a central source, such as uppoer management.
- Day-to-day work is driven by the customer, whose behavior is always unpredictable.
- Technology opens communication lines among groups who were previously isolated in the organizational structure. Distributed systems give remote users new powers. In addition, user-centered design techniques break barriers between builders and users of technical tools, and electronic mail democratizes and speeds up interpersonal communications.
- Cultural diversity breaks the security of a homogeneous work force.

All of these changes are both constructive and destructive. They constructively increase the flexibility and adaptability of organizations, but they render ineffectual our old coping and management mechanisms. Specifically,

- Individuals, tired of on-going change, show dangerous levels of fear, resistance, territoriality, physical and emotional exhaustion, stress, and decreased productivity.
- Management, accustomed to directing activity, find themselves watching, aghast, as the organization moves in surprising directions.
- Historical assumptions about cause and effect are no longer valid. In such a complex, open system, one cannot predict one effect from a single cause. Rather, a nonlinear system generates many and sometimes surprising effects from multiple causes.

Such an environment is different in kind from the organizational structures of the past. To thrive in such an environment, we must define a new descriptive model that will provide innovative coping and management strategies. Chaos science provides such a model.

3. CHAOS SCIENCE DEFINED

A new physical science has emerged during the past decade. It crosses the lines of traditional scientific investigation, and is known by a variety of names: chaos science, complex systems science, science of nonlinear systems, science of adaptive systems, science of dissipative systems.

In all of its permutations, this science involves the investigation of highly complicated systems that defy the rules of classical Newtonian systems and those of statistically determined random systems. These complex, chaotic systems are unpredictable. No one can determine, in advance, how any one component of the system will behave at any given time. The systems do, however, exhibit evidence of underlying, subtle patterns of behavior. Scientists can anticipate the behavior of the whole, but they cannot anticipate the specific behavior of any part.

Complex, chaotic systems have been identified in many areas of scientific study, including:

- Meteorology
- Fluid dynamics
- Thermodynamics
- Ecology
- Economics
- Biology
- Fractal mathematics
- Human cognitive development

In all of these disciplines, chaotic systems exhibit some standard characteristics. We recognize these same characteristics in organizational systems.

Chaotic systems *defy the rules of Newtonian systems*, such as the predictability of cause and effect. This characteristic of the chaotic system is demonstrated in an organization when one examines the causes for success of a working team. What variable or group of variables can predict the success of a team? No one set is sufficient because it is the nonlinear interrelationships among variables that can make one team succeed and another fail.

Chaotic systems *defy the rules of random systems* because statistics are not applicable to describe behavior. Statistics assume smooth distribution of behavior over a field of interaction, but we all know that organizational behavior does not indicate a smooth distribution of anything. One department may be highly successful in one year and face dismal performance in the next.

Chaotic systems *are unpredictable*. Complex organizations thrive on surprises. Each unexpected event becomes an occasion for innovation and subsequent success. For instance, a failed glue became the basis for 3M's Post-Its product line.

Chaotic systems *exhibit subtle, underlying patterns of behavior*. One cannot predict the behavior of a specific indivdual, but the behavior of a whole group can be anticipated. Though the day-to-day sales of a product varies tremendously, one can still predict the stages in the product's life cycle, from introduction, to maturity, to decline.

These characteristic behaviors of complex systems cannot be managed according to the rules of simple, linear systems. Hierarchical management, specific objectives, long-range planning, compensation for performance, standardized operating procedures, and management control are dysfunctional in a complex, non-linear environment. A different model of organizational behavior is required to work within the complex systems that current changes are introducing into organizations.

Physical scientists have defined some factors that describe the behavior of nonlinear, chaotic systems. These behaviors provide insight into new ways of dealing with organizational behavior. Our research has identified sixteen of these factors, but we will describe only four here:

- Butterfly effects
- Subjectivity
- Boundaries
- Transforming feedback loops

4. MANAGING CHAOS

To be successful, new organizational management techniques must recognize and find ways to manipulate the factors that arise in complex systems. In this section, we will define each of the four factors listed above and explain how each can be used to guide the behavior of complex systems.

4.1 Butterfly Effects

In a complex system, a very small cause can have an enormous effect. This tendency is called "extreme sensitivity to initial conditions" or butterfly effect. In general parlance, this has always been known as the tempest in the teapot. If one expects such behavior from a complex system, what can one do to manage the unpredictable effects? Some suggestions we would make are:

- Don't consider butterflies to be mere chance. Examine where they arise, how frequently they arise, and the nature of the information that results.
- Watch for potential butterflies. Collect data constantly with an expectation that the organization will be sensitive to initial conditions.
- Keep lines of communication open. Know when a butterfly has exploded. It will not go away if ignored.
- Build reliable and flexible communication structures to help adjust the butterfly message if necessary.
- Don't look for the "cause" of the butterfly, examine why it was magnified by the system.
- Reinforce positive and squelch negative butterflies.

4.2 Subjectivity

Modern science has assumed that it was objective, that its observations were universal, valid, and reliable. Subjective observations, which depend on the unique circumstances and perspectives of the observer, were relegated to the realm of the social sciences or humanities. Chaos science destroys this assumption because the observer is an integral part of the system that is being observed. There is no such thing as an objective observer of a complex system. Anyone who observes the system affects it and is affected by it. The necessary subjectivity of the observer is clearly demonstrated in organizations. Managers cannot merely manipulate their employees because they are also an integral part of the daily work. Managers can make the most of their subjectivity if they:

- Are willing to learn anything from anybody. The manager must be changed and evolve, based on the perspectives of the managed.
- Constantly reevaluate policies and procedures to ensure that they are functional, given the immediate needs of the organization and the team.
- Ask questions and listen to the answers to ensure that their participation is constructive for the whole system.
- Hire employees who will challenge them.

4.3 Boundaries

Every complex system includes boundaries between regions. A cold front is a perfect example of a complex system boundary. The most interesting--constructive or destructive--behavior of the system occurs at the boundaries. The manager's primary responsibility in an organization is to manage its boundary conditions. Managers can:

- Focus on the boundaries that are most important. Such a focus will decrease activity at destructive boundaries.
- Open and close boundaries consciously to encourage learning and evolution rather than bigotry and destruction across boundaries.
- Monitor how people respond to external boundaries to recognize how the organization is likely to respond to changes that are beyond their control.
- Leverage internal boundaries of diversity to encourage creative tension and learning.

4.4 Transforming Feedback Loops

Information, energy, and resources move across the boundaries in complex systems. These transfers should result in constructive change on both sides of the boundary. This transfer and subsequent change is called a transforming feedback loop. In organizations, any exchange can be a feedback loop, but the more important question is, "What transformations occur as a result of the transfer?" To encourage and manage transforming feedback loops, managers can:

- Watch the boundaries. Consider the transfers across the boundaries and evaluate the effectiveness of transformations that result.
- Consider the transformations that are desirable.
- Adjust feedback to increase (positive feedback) or to decrease (negative feedback) specific behaviors.
- Control the speed of feedback loops. In communications, faster is not always better. Take time and give time for constructive transformations to occur.

5.0 CONCLUSION

In this paper we have demonstrated the need for a new management paradigm to account for the complex behaviors of nonlinear, chaotic systems. We have introduced the characteristics that identify and determine the behavior of chaotic systems, and we have described some ways that managers can use an understanding of chaos to deal constructively with the behaviors of an organization where change is a way of life, not just a transition to be endured.

The study of chaos in physical systems is in its infancy. It is a new science that requires innovative tools and techniques for investigation. Organizational applications of the science are even less mature. We encourage anyone who participates in organizations to investigate the discoveries of complex systems research and to apply them to their own organizational experiences. We welcome communication from anyone who chooses to pursue this fascinating and fruitful inquiry.

WORK WITH DISPLAY UNITS 92
H. Luczak, A. Çakir and G. Çakir (Editors)

Products to relieve or prevent VDU health problems: Exploitation, Placebos or Prophylaxis ?

Brian Pearce

Senior Research Fellow, Department of Human Sciences, Loughborough University of Technology, Loughborough, Leicestershire, UK.

Abstract
Products which claim to contribute to the health, safety or welfare of VDU users can be beneficial if they prevent adverse health effects or merely reassure. A variety of products which are claimed to protect VDU users from electromagnetic radiation are examined. It is argued that the promotion of some products has done more to cause needless alarm among VDU users than the products themselves have done to 'protect' VDU users.

1. INTRODUCTION

A plethora of products have been, and still are, sold on the basis that they contribute to the health, safety or welfare of VDU users by preventing VDU users experiencing a range of symptoms or by protecting VDU users from allegedly hazardous agents. The range of products includes: aprons and tinted spectacles for VDU users to wear; 'anti-radiation' filters and materials with which to screen VDUs; 'low radiation' terminals; novel keyboards and workstations; and software to control the duration of VDU use. Such products can be viewed as providing a benefit to VDU users and their employers *if* they prevent or relieve adverse health effects. Even if a product is ineffective or unnecessary it can be argued that if it reduces anxieties and concerns or simply makes VDU users or their employers 'feel good', there is some benefit to set against the financial cost. However, it is suggested that the promotion and use of some such products can also have disadvantages.

At the most basic level, if the product is not actually needed or if a product does not actually do that which is claimed, there is a financial loss - money which might have been better spent. Whether or not a product does do that which is claimed, there are sometimes unanticipated side effects which, overall, disadvantage the VDU user when using a product. Such products are operationally ineffective. Inevitably some products will be better than others and provide more 'prevention' or 'relief' or 'protection' per dollar than their competitors. However, it is suggested that the cost/benefit equation needs to be assessed in more than just financial terms.

The promotion techniques used for some products may induce anxiety in previously unconcerned VDU users. A few such products could potentially cause VDU users harm. Some of those responsible for marketing these products can be viewed as having a vested interest in promoting the alleged hazards of using VDUs. It is suggested that some seek to induce anxieties and concerns in VDU users - to exploit VDU users - to sell their products. It is not suggested that all products promoted as preventing or relieving adverse health effects are unnecessary, ineffective, harmful or exploitative. However, it is arguable that the promotion of many products has done more to cause needless alarm among VDU users than the products themselves have done to 'protect' VDU users.

To examine the hypotheses outlined above it is necessary to consider the context within which such products are marketed, the attributes of the products and the manner in which they are promoted. These issues can be considered in terms of a series of questions which might legitimately be asked of any product which purports to contribute to the health, safety or welfare of VDU users: What does it do? Why is it needed? Does it actually do what it is claimed to do? Is it fit for the purpose for which it is sold? Does its use have any adverse side-effects? To whom and how is it promoted? What health messages does the use of the product or its promotion convey? Is it promoted ethically?

Within the space available for this paper it is only possible to consider a limited number of types of product and only one or two products of each type. The products chosen for inclusion in this paper all claim to protect VDU users, in some way, from various types of electromagnetic radiation (EMR) and include some of the most extreme examples of the genre. It should be emphasised that the attributes of the products chosen and the manner in which they are promoted are not necessarily representative of all the products of a particular type. Unfortunately, useful products, promoted ethically, often suffer 'guilt by association'. It should also be noted that the criticisms of the promotion of a product included in this paper does not necessarily imply that the product itself is unnecessary, ineffective or useless.

The principal claim made for many products is that they reduce the exposure of VDU users to various types of EMR. There are a number of different types of product which are intended to reduce exposure to EMR and the reasons put forward why they are needed also vary. A selection of these products, and the claims made for them, are referred to in a book entitled *Electro Pollution* [1] and in an article in *Personal Computer World* by the investigative journalist Duncan Campbell [2]. Some products and their promotion betray the suppliers' woeful lack of knowledge about EMR, while many appear to seek to exploit the lack of knowledge and the concerns of VDU users and their employers, about 'radiation'.

2. PROTECTIVE CLOTHING FOR THE VDU USER

There are a number of suppliers of protective clothing for VDU users. The promotion literature for one, North American, range of 'radiation shielding' undergarments 'Silver Lining' manages to combine concerns about radiation with an element of sexual innuendo. The promotion literature, in the form of a letter from the President of the company, starts: "I share your worry about radiation and electric fields. Silver Lining can shield you from computer and power line electric fields and radio, TV, microwave, and radar radiation. It also eliminates electric shocks and static cling. I make Silver Lining with silver plated nylon mesh, like wedding veils.". The literature goes on to explain the properties of the material and includes the following testimonial: "I also have peace of mind, knowing I am shielded from electric fields, including those of my computer. I am protecting myself inconspicuously from whatever the world dishes out. I also avoid shocks and static cling. Be careful who sees you wearing it, though. It's very exciting.". The promotion literature for Silver Lining focuses on its shielding properties in the non-ionising part of the EMR spectrum and particularly on electric fields, making no mention of magnetic fields.

The promotion of Silver Lining is relatively innocuous compared with a product called the MICROSHIELD smock, promoted in the UK in the late 1980s. The front cover of the promotion brochure depicts a female VDU user, dressed in an apron, sitting in front of a terminal from the front of which are coming multi-coloured rays, below the words "The Danger From Within". Inside, below the heading "The ever present risk of Microwave radiation" the brochure states: "One feature all VDUs have in common is that they emit microwave radiation - which is believed to be harmful to the body.". It should be noted that one feature all the studies on EMR emissions from VDUs have in common is that they have rarely ever suggested that VDUs emit microwaves, let alone at levels which might be dangerous.

Below the heading "No VDU operator should be without one" the brochure suggests that "A MICROSHIELD protective smock should hang by every terminal to be worn at all times by anyone using the terminal. By supplying MICROSHIELD, you will virtually eliminate the microwave radiation risks, as well as reassure your operators that you care for their welfare.". To remind operators to wear their smocks the suppliers thoughtfully provide "terminal screen stickers" with the legend "Be on the safe side, wear your MICROSHIELD". The concluding sentence of the brochure states: "Anyone operating a VDU without MICROSHIELD is running a risk.".

In fact, anyone operating a VDU with a MICROSHIELD smock is probably running a risk! As the brochure makes clear, the smock is made out of a fabric woven from nickel coated, polyester fibres. According to a standard text on contact dermatitis [3] "In many countries nickel is the commonest sensitiser in women ...". A significant proportion of the women who wore a MICROSHIELD smock would run the risk of developing an allergic reaction to the product.

In 1985, this product was the subject of successful complaints to the Advertising Standards Authority and to the Code of Advertising Practice Committee, self-regulatory bodies of the British advertising industry. The latter Committee "found the approach taken by the advertiser to be capable of causing unwarranted anxiety and unnecessary concern, and consequently an unjustifiable play on fear.". The findings of the Committee concluded: "The Committee issued a formal request that the advertiser withdraw the leaflet, and refrain from using a similar approach in any future advertising material, until and unless any dangers posed from VDUs were fully established and could be shown to be diminished by the use of the advertised product.".

It was not long, however, before a protective smock for VDU users called Microshield™ was again being marketed in the UK, using a very similar approach, though a different company appeared to be responsible. A further complaint was made to the Code of Advertising Practice Committee in 1988, and again it was upheld. Subsequently, the claims made for the Microshield smock and the people responsible for its promotion were investigated by the BBC's consumer affairs programme *Watchdog*. In a programme broadcast on national television on the 23rd January 1989 it was demonstrated not only that the product was useless, but also that those responsible for promoting both versions of the Microshield smock had been exposed, some years earlier on national television, for misrepresenting the capabilities of a do-it-yourself mammography kit. The programme also noted that one of those responsible for the Microshield smock had a criminal conviction for forging letters of credit.

A news story in the trade magazine *Office Secretary* [4] provides the closing comment on this product and those responsible for its promotion: "Following a campaign which advertised Microshield smocks, which were said to protect pregnant women from 'harmful' emissions from VDUs, the marketing company has been prosecuted by Trading Standards officers. East Sussex Trading Standards Office took the director of the now defunct company to Brighton Magistrates Court where he was found guilty of supplying misdescribed articles and fined £1,014."

3. RETROFIT 'ANTI-RADIATION' FILTERS

There are numerous products on the market which fit over the screen of the VDU and allegedly improve the lot of the VDU user. The rationale for the vast majority of these filters is that they reduce glare and reflections and enhance contrast, thereby reducing the visual symptoms experienced by VDU users. However, in addition, a significant proportion of these filters are also claimed to dissipate static fields and to attenuate various types of EMR. The EMR attenuation claimed for some of these products could be achieved equally well by a plain sheet of glass, while other EMR attenuation claims are scientifically untenable, irrespective of the materials from which they are made. Where the promotion literature focuses on the EMR attenuation properties of a filter it is usually implied that the VDU is a 'radiation' hazard and the cause of adverse reproductive outcomes.

A product, originating in Canada, is claimed to be: "the ultimate in radiation protection and glare reduction for VDTs". Those in the UK seeking further information on the product, around 1989, were provided with a collage of numerous press cuttings under the heading "Computer Radiation: A Worldwide Concern!". Like many similar products the promotion literature includes references to the findings of just one of the ten or so epidemiological studies on VDU use and reproductive outcome: "The most stunning news comes from a recent study by the Kaiser Permanente Medical Group, Inc. which shows that the ratio of miscarriages to live births was 80% higher for heavy users of VDTs than for nonusers.".

The findings of the Kaiser Permanente study are so often misrepresented in product literature that it is worth quoting at length from the abstract of the full report in the *American Journal of Industrial Medicine*: "One possible explanation for these findings is that women who had adverse pregnancy outcomes may have overreported their exposures to VDTs and/or women with normal births may have underreported theirs. The findings may also be due to unmeasured factors confounded with high VDT use such as poor ergonomic conditions or job related stress. That VDTs themselves are hazardous to the pregnant operator remains a possibility. Our results underscore the need for large cohort studies of working women that will provide objective measures of VDT exposures, ergonomic factors, and stress." [5]. The full report of this study refers briefly to ionizing and non-ionizing radiation from VDTs and notes the current interest in "low frequency magnetic radiation" and that: "The highest nonionizing radiation emissions are from the back, sides and even tops of the machine, not the front".

The brochure for "the ultimate in radiation protection" includes the claim that: "Non-ionizing radiation blocked by more than 99.99%". While this filter may attenuate the electric component of some types of non-ionizing radiation emitted from the screen, it won't have any effect on the magnetic component and it clearly has no effect on the emissions from the back, sides and top of the terminal. While the product claims "to attenuate, eradicate and dissipate more forms of radiation from a VDT than any other product in the world" it clearly cannot attenuate the one type of EMR which has recently generated the most interest, the pulsed magnetic component of ELF.

4. VDUs WITH REDUCED EMR EMISSIONS

The Safe Computing Company Inc, based in the USA, supplies a most remarkable computer monitor, if its sales literature, available at WWDU '89 in Montréal, is to be believed. Their product 'The Safe Monitor™' is evidently "The world's first and only computer monitor that emits no radiation to the user - so you can use your computer safely.". This statement appears immediately below a photograph of an apparently pregnant VDU user. Quite how the user is supposed to see the image on the screen if there is no radiation, and therefore no light, emitted, is not explained! The rationale for this product is explained thus: "Because we believe that VDT radiation plays a role in reproduction problems, we developed the Safe Monitor™, which emits no measurable radiation to the user. We feel the Safe Monitor™ is inherently safer than other VDTs, especially for women in their child-bearing years.".

The pamphlet promoting the Safe Monitor™ suggests that "A breakthrough study published in 1988 conclusively linked VDT use to miscarriages." and includes carefully selected quotes from the Kaiser Permanente study [5]. The pamphlet also describes the various types of radiation emitted by VDUs, emphasising the difference between 'Electric Radiation' and 'Magnetic Radiation', but neglecting to mention visible light which is also part of the EMR spectrum. The pamphlet then explains why screens and aprons, "the two types of product on the market that attempt to convince the public that they stop VDT radiation", are ineffective: "While some screen manufacturers make wild claims about how much radiation they stop, the truth is that screens only block the electric radiation, and do not block the magnetic radiation. In addition, the electric radiation is only stopped as it comes directly at the user, through the display. The screens do nothing to stop the high levels of radiation emitted from the back, top, and sides of the VDT.". The pamphlet is equally critical of aprons: "- the electric radiation is only reduced directly behind the apron, and the magnetic radiation isn't blocked at all, because it travels in circles and goes around the apron.".

There is a certain irony in the moral tone adopted for one of the conclusions in the pamphlet promoting the Safe Monitor™: "The next time you hear about one of these shielding devices, you should wonder if it is really doing a good job of shielding all the radiation, or is it misleading the public by giving them a false sense of security?".

Possibly one of the most questionable advertisements for any 'low emission' VDU was that placed by EIZO (UK) LTD in two of the UK's national newspapers, *The Times* and the *Independent*, in November 1991. Below a large photograph of a foetus sucking its thumb were the words "If you're not using the right computer screen, it's not just your work that could suffer.". The carefully worded 'small print' below this emotive message suggests: "An unpleasant thought, certainly. But there is evidence to suggest that working with some computer screens can put the unborn child at risk.". The text goes on to imply that the results of the Kaiser Permanente study, the European Directive 90/270/EEC and the Swedish MPR 2 guidelines all support the need to change to EIZO screens. Phrases such as "Although the evidence is not conclusive, experimental work in this area continues." do not mitigate the basic health message conveyed by this advertisement. It is clearly directed at VDU users and seeks to exploit their fears and concerns.

This advertisement was the subject of a number of complaints to the Advertising Standards Authority (ASA). The complainants questioned the basis of the claims made in the advertisement and considered the approach used to be an unacceptable appeal to fear. The ASA upheld the complaints. The decision published on the 10th June 1992 concluded: "The Authority noted the advertisers' comments but did not consider that the level of uncertainty warranted the use of such an evocative photograph or such an emphasis in the accompanying copy on limited findings. The Authority concluded that the approach was an unacceptable appeal to fear and the advertisers were requested to seek guidance in the preparation of future advertisements.". Although the decisions of the ASA are not legally enforceable and, as illustrated earlier, can be ignored by unscrupulous advertisers it is extremely unlikely, following this ruling, that any UK advertising medium would be prepared to carry a similar advertisement for this product, in the future.

5. DEVICES WHICH ALLEGEDLY NEUTRALIZE RADIATION

One of the more bizarre products available to VDU users is a 'radiation eating' cactus - Cereus Peruvianus. According to a story in a (UK) trade magazine *Computer Talk*: "A rare Mexican cactus could hold the answer to all our fears about the dangerous radiation emission from VDU screens." [6]. The news story goes on to quote the supplier of the product in the UK: "I am not saying that VDUs constitute a major hazard to the health of operators, just that they do contribute to the total load of electromagnetic radiation to which we are all subjected. Taking precautions when using them really makes sense and the cactus does seem to make a difference.". However, Coghill [1] finds this cactus harmless but ineffective: "No one seems to be trying to make capital out of this little plant, and even if it doesn't work, it can do no harm to have a cactus by your screen. I have one here while I write, and it is quite comforting! However, a quick check with the meters tells me that the E-field a foot away is about 10 V/m and is modified down to 8 V/m by the cactus (as it would be by any opaque object), while the H-field's vertical component is fluctuating around 50 nT minimum whether the plant is there or not."

6. CONCLUSIONS

The existence of a market for such products can be viewed as a natural consequence of the lack of a clear, international consensus on the interpretation of the available scientific data concerning the biological effects of exposure to various types of EMR emitted by VDUs. However, in the UK, the Health and Safety Executive's most recent guidance on the use of display screen equipment [7] states, when referring to EMR emissions from VDUs: "There is no need for users to be given protective devices such as anti-radiation screens," [Annex A, Page 38] and "No special protective measures are therefore needed to protect the health of people from this radiation." [Annex B, Page 42].

Few would question the principle that electric and magnetic fields should be As Low As Reasonably Achievable (ALARA). However, this raises questions such as: What is reasonable? and How can lower levels be achieved? What are the benefits and disadvantages? For example, some methods of EMR attenuation can degrade image quality. Providing VDUs with reduced EMR emissions might well be a reasonable way forward. Dressing up VDU users in potentially hazardous smocks or applying ineffective, anti-radiation screens to VDUs is surely not reasonable and achieves little. Promoting such products with alarmist advertising merely increases the perception of risk unnecessarily and callously seeks to exploit the fears and concerns of VDU users.

References

[1] R. Coghill, Electro Pollution: How to protect yourself against it. Thorsons Publishing Group, Wellingborough, England. 1990.

[2] D. Campbell, VODS up, Doc? Personal Computer World. December, 1989. pp 144-149.

[3] E. Cronin, Contact Dermatitis. Churchill Livingston Inc. USA 1980.

[4] Campaign was misleading. Office Secretary. Summer, 1990. pp 14.

[5] M. K. Goldhaber, M. R. Polen, and R. A. Hiatt, The risk of miscarriage and birth defects among women who use visual display terminals during pregnancy. American Journal of Industrial Medicine, 13, 1988. pp 695-706.

[6] Desk-top cactus cures VDU blues. Computer Talk November 5-November 18, 1990. pp 3.

[7] Health and Safety Executive, Display screen equipment work: Guidance on Regulations, L 26. HMSO, London. 1992.

WORK WITH DISPLAY UNITS 92
H. Luczak, A. Çakir and G. Çakir (Editors)

U.S. POLICY APPROACHES TO REGULATING THE OCCUPATIONAL USE OF VIDEO DISPLAY UNITS

DENNIS J. MCINTOSH, Executive Director, Center for Office Technology

I. INTRODUCTION

The issue of whether regulations are needed to protect U.S. workers who use video display units (VDUs) in their daily work attracted growing interest in the public, among the media, and among policymakers at local, state and federal levels during the 1980s. A variety of complaints ranging from increased stress to eyestrain and cumulative trauma disorders (CTD) have been attributed by some to the millions of VDUs that were deployed in U.S. offices over the last ten years. However, enactment of regulations governing the private sector occupational use of VDUs would mark a significant change in U.S. safety regulatory policy. Most of the tens of millions of U.S. workers who use VDUs regularly are white collar office workers (most of whom are not members of a labor union), and currently these workers are subject to virtually no state or federal workplace safety and health regulations directed specifically at their work. Extension of safety and health regulations to them would dramatically expand the scope of U.S. occupational safety and health regulation.

II. PRIMARY U.S. VDU POLICY OPTIONS

Efforts to regulate the occupational use of VDUs in the United States, which began in the early 1980s, have assumed several forms depending upon the political jurisdiction in which they have been considered. VDU policy has been considered in the United States Congress; at the U.S. Occupational Safety and Health Administration (OSHA); in state legislatures; at state occupational safety and health commissions; in county boards of supervisors; and in city councils. VDU regulations have been adopted by some state and local agencies for their own public sector employees. Also, some labor unions have negotiated contract provisions intended to protect their VDU worker members.

Advocates of adoption of VDU regulatory proposals typically have included labor unions representing VDU and other office workers; other office workers' advocacy groups (such as 9 to 5 National Working Women's Organization); and some public health officials. Opponents and skeptics of the need for VDU regulations have included state and local Chambers of Commerce and other traditional business representatives; trade associations representing computer and office equipment manufacturers; and specialized coalitions of employers and VDU manufacturers[1].

In order to better understand the debate over VDU policy in the United States it is important to distinguish among the various types of VDU policies that have been considered. The primary VDU policy options are described below and examples of some policy options are provided.

A. Prescriptive VDU Standards

The most common VDU regulatory proposal would address vision and musculoskeletal concerns (concerns about electromagnetic fields from VDUs seldom have been addressed in VDU proposals) by "prescribing" minimum equipment design standards for VDU workstations, rest breaks at specified intervals for VDU workers, and, in some cases, medical benefits such as eye examinations and corrective lenses.

Only two prescriptive VDU standards applicable to the private sector have been adopted in the United States: by Suffolk County, New York, in 1988, and by the City of San Francisco, California in 1990[2]. The San Francisco ordinance contains detailed equipment standards and requirements for work breaks and VDU ergonomics training. The Suffolk County law contains VDU equipment and workstation design and use standards, work rules, and mandatory eyecare benefits for VDU workers. Both the San Francisco and the Suffolk County VDU ordinances were overturned by state courts on the grounds that neither the City and County of San Francisco nor the County of Suffolk possessed the legal authority under their respective state constitutions to regulate the private sector occupational use of VDUs[3].

Another type of prescriptive VDU standard would "codify" all or a portion of a specific VDU design standard, such as the ANSI/HFS 100-1988 standard for VDUs. For example, California Assembly Bill 644, introduced into the California state legislature in 1991 by Rep. Hayden, would require California employers to ensure that, after a certain future date, all VDUs and related workstation equipment conform to the applicable provisions of the ANSI/HFS 100-1988 standard for VDUs. The bill also would mandate alternative work breaks for VDU workers and require employers to provide VDU workers with training in VDU ergonomics and education in detection of CTDs[4].

B. Data on State VDU Legislative Proposals

The following table depicts VDU measures introduced into state and local legislatures or proposed as executive orders from 1981 through 1992, with totals by year and outcome. The table indicates that state interest in VDU regulatory proposals began in the early 1980's, reached a peak in 1986 with 20 states considering VDU-related legislation, declined late in the decade and rose again in 1991. Although at least 238 proposals have been introduced into state and local legislatures over the last decade, only 14 became law, and only one state law, the state of Maine's VDU training law, currently applies to private sector VDU workers.

Table 1
State, County/City VDU Legislative Proposals and Adopted Legislation, by Year

Year	Total States	Total Bills/Ex Orders	Passed	County/ City Bills	Passed
1981	1	1			
1982	2	2			
1983	6	12			
1984	13	28			
1985	20	34	1	1	
1986	12	19			
1987	13	25		1	1
1988	9	11	1	3	2
1989	13	16	2	3	1
1990	9	20		1	1
1991	18	41	3	1	1
1992	13	19	1		
Total	(a)	228	8	10	6

(a) This column depicts the number of different states that considered VDU bills each year; many states considered such bills in more than one year.

C. General Industry Ergonomic Hazard Standards

Recently, federal and state regulatory agencies have expressed interest in addressing CTD hazards wherever they are thought to occur in the workplace. "General industry ergonomic hazard" standards, as they have been termed, would require employers to evaluate jobs and workstations for potential CTD hazards and attempt to reduce or eliminate CTD hazards that are identified. These standards are also known as "performance" standards because they establish general and flexible requirements for investigating and correcting hazards, in contrast to "prescriptive" standards which contain exact equipment specifications and working conditions. General industry ergonomic hazard standards may encompass concerns that some have associated with intensive use of VDUs. On August 3, 1992, the U.S. Occupational Safety and Health Administration (OSHA) issued an Advanced Notice of Proposed Rulemaking (ANPR) for a general industry ergonomic hazard standard[5].

D. VDU Training/Education Programs

In 1989 the state of Maine adopted a law requiring employers to provide employees training on ergonomic principles in the use of VDUs. This is the only VDU law in the U.S. currently applicable to the private sector.

E. Voluntary VDU Guidelines

Several local jurisdictions have developed VDU programs that call for voluntary employer adherence to VDU guidelines that typically are prescriptive in nature. Some of the guidelines also include training and education provisions.

F. VDU-related Safety/Health Research Programs

Several states have adopted legislation to investigate or research alleged VDU-related safety and health concerns. For example, the state of Minnesota adopted legislation in 1992 directing the Commissioner of Labor to investigate ergonomic hazards associated with occupational use of VDUs and to report to the state legislature by the end of 1992.

G. Public Sector VDU Worker Regulations

A few state and local agencies have adopted VDU regulations for their respective workers. These regulations have come in the form of state executive orders, municipal directives, and agency procurement policies.

III. DISCUSSION OF PROPOSED VDU POLICIES

Although it is impossible to know for certain why so few of the hundreds of VDU regulations proposed have been adopted, the following factors may have contributed to the reluctance of most states and localities to adopt VDU regulations.

1. It may be difficult for some to believe that serious safety and health risks may exist in the office. Federal statistics indicate that the rate of death and serious injury—including CTD —in the office environment is extremely low in comparison with other work environments.

2. The concerns associated with VDUs have changed over the decade, making it difficult to achieve consensus on the alleged risks. VDUs were thought to cause cataracts or eye damage; then VDUs were blamed for miscarriages; and recently, VDUs have been blamed for causing CTD. Broad agreement has not been reached on any of these claims.

3. Scientific evidence of a causal relationship between VDU ergonomic factors and CTD is complicated and incomplete. Dose/response relationships between repetitive keyboarding and the development of hand/wrist CTDs have not been clearly identified, and statistical relationships between VDU ergonomic factors and confirmed cases of CTD are not strong. Most importantly, little more than anecdotal evidence exists to demonstrate that implementing VDU ergonomic standards will actually reduce the incidence of diagnosed CTD among VDU workers.

4. State legislators have expressed reservations about adopting comprehensive regulations over tens of millions of office workers, which would create new enforcement burdens for state governments.

5. In the last three years, as the U.S. economy has slowed, policymakers have expressed growing reservations about adopting substantial new business regulations that may excessively burden businesses or discourage new businesses from locating in a particular state.

IV. CONCLUSION: VDU REGULATORY PROSPECTS IN THE REMAINDER OF THE DECADE

Several new developments indicate that regulations affecting VDUs may be adopted at the federal level or at least in some states in the next several years.

- The U.S. OSHA issued its Advanced Notice of Proposed Rulemaking (ANPR) for an ergonomic management standard that may include provisions applicable to VDUs.
- In 1992, legislation mandating OSHA's adoption of a CTD standard was approved by committees in both the House and Senate. Such legislation may be reintroduced into the new Congress.
- The California Occupational Safety and Health Administration (Cal OSHA) is preparing to recommend adoption of a general industry ergonomic hazard standard. The culmination of more than two years' work, Cal OSHA's recommendation likely will receive serious consideration by the California Standards Board and will attract the interest and attention of safety and health officials in other states.
- Several hundred lawsuits have been filed against U.S. VDU manufacturers by individuals claiming injury as a result of using the VDU. These lawsuits have rekindled publicity about health and safety concerns some have associated with occupational use of VDUs.

None of these factors alone is sufficient to ensure that VDU regulations will be adopted on the federal or state level, but they indicate a growing likelihood that some form of regulation affecting VDUs will be adopted in the next several years. States have not chosen to adopt regulations covering VDUs alone, so VDUs more likely will be regulated under a general standard intended to control CTD. Whether adoption of such regulations will resolve public or political concerns surrounding VDUs remains to be seen.

---

[1] The Center for Office Technology (COT) has questioned the need and efficacy of most VDU regulatory proposals. COT believes there is insufficient reliable research on which to form a health-based standard with which companies might comply.

[2] Part II, Chapter 5, Article 23, Sects. 1301-1315, San Francisco Municipal Code; ordinance no. 405-90, file no. 118-09-5, adopted 17 December, 1990; see amendments related thereto adopted 7 January, 1991. As noted elsewhere in this article, the state of Maine adopted a VDU law that applies to the private sector, it contains no prescriptive requirements, only training provisions.

[3] <u>C & T Management Services, Inc., doing business as Data Processing Accounting Services, and Zack</u>

Electronics, Inc. v. City and County of San Francisco. Case No. 936661, Superior Court for the State of California, City and County of San Francisco; ILC Data Device Corp., Lumex, Inc., Micra Corp., Applies Digital Data v. County of Suffolk, New York Supreme Court, Appellate Div., Second Depart., No. 90-01134.

[4] This bill was adopted by the California Assembly but not by the State Senate and, thus, it did not become law.

[5] Federal Register, Vol. 57, No. 149, Monday, August 3, 1992, p. 34192; 29 CFR Part 1910, Docket No. S-777, Ergonomic Safety and Health Management.

WORK WITH DISPLAY UNITS 92
H. Luczak, A. Çakir and G. Çakir (Editors)
1993 Elsevier Science Publishers B.V.

Introducing Teleworking

Antony J Chapman[a], Sarah Heywood[a], Sylvie Collins[a] and Barbara Dooley[b]

[a]University of Leeds, Department of Psychology, Leeds LS2 9JT, United Kingdom

[b]University College Dublin, Ireland

1.0 INTRODUCTION

Advances in information and telecommunications technologies are impacting substantially on the ways in which work is conceived, managed and conducted. Although most changes have been manifested within established organizational frameworks, further changes in work practices, such as *teleworking*, can themselves facilitate an unfolding of flexibility in organizational arrangements.

Telework has been under discussion for more than two decades, but in practice its adoption as a way of working has been gradual. Seemingly, however, with the rapid development of telematic systems, we have reached a watershed. Amongst policy makers and strategy planners there are forecasts of a rapid growth in flexible work-practices with home-based teleworking by no means unusual at the end of the century.

No single definition of teleworking is accepted universally -- 'telecommuting', 'remote work' and 'location independent work' are just some of the various terms which are used interchangeably -- but, nonetheless, it is generally agreed that telework embodies (a) the performance of work at a location independent from the location of employers or contractors (and usually at a distant location) and (b) the use of telecommunications/telematics as an enabling factor.

Those teleworkers who are home-based are differentiated from other, more conventional homeworkers -- for example, craft designers, architects or artists -- in that, generally, teleworkers have some Information Technology (IT) skills. In particular they are usually 'computer literate'; and most teleworkers depend on visual display units (VDUs) -- hence, the term '*tele*work'.

Occupations across a broad spectrum may be transformed or evolved for teleworking, both full-time and part-time. Prospects for part-time work may be particularly enhanced through telework allowing for employment at home or close to home. While home-based work is for the moment the most salient form of telework, there are already many other forms, which vary for instance in their degree of decentralization: There are satellite work centres, where a unit or department within an organization is geographically separated from the central office but where contact through telecommunication systems is available easily. There are 'neighbourhood offices', 'telecottages' or 'telesteads', providing electronic/IT facilities for various users within a locality, where, for example, freelance workers may rent facilities. There are forms of mobile-work, where individuals using IT may link with colleagues, perhaps office-based, while in transit or with clients.

Telework is perceived as offering many societal and economic benefits. Where regions have high and long-term unemployment, and especially where there is a consequential risk of depopulation and political marginalization, teleworking offers fresh prospects for the economy and infrastructure. Attention has turned particularly to advantages which may accrue to regions which have been formerly dependent upon traditional agricultural concerns, now in decline.

Much of telework's enormous potential derives from the possibilities offered for diversification and new jobs. It challenges the need for people who work collaboratively to be physical proximate. In other words, at least part of a team or partnership might reside in a rural area though undertaking work for an organization which has its plant, offices and headquarters in areas of relatively dense population. Hence a less-favoured, rural region may again plan to retain its young and talented people; and, at a societal level, this will help secure cultural diversification, including minority languages. Indeed, teleworking may cause migratory, rural-to-urban trends to be reversed. Some folk are already being tempted to reside in rural areas where, until the availability of telematic systems, they could not envisage using their professional skills to sufficient financial advantage.

Other tangible advantages attaching to the successful introduction and maintenance of telework initiatives are: (a) reductions in central office overheads; (b) increased productivity and motivation; (c) recruitment and retention of personnel who have scarce skills and/or who are unable to work in conventional workplace settings (e.g., individuals with mobility problems); (d) flexibility in terms of working hours (as well as location); (e) reduction in commuting time; (f) pollution reduction (e.g., through reduced transportation); and (g) work, leisure and family life can be combined more efficaciously.

As already intimated, however, and notwithstanding the substantial advantages apparently on offer, teleworking has not yet captured employer-investment and employee-imagination to the degree generally expected. The necessary impetus may have arrived, in the form of further improvements in telematics coupled with better-value-for-money hardware and software. Our view is decidedly less optimistic; *viz* there are significant psychological and organizational issues to be resolved before technology can be exploited to an optimal level for telework to become commonplace.

Many of the dimensions which undermine employee enthusiasm for telework are conspicuously psychological, whether they bear principally on the individual, management or the organization: (a) many teleworkers report physical and social isolation; (b) typically there are poor promotion opportunities; (c) the flow of work can be uncomfortably intermittent; (d) there are pronounced conflicts between work roles and home roles; (e) job security is often minimal; (f) a reduced skill variety is not uncommon; (g) working environments are of relatively poor quality; and (h) there is low pay and restricted benefits.

Trades Unions sometimes do not trust particular telework arrangements because of the potential for employee manipulation; and prospects for exploitation are at least implicit, and some explicit, in the issues pertaining to employment status, just listed. Managers, too, are sometimes resistant to the introduction of telework into their own portfolios of responsibilities. Indeed, some telework researchers have cited managerial resistance as the main cause of slow progress towards organizational change. Many established managers are not well acquainted with new technology, and they are concerned about losing control and authority if staff are remote workers.

The remainder of this essay overviews psychological aspects of teleworking in order to expose the likely barriers to telework up-take. The analysis is in organizational-psychological terms, with a focus on the individual, either as employee or as manager, and as a member of cultural, social, and familial groups. Attention is also given to technology and the tasks which comprise work.

2.0 ORGANISATIONAL AND PSYCHOLOGICAL FACTORS

There follows a critique and synthesis of some of the more prominent factors which define success in teleworking. They include job satisfaction, motivation, commitment, performance, selection and training, social isolation, family-role and work-role conflicts, and individual differences such as gender.

If *job satisfaction* is defined as an emotional response to a job situation, then a satisfied worker is one who responds with positive affect more than with negative affect to the job and job-related experiences. In teleworking, many sources can be expected to generate dissatisfaction, although in aggregate the negative perceptions and negative experiences are not likely to negate nor perhaps to diminish seriously the satisfaction which emanates from augmented levels of autonomy and flexibility.

The teleworker may feel disadvantaged in promotion procedures, being forgotten or uninformed when new vacancies arise as well as relatively deprived of performance feedback and access to programmes of staff development. Professional teleworkers tend to report that frequent contact with those in authority is necessary for career advancement. Dissatisfaction also results when the teleworker believes that office-based employees are being paid more for similar work, and this may be a particularly acute factor in the telework context since pay is often closely associated with performance and since job security may be particularly tenuous. Conflicts between work and non-work roles may also be especially acute in telework, where family life and work may occur in very close proximity and where other forms of social contact, normally allied to work hours, are likely to be drastically impoverished.

To begin teleworking the individual's *motivation* must be high. In general work motivation is influenced by conditions affecting the production, direction and maintenance of work-related behaviours. On the one hand, the individual may initially be attracted by notions of flexible work practices, autonomy, and freedom from regular commuting; and, on the other hand, s/he may turn to telework through lack of other opportunities, perhaps in work options and perhaps because of life-style demands (such as mobility restrictions). The original reasons for teleworking and initial levels of motivation are thought to affect the individual's motivation to continue, or persevere, as a teleworker. Nonetheless the individual's motivation can be sustained/strained by the employer's regard/disregard for the quality of the teleworker's working-life; due attention must be given to reviewing performance with a view to identifying the individual's training needs, commensurate with changes in work to be undertaken and personal and professional development.

Working remotely is presumed by many to impact negatively on the employee's *commitment* to an organization and identification with it. An existing organizational culture may not be readily communicable to the teleworker, nor even conducive to teleworking where, for example, a marked degree of autonomy may be prized. The pioneers and champions of teleworking characteristically place key life-style considerations far ahead of employing organizations in their hierarchies of commitment. Then again some commentators believe that telework inspires singular loyalty to employing organizations because the teleworker appreciates the trust invested in him/herself and finds invaluable the flexibility afforded for other needs and demands.

The *training* of teleworkers tends to be more exclusively direct and formal than for office-based workers. The initial introduction to the job is at one and the same time more focused and more limited, and the teleworker's distinctness is then accentuated through the paucity of incidental 'on-the-job' learning with others on the organization's prime territory. Relative to office-based contemporaries the teleworker's narrow training is debilitating to the extent that typically s/he acquires a more confined range of skills; and the absence of a general induction to the organization does little to inculcate a sense of belonging. However, the teleworker's independence and the focus on self-contained tasks is of relative benefit in reducing the potential for *role ambiguity* and *role conflict*. Then again, teleworkers make extensive use of VDUs and some work in rather casually arranged and modest environments where it is not obvious that *health and safety* issues are properly addressed.

Various psychological and demographic variables are important in determining teleworking viability and success; for example, gender, personality, employment status, union membership, whether full-time or part-time work is sought, employee involvement in initiating teleworking, and the general 'marketability', skills and experience of the employee. Sets of difficulties invariably arise for the individual because channels for interaction with colleagues are significantly constricted or non-existent. Difficulties may, for instance, take the form of reduced personal and professional feedback, scant identification with the organization, social isolation, and communication problems. To a degree the impact of these difficulties may be mitigated if the teleworker's supervisor adopts appropriate managerial styles as circumstances demand. (Section 4.0). Whatever the manager's sensitivities and adaptability, however, there are areas of difficulty over which s/he can expect to have little impact, particularly those involving familial, cultural and other social groups in relation to role conflicts and stress.

Whether teleworking, for the near future, is anything like a panacea enabling *disabled* folk to secure permanent and appropriately-rewarding work is rather doubtful. Much of the speculation so far is glib, and some may be insidious, going beyond what some organizations, under present legislation, may intend to deliver. While telework may indeed be a practical way of enabling disabled individuals to secure permanent jobs, full- or part-time, the individual may very well experience greater and intolerable social isolation and the employer may declare that financial investment and costs are prohibitive. However, there may be legislation and financial incentives to help alter employers' attitudes and practises. Also non-profit making organizations may become increasingly influential through bearing some of the training costs. Already, for example, "Abilities" (UK) and "Ability Enterprise" (Ireland) train disabled people in flexible work practices.

3.0 ORGANISATIONAL STRUCTURE

Organizational structure may be defined as the system of authority and reporting relationships which co-ordinates an organization's activities. Consideration of structure is particularly important in telework because one effect of teleworking, when it is at more than just the margins, is to decentralize the organization and thereby to influence structure fundamentally. The degree of formal structuring of an organization embodying telework should be contingent on the type of teleworking and the circumstances in which it is done. A formal structure may be best suited for dispersed home-based workers, whereas a more adaptive, organic structure may be more appropriate for telecottage arrangements. The organic structure is characterized by being relatively open to environmental influences and less formalized in its activities, with more dispersed and multiple authority structures, shared responsibilities, loosely-defined tasks and functions, few written and formal procedures, and decentralized decision-making. In the organic structure the individual has authority according to the perceived expertise and knowledge which s/he brings to bear on any particular task, rather than according to his/her job-description or job-title.

The number of subordinates whom a telework-supervisor can supervise optimally varies according to key organizational aspects of the telework operation, for example according to whether it is decentralized-homebased, decentralized-downsized or third-party-telecottage. Home-based teleworking can normally be expected to function best when the link to the supervisor is direct. There is then efficient control of the decentralized worker who, in turn, has an appropriate perception of his/her place in the organization's hierarchical structure, *vis-a-vis* authority, responsibility and accountability. As organizations move into telework there is a tendency for established managers to endeavour retaining a hierarchical and formalized structure. They recognize a potential loss of control as 'remote workers' are recruited, and they perceive that the superior-subordinate model is placed under threat. Many teleworkers, particularly those who are not home-based, might be seeking a more dynamic and adaptive form of leadership, rather than line-management and control. In fact managers can find that they have greater information, if not control, with regard to teleworked jobs, through having access to the system on which tasks are being conducted. In contrast, the teleworkers while usually gaining autonomy and freedom from the **workplace** often find that they have sacrificed some independence with regard to **work tasks**.

To engage successfully in teleworking an organization has first to specify clearly its mission and objectives and, therefore, its activities. In so doing work-roles can be stipulated with some precision at the level of the individual, and hence there is less prospect of the teleworker experiencing serious role conflict and role ambiguity. Correspondingly the most effective channels of communication are generally those fashioned at an early juncture. It is also crucial that top-management is supportive and committed, and open to change and innovation. It has to specify needs which are best met through telework and fund accordingly, both at the outset and subsequently. Appropriate start-up investment is essential for training and equipment. Above all, as in virtually all organizations, the top-management must ensure availability of information if staff are to be optimally effective and loyal.

There is allusion in the above text to some of the possible benefits of teleworking. For the organization the benefits include: (a) the recruitment and retention of personnel with scarce skills; (b) a drop in employee turnover; (c) enhanced motivation and improved productivity; (d) increased flexibility in the assignment of work; and (e) contraction in central office overheads. At the societal level, the present thrust towards teleworking is largely identified, at least in the European Community, with the development of rural areas. As for obstacles many commentators agree that traditional organizational structures, with their concomitant cultures and management attitudes, comprise the main sources of hindrance.

4.0 MANAGERIAL CONCERNS

A *task-oriented/goal-setting managerial style* may be entirely suitable for supervising workers at a distance. It is a style in which there is emphasis on the regular control of results and constructive feedback. A more *people-orientated* style, where the manager is attentive to the subordinate's needs and relationships, is particularly difficult to apply when little face-to-face contact is possible. In the former approach, when applied to telework (and then known as *tele-management*), there is a setting of specific goals and measurement of output. Those processes reduce uncertainty and ambiguity in the teleworker, and for many that is associated with elevated job satisfaction and motivation. When *selecting* telework-supervisors it is obviously important to consider whether candidates can adopt an appropriate 'management-by-objectives' style for teleworkers while adopting other styles, as necessary, for those with whom there is more personal contact.

In telework it might seem that there is little need for continual interpersonal communication. In formal communications teleworker-interaction is thought to be little affected by the distances between interactants, but the quantity and quality of informal interaction is greatly reduced for the individual teleworker. However, even disregarding any gregarious facets of *homo sapiens*, it is evident that teleworkers require effective communication channels for their work. The manager must specify how teleworkers are to communicate through those channels with other members in the organization, both remote and office-based.

The telework-manager must also be comfortable with a measure of decentralized decision-making. If decentralization means allowing participation in decision-making processes it should raise employee motivation and commitment. Plainly distant locations no longer imply slow communications. Telephones, fax-machines and computer-mediated forms of communication (e.g., 'e-mail'), are available to teleworkers generally, and they enable rapid consultation and transmission of information. They are also useful for conveying aspects of company culture.

5.0 ORGANISATIONAL CULTURE

There is widespread recognition that the culture which pervades an organization can have a substantial impact on the success of a teleworking initiative. A climate of mutual trust between workers and management must be firmly established before teleworking is introduced. An organization announces, or perhaps unwittingly discloses, aspects of its culture in various ways. The culture is imparted to new members of the organization through explicit and implicit processes of *socialization*, starting from the employee's first contact, and elements are established and/or reinforced through rituals, myths, stories and so forth. From an organization's viewpoint there is something to be said for selecting teleworkers from the existing work-force because issues to do with conveying culture and climate, and building loyalty, may not arise. Large organizations may be able to appoint teleworkers from existing staff: that is, from members of staff who have demonstrated their commitment to the organization and who are trusted by existing management and *vice versa*. When this is not possible, a period of socialization is recommended for new entrants before they begin to telework.

6.0 TECHNOLOGY AND TASKS

Technology, within a systems model, is about transforming inputs into outputs, and it incorporates both machines and procedures. *Tasks* are performed by people to achieve the demands of their work. Teleworking uses technology and is expected to impact on jobs in that the teleworkers will increasingly seek tasks requiring greater control, greater cognitive acumen, high responsibility and little face-to-face interaction. Teleworking is not exclusively suitable for tasks requiring low-level skills, any more than it is especially suitable for high-level skills. Many professional jobs and many unskilled jobs can be undertaken as telework.

7.0 CONCLUSION

Although substantial technological progress has been made to advance teleworking, psychological problems remain to be recognized and resolved before teleworking becomes widespread. This paper has identified some broad individual, social and organizational issues which may impede the introduction of teleworking until they are given due regard by employing organizations.

WORK WITH DISPLAY UNITS 92
H. Luczak, A. Çakir and G. Çakir (Editors)

Procedure to bring into force the Council Directive on the minimum safety and health requirements for work with display screen equipment

A. Rückert

Federal Ministry of Labour and Social Affairs
Postfach 14 02 80, D - 5300 Bonn-Duisdorf, Federal Republic of Germany

Abstract

The EC Council Directive on work with display screen equipment regulates the safety and health requirements for the employees. New important aspects of the directive as well as the way the Federal Republic of Germany plans to translate it into national law are described.

1 INTRODUCTION

Work with display screen equipment concerns an increasing number of employees. From a few hundred screens in the 50s the number of display units has meanwhile developed into a stock of about 2 million in the Federal Republic of Germany alone. According to forecasts one in two employees will work with display screen equipment by the end of this decade.

Work with display screen equipment becomes increasingly important for the planning, carrying out and control of work tasks. This is true for industry, research and administration but also for the service sector. Such work tasks include word processing data input and output programming, computer-aided design, process control and monitoring.

2 EC ASPECT

In the framework of its action programme on safety, hygiene and health work the EC Commission adopted a package of occupational safety and health directives under Article 118 a of the Single European Act. This package includes the Display Screen Equipment Directive or, to use its full title, the Council Directive on the minimum safety and health requirements for work with display screen equipment. It is the 5th individual directive under the EC framework Directive on Occupational safety and health. It regulates safety and health requirements for work with display screen equipment to be met in the establishments; it is not a single market directive on the marketing of display units.

3 WORK WITH DISPLAY SCREEN EQUIPMENT

The EC Directive on work with display screen equipment illustrates in particular the EC's broad view of safety and health at work. In Germany one is familiar with this far-reaching view of safety and health at work since it is embedded in the Law on company doctors, safety engineers and other occupational safety advisers. This Law lays down the tasks to be performed by company doctors and occupational safety advisers. By means of preventive measures the EC intends to protect workers against health hazards in relation to all aspects concerning work. One of the most important principles in this context is the adaption of work to humans.

In case of display screen work, for example, a work-station design not adapted to the human body dimensions and the scope of movement, a poor legibility of the screen or source documents lead to unfavourable working postures of the employees. Repetitive short-cyclical movements in a quick sequence, for example when the keyboard is used for the input of data, may cause health problems in the region of the hands or/ and forearms.

The need to frequently turn from the screen to the source document and the keyboard and vice-versa together with the need to adjust to differing contrasts and levels of brightness and different visual distances may lead to considerable eye strain.

Shortcomings in the dialogue design of the software may cause an increased mental strain for the employees. The way in which the stressful factors which have been mentioned by way of example act upon employees, however, have to be assessed in the overall context of the work with display screen equipment.

They may give rise to health problems of the employees which, unless they are detected and eliminated at an early stage by an ergonomic design of work may lead to psychosomatic syndromes.

4 NEW ASPECTS OF THE EC DIRECTIVE ON DISPLAY SCREEN WORK

From a German point of view it is a new development that by means of this directive the subject-matter to be regulated has been raised to the level of a law. So far, there have been no legal provisions on work with display screen equipment in the Federal Republic of Germany.

Further important aspects of the directive are the following:

- Compared with existing sets of instruments applicable to work with display screen equipment the EC directive has a wide scope of application.

- Employers are obliged to analyze the work with display screen equipment, in order to evaluate the safety and health conditions to which they give raise for their employees (particularly as regards physical problems, problems of mental stress and possible risks to eyesight). On basis of these evaluations the measures necessary to prevent any health impairments have to be taken. In Germany these analyses could be done by the company doctors and safety advisers of the establishments.

- The display screen workstation is defined in a very comprehensive way. It comprises not only working equipment (display screen keyboard, printer, work desk, work chair and so on) but also work environment (physical, in terms of work organization, social) and the software determining the operator/computer interface.

- The directive also includes requirements for the daily work routine with display screen equipment.

- Employees are given the right to have an appropriate eye and eyesight test.

- The Annex includes minimum requirements for the design of the working equipment, of the work environment and the operator/computer interface in case of work with display screen equipment. The requirements are very general and have to be specified in order to be applied in the establishments.

5 TRANSLATION INTO NATIONAL LAW

In Germany it is planned to translate the whole directive into national law by means of a new Ordinance of the Federal Government. It will be applicable to all employees. Such an Ordinance will essentially provide for the same level of protection as the directive. It will lay down all minimum requirements mentioned therein - from the analysis of workstations to the daily work routine, the design of the hardware and software and the work environment. If necessary, it will specify these requirements. The Ordinance will not be restricted to certain fields of application or work. This is why such an Ordinance does not contain any numerical figures with regard to frame frequency, size of characters, noise, for example.

It is planned to use the new Law on Safety and Health at Work as a basis for the Ordinance. This law is meant to implement the EC Framework Directive on Occupational safety and health. This legislative project is a step towards a more comprehensible and harmonised legislation on occupational safety and health in the Federal Republic of Germany. It fulfils the mandate laid down in Article 30 of the Unification Treaty, namely to newly regulate occupational safety and health in accordance with the requirements of today. The planned Ordinance on Work with Display screen Equipment will be discussed with Federal States, employers, trade unions, technical institutes and associations and others.

Furthermore, the concept includes to give the Industrial Professional Associations the possibility to specify the Ordinance on Work with Display Equipment for the individual branches in their accident prevention regulations. If necessary, they could supplement it by more far-reaching provisions. Preparatory work in the form of collecting material is being made by working groups of the Central Agency for Accident Prevention and Occupational Medicine of the Central Federation of Industrial Professional Associations. Thus it will be relatively easy to adjust the defined provisions to the technical developments and other scientific findings.

6 REFERENCES

Richtlinie des Rates vom 29. Mai 1990 über die Mindestvorschriften bezüglich der Sicherheit und des Gesundheitsschutzes bei der Arbeit an Bildschirmgeräten, ABl. EG L 156 vom 21. Juni 1990, S. 14

WORK WITH DISPLAY UNITS 92
H. Luczak, A. Çakir and G. Çakir (Editors)

European Regulations for Work With VDU

Francis Gattegno,

Eurobit, France

Relationship between VDU Directive and Technical specifications for industrial products

Employers, at dawn of 1993, will be puzzled to achieve their obligations towards the VDU Directive minimal requirements laid down in their national laws transposing the EC social Directive.

The issue, as regarded by *employers*, can be worded as follows: can I assure, when buying pieces of equipment that the workplace and the working conditions will be in compliance with the law?

The second issue comes from potential discrepancies between member states requirements when transposing the Directive and setting levels of requirements much higher than the *minimal* ones laid down in the Directive.

Manufacturers, providing specific equipment are not in a position to guarantee any *compliance* to legislation which may be applied differently from one country to another, from one employer to another...

The standards mandated to CEN by DG XIII of the EC Commission, determine harmonized specifications which could potentially meet the *essential requirements* of a New approach Directive on VDUs. Note that such a Directive does not exist, and is not even envisaged.

In February 1992, DG XIII requested DG V, to make a link between the VDU Directive and ergonomics standards. This could be a good solution to provide a presumption of compliance, to regulate the social levels among countries and avoid gaps which could harm the achievement of the social Directive and could lead to negative economical impact.

Manufacturers believe that the Annex of the Directive should be removed when the relevant parts of the European standard are available, and that reference to this standard should be then specified.

Will be discussed in this paper concerns related to the applicability of the annex; how the EN 29241 standard can provide adequate solutions to the above issues; how compliance statement can be debated in regard to each part of the standard and for the total document.

I) Applicability of the Annex

The Preliminary remark is essential to make sure that the application of the Directive could be based on the analysis of the tasks by the employer (article 3 of the Directive 90/270).

The assessment of compliance to the Directive clauses depends upon the interpretation that will be made by the various actors. The clause "Characters well defined and clearly formed" is subject to interpretation. User can easily get a good display and degrade its ergonomics characteristics by his (her) usage.

Recommendations from country social affairs may interpret the Directive in a way which leads to create conflict with standard specifications: e.g. "flicker free screens" are nearly impossible to technically achieve for 100 % of the population as being dependent on personnel perception ability. Moreover it is impossible to predict the 100 %.

Glare can be solved by antireflective treatment built in the product or by all installation means which are at the user disposal. But how to control compliance to the minimal requirements?

II) EN 29241 as an adequate foundation for Directive compliance

It is of great importance that International standards, accepted at European level as ENs provide all the warranties of technical accuracy, reproducibility and liable results, all throughout the various countries and companies. International Companies need to have the same confidence on the products they buy to achieve the social aim of the Directive. The ergonomics standard, with its 3 first parts published and the 14 others in preparation, provide the whole set of technical information to buy the relevant equipment and install it in reliable manner.

III) Compliance to EN 29241: each part or total standard

Compliance is the key issue to be settled with the standard; manufacturer's declaration provide assurance of standard compliance to employers, work councils, users.

Generally, products from most of the manufacturers offer good quality screens in terms of ergonomics. These are designed to meet the user's requirements on comfort, safeness and productivity.

New technologies are now available on the market place and progress is even developing at an increasing pace. Standards are expected to evolve at same speed. A few parts are under the responsibility of the manufacturer, others belong to the employer responsibility, others are user oriented.

References

Council Directive 29 May 1990, JOCE: L 156 dated 21.6.90. On the minimum safety and health requirements for work with display screen equipment (fifth individual Directive within the meaning of Article 16 of Directive. 87/391/EEC).

ISO 9241 Ergonomic requirements for office work with visual display terminals 1992.

SOGITS N591: Following-up of BC-IT-73 VDT (Ergonomics of video terminals) 24 February 1992.

WORK WITH DISPLAY UNITS 92
H. Luczak, A. Çakir and G. Çakir (Editors)

The Gender Gap in I.T. in Britain

A. Durndell

Dept. of Psychology, Glasgow Polytechnic, Cowcaddens Road, Glasgow, Scotland G4 0BA

Abstract

University entrants, who had enrolled for business or natural science subjects in 1986 or 1989, were studied to assess the persistence of the gender gap in I.T. and computing. Whilst 1989 entrants were more knowledgeable about I.T., the gender gap in favour of males persisted. Reported use of computers, particularly a students own computer, was higher in 1989, but again the gender gap persisted. The 1989 entrants were asked why they had chosen not to study computer studies, using open ended and fixed answer questions. Whilst gender differences did occur, gender similarity was more apparent. A negative image of the computer specialist interacting with a terminal all day was very important.

Introduction

Interest in the relatively low level of female participation in education in computing within the U.K. is now widespread. The official university statistics [1] have documented a generally rising trend of female participation in university education in most subjects over the past decade. Computer studies is unique, however, in that the proportion of home undergraduate UK admissions that are female has dropped from 25% to 11% over this period. The situation has become sufficiently critical, linked to a shortage of computer related skills and the demographic decline in school leavers, that the Minister of Education has come out in favour of special measures to attract females into technological areas, and supports the compulsory inclusion in teacher training courses of the understanding of gender based stereotypes and awareness of equal opportunity issues [2]. Discussion at the GASAT (Gender and Science and Technology) 1990 conference [3] revealed that a declining female participation in computer studies appeared to be an international trend, at least within northern Europe. (The trend is not universal though, take for example Singapore [4] where approximately half of computer studies students are female).

Research carried out in schools [5] helps to address these questions, but the focus here is on the important choice point of entry into higher education. A sequence of studies has been carried out on newly enrolled university students covering successive intakes to a number of courses from 1986. The first study [6] indicated that a gender gap existed in the use of, ownership and experience of computers reported by these students, with males typically reporting more contact with computers than females. This gender gap was also found in an I.T. quiz test result, with the males on average outscoring females across almost all course groups. Attitudes to computing were in general similar for both genders, with computing perceived as an important part of the future. It was also found that female computer specialists were not perceived as unfeminine [7].

The second study [8] tended to show that the motives of computing students of both genders about their choice of subject were similar (cf. [9]), whilst some general support for the 'we can I can't' idea [10] was uncovered. The third study [11] targetted business and natural science students, and by asking them why they had chosen not to study computer studies, was able to describe the very severe image problem of computer studies. This effected males and females, but with a larger effect on females. A computer specialist was perceived to be cut off from humans and to spend most of their time interacting with machines. It seemed to be this inhumanity, rather than any direct nonfeminine image, that was very damaging to computer studies. However, as females stereotypically are more concerned with human relations than males are, a gender differentiated effect is not surprising.

For the next study in this series the investigation of why business and natural science students avoided computer studies was continued with an extended questionnaire: This was combined with a comparison between students enrolling in 1986 and 1989 of their I.T. knowledge and their experience and use of computers.

The main questions to be investigated were (1) whether there had been a general increase in computer use and I.T. knowledge, and whether gender differences in these areas had decreased over time; and (2) how important the 'sitting at a terminal screen' image was in choice to avoid computer studies, whether it was gender differentiated, and in addition questions of confidence, specialisation and male hostility, vis a vis choice to avoid computer studies.

Method

The 1989 sample comprised 127 female and 78 male students enrolling for their first year at a Scottish university. They were targetted because they had selected to study degree subjects which would provide reasonable numbers of male and female business or natural science students who might be qualified to study computing.

The 1989 sample were presented with a questionnaire as part of their enrolment programme, administered in a group situation by a researcher who was not to be one of their tutors. A promise of confidentiality was given and an assurance that this was a research exercise and that no information on an individual would be passed on to the course organiser. Filling in the questionnaire took about a half an hour.

The questionnaire initially requested background information on age and sex, and asked an open ended question - 'why did you choose to study on this course?', followed by a request to write in their answer on the front page. Page 2 reproduced exactly an I.T. quiz utilised in 1986 [6]. Respondents were asked to match 12 items (such as 'bit', 'cursor', 'rom') with the appropriate definitions out of 17 presented (such as 'the physical devices which comprise a computer', 'a method of logging incoming data', 'a device used to interface a digital computer to a telephone line' etc.). The first example was completed in advance, and the respondents were invited to omit items that they could not answer.

On the third page respondents were asked whether they had ever considered studying a course comprised mainly of computer studies, and then presented with a subsequent open ended question 'if yes, why are you <u>not</u> intending to study computer studies now?', or 'if no, why do you think that you never considered this?'.

After allowing space for the above answer, respondents were asked various questions (taken from the 1986 study) about their use and experience of computers in the last two years. Finally on page 4 they were presented with a 5 point scale going from 1 - of no importance to me - through to 5 - very important to me. They were then asked how important to them were a series of items in their decision not to study computing, each item to be evaluated for themselves using the 5 point scale. The scale was similar to that used in 1988 [8], with a number of modifications following on from that study (such as the addition of an item about sitting in front of a terminal and another on the specialisation of computing courses).

Results

(1) Comparisons between 1986 and 1989: For these results, students on the target courses aged 16-18 years old in 1986 or 1989 respectively were extracted from the two sets of data so that only recent school leavers were compared. This yielded 52 males and 85 females from 1986, and 53 males and 105 females from 1989. Tables 1 and 2 show the results respectively obtained for experience of computers, where chi squared analysis was used, and for the I.T. quiz, where 't' tests were used.

Table 1 % reporting experience of computing in previous two years, 16-18 year old university entrants, by gender and year of intake

	1986			1989		
	M	F	total	M	F	total
used computer at school	42	52	48	67	61	63
used own computer	24*	9*	14	49*	18*	29
used family computer	24	29	27	26	38	34
used friend's computer	65*	46*	53	50*	31*	38

* Gender difference p< 0.05, M=male, F=female

Table 2 IT quiz score, 16-18 year old university entrants, by gender and year of intake

	Female mean	Male mean	Male-female difference
1986	2.54*	4.60*	2.06
1989	4.10*	6.02*	1.92
improvement 1986-1989	1.56	1.42	

* Gender difference p< 0.01

(2) Open ended material: 10% of the subjects volunteered comments that were hostile to sitting in front of a screen all day, 13% wrote of their negative and boring school experience of computing and 12% said that computing courses were too specialised. 28% of females as opposed to 8% of males volunteered that they had had little or no experience of computing. Those students who had considered studying computing gave similar responses to those who had not. Some illustrative comments were: 'thought of sitting at a terminal all day does not appeal in the slightest', 'put off by school teaching of computing', 'thought of being obligated to sit at a VDU all day is mind numbing', 'don't want to be hemmed in behind desk staring at green screens and pressing buttons', 'boring people who cannot socialise'.

(3) Statistical results: 14 items were evaluated by subjects for their importance in student choice not to study computer studies, and were analysed by gender. Few significant differences were found, with gender similarity predominant. *'I do not want to be sitting in front of a computer all day'* was most important, followed by *'the subject matter would not be interesting'* and *'I am more interested in people than objects'*. *'Computing has a rather unfeminine image'* was least important.

Discussion

The comparisons between 16-18 year olds in 1986 and 1989 in Tables 1 and 2 show virtually no closing of the gender gap, within a context of increasing use and knowledge about computers. The overall reported use of computers at school and of a family computer have increased and the use of the students' own computer has doubled. Reported use of a friends computer has reduced, perhaps because of the wider ownership reducing the need to borrow or indulge in 'social' computing. However, gender differences have remained, with males remaining more than two and a half times more likely than females to report using their own computer and much more likely to report use of a friends' computer, whilst females were more likely to report using a family computer. Students of both genders entering higher education appeared to arrive with considerably more computer based knowledge in 1989 than in 1986, but the gender gap with males scoring higher than females has remained almost unchanged in its absolute size. These results are consistent with the very low female participation in computer studies courses.

Whilst accepting the warning of Henwood [12] that the reasons for choice of courses are very complex and often contradictory, nonetheless the image of computing does seem to have an important role. In relation to gender, it is not a directly unfeminine image, but rather one mediated through a gender connected series of images about sitting in front of screens, interacting with machines rather than people and being bored with this. This leads to 'we can I do not want to' rather than 'we can I can't', and affects males as well as, though less than, females. An important question is whether this image has any base in reality. Do computer professionals spend very large amounts of time working on a terminal as opposed to interacting with people? Many computer professionals would no doubt emphasise the importance of interpersonal skills, and employer demands seem to be particularly for business skills including interpersonal skills [13], but out of necessity does not a specialist in computing have to interact more than most people with a machine?

The evidence of the lack of closure of the gender gap in use and knowledge of I.T., within a context of a general rise in computer awareness, indicates a lack of progress on gender questions.

The effects of the introduction of I.T. oriented courses in schools in Britain, both across the curriculum and in the core curriculum, have not yet been able to work through to higher education, but the omens are not too good. Some single sex tuition may be helpful (cf. [14]). A variety of other strategies are being tried out (cf. [3]), such as computing workshops for girls, providing female role models from the computer industry, and attempts to show that female (and male!) computer specialists can be quite normal people. Inservice training for teachers is obviously also important, as would it be for higher education to develop more flexible and mixed courses to attract females into computing. City Polytechnic [15], for example, has been successful in this fashion, and may be providing graduates with the range of skills - business, interpersonal and I.T.- that employers require.

References

1. UCCA, 26th Annual Report 1987/1988. UCCA, Cheltenham. (1989)
2. MacGregor, J., Keynote Speech, to Women into Computing 1990 Conference, University of East Anglia, (1990).
3. Granstam, I. (Ed.), Contributions GASAT 1990. Jonkoping University, Jonkoping, Sweden (1990).
4. Kheng, L.G., WIT: The Singaporean Way. Computer Bulletin, **2**, 18-21 (1990).
5. Siann, G., MacLeod, H., Glissov, P. & Durndell, A., The effect of computer use on gender differences in attitudes to computers. Computers and Education, **14**, 183-191 (1990).
6. Durndell, A., MacLeod, H. & Siann, G., A survey of attitudes to, knowledge about and experience of computers. Computers and Education, **11**, p167-175 (1987).
7. Siann, G., Durndell, A., MacLeod, H. & Glissov, P., Stereotyping in relation to the gender gap in participation in computing. Educational Research, **30**, p98-103 (1988).
8. Durndell, A., Siann, G., & Glissov, P., Gender differences and computing in course choice at entry into Higher Education. British Educational Research Journal, **16**, p147-162 (1990).
9. Kolmos, A., Women and men in engineering education - different approaches? In Granstam, I. (Ed.) Contributions GASAT 1990. Jonkoping University, Jonkoping, Sweden (1990).
10. Sanders, J., Closing the computer gap in school. In Daniels, J.Z. & Kahle, J.B. (Eds.) Contributions to the 4th GASAT Conference. National Science Foundation, University of Michigan, U.S.A. (1987).
11. Durndell, A., Why do female students avoid computer studies? Research in Science and Technological Education, **8**, 163-170 (1990).
12. Henwood, F., Young women and the culture of software engineering. Paper presented at Women into Computing 1990 Conference, University of East Anglia, U.K. (1990).
13. Virgo, P., Gender and computing in the 1990's. Paper presented to SIACE Conference on Bridging the Skills Gap: Women and Education in Scotland, Strathclyde University, U.K. (1989).
14. Glissov, P., The gender gap in computer use: Pupil motivation and attitudes in secondary education. Women into Computing 1990 Conference Proceedings, WIC, University of East Anglia (1990).
15. Ward, J., City Poly solves conundrum of how to get women to do computing courses. Women into IT Newsletter, **March**, 12 (1990).

WORK WITH DISPLAY UNITS 92
H. Luczak, A. Çakir and G. Çakir (Editors)

Socio-political aspects of RSI

G. Bammer[a] and B. Martin[b]

[a]National Centre for Epidemiology and Population Health, Australian National University, GPO Box 4, Canberra ACT 2601, Australia

[b]Department of Science and Technology Studies, University of Wollongong, Wollongong NSW 2522, Australia

Abstract

We discuss three avenues for insight into the socio-political dimensions of work-related musculoskeletal problems or RSI, namely the social construction of medical knowledge, social problems as social movements and the politics of research. Each approach leads to a different set of characteristic insights and is primarily useful for a particular set of purposes and groups.

1. INTRODUCTION

Work-related musculoskeletal problems have most commonly been approached using standard ergonomic and epidemiological techniques. More recently there has been growing recognition that these disorders have an important socio-political dimension which determines the context in which other explorations take place. In this paper we offer three insights into socio-political issues and use the Australian experience of so-called 'repetition strain injuries' or 'RSI' as an illustration. The insights we discuss are the social construction of medical knowledge, the relationship between the recognition of a problem and a social movement, and the politics of research.

2. THE SOCIAL CONSTRUCTION OF MEDICAL KNOWLEDGE

Research into musculoskeletal problems faces the constant challenge of definition of what it is that is being examined. This reflects the uncertainties in diagnoses and underlying pathophysiology. It helps explain why there are important differences in, for example, the prevalence of symptoms and signs depending on whether they are measured by self-completion questionnaires, interviews or medical examinations. These uncertainties are not only intellectual challenges but are also important for the ability of affected individuals to understand and manage their condition. This ability can be significantly undermined by disagreements about pathophysiology. The same disagreements however are a delight for social scientists as they provide a direct window for observing the social construction of medical knowledge.

Disagreements allow first hand observation of the challenge to the conventional belief that the physical realities of health and disease are revealed unproblematically by clinical examinations, supplemented by biochemical and other scientific methods of assessment of evidence. With regard to RSI there are two basic contests. One is between the views that these disorders are primarily physically based and that they are psychogenic and/or hysterical (for more detail see Bammer and Martin, 1988). In this debate those critical of the view that these disorders are physically based have highlighted what might otherwise have been ignored, namely how diverse symptoms and the social phenomenon of RSI have been interpreted and organised into a traditional medical injury model, with inadequacies and loose ends being dropped along the way. The other debate is within the view that these disorders are primarily physically based and is a contest between which signs and symptoms are meaningful and how they can be best explained. This debate partly revolves around issues of reproducibility, specificity, sensitivity and validity. One of us (GB) is involved in co-ordinating a set of working papers which aim to promote discussion about and possible resolution of competing explanations (Quintner and Elvey, 1991; Cohen et al., 1992; Fry 1992).

The sociology of medical knowledge is founded on deconstructing, and thereby opening to social explanations, the origins, development and deployment of medical knowledge. By its very nature such analysis threatens the dominant position in a medical debate. In the case of RSI, understandings from the sociology of medical knowledge were brought into play when the dominant position was that RSI is an organic work-related condition and were thereby used to undermine that position. If the dominant position had been that RSI is a form of mass hysteria, a sociology of knowledge analysis would have undermined that claim (for more detail see Bammer & Martin, 1992).

3. SOCIAL PROBLEMS AS SOCIAL MOVEMENTS

This analysis addresses questions such as 'why is it that RSI has received so much attention in Australia?', 'why did the issue not come to the same widespread attention in the USA and the UK until many years later?', 'why is there an emphasis in the USA on carpal tunnel syndrome, which is unmatched elsewhere?', 'why is there a common perception that the problem in Australia has disappeared?'.

When relevant people in society define something as a social problem, it can be transformed into one. This analysis draws heavily on the work of Armand Mauss (1975, 1989), who sees social problems as inseparable from social movements, because the characteristics of social problems are typically those of social movements. Social movements undergo a natural history dependent on their interaction with the surrounding society. Typically this includes incipiency, coalescence, institutionalisation, fragmentation and demise. Particularly at the beginning of a social movement, there are several levels of participants, including principal leaders and organisations, an active membership and a sympathetic public. Changes in participation are important in the natural history. Subjective definitions of reality and the mobilisation of public opinion are also central to understanding social movements.

We have described the value of a social movements explanation in understanding the rise in the RSI 'epidemic' in Australia in the early 1980s elsewhere (Bammer & Martin, 1992). Here we will examine the demise of the epidemic from that perspective.

Not only did the recognition of RSI as a social problem depend on the existence of an RSI movement, but as the movement fragmented and declined the 'problem' was also seen to recede. There are a number of reasons which help explain why social movements decline. Unless the movement is institutionalised, for example through jobs or laws, many participants will drop out or move on to other issues. Key activists, in particular, become burnt out after years of campaigning. The role of the media is also important. Media interest in issues is often short-lived and a movement must provide increasingly dramatic stories to maintain media coverage. Finally opposition to and accommodation of the movement are crucial. Overt opposition can thwart movement initiatives, reduce morale, and lead to disillusionment; accommodation or co-option involves addressing the problem, often in a limited fashion, and removing its urgency or saliency.

Each of these factors played a role in the decline of the RSI movement in Australia. As the number of RSI claims stabilised and declined, the opponents of RSI mobilised. They were effective in capturing and silencing the debate. For example, in line with the view of opponents that the 'epidemic' was being fuelled by discussion about it, *The Medical Journal of Australia*, which was the main forum for the debate, decided not to publish papers about RSI for an 18 month period beginning in September 1987. The federal government ceased routinely publishing statistics about the number of cases amongst its employees at about the same time. Although new cases continue to be reported, there is little media attention to the problem and hence a perception in many quarters that it has gone away. Workers' compensation entitlements have been and continue to be reduced. A landmark court case by a worker with RSI against the federal government was lost, partly because the federal government argued that RSI was not an organic injury (Campbell, 1988). On the other hand, a number of measures were also introduced to mitigate the problem. There was widespread introduction of so called 'ergonomic' furniture and equipment. Moves towards industrial democracy were enhanced and, in the office environment in particular, job redesign to increase task variety was common. Worker awareness of RSI and likely risk factors was greatly increased, leading to earlier reporting and intervention. There was an increased emphasis on rehabilitation. While many people previously sympathetic to the problem have 'burnt out' and moved on, there is a residual network of sympathetic doctors, researchers and support groups (see also Bammer 1990a & b).

The social problems as social movements perspective is useful in understanding the widespread public attention given to RSI in Australia in the mid-1980s and its subsequent decline. This situation was unique. More recently there has been public recognition of these disorders in the UK and the USA but it has not replicated the intensity of the Australian situation. Despite its value, a social movement explanation tends to delegitimate RSI because it is commonly assumed—except by analysts of social problems—that a real, organic condition will be recognised as a social problem without the entrepreneurial activities of a social movement. In principle, the description of RSI as a social movement should not legitimate or delegitimate the reality or importance of RSI.

4. THE POLITICS OF RESEARCH

Research, intentionally or not, may influence political debates. The choice of what is studied and how leads to partisanship, which can be intentional or de facto (Scott et al., 1990). As illustrated above, bringing the sociology-of-medical-knowledge and the social-problems-as-social-movements perspectives to bear on RSI tends to delegitimate the claims that it is a 'real' problem. Given that partisanship is built into the choice of theoretical framework and the choice of where and when to apply it, it is futile to try to eliminate partisanship, de facto or otherwise. Instead partisanship needs to be recognised and accepted, along with the understanding that there is no single road to 'truth'.

This highlights the limitations of research based on positivism and reductionism and the need for new approaches. Participatory action research is one model which may be useful. This begins with the premise that no social enquiry is possible unless it is effectively value driven. Participatory action research emphasises investigation which is driven by the interests of those whose problems or situations give rise to the research questions. This connection between researcher and researched (where the researched often become the researchers) allows social realities to be better understood and explained (Wadsworth, 1984; see also pamphlets of the Action Research Issues Centre, Melbourne).

Another model of research which may be useful is being developed by one of us (GB) and has two elements. One is that it is problem centred and brings a range of disciplinary perspectives to bear on the problem. The second is that is consultative and collaborative with all relevant interest groups.

5. CONCLUSIONS

We have illustrated several approaches to the social analysis of RSI. Each approach leads to a different set of characteristic insights and is primarily useful for a particular set of purposes and groups. One implication of this is that anyone undertaking a social analysis of RSI should carefully choose the approach which is most useful for their own purposes. A second implication is that it is important to scrutinise approaches used by others, taking note of the groups to which they are most useful. There are no neutral methods in this enterprise.

6. REFERENCES

Bammer G 1990a The epidemic is over ... or is it? *Australian Society 9(April)*: 22-24.

Bammer G 1990b Occupational disease and social struggle: the case of work-related neck and upper limb disorders. NCEPH Working Paper Number 20. Canberra: National Centre for Epidemiology and Population Health.

Bammer G & B Martin 1988 The arguments about RSI: an examination. *Community Health Studies 12*: 348-358.

Bammer G & B Martin 1992 Repetition strain injury in Australia: medical knowledge, social movement and de facto partisanship. *Social Problems 39*: 219-237.

Campbell, SA 1988 Taxing work: Susan Cooper's RSI case. Paper presented at the National Conference of Social Science Research on Occupational Health and Safety: Past Present and Future, Adelaide, August.

Cohen ML, Arroyo JF & GD Champion 1992 The relevance of concepts of hyperalgesia to 'RSI'. In Bammer G (ed) *Discussion papers on the pathology of work-related neck and upper limb disorders and the implications for diagnosis and treatment.* NCEPH Working Paper Number 31. Canberra: National Centre for Epidemiology and Population Health.

Fry HJH 1992 Overuse syndrome and the overuse concept. In Bammer G (ed) *Discussion papers on the pathology of work-related neck and upper limb disorders and the implications for diagnosis and treatment.* NCEPH Working Paper Number 32. Canberra: National Centre for Epidemiology and Population Health.

Mauss AL 1975 *Social problems as social movements.* Philadelphia: JP Lippincott.

Mauss AL 1989 Beyond the illusion of social problems theory. In Holstein JA & G Miller (eds) Perspectives on social problems Volume 1. Greenwich, Connecticut: JAI Press, 19-39.

Quintner J & R Elvey 1991 The neurogenic hypothesis of RSI. In Bammer G. (ed) *Discussion papers on the pathology of work-related neck and upper limb disorders and the implications for diagnosis and treatment.* NCEPH Working Paper Number 24. Canberra: National Centre for Epidemiology and Population Health.

Scott P, Richards E & B Martin 1990 Captives of controversy: the myth of the neutral social researcher in contemporary scientific controversies. *Science, Technology, and Human Values 15*: 474-494.

Wadsworth Y 1984 *Do it yourself social research.* Collingwood, Victoria: Victorian Council of Social Service & Melbourne Family Care Organisation; in association with Sydney: Allen & Unwin.

CLOSING SESSION

WORK WITH DISPLAY UNITS 92
H. Luczak, A. Çakir and G. Çakir (Editors)

Closing remarks

Holger Luczak*, Ahmet Çakir**

* Technische Universität Berlin, Institut für Arbeitswissenschaft, Ernst-Reuter-Platz 7-9, D - 1000 Berlin 12, F.R. Germany

** ERGONOMIC Institute for Social and Occupational Sciences, Research Co., Ltd. Soldauer Platz 3, D - 1000 Berlin 19, F. R. Germany

Closing remarks of an event, like WWDU'92 imply at least 3 components:
- a grateful recognition of the supporters of the conference,
- a short scientific balance of the conference programme, and
- a personal view of events and outcomes.

1. THANKS

Turning to the thanks for our Berlin WWDU support structures, we take the freedom to criticize at first: In 1988 when we decided for the congress here West-Berlin seemed to be a good place for international congresses and for congress-organizers. Considerable amounts of comfortable and cheap hotel capacity - at 1/3 of todays price level, a conference center with really acceptable delivery and total support packages, an iron curtain which separated the customers into convertible currency payers in West-Berlin and into non-convertible currency payers in East-Berlin, and last not least a government in West-Berlin, who by political reasons promised several hundred thousand marks of subsidies to persons who managed to secure an international scientific conference for West-Berlin. During the preparation of our conference the situation changed totally: Within the two years after unification all prices relevant to conference organization doubled or tripled, and all public local subsidies broke down to zero. If zero had been the initial basis for our calculations, all right, but in this way we started our conference preparation with a calculatory advance deficit of between 200 and 300 thousand marks. We confess, that in 1990 we had the impression, that the conference would ruin us, because promised Berlin subsidies did not come in.

The situation changed with respect to stability by at least 3 events, which we gratefully acknowledge:

The first positive event was, that the *Deutsche Forschungsgemeinschaft*, that is our national research foundation, gave a grant of seed money for the printing and distribution of "Calls for Papers and Participation", as well as for the travel expenses of the international scientific advisory committee. My application was decided on positively, which means, that the reviewers and the senate of this high ranking body in the German scientific sphere took seriously the scientific field and approach of WWDU, and that the presented planning of the conference was evaluated as feasible and sound.

The second positive event was that our Federal Minister of Labour, Dr. Blüm, took over the patronage over the conference, which means that under the practical and political view the possible results were evaluated as so important for work design, work protection, and occupational health, that Dr. Blüm gave his name and a certain guarantee for financial catastrophes, if the conference should run into the red zone of financial figures.

The third positive event was that in our capitalist system, several companies found that it was an interesting idea to sponsor the conference and to advertise their firm and their products in the "Calls" and in the "Programmes". By the way, these companies belonged to the market leaders in Europe in software products, keyboards and visual displays, office equipment and lighting. So WWDU found the interest of the economic and efficiency-oriented sphere of our society as an important factor for applied research and the development of products.

As you perhaps know from physics and mechanics, a mechanical construction, built on 3 fundamental points, is especially stable. We gratefully acknowledge this stability as basis for our preparation work, stability given by

* the research foundation,
* the political patron, and
* the sponsors.

In addition to this financial acknowledgement much of the success of the conference can be assigned to our *co-sponsoring organizations*, that are mostly scientific societies of different character, which helped us with different kinds of support, mostly with the distribution of information material.

The quality of the conference programme was influenced to a great extent by the members of the *scientific advisory committee* and the *organizers of special sessions*. They were partly responsible for the scientific soul of this event, the different sessions.

The hard work in detail was done by the coworkers of the Institut für Arbeitswissenschaft of the Berlin University of Technology and the ERGONOMIC Institute.

2. SCIENTIFIC BALANCE

What then was the scientific output of all these helping inputs? Do not expect a total scientific balance of the conference. But we will try to emphasize some points, which seem to be not only interesting in scientific terms, but in practical terms of having some significance for human working conditions and the individual worker, too.

The newest occupational health research results, partially backed by extensive epidemiological studies, referring to radiation, eye fatigue, stressors and diseases of the musculoskeletal apparatus and the medical surveillance of workers with display units were presented at this conference. To a certain extent we found stable ground in the swamp of fears, doubts and preventive measurements.

l studies of relevance for design improvements were reported.

The support of the human operator by intelligent user surfaces and interfaces was demonstrated by experimental results; the latest developments in input devices including virtual reality as well as multi-media, multi-screen and multi-language human computer interaction were found at this congress.

Concepts of groupwork and organizational stress in combination with its psychophysical and psychophysiological evaluation was brought to new levels of insight. Especially the problem of stress-strain-regulation, adaption and long-term effects in recovery and recreation were brought into focus. So new doors have been opened in stress-strain-research.

Another remarkable development is that of computer tools which are subsumed under the "CAx" and "Hyper"-heading. Hypertext and hypermedia as well as applications of computer aided techniques for knowledge acquisition, knowledge structuring and knowledge use for decisions and working processes were reported and discussed in different contexts.

Without wanting to rank all this scientific and technological output I personally found that some very new and stimulating sessions were organized on themes, which we had not yet heard much about: As examples for many other stimulating and convincing approaches I name the work environment approach to the "*sick building syndrome*", I pronounce "*Kansei engineering*", the Japanese prescription and remedy for a successful work design in industry, I emphasize "*Error management*", an important concept and approach for the improvement of software systems and for an increase of performance. Anybody who works with computers knows that the "debugging" efforts often exceed a tolerable level. I mention also the Swedish concept of fighting against "*electronic smog*", and the approach of "*chaos theory*" as an incentive for an organizational development in the future.

Aside from these developments, which have newly begun, we can observe a certain stability in occupational and public health findings, which allow the state authorities to formulate clear- cut work protection laws, which allow standardization offices in Europe and worldwide to decide on product and performance criteria of Work With Display Units.

3. PERSONAL PERSPECTIVE

But what are my personal impressions of all this stuff? As ergonomist with an education in engineering and with the respective scientific background I tend to have a positive perspective on development processes for new working conditions and new technical equipment at the workplace. Innovation - besides research and development - sounds very good in the ears of engineers.

So in our "First Announcement" - 3 years ago - until the present programme we tried to propagate this positive perspective by calling for pluridisciplinary approaches

* to support the human ability to combine and process information by tools and techniques in all areas of human industry, both for experts and for novices

* to reduce health hazards by preventive research and measurements in all areas of information technology

* to endeavour to provide innovative solutions in workplace design and the complex and flexible arrangement of individual workers in new organizational and management concepts.

This positive perspective is not shared by all researchers in our scientific area. Taking into account our conference outcome, fatigue, health hazards, complaint studies, environmental dangers, work stress and strain risks and other concepts and terms with a pejorative tendency were highlighted in presentations and discussions. No doubt, criticism is necessary as a prerequisite for demonstrating improvements for a situation. But is it really necessary to follow Leonardo da Vinci in his pessimistic formulation: "The works of man will be the cause of his death!"?

Please be reminded that via "displays" and the technology behind them, you can communicate with your family from Berlin to almost any place of the world, you can consume the masterpieces of theatres and philharmonic orchestras worldwide without being present on site, you could cook your meals with the help of microprocessors and respective controls as well as heat and cool your home with respective interfaces. No doubt that your conference attendance here was dispatched via displays, that your hotel reservation was done that way, that the pilot of your flight used displays to stabilize the aircraft, that the air traffic controller could not have found a safe route without them, and that even your doctor would be quite helpless in diagnosing the causes of your sickness symptoms without a display of measurements.

But good servants - like display technology - can cause dependencies - like drugs. Not only for the kids with respect to television and video games; what is the researcher or manager without his laptop, PC or electronic notebook? Helpless! The more efficient and the more reliable those servants are, the more dependent we become. A Lord without his butler had better stay in bed instead of taking the risk of getting up.

But servants cannot only make dependent, sometimes they are more intelligent, more efficient, more humorous than their masters. What would Faust have been without his Mephisto, or Don Quichote without Sancho Panza. The great works of world literature show us that servants and masters sometimes change their role.

Are we dominated by our servants? Have they become the masters? Should we chase them away immediately?

Clearly not!

Unfortunately we find in the human character the specific trait to search for scapegoats for developments which have gone the wrong way. Before a minister of state quits his service against his will, he will find a guilty person in his administration. When God accused Adam for the "Fall of Man", Adam shifted the responsibility to Eve, and she accused the snake.

So a critical evaluation of display technology - as well as technology development as a whole - can have several reasons:

1. *Firstly* higher risks could have been generated or have become visible, which means that our servant makes mistakes, becomes unreliable, or has hidden deficits with unwanted side-effects. We think the discussion around unreliable and unfriendly software packages has a lot to do with this phenomenon. Frequently, the real reason or cause lies in the labour market with risks of loosing an old-

fashioned job, a deficit in qualification and training procedures, or in a maladapted organization of work, when computers are introduced. Thus, the bad reputation of CIM - Computer Integrated Manufacturing - for instance is due to the misunderstanding, that the integration is done quasi automatically by the computer network. The inverse seems to be the right argumentation; at first an integration of working processes has to be performed by an appropriate organization, and then an integration of information flows by a computer network in the sense of a CIM, CAM or CAD concept may be useful and helpful. Thus the deficit frequently lies not in the "servants" - the "master" did not spend enough mental capacity on the adaption of his problem field to the possibilities of the "servant".

2. *Secondly* the society becomes aware of problems, whose generation or at least amplification is assigned to display technology with only a very weak cause to effect relationship. The technological equipment becomes the whipping boy, technology criticism has a substitute function. Lets take the RSI problems for example: Nobody can sit in a definite posture with highly repetitive one sided manual movements for 8 hours a day 7 days a week, up to... a whole working life without complaints about his bodily functions, neither in manual assembly, nor in handling and operating a punching machine, nor in a-data entry task at a keyboard.
3. *Thirdly* we are experiencing a renaissance of something like an anti-technology cultural criticism. The change of the world, of life, and of values is assigned to technological development with a pejorative undertone, especially in "Work With Display Units" in all facets. Many literary contributions to the situation of our age presume a strong participation and responsibility of natural sciences and technology for a crisis of civilization. Two lines of arguments can be identified:
   * The one line argues: Natural sciences and technology have a special responsibility, thus they need a new ethic and a new orientation!
   * The other line emphasizes: Natural sciences and technology have side-effects, which have to be controlled early and fiercely!

   These arguments are based logically on two causal relationships:
   * The first saying: Ethics has to do with human action. The possibilities of action of man are increased considerably by technology. Thus technical action has to be ruled by ethical restrictions. Thus an outstanding responsibility of engineers is given.
   * The other argument taking into account the time lags: Industrially produced goods of the present time, based on investment decisions dating from yesterday and the technological innovations of the day before yesterday, will be confronted with countermeasures tomorrow, which become efficient perhaps the day after tomorrow.

We strongly believe, that in this field of making ethical imperatives more concrete and in this period of time between yesterday and tomorrow the conference WWDU plays its specific role as a link between human sciences and technological development, and as a link between the failures of the past and the corrections of the future.

AUTHOR INDEX

AUTHOR INDEX

www.ingramcontent.com/pod-product-compliance
Ingram Content Group UK Ltd.
Pitfield, Milton Keynes, MK11 3LW, UK
UKHW020225290926
15470UKWH00001B/377

9 780444 897596